# Fertility and Reproductive Medicine

# Fertility and Reproductive Medicine

Proceedings of the XVI World Congress on Fertility and Sterility, San Francisco, 4–9 October 1998

*Editors:*

**Roger D. Kempers, M.D.**
Professor Obstetrics and Gynecology, Emeritus
Mayo Medical School and Mayo Clinic
Rochester, MN, USA

**Jean Cohen, M.D.**
Directeur de Centre de Sterilite
Hospital de Sevres
Paris, France

**Arthur F. Haney, M.D.**
Roy T. Parker Professor and Director
Department of Obstetrics and Gynecology
Duke University Medical Center
Durham, NC, USA

**J. Benjamin Younger, M.D.**
Professor Emeritus
Department of Obstetrics and Gynecology
University of Alabama School of Medicine
Birmingham, AL, USA

**1998**

**ELSEVIER**

**Amsterdam – Lausanne – New York – Oxford – Shannon – Singapore – Tokyo**

ELSEVIER SCIENCE B.V.
Sara Burgerhartstraat 25
P.O. Box 211, 1000 AE Amsterdam, The Netherlands

First edition 1998

Library of Congress Cataloging in Publication Data
A catalog record from the Library of Congress has been applied for.

International Congress Series No. 1183
ISBN: 0 444 50068 5

⊗ The paper used in this publication meets the requirements of ANSI/NISO Z39.48-1992 (Permanence of Paper).

Printed in the Netherlands

# Preface

On the occasion of the 30th anniversary of the International Federation of Fertility Societies (IFFS), it's XVI World Congress of Fertility and Sterility is being held jointly with the 54th Annual Meeting of the American Society for Reproductive Medicine (ASRM). The Scientific Program Committee of this World Congress grasped the opportunity to organize an outstanding scientific program with great enthusiasm. Reproductive Medicine continues its explosive expansion. Seminal advances in molecular and cellular biology continue to unfold and have been followed with remarkable rapidity by application to clinical infertility management. In order to provide the most current scientific information to the meeting participants, a major feature of this Scientific Congress has been the bringing together of a group of recognized authorities at the cutting edge of their specific fields in basic and clinical research in Reproductive Medicine to share their current studies and challenges. The manuscripts derived from these presentations have been compiled into this book of the Proceedings of the XVI World Congress. While a number of the chapters included are from Key Note lectures, most are part of the Trilogy format of the meeting. According to the focus or emphasis of the presentations, the trilogies have been assigned to one of three categories — Review, Practice, or Research. The result has been an excellent blending of contemporary research and clinical information. Articles in the Review section range from updates on current investigation in polycystic ovarian disease (PCOD), to microlaparoscopy technology for tubal factor infertility, and legal and ethical considerations of assisted reproductive technology. Articles in the Practice section include the latest clinical studies in ovulation induction regimens, the most effective management of the different stages of endometriosis, and the most current recommendations for the management of menopause. Articles in the Research section report on a wide variety of investigations which include research on the role of glycodelins with immunosuppressive properties in implantation and placentation, reports on the rapid progress in defining genes on the Y chromosome and the implications of their deletions on male infertility, and studies increasing our understanding of androgen receptor structure and function.

The editors wish to thank all of the contributing authors for the quality and timeliness of their reports, which have greatly facilitated our task. The collaborative effort has produced a comprehensive and integrated text on a wide range of current topics in reproductive medicine. It will be a valuable addition to the personal libraries of gynecologists, urologists, endocrinologists, basic scientists, and allied health professionals including those in laboratory medicine, physicians in training, and educators alike.

Roger D. Kempers MD
Jean Cohen MD
Arthur F. Haney MD
J. Benjamin Younger MD

## Editorial Advisory Board

We wish to thank Serono Laboratories, Inc. for their generous support which partially subsidized this publication.

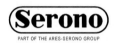

PART OF THE ARES-SERONO GROUP

# Contents

## Psychological approach and medical management of male sexual dysfunction

## Challenges in reproduction

## Infection and reproduction

## Ovulation induction

## Epidemiological controversies in reproduction

# KEYNOTE LECTURES

# Cloning Dolly: implications for human medicine

Keith H.S. Campbell

*PPL Therapeutics, Roslin, Midlothian, UK*

**Abstract.** The demonstration that live offspring can be obtained from embryonic-, foetal- and adult-derived cultured cell populations [1,2] has not only answered one of the fundamental questions of developmental biology but also provided potential applications in a range of human therapeutic fields. The birth of "Dolly" was the first demonstration of "nuclear equivalence" in adult cells from any species, proving that somatic nuclei contain all of the genetic material required for production of a viable animal by nuclear transfer and demonstrating that the differentiated phenotype (at the nuclear level) can be reversed. The technology developed during these studies not only provides a route for the precise genetic modification of farm animal species but also provides a basis for renewing our efforts to understand cellular differentiation which may lead to a range of novel therapies for the treatment of human diseases.

This paper will review the background to nuclear transfer and the production of Dolly, the potential benefits of this technology and the potential for future human therapeutic uses.

**Keywords:** cell cycle, cloning, human therapeutics, nuclear transfer.

## Introduction

The technique of nuclear transfer was originally proposed by Spemann [3] as a method of studying cellular differentiation. By transferring nuclei from increasingly advanced developmental stages to an egg from which the genetic material had been removed, any restrictions on development due to loss or irreversible inactivation of the genome would be elucidated. These experiments were carried out by Briggs and King [4] who obtained development using embryonic blastomeres as nuclear donors and then by Gurdon who produced adult frogs after transferring nuclei from tadpole intestinal epithelial cells [5], however, no adults were produced where somatic nuclei from adult animals were used as nuclear donors [6]. In mammals the techniques for embryo reconstruction were not developed until the early 1980s when McGrath and Solter [7] demonstrated pronuclear exchange in mouse zygotes. Subsequently Willadsen [8] produced live lambs after transferring nuclei from 8–16 cell sheep embryos to enucleated MII oocytes.

## Methodology of nuclear transfer

In mammalian species enucleated MII oocytes have now become the recipient

---

*Address for correspondence:* Keith Campbell PhD, PPL Scotland, Roslin Midlothian EH25 9PP, UK.
Tel.: +44-131-440-4888. Fax: +44-131-440-4888.

cell of choice, this is due to the lack of development obtained when using enucleated zygotes (i.e., in cattle [9] and pig [10]). This restriction may be due to the removal of zygotic factors which are essential for early development which may be associated with the pronuclei. MII oocytes to be used as nuclear donors may be obtained from a variety of sources dependent upon species. In ruminants, particularly cattle, oocytes may be aspirated from ovarian follicles following slaughter and matured in vitro. Additionally matured oocytes may be flushed from the oviducts of donor animals following superovulation regimes, and immature oocytes may be aspirated from follicles in vitro or following ovariectomy. Having obtained a suitable donor oocyte, the genetic material located on the meiotic spindle is removed by microsurgery. Briefly a small amount of cytoplasm is aspirated from directly beneath the first polar body using a fine glass pipette. Fluidity of the cell membranes allows both the oocyte and the aspirated karyoplast to reseal following manipulation. The enucleation procedure can be monitored by staining the aspirated karyoplast with a DNA-specific fluorochrome, e.g., Hoechst 3332. Following enucleation the genetic material from the donor cell is introduced into by fusion of the donor cell (karyoplast) to the enucleated oocyte (cytoplast). In farm animal species electrofusion has become the method of choice although viral and chemical methods have been used, which have proved less reproducible and in the case of chemical fusion may be toxic. At this point the reconstructed embryo is able to begin development, however, many factors are involved in the successful development of such reconstructed embryos. These include other techniques associated with the methods of activation (induction of fertilisation responses), culture and in addition biological factors relating to both the cytoplast and the karyoplast (for reviews see [11,12]). Of great importance for successful development is coordination of the nuclear and cytoplasmic cell cycle phases of both donor and recipient cells (for a review see [13]).

## Cell cycle coordination in nuclear transfer reconstructed embryos

The cytoplasm of the enucleated oocyte remains arrested at MII in the absence of genetic material until an activation stimulus is applied. In all eucaryotic cells the onset of mitosis and meiosis is controlled by a cytoplasmic kinase activity termed MPF (mitosis-/meiosis-/maturation-promoting factor). MPF kinase activity increases during the G2 phase of the cell cycle and causes dissolution of the nuclear membrane, chromatin condensation and changes in the cytoskeleton. The kinase activity of MPF is maximal at the metaphase of the mitotic/meiotic division after which it declines rapidly allowing decondensation of the chromosomes and reformation of the nuclear membrane. In MII oocytes, MPF activity remains at high levels stabilised by a second factor termed CSF (the product of the c-mos proto-oncogene) until fertilisation or activation. When donor nuclei are transferred into this cytoplasmic environment they respond to the MPF and undergo nuclear envelope breakdown (NEBD) and precocious chromosome condensation. As the majority of nuclei would unlikely be about to enter mitosis at the time of transfer this has been termed PCC or premature chromosome condensation. The effects of PCC on the donor nucleus are dependent upon its cell cycle stage at the time of transfer. Nuclei in the G1 phase (prior to the DNA synthetic period or S-phase) or in then G2 phase (post-S-phase) form single or double chromatids, respectively, and suffer no apparent DNA damage. In contrast, the chromatin of nuclei which are undergoing DNA synthesis (S-phase) has a typical "pulverised" appearance and suffers large amounts of DNA damage.

NEBD due to MPF has a second effect, during a single cell cycle the nucleus must replicate all of its DNA once but only once. Failure to replicate a portion of the DNA or to replicate a portion more than once will lead to aneuploidy in the resultant daughter cells and affect development. Central to the control of DNA replication is the maintenance of an intact nuclear envelope. Thus when nuclei are transferred to MII oocytes with high MPF, NEBD occurs and a DNA replication occurs in all donor nuclei regardless of their cell cycle phase at the time of transfer. Only those nuclei which were diploid or pre-S-phase at the time of transfer will give rise to daughter cells of the correct ploidy. Alternatively, if the MII oocyte is activated and MPF activity has declined prior to cell fusion, then no NEBD or PCC occur. Nuclei from G1, S or G2 stages of the cell cycle undergo coordinated replication and give rise to diploid daughter cells. When using donor cells at unknown stages of the cell cycle then the use of such preactivated oocytes or "universal recipients" is advocated. In contrast if nuclei can be selected or maintained in a pre-S, diploid stage then these may be transferred to MII oocytes with high MPF activity.

When working with early embryonic blastomeres as donors of genetic material both the cell cycle phase of the nucleus and the developmental stage of the embryo donor have been shown to have an effect upon development during early embryonic development little or no transcription occurs from the zygotic nucleus. At later stages the zygotic nucleus becomes transcriptionally active and assumes developmental control. In early studies in nuclear transfer there was an apparent association between those species in which zygotic transcription occurs at a later stage and the stage at which successful development can be obtained. In those species where transcription occurs later, development from later developmental stages has been possible. This was interpreted in two ways; firstly, that in species where zygotic transcription occurs early, then the donor blastomeres were more differentiated. In contrast when zygotic transcription occurs later during development the donor blastomeres are less differentiated. An alternative explanation is that in those species which initiate transcription at a later developmental stage, then following nuclear transfer the donor nucleus is able to undergo more mitotic divisions in the absence of transcription and therefore, to interact with maternal factors controlling development to a greater extent. Studies examining development from different donor recipient cell cycle combinations have identified a possible window of opportunity for maximal development within the donor cell cycle. Donor cells transferred in late G2-phase, during M or early G1-phases promote a greater frequency of development. This may be due to changes in the donor chromatin which may result in the dissociation of factors involved with transcription. In turn, this may facilitate the association of maternal factors which are important for the temporal and spatial pattern of gene expression required for successful development.

## Nuclear transfer from cultured cell populations

Until recently development of mammalian nuclear transfer reconstructed embryos was restricted to the use of donor genetic material from early embryos. Although this technique has a number of applications both on a scientific and a technological level, it was the goal of many scientists to obtain development of nuclear transfer embryos from cells which could be maintained in culture. Many reports suggested that specific "pluripotent" cell types (e.g., embryonic stem cells (ES)) would be required, however, in farm animal species such cell populations have as yet not been identified and in the mouse no development has been reported (for a review see [14]).

Previous reports from our laboratory demonstrated that offspring can be obtained by nuclear transfer using inner cell mass cells of blastocyst stage embryos in both cattle and sheep. Rather than try to isolate a "pluripotent" ES-like cell line we followed the ability of blastocyst derived cells to produce live off-spring when placed into culture and used as donors of genetic material for nuclear transfer. Due to the seasonal nature of ovine reproduction these experiments were initiated over the winter of 1993—94. To avoid the need for synchronisation of the donor cell cycle, nuclear transfer embryos were reconstructed using preactivated enucleated MII oocytes as recipients. During early passages (P1—P3) live offspring were obtained, however, on continued culture (P6—11) of and subsequent embryo reconstruction during the winter of 1994—95 no further off-spring were obtained. Immunofluorescent analysis of this cell population demonstrated the presence of A type lamins, cytokeratin and vimentin which are associated with differentiated cells [13].

An alternative to selecting a cell type which may be successful at controlling development in nuclear transfer embryos is to modify the donor chromatin structure prior to embryo reconstruction. Previously this paper has discussed the cell cycle in relation to growing cells, an additional cell cycle phase termed G0 is found in cells which have exited the cell cycle in response to a number of conditions. Such cells are said to be quiescent and the G0 stage has been implicated in cellular differentiation. G0 cells are arrested in a post-M, pre-S-phase state with a diploid DNA content and may therefore be transferred to MII oocytes with high MPF activity. In our experiments cells were induced into a quiescent state by serum starvation. Quiescent donor nuclei were transferred to MII oocytes at the time of activation, prior to activation and following activation. Live lambs (five in total) were obtained from all combinations, unfortunately two of these died within minutes of birth and one-third at 10 days following birth with a range of congenital abnormalities [13]. The remaining two lambs remain healthy and both have proved to be fertile. To confirm and extend these studies they were subsequently repeated using a male day 9 embryo derived cell population, primary foetal fibroblasts from a day 26 foetus and a mammary epithelial cell line isolated from a 6-year-old ewe. Live offspring were obtained from each of these cell populations.

The potential role of quiescence in successful development of nuclear transfer reconstructed embryos using cultured cell populations is presently unclear. The use of a diploid cell line allows coordination of donor and recipient cycles, the use of MII oocytes maximises the number of mitotic events which the donor nucleus passes through in the absence of transcription, changes in the donor cell including a reduction in transcription, a reduction in translation, active degradation of unnecessary mRNA and chromatin condensation are factors which may facilitate interaction of the donor chromatin with maternal factors in the recipient oocyte cytoplasm.

## Implications of nuclear transfer from cultured cells

Nuclear transfer using embryonic blastomeres as nuclear donors has a number of applications in agriculture and research for multiplication of elite embryos or for the production of multiple copies for research purposes. However, these applications are limited by the number of donor cells available and the efficiency of the process. The use of cultured cell populations can increase the number of animals which may be produced from an elite embryo, foetus or adult. In addition the storage of frozen cell populations may prove useful in the preservation of genetic resources in a number of species. However, in the short term, the major implication of the use of cell populations that may be maintained in culture prior to their use as nuclear donors is the provision of a route for the precise genetic modification of farm animal species. Previously transgenic farm animals were produced by pronuclear injection and this route to genetic modification will be discussed in relation to nuclear transfer, and subsequently specific applications of genetic modification for human therapeutic use will be cited.

## Advantages of nuclear transfer for genetic modification of farm animal species

The addition of genetic material or production of a transgenic animal can be achieved by the injection of the required gene into the pronucleus of a zygote. Although this technique has been applied successfully in a number of species including mice, rabbits, pigs, sheep, goats and cattle (for a review see [15]), there are a number of disadvantages. Integration does not always occur during the first cell cycle resulting in the production of mosaic embryos [16]. Integration occurs at random within the genome resulting in variable expression of the gene product. At present only simple gene additions may be performed. The selection of transgenic embryos prior to their transfer is hampered by mosaicism [17]. The production of the required phenotype coupled to germ line transmission may require the generation of several transgenic lines. Multiplication of the required phenotype or its dissemination into the population is restricted by breeding programmes.

In contrast the production of offspring from a single cell, or cloned population offers significant advantages. Genetic modification can be performed in culture and the modified cells selected prior to animal production. It will be possible to remove (knockout) as well as to add genes. Also, precise modification of control regions or addition of genes to specific regions of the genome (knocking) will be facilitated. The production of an animal from a single nucleus removes the problems associated with mosaicism, all of the cells within the resultant animal will contain the modification which will be transmitted through the germ line. All of the animals produced will be transgenic and flock or herd generation can be accelerated by producing multiple copies from the cultured cells. The experiments which lead to "Dolly" involved the use of mammary epithelial cells. The use of this cell line was related to the potential screening of transgenic cells for milk production in vitro prior to animal production. Thus it may be possible to predict expression level and select the highest expressing cell populations prior to animal production.

In order to carry out these modifications the cultured cell populations must be amenable to transfection and selection in culture and maintain their ability to be used for successful nuclear transfer. We have previously demonstrated that foetal fibroblasts are suitable for this purpose with the production of "Polly" a nuclear transfer lamb transgenic for human factor IX derived from a transfected, selected cell population [18]. These experiments also demonstrated that the efficiency of animal production was increased over 2-fold, in terms of total animals used, as compared to pronuclear injection. The generation of animals carrying multiple genetic modifications requires the sequential addition and removal or modification of specific genes. In culture primary cell populations have a finite life span, however, by rederiving cell populations from embryos, foetuses or offspring produced by nuclear transfer it will be possible to extend the period that cells can be maintained in culture to carry out these modifications.

## Uses of genetic modification in human medicine

The ability to carry out precise genetic modification on cells in culture not only provides a method for the improvement of present transgenic technology but also facilitates previously improbable genetic modifications. Transgenic animals can play a role in a range of human therapies and these will be discussed in relation to present and future therapies.

### *Biopharmaceuticals*

The production of human proteins in transgenic animals. Human proteins may be produced in a range of tissues and bodily fluids including blood, urine and milk. Although each of these may play a particular role the value of biopharmaceutical production in transgenic animals lies in the high volume which can potentially be produced at relatively low cost. To this end the production of proteins in the milk of sheep, goats and cattle provides a useful route, although for products required in small amounts transgenic rabbits may also be used. A range of therapeutic proteins are being produced in the milk of transgenic animals including α-1-antitrypsin (for treatment of cystic fibrosis) factor IX (for treatment of haemophilia B) (for a review see [19]). Nuclear transfer will facilitate the removal of endogenous genes to aid purification, for example, the replacement of bovine serum albumin with human serum albumin (HAS) in order to produce large amounts of HSA for the treatment of burns.

*Nutraceuticals*

The modification of animal milk to enhance nutritional value, removal of allergens (e.g., β-lactoglobulin in cattle).

*Xenotransplantation*

The use of animal organs and other tissues for human transplantation: physiologically pig organs are similar to humans and are considered suitable for transplantation. However, there is a major problem with organ rejection. Although all of the mechanisms which are involved in this rejection are not completely understood, it is known that a major antigen involved is α-1,3,galactose. This is present on pig cell but is not found in humans who therefore mount an immune response. Nuclear transfer from cultured cells will facilitate knockout of the pig gene coding for α-1,3-galactosyl transferase. Potential organs and tissues for transplantation include the heart, lungs, kidneys, liver and islets (treatment of diabetes) (for a review see [20]).

*Disease models*

At the present time many of the animal models available for the study of human genetic disorders are only available in mice. This species may not manifest the same clinical symptoms as in humans. Nuclear transfer technology will allow the production of disease models in species which are physiologically more similar to the human in order to follow disease progression or to assess the benefits of any potential new therapies (including gene therapy). An example of this is cystic fibrosis; in mice this disease manifests in the gut and not the chest.

**Examples with indirect effects on human health**

Genetic modification of farm animals may be used to improve various production or nutritional traits. In addition improvement of animal health by the introduction of genes for disease resistance or removal of genes for disease susceptibility (i.e., PrP gene involved in scrapie and BSE) may have long-term implications for human health.

## Other uses of nuclear transfer technology

The production of "Dolly" by nuclear transfer from an adult somatic cell demonstrates that the differentiated state of the genetic material may be reversed. In humans there are many diseases or traumas which result in the loss of specific cell types or tissues. Nuclear transfer offers a route whereby the phenotype of a single differentiated cell may be removed and undifferentiated cells produced. With a greater understanding of cellular differentiation it may be possible to remove cells from a patient, produce undifferentiated cells by nuclear transfer and then to differentiate these cells in culture to specific phenotypes. Such cells may be then be returned to the patient avoiding the problems of rejection due to mismatching of tissue types. Such cells may be used to replace lost populations such as in nerve damage or Parkinson's disease, possibly as a treatment for immune disorders, leukaemias and other blood diseases or as a vector for gene therapy.

## References

1. Campbell KHS, McWhir J, Ritchie WA, Wilmut I. Sheep cloned by nuclear transfer from a cultured cell line. Nature 1996;380:64—66.
2. Wilmut A, Schnieke E, McWhir J, Kind AJ, Campbell KHS. Viable offspring derived from fetal and adult mammalian cells. Nature 1997;385:810—813.
3. Spemann H. Embryonic Development and Induction. New York: Hafner Publishing Company, 1938;210—211.
4. Briggs R, King T. Changes in the nuclei of differentiating cells as revealed by nuclear transfer. J Morph 1957;10:269—312.
5. Gurdon JB. The developmental capacity of nuclei taken from intestinal epithelium cells of feeding tadpoles. J Embryol Exp Morphol 1962;10:622—640.
6. Gurdon JB. Adult frogs from the nuclei of single somatic cells. Devel Biol 1962;4:256—273.
7. McGrath J, Solter D. Nuclear transplantation in the mouse embryo by microsurgery and cell fusion. Science 1983;220:1300—1302.
8. Willadsen SM. Nuclear transplantation in sheep embryos. Nature 1986;320:63—65.
9. Robl JM, Prather R, Barnes F, Eyestone W, Northey D, Gilligan B et al. Nuclear transplantation in bovine embryos. J Animal Sci 1987;64:642—647.
10. Prather RS, Sims MM, First NL. Nuclear transplantation in early pig embryos. Biol Reprod 1989;41:414—418.
11. Campbell K, Wilmut I. Recent advances on in vitro culture and cloning of ungulate embryos. Proceedings, 5th World Congress on Genetics Applied to Livestock Production, University of Guelph, Guelph, Ontario, Canada, vol 20, 7—12 August 1994.
12. Campbell KHS, Wilmut I. Nuclear transfer. In: Clark AJ (ed) Animal Breeding: Technology for the 21st Century. Amsterdam: Harwood Academic Publishers, 1998;47—62.
13. Campbell KHS, Loi P, Otaegui PJ, Wilmut I. Cell cycle co-ordination in embryo cloning by nuclear transfer. Rev Reprod 1996;1:40—46.
14. Campbell KHS, Wilmut I. Totipotency or multipotentiallity of cultured cells: applications and

progress. Theriogenology 1997;47:63—72.

15. Wall RJ. Transgenic livestock: progress and prospects for the future. Theriogenology 1996;45:57—68.

16. Burdon TG, Wall RJ. Fate of microinjected genes in preimplantation mouse embryos. Molec Reprod Devel 1992;33:436—442.

17. Rusconi S. Transgenic regulation in laboratory animals. Experientia 1991;47:866-877.

18. Schnieke AE, Kind AJ, Ritchie WA, Mycock K, Scott AR, Ritchie M, Wilmut I, Colman A, Campbell KHS. Sheep transgenic for human factor IX produced by transfer of nuclei from transfected fetal fibroblasts. Science 1997;278:2130—2133.

19. Garner I, Colman A. Therapeutic proteins from livestock. In: Clark AJ (ed) Animal Breeding: Technology for the 21st Century. Amsterdam: Harwood Academic Publishers, 1998;215—228.

20. White D, Langford G. Xenografts from livestock. In: Clark AJ (ed) Animal Breeding: Technology for the 21st Century. Amsterdam: Harwood Academic Publishers 1998;229—243.

# The Y chromosome and male infertility

David C. Page[1,2], Raaji Alagappan[1,2], Laura G. Brown[1,2], Bruce Lahn[1,2], Doug Menke[1,2], Loreall Pooler[1,2], Tomoko Sawai-Kawaguchi[1,2], Richa Saxena[1,2], Helen Skaletksy[1,2], Chao Sun[1,2], Zhao Lan Tang[1,2], Charles Tilford[1,2], Robert Oates[3], Sherman Silber[4], Steve Rozen[1,2] and Jeremy Wang[1,2]

[1] *Howard Hughes Medical Institute, Whitehead Institute, and* [2] *Department of Biology, Massachusetts Institute of Technology, Cambridge, Massachusetts;* [3] *Department of Urology, Boston University School of Medicine, Boston, Massachusetts; and* [4] *St. Luke's Hospital, St. Louis, Missouri, USA*

**Abstract.** Using our comprehensive map of the Y chromosome, we determined that deletion of the AZFc region is the most common molecularly defined cause of spermatogenic failure. We speculate that AZFc is involved in the generation or maintenance of spermatologonial stem cells. The DAZ gene cluster, which is located in the AZFc region, is expressed in spermatogonia and encodes a putative RNA-binding protein. Absence of DAZ funtion may cause the spermatogenic failure observed in men with AZFc deletions. We have shown that most Y genes are members of Y-amplified families expressed specifically in testes. This suggests that the Y chromosome may have acquired a specialized role in male germ cell development during evolution.

**Keywords:** AZF, DAZ, evolution, germ cell development, male infertility, spermatogneia, Y chromosome.

Two characteristics distinguish the Y chromosome from all other chromosomes in the nuclei of human cells: it is specific to males, and the bulk of the chromosome does not undergo recombination. It is also among the smallest of human chromosomes, with its euchromatic or functional portion spanning roughly 30 million base pairs of DNA, or about 1% of the human genome. In 1992, our laboratory reported comprehensive physical maps of the human Y chromosome [1,2]. These maps incorporated hundreds of PCR-detectable Y-DNA landmarks, sometimes referred to as sequence-tagged sites (STSs). We continue to refine these maps, which we anticipate will provide a framework for determining the DNA sequence of the Y chromosome.

Investigators in many countries have used these maps, and the STSs on which they are based, to explore the hypothesis that some cases of spermatogenic failure are caused by Y chromosome defects [3]. These studies have demonstrated that deletion of a particular segment of the Y chromosome, a segment often referred to as the AZFc region, is the most common molecularly defined cause of spermatogenic failure [4—16]. Our laboratory has found that the AZFc region of the Y chromosome is deleted de novo in 13% of men with nonobstructive azoospermia ([4] and unpublished results), and in a smaller percentage of men with severe oligozoospermia ([5] and unpublished results). These deletions define a region in

14

which should be found one or more genes required for spermatogenesis, hence the name azoospermia factor, or AZF. Though infertile, AZFc-deleted men are otherwise healthy, suggesting that AZFc is a "pure sterile" locus required only for germ cell development. In the absence of AZFc, spermatogenic output is greatly diminished, and in some cases the testes contain no germ cells [4]. We speculate that AZFc facilitates differentiation of primordial germ cells into spermatogonial stem cells or influences the destiny of these stem cells, which in normal males confront three alternative fates: proliferation, degeneration, or differentiation. AZFc deletions encompass a cluster of virtually identical DAZ (deleted in azoospermia) genes [4,17], which are expressed specifically in spermatogonia (and their immediate descendants, primary spermatocytes) and encode a putative RNA-binding protein [4,18]. The absence of DAZ may cause the severe spermatogenic defects observed in men in whom the gene cluster is deleted. In fruit flies and in mice, a gene homologous to DAZ is required for male germ cell development [19,20]. We are exploring the possibility that DAZ is AZFc.

Though less frequent than deletions of the AZFc region, de novo deletions of other portions of the Y chromosome are also observed in some men with severe spermatogenic defects, and in these Y regions investigators around the world are searching for genes that play critical roles in male germ cell development. Indeed, we have systematically searched the whole of the Y chromosome for transcription units and have discovered that the majority of genes are members of Y-amplified families expressed specifically in testes [21]. (Most other human Y genes are shared with the X chromosome and are ubiquitously expressed.) The association of Y deletions with male infertility, and the abundance of testis-specific gene families, suggest that, over evolutionary time, the Y chromosome may have acquired a specialized role in male germ cell development.

## References

1. Vollrath D, Foote S, Hilton A et al. The human Y chromosome: A 43-interval map based on naturally occurring deletions. Science 1992;258:52—59.
2. Foote S, Vollrath D, Hilton A, Page DC et al. The human Y chromosome: Overlapping DNA clones spanning the euchromatic region. Science 1992;258:60—66.
3. Tiepolo L, Zuffardi O. Localization of factors controlling spermatogenesis in the nonfluorescent portion of the Y chromosome long arm. Hum Genet 1976;34:119—124.
4. Reijo R, Lee TY, Salo P et al. Diverse spermatogenic defects in humans caused by Y chromosome deletions encompassing a novel RNA-binding protein gene. Nature Genet 1995;10: 383—393.
5. Reijo R, Alagappan RK, Patrizio P, Page DC. Severe oligozoospermia resulting from deletions of azoospermia factor gene on Y chromosome. Lancet 1996;347:1290—1293.
6. Vogt PH, Edelmann A, Kirsch S et al. Human Y chromosome azoospermia factors (AZF) mapped to different subregions in Yq11. Hum Mol Genet 1996;5:933—943.
7. Nakahori Y, Kuroki Y, Komaki R et al. The Y chromosome region essential for spermatogenesis. Horm Res 1996;46(Suppl 1): 20—23.
8. Qureshi SJ, Ross AR, Ma K et al. Polymerase chain reaction screening for Y chromosome

microdeletions: A first step towards the diagnosis of genetically-determined spermatogenic failure in men. Molec Hum Reprod 1996;2:775—779.

9. Najmabadi H, Huang V, Yen P et al. Substantial prevalence of microdeletions of the Y-chromosome in infertile men with idiopathic azoospermia and oligozoospermia detected using a sequence-tagged site-based mapping strategy. J Clin Endocrinol Metab 1996;81:1347—1352.

10. Simoni M, Gromoll J, Dworniczak B et al. Screening for deletions of the Y chromosome involving the DAZ (deleted in AZoospermia) gene in azoospermia and severe oligozoospermia. Fertil Steril 1997;67:542—547.

11. Pryor JL, Kent-First M. Muallem A et al. Microdeletions in the Y chromosome of infertile men. N Engl J Med 1997;336:534—539.

12. Kremer JA, Tuerlings JH, Meuleman EJ et al. Microdeletions of the Y chromosome and intracytoplasmic sperm injections: From gene to clinic. Hum Reprod 1997;12:687—691.

13. Girardi SK, Mielnik A, Schlegel PN. Submicroscopic deletions in the Y chromosome of infertile men. Hum Reprod 1997;12:1635—1641.

14. Vereb M, Agulnik AI, Houston JT, Lipschultz LI, Lamb DJ, Bishop CE. Absence of DAZ gene mutations in cases of non-obstructed azoopsermia. Molec Hum Reprod 1997;3:55—59.

15. van der Ven K, Montag M, Peschka B et al. Combined cytogenetic and Y chromosome microdeletion screening in males undergoing intracytoplasmic sperm injection. Molec Hum Reprod 1997;3:699—704.

16. Foresta C, Ferlin A, Garolla A, Rossato M, Barbaux S, De Bortoli A. Y-chromosome deletions in idiopathic severe testiculopathies. J Clin Endocrinol Metab 1997;82:1075—1080.

17. Saxena R, Brown LG, Hawkins T et al. The DAZ cluster on the human Y chromosome arose from an autosomal gene that was transposed, repeatedly amplified and pruned. Nature Genet 1996;14:292—299.

18. Menke DB, Mutter GL, Page DC. Expression of DAZ, an azoospermia factor candidate, in human spermatogenia. Am J Hum Genet 1997;60:237—241.

19. Eberhart CG, Maines JZ, Wasserman SA. Meiotic cell cycle requirement for a fly homologue of human deleted in azoospermia. Nature 1996;381:783—785.

20. Ruggiu M, Speed R, Taggart M et al. The mouse Dazla gene encodes a cytoplasmic protein essential for gametogenesis. Nature 1997;389:73—77.

21. Lahn BT, Page DC. Functional coherence of the human Y chromosome. Science 1997;278:675—679.

Fertility and Reproductive Medicine.
R.D. Kempers, J. Cohen, A.F. Haney and J.B. Younger, editors.

# Transgenic models in the study of reproduction

Martin M. Matzuk

*Departments of Pathology, Molecular and Human Genetics, and Cell Biology, Baylor College of Medicine, Houston, Texas, USA*

**Keywords:** development, ovary, reproduction, TGF-β superfamily, transgenic.

In mammals, there are approximately 100,000 genes which govern the development of an organism. For development to proceed normally, there must be coordinate interaction of thousands of these gene products in any given cell of the organism. Beginning with fertilization, precise expression of these gene products is required during embryonic, fetal, postnatal, and adult development. Aberrant synthesis of even one of these gene products can be disastrous — birth defects, cancer, infertility, and even death are all possible when this developmental program is altered. To fully understand these processes in humans, it is necessary to have physiological models that closely mimic developmental events which occur during the creation of a human being.

It is now possible to manipulate the mammalian germline to generate transgenic mice that either overexpress a wild-type or mutant gene or lack a functional copy of an endogenous gene [1,2]. In particular, the rapid advances in embryonic stem cell technology to generate mice functionally deficient in specific gene products (i.e., knockout mice) has allowed investigators to address the unique and essential functions of these gene products in vivo. Research in my laboratory is defining some of the critical genes involved in both normal and abnormal mammalian development with particular emphasis on genes involved in reproductive development and function (Table 1). Several of these genes will be described below.

## Functional analysis of the transforming growth factor β superfamily signal transduction

The transforming growth factor β (TGF-β) superfamily is the largest family of extracellular signaling proteins. Homology based cloning approaches have resulted in the identification of TGF-β-like factors in such diverse species as *C. elegans*, *Drosophila*, and *Xenopus* and have extended the number of mammalian members to over 30. These proteins, synthesized as prepropeptides and processed

*Address for correspondence:* Prof Martin M. Matzuk MD, PhD, Departments of Pathology, Molecular and Human Genetics, and Cell Biology, Baylor College of Medicine, Houston, TX 77030, USA.

*Table 1.* Knockout models created by Matzuk and colleagues which have birth defects or reproductive findings.

| Knockout mouse model | Phenotype | References |
|---|---|---|
| Activin/inhibin βA | Neonatal lethal; craniofacial defects (cleft palate, lack of whiskers, and tooth defects) | [3,4] |
| Activin/inhibin βB | Large litters but delayed parturition; nursing defects; eyelid closure defects at birth | [5] |
| Follistatin | Neonatal lethal; craniofacial defects, growth retardation, and skin defects | [6] |
| Activin receptor type II | Infertility in females due to folliculogenesis defect; delayed fertility in males; small gonads; 25% of mice die neonatally secondary to mandible defects | [7] |
| Inhibin α | Infertility in females; secondary infertility in males; granulosa/Sertoli cell and adrenal tumours; cachexia-like syndrome | [8–10] [10a] |
| Inhibin α/Müllerian inhibiting substance double mutants | Males develop early onset testicular Leydig cell tumors and demonstrate earlier development of Sertoli/granulosa cell tumors | [11] |
| Growth differentiation factor 9 | Infertile; defect in folliculogenesis at one-layer follicle stage | [12] |
| Follicle stimulating hormone β subunit | Female infertility; folliculogenesis block prior to antral follicle stage; males fertile but decreased testis size | [13,14] |
| Oxytocin | Nursing defect | [15] |
| Mouse atonal homolog 1 (Math1) | Neonatal lethal; absence of external germinal layer in cerebellum | [16] |
| FKBP12 | Majority of mice die between E14.5 and birth due to cardiomyopathy and neural tube defects | [17] |
| Superoxide dismutase I | Reduced fertility; increase in embryonic lethality | [18] |

into dimeric proteins, are structurally related in their mature, carboxy-terminal region. Several members of the TGF-β superfamily, such as the inhibins and activins, Müllerian inhibiting substance (MIS), bone morphogenetic proteins 8a and 8b, and growth/differentiation factor-9 (GDF-9), are implicated as important regulatory factors in mammalian reproduction. Many of these ligand family members and downstream signaling proteins have been mutated using embryonic stem (ES) cell technology [10,19] (Table 2). Our laboratory has studied mice with mutations in TGF-β superfamily ligands (e.g., activins βA and βB, inhibin α, MIS, and GDF-9), binding proteins (e.g., follistatin, an activin-binding protein), receptors (e.g., activin receptor type II), and putative downstream proteins (e.g., the FK506-binding protein, FKBP12). Among the models we have created are several lines of mice which die perinatally. For example, mice with mutations in the activin βA and follistatin genes have cleft palate, a common birth defect in humans of unknown etiology [3,6]. These mice also demonstrate defects in whisker development, and the activin βA-deficient mice have complete absence of incisors and lower molars [3,4]. In addition, mice with mutations in another related gene, the activin receptor type II gene, were discovered to have skeletal

*Table 2.* Mouse TGF-β superfamily ligand, binding protein, receptor, or signal transducer mutants.

| Knockout mouse model | Phenotype | References |
|---|---|---|
| Activin/inhibin βA | Perinatal lethal; craniofacial defects (i.e., cleft palate and lack of whiskers and incisors) | [3,6,7,11] |
| Activin/inhibin βB | Viable; eyelid defects and reproductive abnormalities in females | [5,20] |
| BMP-2 | Embryonic lethal; failure to close proamniotic canal; defective cardiac development | [21] |
| BMP-4 | Embryonic lethal; most show no mesoderm differentiation | [22] |
| BMP-5 (*short ear*)[a] | Viable; skeletal and cartilage abnormalities | [23] |
| BMP-7 | Perinatal lethal; kidney disgenesis and anophthalmia; skeletal patterning defects | [24, 25] |
| BMP-8A | Viable; some male infertility due to germ cell degeneration; epididymal epithelial degeneration in a small percentage of males | [26] |
| BMP-8B | Viable; male infertility due to germ cell depletion | [27] |
| GDF-5 (*brachypodism*)[a] | Viable; bone defects in the limbs | [28] |
| GDF-8 (*myostatin*) | Viable; increased muscle mass via muscle cell hypertrophy and hyperplasia | [29] |
| GDF-9 | Viable; female infertility; folliculogenesis arrested at one layer primary follicle stage | [12] |
| GDNF | Perinatal lethal; required for proper kidney development including heterozygotes; lack enteric nervous system | [30—32] |
| Inhibin α | Tumor-suppressor role for inhibin; gonadal and adrenal tumors | [8,9] |
| MIS | Viable males develop uteri; Leydig cell hyperplasia and infertility in males | [33] |
| Nodal (413-d mutant)[b] | Embryonic lethal; arrest at early gastrula stage; no primitive streak | [34—36] |
| TGF-β1 | > 50% die during embryogenesis; survivors develop inflammatory disorders and die within 1 month | [37,38] |
| TGF-β2 | Perinatal lethal; defects in many neural crest derived tissues | [39] |
| TGF-β3 | Perinatal lethal; cleft palate; delayed lung development | [40,41] |
| Follistatin | Perinatal lethal; shiny skin; craniofacial defects, rib defects | [3,6,7,11] |
| Activin receptor type IB | Embryonic lethal; disrupted primitive streak | [42] |
| Activin receptor type II | 25% die perinatally from craniofacial defects; males have delayed fertility; females are infertile | [7,10] |
| Activin receptor type IIB | Perinatal lethal; left-right and anteroposterior axis defects | [43] |
| Bmpr Type I Receptor (*ALK-3* or *Brk-1*) | Embryonic lethal; no mesoderm formation | [44] |
| c-RET (GDNF receptor) | Perinatal lethal; required for proper kidney development including heterozygotes; lack enteric nervous system | [45] |

*(contd.)*

*Table 2.* Continued.

| Knockout mouse model | Phenotype | References |
|---|---|---|
| MIS type II receptor | Phenocopy of MIS ligand-deficient mice | [46] |
| TGF-β receptor type II | Phenocopy of lethal TGF-β1-deficient embryos; disrupted hematopoeisis and vasculogenesis in the yolk sack | [47] |
| SMAD2 | Embryonic lethal; no embryonic mesoderm formation; lack anteroposterior axis | [48] |
| SMAD4 (*DPC4*) | Embryonic lethal; defective visceral endorm leading to gastrulation defect | [49,50] |

[a]*Short ear* and *brachypodism* are induced mutations which have been identified as mutations in the BMP-5 and GDF-5 genes, respectively. [b]The 413-d mutant is a retrovirally induced recessive lethal mutation in the nodal gene.

and facial abnormalities [7] which mimic the human Pierre-Robin syndrome; human newborns with this syndrome have hypoplasia of the mandible, leading to respiratory distress which must be surgically corrected immediately. In addition, we have shown that 100% of mice lacking the FK506-binding protein, FKBP12, have dilated cardiomyopathy and ventricular septal defects [17] which mimic a human congenital heart disorder, noncompaction of left ventricular myocardium. A smaller percentage of the FKBP12 mutants also have neural tube defects leading to exencephaly. FKBP12 was shown to previously interact in vitro with the cytoplasmic domains of type I receptors of the TGF-β superfamily. However, physiological studies using cells derived from FKBP12-deficient embryos demonstrate that FKBP12 is dispensable for TGF-β-mediated signaling. Alternatively, we showed that FKBP12 modulates the calcium release activity of both skeletal and cardiac ryanodine receptors. These above-mentioned transgenic models have helped clarify the roles that these proteins play in the signal transduction of this large superfamily.

**The inhibin α knockout mouse — a model for studying gonadal tumor development**

Ovarian cancer has the highest fatality rate of any gynecologic malignancy and is the fourth leading cause of cancer death in women. Testicular cancer is the most common malignancy in males between the ages of 15 and 34. Similar to other malignancies, ovarian and testicular cancers arise through multiple genetic alterations. One reason for the complexity of ovarian and testicular cancers is that normal ovarian and testicular function is modulated by extragonadal (e.g., follicle-stimulating hormone (FSH) and luteinizing hormone (LH)) and intragonadal regulators (e.g., steroids and gonadal peptides). Among the gonadal peptides that play a critical role in both FSH regulation and intragonadal regulation are the inhibins and activins (functionally antagonistic proteins which share common β subunits), follistatin, (an activin-binding protein which antagonizes activin function), and Müllerian inhibiting substance (MIS). Using embryonic stem (ES) cell technology, we have generated a transgenic mouse with a genetic lesion which is clearly central to the development of ovarian and testicular cancers. Mice lacking the α:β heterodimeric TGF-β family member inhibin via a knockout of the α subunit develop ovarian and testicular tumors in the adolescent stage which resemble juvenile granulosa cell tumors which arise in young human females [8]. The development of these ovarian and testicular tumors is rapidly followed by a cancer cachexia-like (wasting) syndrome [9] which mimics the human cancer cachexia syndromes that accompany the development of cancer in many human patients. In inhibin-deficient mice with gonadal tumors, we have demonstrated that activins are secreted from the tumors leading to a dramatic elevation in the serum activin levels [9]. By generating mice deficient in both inhibin and activin receptor type II (ActRII), we have shown that activin signaling through ActRII causes the cancer cachexia-like syndrome [10a]. We have also generated other mice with multiple genetic lesions to further understand the genetic and physiological events involved in granulosa/Sertoli cell tumor development. In particular, we utilized the hypogonadal (*hpg*) mouse to further study tumor development in our model system. *hpg/hpg* mice have a null mutation in the gonadotropin-releasing hormone (GnRH) gene leading to suppressed FSH and LH levels. Mice deficient in both GnRH and inhibin fail to develop ovarian or testicular tumors demonstrating that FSH and/or LH are required for the formation and/or progression of both the ovarian and testicular cancer in the inhibin-deficient mice [51]. Future studies using this important inhibin knockout mouse model will continue to lead to a better understanding of the physiological and genetic events required for ovarian and testicular cancer development and cancer cachexia-like syndromes.

**Mouse models to study reproductive function**

The hypothalamic-pituitary-gonadal axis is a complex network that requires in vivo analysis to define function. The generation of knockout models lacking key components of this axis have advanced research on mammalian reproduction. Several genes essential for sex determination and establishment and maintenance of the reproductive system have been addressed using transgenic mouse technology [52–54]. These models have given many valuable clues to understanding the function of those genes in vivo. In addition to the developmental and cancer models, we have generated several mouse models which have reproductive defects. Female mice deficient in growth differentiation factor 9 (GDF-9), follicle stimulating hormone (FSH), and activin receptor type II (ActRII) are infertile due to blocks at specific stages of folliculogenesis (Table 1 and Fig. 1). As shown, absence of GDF-9 results in a block in folliculogenesis at the one layer primary follicle stage [12] whereas absence of FSH blocks folliculogenesis at the multi-layer preantral follicle stage [13]. The GDF-9 knockout studies have defined GDF-9 as the first oocyte-derived growth factor required for somatic cell func-

22

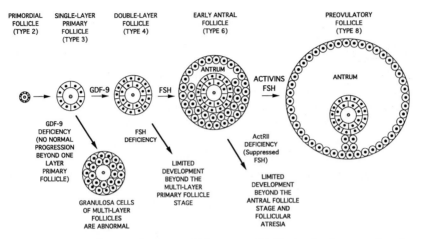

*Fig. 1.* Schematic diagram showing multiple stages of follicular development. Based on the mouse models generated by our group, GDF-9, FSH, and activins play essential functions at various times in follicular development. As shown, absence of GDF-9, FSH, and ActRII in these mouse models results in different blocks in folliculogenesis.

tion in vivo. We have also used the FSH knockout mice to understand the intra-ovarian function of IGF-I in the ovary [14]. Besides the developmental defects described above, adult mice lacking activin receptor type II have a later block in folliculogenesis at the early antral follicle stage [7]. Furthermore, both the FSH-deficient and ActRII-deficient male mice have decreased testis size demonstrating in vivo that FSH and activins are important mitogens for Sertoli cell growth [7,13].

We and others have also produced mice lacking oxytocin and shown that these mice continue to deliver in the absence of oxytocin but fail to nurse their offspring [15,55]. Likewise, mice lacking the activin/inhibin βB subunit have nursing defects and in addition have delayed parturition [5,20]. Other models created by our group and others which have reproductive defects in females, males, or both sexes will allow investigators to more fully understand the relationship of these many proteins in reproductive development and function.

### Acknowledgements

Research in the Matzuk Laboratory has been supported by grants from the National Institutes of Health, Genetics Institute, and Metamorphix.

### References

1. Capecchi MR. Targeted gene replacement. Sci Am 1994;270:52—59.
2. Camper SA, Saunders TL. Kendall SK, Keri RA, Seasholtz AF, Gordon DF, Birkmeier TS, Keegan CE, Karolyi IJ, Roller ML, Burrows HL, Samuelson LC. Implementing transgenic and

embryonic stem cell technology to study gene expression, cell-cell interactions and gene function. Biol Reprod 1995;52:246—257.

3. Matzuk MM, Kumar TR, Vassalli A, Bickenbach JR, Roop DR, Jaenisch R, Bradley A. Functional analysis of activins in mammalian development. Nature 1995;374:354—356.

4. Ferguson CA, Tucker AS, Christensen L, Lau AL, Matzuk MM, Sharpe PT. The role of activin signalling in patterning of the murine dentition. Genes Devel 1998;(In press).

5. Vassalli A, Matzuk MM, Gardner HAR, Lee K-F, Jaenisch R. Activin/inhibin βB subunit gene disruption leads to defects in eyelid development and female reproduction. Genes Devel 1994;8:414—427.

6. Matzuk MM, Lu H, Vogel H, Sellheyer K, Roop DR, Bradley A. Multiple defects and perinatally death in mice deficient in follistatin. Nature 1995;374:360—363.

7. Matzuk MM, Kumar TR, Bradley A. Different phenotypes for mice deficient in either activins or activin receptor type II. Nature 1995;374:356—360.

8. Matzuk MM, Finegold MJ, Su JJ, Hsueh AJW, Bradley A. α-Inhibin is a tumor suppressor gene with gonadal specificity in mice. Nature 1992;360:313—319.

9. Matzuk MM, Finegold MJ, Mather JP, Krummen L, Lu H, Bradley A. Development of cancer cachexia-like syndrome and adrenal tumors in inhibin-deficient mice. Proc Natl Acad Sci USA 1994;91:8817—8821.

10. Matzuk MM, Kumar TR, Shou W, Coerver KA, Lau A, Behringer RR, Finegold MJ. Transgenic models to study the roles of inhibins and activins in reproduction, oncogenesis, and development. Recent Progress Horm Res 1996;51:123—157.

10a. Coerver KA, Woodruff TK, Finegold MJ, Mather J, Bradley A, Matzuk MM. Activin signaling through activin receptor type II causes the cachexia-like symptoms in inhibin-deficient mice. Molec Endocrinol 1996;10:534—543.

11. Matzuk MM, Finegold MJ, Mishina Y, Bradley A, Behringer RR. Synergistic effects of inhibins and Müllerian-inhibiting substance on testicular tumorigenesis. Molec Endocrinol 1995;9: 1337—1345.

12. Dong J, Albertini DF, Nishimori K, Kumar TR, Lu N, Matzuk MM. Growth differentiation factor-9 is required during early ovarian folliculogenesis. Nature 1996;383:531—535.

13. Kumar TR, Wang Y, Lu N, Matzuk MM. Follicle stimulating hormone is required for ovarian follicle maturation but not male fertility. Nature Genet 1997;15:201—204.

14. Zhou J, Kumar T, Matzuk M, Bondy C. Insulin-like growth factor I regulates gonadotropin responsiveness in the murine ovary. Molec Endocrinol 1997;11:1924—1933.

15. Nishimori K, Young LJ, Guo Q, Wang Z, Insel TR, Matzuk MM. Oxytocin is required for nursing but is not essential for parturition or reproductive behavior. Proc Natl Acad Sci USA 1996;93:11699—11704.

16. Ben-Arie N, Bellen HJ, Armstrong DL, McCall AE, Gordadze PR, Guo Q, Matzuk MM, Zoghbi HY. *Math1* is essential for genesis of cerebellar granule neurons. Nature 1997;390: 169—172.

17. Shou W, Aghdasi B, Armstrong DL, Guo Q, Bao S, Charng M-J, Mathews LM, Schneider MD, Hamilton SL, Matzuk MM. FKBP12-deficient mice display cardiac defects and altered ryanodine receptor function. Nature 1998;391:489—492.

18. Matzuk MM, Dionne L, Guo Q, Kumar TR, Lebovitz RM. Analysis of superoxide dismutase 1 and 2 in ovarian function using knockout mice. Endocrinology 1998;(In press).

19. Lau AL, Shou W, Guo Q, Matzuk MM. Transgenic approaches to study the functions of the transforming growth factor β superfamily members. In: Aono T, Sugino H, Vale WW (eds) Inhibin, Activin, and Follistatin. New York: Springer, 1997;220—243.

20. Schrewe H, Gendron-Maguire M, Harbison ML, Gridley T. Mice homozygous for a null mutation of activin βB are viable and fertile. Mechan Devel 1994;47:43—51.

21. Zhang H, Bradley A. Mice deficient for BMP2 are nonviable and have defects in amnion/chorion and cardiac development. Development 1996;122:2977—2986.

22. Winnier G, Blessing M, Labosky PA, Hogan BLM. Bone morphogenetic protein-4 is required

for mesoderm formation and patterning in the mouse. Genes Devel 1995;9:2105—2116.

23. Kingsley DM, Bland AE, Grubber JM, Marker PC, Russell LB, Copeland NG, Jenkins NA. The mouse short ear skeletal morphogenesis locus is associated with defects in a bone morphogenetic member of the TGF beta superfamily. Cell 1992;71:399—410.

24. Dudley AT, Lyons KM, Robertson EJ. A requirement for bone morphogenetic protein-7 during development of the mammalian kidney and eye. Genes Devel 1995;9:2795—2807.

25. Luo G, Hofmann C, Bronckers AL, Sohocki M, Bradley A, Karsenty G. BMP-7 is an inducer of nephrogenesis, and is also required for eye development and skeletal patterning. Genes Devel 1995;9:2808—2820.

26. Zhao GQ, Liaw L, Hogan BL. Bone morphogenetic protein 8A plays a role in the maintenance of spermatogenesis and the integrity of the epididymis. Development 1998;125:1103—1112.

27. Zhao GQ, Deng K, Labosky PA, Liaw L, Hogan BL. The gene encoding bone morphogenetic protein 8B is required for the initiation and maintenance of spermatogenesis in the mouse. Genes Devel 1996;10:1657—1669.

28. Storm EE, Huynh TV, Copeland NG, Jenkins NA, Kingsley DM, Lee SJ. Limb alterations in brachypodism mice due to mutations in a new member of the TGF beta-superfamily. Nature 1994;368:639—643.

29. McPherron AC, Lawler AM, Lee SJ. Regulation of skeletal muscle mass in mice by a new TGF-beta superfamily member. Nature 1997;387:83—90.

30. Moore MW, Klein RD, Farinas I, Sauer H, Armanini M, Phillips H, Reichardt LF, Ryan AM, Carver MK, Rosenthal A. Renal and neuronal abnormalities in mice lacking GDNF. Nature 1996;382:76—79.

31. Pichel JG, Shen L, Sheng HZ, Granholm AC, Drago J, Grinberg A, Lee EJ, Huang SP, Saarma M, Hoffer BJ, Sariola H, Westphal H. Defects in enteric innervation and kidney development in mice lacking GDNF. Nature 1996;382:73—76.

32. Sánchez MP, Silos SI, Frisen J, He B, Lira SA, Barbacid M. Renal agenesis and the absence of enteric neurons in mice lacking GDNF. Nature 1996;382:70—73.

33. Behringer RR, Finegold MJ, Cate RL. Müllerian-inhibiting substance function during mammalian sexual development. Cell 1994;79:415—425.

34. Conlon FL, Barth KS, Robertson EJ. A novel retrovirally induced embryonic lethal mutation in the mouse: assessment of the developmental fate of embryonic stem cells homozygous for the 413.d proviral integration. Development 1991;111:969—981.

35. Zhou X, Sasaki H, Lowe L, Hogan BL, Kuehn MR. Nodal is a novel TGF-β-like gene expressed in the mouse node during gastrulation. Nature 1993;361:543—547.

36. Collignon J, Varlet I, Robertson EJ. Relationship between asymmetric *nodal* expression and the direction of embryonic turning. Nature 1996;381:155—158.

37. Shull MM, Ormsby I, Kier AB, Pawlowski S, Diebold RJ, Yin M, Allen R, Sidman C, Proetzel G, Calvin D et al. Targeted disruption of the mouse transforming growth factor-beta 1 gene results in multifocal inflammatory disease. Nature 1992;359:693—699.

38. Kulkarni AB, Huh CG, Becker D, Geiser A, Lyght M, Flanders KC, Roberts AB, Sporn MB, Ward JM, Karlsson S. Transforming growth factor beta 1 null mutation in mice causes excessive inflammatory response and early death. Proc Natl Acad Sci USA 1993;90:770—774.

39. Sanford LP, Ormsby I, Gittenberger-de Groot AC, Sariola H, Friedman R, Boivin GP, Cardell EL, Doetschman T. TGFbeta2 knockout mice have multiple developmental defects that are non-overlapping with other TGFbeta knockout phenotypes. Development 1997;124:2659—2670.

40. Kaartinen V, Voncken JW, Shuler C, Warburton D, Bu D, Heisterkamp N, Groffen J. Abnormal lung development and cleft palate in mice lacking TGF-β3 indicates defects of epithelial-mesenchymal interaction. Nat Genet 1995;11:415—421.

41. Proetzel G, Pawlowski SA, Wiles MV, Yin M, Boivin GP, Howles PN, Ding J, Ferguson MWJ, Doetschman T. Transforming growth factor-β3 is required for secondary palate fusion. Nat Genet 1995;11:409—414.

42. Gu Z, Nomura M, Simpson BB, Lei H, Feijen A, van den Eijnden-van Raaij J, Donahoe PK, Li E. The type I activin receptor ActRIB is required for egg cylinder organization and gastrulation in the mouse. Genes Dev 1998;12:844—857.

43. Oh SP, Li E. The signaling pathway mediated by the type IIB activin receptor controls axial patterning and lateral asymmetry in the mouse. Genes Dev 1997;11:1812—1826.

44. Mishina Y, Suzuki A, Ueno N, Behringer RR. Bmpr encodes a type I bone morphogenetic protein receptor that is essential for gastrulation during mouse embryogenesis. Genes Dev 1995;9: 3027—3037.

45. Schuchardt A, D'Agati V, Larsson BL, Costantini F, Pachnis V. Defects in the kidney and enteric nervous system of mice lacking the tyrosine kinase receptor Ret. Nature 1994;367:380—383.

46. Mishina Y, Rey R, Finegold MJ, Matzuk MM, Josso N, Cate RL, Behringer RR. Genetic analysis of the Müllerian-inhibiting substance signal transduction pathway in mammalian sexual differentiation. Genes Dev 1996;10:2577—2587.

47. Oshima M, Oshima H, Taketo MM. TGF-beta receptor type II deficiency results in defects of yolk sac hematopoiesis and vasculogenesis. Dev Biol 1996;179:297—302.

48. Waldrip WR, Bikoff EK, Hoodless PA, Wrana JL, Robertson EJ. Smad2 signaling in extraembryonic tissues determines anterior-posterior polarity of the early mouse embryo. Cell 1998;92:797—808.

49. Sirard C, de la Pompa JL, Elia A, Itie A, Mirtsos C, Cheung A, Hahn S, Wakeham A, Schwartz L, Kern SE, Rossant J, Mak TW. The tumor suppressor gene Smad4/Dpc4 is required for gastrulation and later for anterior development of the mouse embryo. Genes Dev 1998;12:107—119.

50. Yang X, Li C, Xu X, Deng C. The tumor suppressor SMAD4/DPC4 is essential for epiblast proliferation and mesoderm induction in mice. Proc Natl Acad Sci USA 1998;95:3667—3672.

51. Kumar TR, Wang Y, Matzuk MM. Gonadotropins are essential modifier factors for gonadal tumor development in inhibin-deficient mice. Endocrinology 1996;137:4210—4216.

52. Nishimori K, Matzuk MM. Transgenic mice in the analysis of reproductive development and function. Rev Reprod 1996;1:203—212.

53. Sassone-Corsi P. Transcriptional checkpoints determining the fate of male germ cells. Cell 1997;88:163—166.

54. Elvin JA, Matzuk MM. Mouse models of ovarian failure. Rev Reprod 1998;(In press).

55. Young WS, Shepard E, Amico J, Hennighausen L, Wagner KU, LaMarca ME, McKinney C, Ginns EI. Deficiency in mouse oxytocin prevents milk ejection, but not fertility or parturition. J Neuroendocrinol 1996;8:847—853.

# Is ICSI the ultimate ART procedure?

André Van Steirteghem[1], Anick De Vos[1], Catherine Staessen[1], Greta Verheyen[1], Ayse Aytoz[1], Maryse Bonduelle[2], Herman Tournaye[1] and Paul Devroey[1]

*Centers for [1]Reproductive Medicine, and [2]Medical Genetics, Dutch-speaking Brussels Free University, Brussels, Belgium*

**Abstract.** Since its first clinical success in 1992 intracytoplasmic sperm injection (ICSI) is now the widely accepted assisted reproductive technology for couples with severe male-factor infertility using ejaculated, epididymal or testicular sperm. The results of several thousands of ICSI cycles indicate that the results of ICSI in terms of fertilization, embryo cleavage and implantation are similar to the results of conventional IVF in couples with tubal or idiopathic infertility. An important issue regarding ICSI is its safety. Current results of a prospective follow-up of ICSI pregnancies and children indicated a slight but significant increase in foetal sex chromosome anomalies and de novo autosomal translocations. The incidence of 46 major congenital malformations in 1,966 children born alive (2.3%) is similar to that found in national registries or ART surveys. The issue of using immature male germ cells such as round spermatids in ICSI remains unresolved and includes reliable identification of the round spermatids, defining the target group for ICSI with round spermatids and assessing its safety. The question whether the indications of ICSI should be extended to patients with nonmale infertility awaits the outcome of randomized controlled trials comparing IVF and ICSI including the health of the children. ICSI is now most often used in preimplantation genetic diagnosis in order to avoid contamination by extraneous DNA in polymerase chain reaction procedures.

**Keywords:** children, fetal karyotype, ICSI, indications, male infertility.

## Introduction

In the mid-80s it became clear that conventional IVF had limitations in the alleviation of long-standing andrological infertility. A substantial member of treatment cycles did not result in embryo transfer and couples were not accepted for IVF if the semen parameters were too impaired. The initial attempts to assist the fertilization by zona drilling, partial zona dissection or subzonal insemination were associated with erratic but generally low normal fertilization rates and live-birth rates. In 1992, our group reported the first pregnancies and births to result from replacement of embryos generated by ICSI, which involved injection of a single spermatozoon through the zona pellucida directly into the oocyte [1]. The ICSI experience has been that the fertilization rate is considerably better than after other assisted fertilization procedures and that ICSI also leads to the production of more embryos able to achieve implantation. Since July 1992, ICSI was the only procedure used when assisted fertilization is necessary [2].

*Address for correspondence:* Prof André Van Steirteghem, Center for Reproductive Medicine AZ-VUB Laarbeeklaan 101 B-1090 Brussels, Belgium. Tel.: +32-2-477-50-50. Fax: +32-2-477-50-60.

This review reports on the current indications, outcome and limitations of ICSI. The possibility of using ICSI for less severe male-factor infertility, tubal and idiopathic infertility or preimplantation genetic diagnosis will also be discussed.

## Current ICSI indications

The majority of couples with severe male factor infertility can be treated by ICSI, which requires only one spermatozoon with a functional genome and centrosome for the fertilization of each oocyte. ICSI can also be used with spermatozoa from the epididymis or testis when there is an obstruction in the excretory ducts. If a patient is azoospermic because of extremely reduced germ cell production, ICSI can be used if enough spermatozoa can be retrieved in testicular tissue samples. The current indications of ICSI are summarized in Table 1.

Artificial insemination with donor sperm (AID) is currently only used when ICSI with sperm from the ejaculate, the epididymis or the testis could not be applied or failed and in men, who prefer AID above other procedures because of financial, psychological, ethical or genetic considerations.

## Current ICSI results

A recent literature survey on 14 retrospective case studies and the reports of ESHRE Task Force on ICSI have analyzed the results of ICSI [3—5]. As an exam-

*Table 1.* Current indications for ICSI.

Ejaculated spermatozoa
  Oligozoospermia
  Teratozoospermia ($\leqslant 4\%$ normal morphology using strict criteria — caveat for globozoospermia)
  Asthenozoospermia (caveat for 100% immotile spermatozoa)
  High titers of antisperm antibodies
  Repeated fertilization failure after conventional IVF
  Autoconserved frozen sperm from cancer patients in remission
  Ejaculatory disorders (e.g., electroejaculation, retrograde ejaculation)

Epididymal spermatozoa
  Congenital bilateral absence of vas deferens (CBAVD)
  Young syndrome
  Failed vaso-epididymostomy
  Failed vasovasostomy
  Azoospermia after bilateral herniorraphy
  Obstruction of both ejaculatory ducts

Testicular spermatozoa
  All indications for epididymal spermatozoa
  Extensive scar tissue preventing aspiration of spermatozoa from the epididymis
  Azoospermia caused by testicular failure
  Necrozoospermia

ple of results of ICSI the 7 years of ICSI practice at the Brussels Free University (VUB) Center for Reproductive Medicine will be summarized.

Between January 1991 and December 1997 almost 7,400 ICSI cycles involving almost 74,500 metaphase-II oocytes were carried out and evaluated in our center.

A total of 7,610 ICSI cycles were scheduled in couples with long-standing infertility. The ICSI procedure could not be carried out in 236 cycles (3.1%) because there were no cumulus-oocyte complexes or metaphase-II oocytes (106 cycles), or because no spermatozoa were available for the microinjection procedure (130 cycles). The latter condition occurred especially in patients with nonobstructive azoospermia who were scheduled for ICSI with testicular spermatozoa.

The ICSI procedure was performed with spermatozoa from the ejaculate in 6,397 cycles (86.8%), with freshly collected epididymal spermatozoa in 161 cycles (2.2%), with frozen–thawed epididymal spermatozoa in 130 cycles (1.8%) and with testicular spermatozoa in 686 cycles (9.2%).

After controlled ovarian stimulation using in most cycles GnRHa-hMG-hCG a total of 92,838 cumulus-oocyte-complexes (COCs) were retrieved during 7,610 cycles, i.e., a mean of 12.2 COCs per cycle. Cumulus and corona cells were removed by means of a combination of enzymatic and mechanical procedures. Microscopic observations revealed that 95.0% of the COCs contained an oocyte with an intact zona pellucida, 81.5% contained metaphase-II oocytes that had extruded the first polar body, 9.8% contained germinal-vesicle stage oocytes and 3.7% contained metaphase-II oocytes that had undergone breakdown of the germinal vesicle but had not yet extruded the first polar body (metaphase-I oocytes). The distribution of oocytes with different nuclear maturity was quite variable from patient to patient. ICSI was only carried out on metaphase-II oocytes.

Semen assessment of freshly ejaculated sperm used in 6,180 cycles revealed that all three semen parameters (sperm density, motility and morphology) were abnormal in 44.0% of the cycles, two semen values were abnormal in 30.4% of the cycles, one semen value was abnormal in 18.4% of the cycles and all three semen values were normal in 7.2% of the cycles. Most of the couples with normal semen values had previously undergone conventional IVF treatments without success.

In total, ICSI was performed in 7,374 cycles on 74,520 metaphase-II oocytes (a mean of 10.1 metaphase-II oocytes per cycle). Sixteen to 18 h after ICSI, oocytes were inspected for intactness and fertilization. The number of intact oocytes was 67,708 (90.9% of the oocytes that received injections), i.e., a damage rate of 9.1% of the injected oocytes. The mean number of successfully injected oocytes was 9.2 per treatment. Oocytes were considered to be normally fertilized when two individualized or fragmented polar bodies were present together with two clearly visible pronuclei containing nucleoli. Normally fertilized oocytes resulted from 72.2% of the successfully injected oocytes, 65.6% of the injected metaphase-II oocytes and 52.6% of the retrieved COCs. Abnormal fertilization occurred as one-pronuclear (PN) oocytes in 2.8% (2090) of the injected metaphase-II oocytes, and 3.7% (2741) of the injected metaphase-II oocytes revealed three pronuclei. If such abnormally fertilized 1-PN or 3-PN cleave further they are not transferred.

Damage and pronuclear status after ICSI were analyzed for all four types of sperm (ejaculated, fresh and frozen–thawed epididymal, and testicular) used in performing ICSI (Table 2). The percentages of oocytes that remained intact after ICSI varied between 89.8 and 92.3% and was similar for the four types of spermatozoa. The percentage of oocytes fertilized normally (two pronuclei) varied between 56.6 and 67.0%. The normal fertilization rate for ICSI was higher when ejaculated sperm was used than when other types of sperm were used. The percentage of oocytes with one pronucleus after ICSI varied between 2.6 and 4.2%. The percentage of oocytes with three pronuclei after ICSI varied between 3.3 and 4.9%. Abnormal fertilization occurred to a similar extent in the four different groups of spermatozoa. The exceptional circumstances by which no injected oocytes fertilized normally were associated with only very few metaphase-II oocytes being available for ICSI, only totally immotile spermatozoa being available for the injection, gross abnormalities present in the oocytes, round-headed spermatozoa being injected or all oocytes being damaged in the injection procedure. In this case, most of the patients achieved fertilization in subsequent cycles [6,7].

Embryo cleavage is evaluated after a further 24 h of in vitro culture. The cleaving embryos are scored according to equality of size of the blastomeres and proportion of anucleate fragments as excellent type-A embryos (no anucleate fragments), good-quality, type-B embryos (between 1 and 20% of the volume filled with anucleate fragments) and fair-quality, type-C embryos (between 21 and 50% of the volume filled with anucleate fragments). Cleaved embryos with less than one-half of their volume filled with anucleate fragments are eligible for transfer. Supernumerary embryos with less than 20% anucleate fragments are cryopreserved on day 2 or 3 after oocyte retrieval. The total number of embryos of sufficient quality to be transferred, i.e., those with less than 50% anucleate fragments was 39,135: 80.0% of the two-pronuclear oocytes, 57.8% of the successfully (intact) oocytes, 52.5% of the injected metaphase-II oocytes and 42.2% of the retrieved cumulus-oocyte complexes. The percentages of 2-PN oocytes

Table 2. Sperm origin, oocyte damage and pronuclear status after ICSI.

| | Ejaculated semen | Epididymal | | Testis |
|---|---|---|---|---|
| | | Fresh | Frozen – thawed | |
| No. of cycles | 6397 | 161 | 130 | 686 |
| No. of oocytes that received ICSI | 63645 | 1877 | 1374 | 7624 |
| Percentage of intact oocytes | 90.9 | 89.8 | 92.3 | 90.8 |
| Percentage of injected oocytes with | | | | |
|     one pronucleus | 2.6 | 4.0 | 3.2 | 4.2 |
|     two pronuclei | 67.0 | 59.8 | 57.3 | 56.6 |
|     three or more pronuclei | 3.7 | 4.9 | 4.8 | 3.3 |

developing into excellent, good-quality and fair-quality embryos for the different types of spermatozoa used for ICSI are summarized in Table 3. A higher percentage of good-quality embryos was obtained in the group of ejaculated spermatozoa. The percentages of embryos actually transferred or frozen as supernumerary embryos was similar for the four types of spermatozoa and varied between 59.6 and 65.7% of the two-pronuclear oocytes.

Embryo replacement of at least one embryo was possible in 6,834 of the 7,374 treatment cycles with ICSI (92.7%). This may be considered a high transfer rate because it represents couples with previous fertilization failure in conventional IVF, ejaculated sperm too poor to be included in IVF, or men with obstructive or nonobstructive azoospermia. As indicated in Table 4, the transfer rate was similar across the four groups of sperm used for ICSI; the transfer rate varied from 86.2 to 93.0% of the 6,834 embryo replacements; 6,758 transfers were with known serum hCG outcome. For the other 76 transfers (61 in the ejaculated sperm group, four in the frozen–thawed epididymal sperm group and 11 in the testicular sperm group) the serum hCG was unknown. The overall pregnancy rate per transfer with known serum hCG outcome and the pregnancy rate per number of embryos transferred were similar for the four types of spermatozoa. Especially high pregnancy rates were observed when elective transfer of two or three embryos was performed [8,9]. The pregnancy rate per cycle with known serum hCG outcome varied from 27.8 to 39.8%. Delivery rates per transfer with known outcome until delivery were calculated for the ICSI treatment cycles performed from 1991 to 1996. All but 68 (55 in the ejaculated semen group, two in the fresh epididymal spermatozoa group and 11 in the testicular spermatozoa group) embryo replacements with positive serum hCG resulted in a known pregnancy outcome. Delivery rates per transfer with known pregnancy outcome varied from 22.3 tot 29.2%.

## Outcome of ICSI

When assisted fertilization procedures (initially PZD and SUZI, since 1991 ICSI)

Table 3. Sperm origin and embryo development after ICSI.

| | Ejaculated semen | Epididymal | | Testis |
| --- | --- | --- | --- | --- |
| | | Fresh | Frozen – thawed | |
| No. of two-pronuclear oocytes | 42648 | 1122 | 787 | 4315 |
| Percentage or excellent embryos | 7.0 | 7.9 | 3.9 | 5.9 |
| Percentage of good-quality embryos | 58.3 | 49.4 | 45.2 | 49.7 |
| Percentage of fair-quality embryos | 15.8 | 14.6 | 18.7 | 19.3 |
| Percentage of transferred or frozen embryos | 65.7 | 64.8 | 59.6 | 62.7 |

*Table 4.* Sperm origin and outcome of embryo transfers after ICSI.

| | Ejaculated semen | Epididymal | | Testis |
|---|---|---|---|---|
| | | Fresh | Frozen – thawed | |
| **1991–1997** | | | | |
| No. of cycles | 6397 | 161 | 130 | 686 |
| No. of transfers | 5949 | 149 | 112 | 624 |
| Transfer rate (%) | 93.0 | 92.5 | 86.2 | 91.0 |
| No. of pregnancies | 2128 | 64 | 35 | 201 |
| Pregnancy rate per transfer[a] (%) | 36.1 | 43.0 | 32.4 | 32.8 |
| one embryo | 13.9 | 20.0 | 21.4 | 11.3 |
| two embryos | 24.7 | 33.3 | 17.6 | 27.3 |
| two embryos (elective) | 42.6 | 31.8 | 33.3 | 31.1 |
| three embryos | 38.0 | 43.2 | 31.0 | 32.9 |
| three embryos (elective) | 45.4 | 59.4 | 45.5 | 46.5 |
| more than three embryos | 34.6 | 44.0 | 41.2 | 38.4 |
| Pregnancy rate per cycle[a] (%) | 33.6 | 39.8 | 27.8 | 29.8 |
| **1991–1996** | | | | |
| No. of transfers with known outcome (until delivery) | 4903 | 144 | 95 | 439 |
| No. of deliveries | 1254 | 42 | 26 | 98 |
| Delivery rate per transfer (%) | 25.6 | 29.2 | 27.4 | 22.3 |

[a]With known serum HCG outcome.

were introduced into clinical practice there was major concern about its safety: the procedure is more invasive and spermatozoa are microinjected which could not be used successfully in conventional IVF. There was even more concern when ICSI was carried out with epididymal or testicular spermatozoa: genomic imprinting may be less complete in these sperm and related anomalies may become manifest only at birth or later in life.

Here we summarize the outcome of 2,375 ICSI pregnancies (generated between April 1991 and September 1997) leading to the birth of 1,987 children. This follow-up was carried out by the Centers for Medical Genetics and Reproductive Medicine and has already been partially reported [10–15]. The study included genetic counselling (before ICSI or at 6–8 weeks of pregnancy), prenatal karyotype analysis and a prospective follow-up of pregnancies and the resulting children. Initially, prenatal diagnosis was strongly recommended; currently the couples are informed about the risk factors and left to choose whether or not to have prenatal testing by amniocentesis (for singleton pregnancies) or by chorionic villus sampling (for multiple pregnancies).

There was a genetic risk in 557 out of 1,513 couples attending the genetic counselling session(s). These risks included increased parental age, chromosomal abnormality in parents, monogenic diseases (especially cystic fibrosis), multifactorial diseases and consanguinity.

Abnormal fetal karyotypes were found in 15 of 690 amniocenteses and 13 of 392 chorionic villous samplings. In these 1,082 tests we observed 18 (1.7%) de novo chromosomal aberrations: nine of these (0.8%) were sex-chromosomal aberrations and another nine (0.8%) were autosomal aberrations (trisomies and structural). These figures show that there is a significant increase in sex-chromosomal aberrations, since the 95% confidence limit of this percentage (0.3—1.6%) does contain the aberration percentage (0.19—0.23%) described in the literature with regard to a neonatal population. The incidence of autosomal aberrations is due partly to the increase in trisomies, linked with higher maternal ages. On the other hand, there is also an increase in structural de novo aberrations (0.36% compared to 0.07% in the literature), which is significant. The increase in inherited structural aberrations (one of them being nonbalanced) is, of course, higher than in the general population but was predictable for the individual couples, where the father was carrying the structural anomaly in all but one case.

Regarding the pregnancy loss after prenatal diagnostic procedures in ICSI pregnancies, we compared a group of 460 consecutive ICSI singleton pregnancies with amniocentesis and 360 consecutive ICSI singleton pregnancies without amniocentesis. There was no statistical difference in outcome measured in terms of prematurity, low birth weight, very low birth weight or loss of pregnancy. The same findings were observed in 109 consecutive ICSI twin pregnancies with and 174 ICSI twin pregnancies without chorionic villous sampling [16].

The follow-up of the expected child consisted of a visit to the geneticist-paediatrician at 2 and 12 months of age, and then once a year. A widely accepted definition of major malformations was used, that is, malformations that generally cause functional impairment or require surgical correction. The remaining malformations were considered to be minor. The mean birthweight of 1,966 liveborn children of at least 20 weeks was 2,818 g, the mean length was 47.9 cm and the mean head circumference was 33.5 cm. Prematurity, that is, birth under or at 37 weeks of pregnancy, was observed in 12% of the 1,063 singletons, 59% of the 805 twins and 96% of the 98 triplets. Birthweight under 2,500 g was observed in 8% of the singletons, 52% of the twins and 85% of the triplets. Very low birthweight under 1,500 g was recorded for 2% of the singletons, 5% of the twins and 36% of the triplets. Sex ratio of the males to females was 0.98%.

Major malformations were found in seven interruptions and in four intrauterine deaths, and in a total of 21 stillbirths after 20 weeks of gestation. Major malformations were found in 22 of 1,063 (2.1%) singleton children, 22 of 805 (2.7%) twin children and two of 98 (2.0%) triplet children. This is 46 of 1,966 or 2.3% of all babies born alive. This figure of 2.3% malformation rate is similar to that found in most of the general population national registries and the ART surveys.

Two recent articles report on the development of ICSI children as assessed by the Bayley scales of infant development. An Australian study report on the outcome of almost 100 children conceived by ICSI in comparison to about the same number of children conceived naturally or by conventional IVF techniques. The mental developmental index of the ICSI children seemed to be significantly lower than that of either control group. The development of boys was more retarded than that of girls [17]. In the same issue of Lancet our group reported on the mental development of 201 ICSI and 131 IVF children at the age of 2 years. The overall results for ICSI and IVF children indicated a score no lower than that for the general population. Although there is no indication in our own study that ICSI children have a slower mental development than the general population, a detailed case-control study taking into account parental background is needed to be able to draw final conclusions [18].

The observations on the pregnancies and children should be completed by others and by collaborative efforts such as the ESHRE Task Force on Intracytoplasmic Sperm Injection. In the meantime, before any ICSI treatment is started, couples should be informed on the existing date: the risk of de novo sex chromosomal and structural aberrations, and the risk of transmitting fertility problems to the offspring. Patients should also be reassured that there seems to be no higher incidence of major congenital malformations in children born after ICSI.

## ICSI with immature sperm

In patients with obstructive azoospermia due to germ-cell failure or maturation arrest, recovery of mature testicular spermatozoa or late elongated spermatids in view of ICSI is only possible in about 50% of the patients even when multiple testicular biopsies are taken. None of the clinical parameters, such as testicular volume, semen analysis, serum FSH or testicular histology care reliably predict whether testicular spermatozoa will be found [19]. Recently, there are a few reports in the literature describing ICSI with immature sperm cells such as round spermatids. The fertilization and pregnancy rates, however, generally remain far below those obtained with mature spermatozoa and elongated spermatids. The use of round spermatids in ICSI raises several concerns such as DNA immaturity, genomic imprinting, normality of the centerosome and presence of sperm-derived oocyte-activating factor. Furthermore the correct identification of the round spermatids within a heterogeneous population of testicular cells has not received enough attention. Identification of round spermatids is problematic when conventional Hoffman modulation contrast systems were used on the inverted microscope. If appropriate phase-contrast optics are used on an inverted microscope reliable recognition of the round spermatids in a cell suspension smeared at the glass bottom of a dish is possible. However, exploration of several biopsies from patients with nonobstructive azoospermia showing no spermatozoa after extensive search have never, in our experience, revealed round spermatids. This observation firstly questions whether enough effort is spent in general on searching for mature spermatozoa or later spermatids. Furthermore, its casts some doubt on the existence of the real target group for round spermatid injection. In any case, experimental investigations should precede the introduction of round spermatid injection into the clinical practice of any ART center [20].

## ICSI for other indications than severe male-factor infertility

The question arises whether the ICSI procedure should be extended to other indications than severe male-factor infertility. Is normal fertilization and embryo cleavage better after ICSI than after conventional IVF? Can we avoid unexpected fertilization failures when ICSI is used? If the answers to both questions are positive, the implantation potential of IVF- and ICSI-embryos should be examined. This study should then be completed by answering the ultimate question regarding safety: are there more problems during pregnancy and after delivery when the ICSI procedure instead of conventional IVF has been used?

A few controlled comparisons between conventional IVF and ICSI in patients with moderate male infertility were reported. There appears to be 4 times more chance for an oocyte to be fertilized when ICSI was used instead of IVF. Moreover the risk of fertilization failure was 6 times lower in ICSI [21–24]. Two controlled studies compared IVF and ICSI in couples with tubal or idiopathic infertility. The most striking result was that unexpected fertilization did not occur after ICSI [25,26].

In a series of ongoing controlled studies we have searched for an answer to these questions in couples with tubal, idiopathic and borderline male-factor infertility. Couples, who were infertile because of the above mentioned reasons, were included in these controlled comparisons between conventional IVF and ICSI when at least six cumulus-oocyte-complexes were retrieved; half of the cumulus-oocyte complexes underwent conventional IVF and half of the complexes the ICSI procedure. Primary endpoints of these studies were fertilization and embryo development (morphology and speed of embryo cleavage after 48 h of in vitro culture).

In 50 cycles of couples with tubal infertility and normal sperm parameters and with at least six cumulus-oocyte complexes recovered, half of the oocytes were inseminated by conventional IVF and the others were injected by ICSI. A total of 630 cumulus-oocyte complexes were collected in these 50 cycles; 316 sibling oocytes were inseminated by conventional IVF and the remaining 314 were treated by ICSI. A significantly higher number of oocytes showed two pronuclei after ICSI (68%) than after IVF (57%). Total fertilization failure occurred in four patients (20 oocytes) after conventional IVF and in one patient after ICSI (when only two metaphase-II oocytes could be injected). Although injection and insemination of the oocytes were performed at the same time, 42 h later the embryos after ICSI were at a more advanced stage of development. The best embryos were selected for transfer independently of the insemination procedure, but preferably this involved only one type of embryos. There were 17 (34.7%) positive serum HCG after 49 embryo transfers. Pregnancy and implantation rates were similar between the two groups.

In an ongoing controlled comparison of IVF and ICSI involving patients with idiopathic infertility, we recorded so far similar fertilization rates in 24 treatment cycles with, however, six unexpected complete fertilization failures in conventional IVF. In 20 cycles involving asthenozoospermic semen ($< 5\%$ type A motility) but with enough progressive motile spermatozoa available for IVF, a significantly reduced fertilization rate was observed in conventional IVF (22.9%) as compared to ICSI (63.4%). Unexpected IVF fertilization failures occurred in seven cycles. In 10 of the 20 cycles none of the oocytes fertilized normally after conventional IVF.

The question arises as to whether ICSI will become the procedure of choice for all couples requiring ART. Since the ICSI procedure itself is more invasive, the questions that have arisen on safety issues have to be elucidated. Only when the outcome for ICSI children is similar to the outcome for ICSI children, can one consider a broader use of ICSI.

Preimplantation genetic diagnosis (PGD) is a recent development which became possible thanks to ART and progress in molecular genetics. PGD can be offered to couples at risk of having a child with a genetic disease. Indications for PGD are similar as for prenatal diagnosis by chorionic villus sampling or amniocentesis. PGD is usually carried out by molecular genetic procedures (fluorescent in situ hybridization (FISH) or polymerase chain reaction (PCR)) on one or preferentially two blastomeres from a day 3 cleaving embryo (with usually about two blastomeres). PGD involves genetic counseling and preparation of the couple, ART procedure (conventional IVF or ICSI), biopsy of one or two blastomeres by micromanipulation on a day-three embryo, the diagnostic procedure on the biopsied blastomere(s) and replacement of nonaffected embryos (maximum two or three). In PCR contamination by extraneous DNA may be a problem and could arise during embryo biopsy procedure if sperm DNA is adhering to the zona pellucida. This contamination can be prevented by using ICSI as ART procedure in PGD cycles. This policy is followed worldwide by all centers that practice PGD. The clinical experimental nature of this early form of prenatal diagnosis requires that in case of pregnancy the PGD is confirmed by prenatal diagnosis and that pregnancies and health of children born after PGD are carefully monitored [27].

## Acknowledgements

We are indebted to many colleagues of the Centers for Medical Genetics and Reproductive Medicine: the clinicians, the clinical embryologists, the scientists, the nurses and laboratory technicians. This work is supported by grants from the Fund for Scientific Research-Flanders (FWO-Vlaanderen), the Brussels Free University Research Council and an unconditional educational grant from Organon International.

# References

1. Palermo G, Joris H, Devroey P, Van Steirteghem AC. Pregnancies after intracytoplasmic injection of single spermatozoon into an oocyte. Lancet 1992;340:17—18.
2. Van Steirteghem AC, Nagy Z, Joris H, Liu J, Staessen C, Smitz J et al. High fertilization and implantation rates after intracytoplasmic sperm injection. Hum Reprod 1993;8:1061—1066.
3. Van Steirteghem A, Verheyen G, Tournaye H, Devroey P. Assisted reproductive technology by intracytoplasmic sperm injection in male-factor infertility. Curr Opin Urol 1996;6:333—339.
4. ESHRE Task Force on Intracytoplasmic Sperm Injection. Assisted reproduction by intracytoplasmic sperm injection: a survey on the clinical experience in 1994 and the children born after ICSI, carried out until 31 December 1993. Hum Reprod 1998;13:1737—1746.
5. Tarlatzis B, Bili H. Survey on intracytoplasmic sperm injection: report from the ESHRE ICSI Task Force. In: Devroey P, Tarlatzis B, Van Steirteghem A (eds) Current Theory and Practice of ICSI. Oxford, UK: Oxford University Press, Hum Reprod 1998;13 (Suppl 1):165—177.
6. Liu J, Nagy Z, Joris H, Tournaye H, Smitz J, Camus M et al. Analysis of 76 total fertilization failure cycles out of 2732 intracytoplasmic sperm injection cycles. Hum Reprod 1995;10: 2630—2636.
7. Vandervorst M, Tournaye H, Camus M, Nagy Z, Van Steirteghem AC, Devroey P. Patients with absolutely immotile spermatozoa and intracytoplasmic sperm injection. Hum Reprod 1997;12: 2429—2433.
8. Staessen C, Janssenswillen C, Van den Abbeel E, Devroey P, Van Steirteghem AC. Avoidance of triplet pregnancies by elective transfer of two good quality embryos. Hum Reprod 1993;8: 1650—1653.
9. Staessen C, Nagy ZP, Liu J, Janssenswillen C, Camus M, Devroey P, Van Steirteghem AC. One year's experience with elective transfer of two good quality embryos in the human in-vitro fertilization and intracytoplasmic sperm injection programmes. Hum Reprod 1995;10:3305—3312.
10. Bonduelle M, Legein J, Buysse A, Van Assche E, Wisanto A, Devroey P et al. Prospective follow-up study of 423 children born after intracytoplasmic sperm injection. Hum Reprod 1996;11: 1558—1564.
11. Bonduelle M, Wilikens A, Buysse A, Van Assche E, Wisanto A, Devroey P et al. Prospective follow-up study of 877 children born after intracytoplasmic sperm injection (ICSI), with ejaculated epididymal and testicular spermatozoa and after replacement of cryopreserved embryos obtained after ICSI. In: Van Steirteghem A, Devroey P, Liebaers I (eds) Genetics and Assisted Human Conception. Oxford, UK: Oxford University Press. Hum Reprod 1996;11(Suppl 4): 131—159.
12. Wisanto A, Bonduelle M, Camus M, Tournaye H, Magnus M, Liebaers I, Van Steirteghem AC. Obstetric outcome of 904 pregnancies after intracytoplasmic sperm injection. In: Van Steirteghem A, Devroey P, Liebaers I (eds) Genetics and Assisted Human Conception. Oxford, UK: Oxford University Press. Hum Reprod 1996;11(Suppl 4):121—130.
13. Bonduelle M, Devroey P, Liebaers I, Van Steirteghem A. Commentary: Major defects are overestimated. Br Med J 1997;315:1265—1266. on article by Kurinczuk J and Bower C. Birth defects in infants conceived by intracytoplasmic sperm injection: an alternative interpretation. Br Med J 1997;315:1260—1266.
14. Bonduelle M, Wilikens A, Buysse A, Van Assche E, Devroey P, Van Steirteghem A, Liebaers I. A follow-up study of children born after intracytoplasmic sperm injection (ICSI) with epididymal and testicular spermatozoa and after replacement of cryopreserved embryos obtained after ICSI. In: Devroey P, Tarlatzis B, Van Steirteghem A (eds) Current Theory and Practice of ICSI. Oxford, UK: Oxford University Press. Hum Reprod 1998;13(Suppl 1):196—207.
15. Bonduelle M, Aytoz A, Van Assche E, Devroey P, Liebaers I, Van Steirteghem A. Incidence of chromosomal aberrations in children born after assisted reproduction through intracytoplasmic sperm injection, Editorial, Hum Reprod 1998;13:781—782.
16. Aytoz A, De Catte L, Camus M, Bonduelle M, Van Assche E, Liebaers I et al. Obstetrical out-

come after prenatal diagnosis in pregnancies obtained after in intracytoplasmic sperm injection. Hum Reprod 1998;13:(In press).

17. Bowen J, Gibson F, Leslie G, Saunders D. Medical and developmental outcome at 1 year for children conceived by intracytoplasmic sperm injection. Lancet 1998;351:1529—1534.

18. Bonduelle M, Joris H, Hofmans, K, Liebaers I, Van Steirteghem A. Mental development of 201 ICSI children at 2 years of age. Research Letter. Lancet 1998;351:1553.

19. Tournaye H, Verheyen G, Nagy P, Ubaldi F, Goossens A, Silber S, Van Steirteghem A, Devroey P. Are there any predictive factors for successful testicular sperm recovery in azoospermic patients? Hum Reprod 1997;12:80—86.

20. Verheyen G, Crabbé E, Joris H, Van Steirteghem A. Simple and reliable identification of the human round spermatid by inverted phase-contrast microscopy. Hum Reprod 1998;13:(In press).

21. Hamberger L, Sjögren A, Lundin K, Söderlund B, Nilsson L, Bergh C et al. Microfertilization techniques - The Swedish experience. Reprod Fertil Dev 1995;7:263.

22. Fishel S, Lisi F, Rinaldi L, Lisi R, Timson J, Green S et al. Intracytoplasmic sperm injection (ICSI) versus high insemination concentration (HIC) for human conception in vitro. Reprod Fertil Dev 1995;7:169—175.

23. Calderon G, Belil I, Aran B, Veiga AZ, Gil Y, Boada M et al. Intracytoplasmic sperm injection (ICSI) versus conventional in-vitro fertilization: first results. Hum Reprod 1995;10:2835—2839.

24. Aboulgar M, Mansour R, Serour GI, Amin YM. The role of intracytoplasmic sperm injection (ICSI) in the treatment of patients with borderline semen. Hum Reprod 1995;11:2829—2830.

25. Aboulgar M, Mansour R, Serour GI, Sattar MA, Amin YA. Intracytoplasmic sperm injection and conventional in-vitro fertilization for sibling oocytes in cases of unexplained infertility and borderline semen. J Assoc Reprod and Genet 1996;13:3842.

26. Aboulgar M, Mansour R, Serour GI, Amin YA, Kamal A. Prospective controlled randomized study of in-vitro fertilization versus intracytoplasmic sperm injection in the treatment of tubal factor infertility with normal semen parameters. Fertil Steril 1996;66:753—756.

27. Liebaers I, Sermon K, Staessen C, Joris H, Lissens W, Van Assche E et al. Clinical experience with preimplantation genetic diagnosis and intracytoplasmic sperm injection. In: Devroey P, Tarlatzis B, Van Steirteghem A (eds) Current Theory and Practice of ICSI. Oxford, UK: Oxford University Press. Hum Reprod 1998;13(Suppl 1):186—195.

Fertility and Reproductive Medicine.
R.D. Kempers, J. Cohen, A.F. Haney and J.B. Younger, editors.

# New developments in human embryology offer a new dimension to clinical reproductive medicine

Alan Trounson

*Centre for Early Human Development, Institute of Reproduction and Development, Monash University, Monash Medical Centre, Clayton, Victoria, Australia*

**Abstract.** We have entered a phase of rapid new developments in mammalian embryology that now challenge human reproductive medicine to respond. New methods for the development of human embryos through the entire preimplantation period in vitro provide the basis for exploring new ways of identifying viable and genetically healthy embryos for embryo transfer and cryopreservation. New methods are evolving for the maturation of oocytes and their vitrification that offer new clinical opportunities. Embryos may be successfully multiplied and nuclear transfer techniques offer new therapies for genetic disease and even the potential construction of gametes for patients. The potential production of regenerative cell lines derived from embryonic stem cells are at the beginning and need to be considered in the ethical and legal framework of advancing human medicine.

**Keywords:** artificial gametes, blastocysts, embryonic stem cells, human embryo, nuclear transfer, preimplantation genetic diagnosis.

## Introduction

Developments in human embryology have progressed rather slowly because the majority of embryos were grown to early cleavage stages for transfer to the uterus. In the human, as distinct to many other mammalian species, replacement of two- to eight-cell embryos in the uterine cavity is compatible with their survival and development to term [1,2]. There is a growing recognition of the benefits for growing embryos to the blastocyst stage in culture before transfer to the uterus [3,4] and a renewal of interest in determining more appropriate culture conditions for the growth and development of embryos throughout the whole preimplantation period in vitro. This provides the opportunity to explore a new range of options that have very important clinical implications for reproductive medicine. These opportunities involve infertile couples and those couples who are carriers of serious genetic disorders. In addition, the use of human embryonic stem (ES) cells for transplantation [5] may offer the opportunity to correct a wide range of pathologies and injuries if we are able to control their differentiation pathways, expand the regenerative stem cell populations and prevent their rejec-

---

*Address for correspondence:* Alan Trounson, Centre for Early Human Development, Institute of Reproduction and Development, Monash University, Monash Medical Centre, 246 Clayton Road, Clayton, Vic. 3168, Australia.

tion after implantation. This paper explores these issues for the present and future of human medicine.

## The culture of human embryos throughout the entire preimplantation period

The evolution of more appropriate culture media and conditions for allowing human zygotes to express their full developmental potential has been a major advance in clinical embryology. It has been claimed for some time that the coculture of human embryos with human fallopian tube epithelial cells [6] or other cell types [7,8] is necessary to obtain the full potential of their development. However, this has been questioned by others [9—11] who were able to show at least equivalent rates of development to blastocysts in media without feeder cells. Indeed high rates of development of viable blastocysts were shown by Scholtes and Zeilmaker [12] in biphasic culture conditions of Earle's medium and Hams F10 (without hypoxanthine and thymidine) with added 8.8% pasteurized plasma protein. In this study, implantation rates were in excess of 20% when embryos were blastocysts by day 5 of culture.

The design of a cell-free culture system for human embryos to the blastocyst stage reported by Jones et al. [3] utilizes a brief insemination period (1 h) to avoid the adverse effects of exposure of the zygote to large numbers of live, dying and degenerating spermatozoa [13]. Antibiotics and pH indicators were also removed from embryo culture media because of their possible inhibition of cleavage and development [14]. It has also been known for some time that the zygote requires pyruvate for energy utilization in the TCA cycle. The preferential requirement for pyruvate continues in the cleavage stage embryo up until the morula stage. The preference for pyruvate changes with increasing glycolysis and a rapid conversion to utilization of glucose [15,16]. The presence of high levels of glucose and phosphate during early cleavage divisions can be detrimental to embryo development and even inhibit the development of aerobic glycolysis and the utilization of the pentose phosphate pathway at compaction and blastulation. Given the repetitive observation of these differences, the use of biphasic or triphasic media more suited to the metabolic needs of the stage of embryogenesis, is compelling. Moreover, the presence of serum in culture media for embryos is undesirable because of the significant perturbations in embryo metabolism with excessive lactate production, reduced oxidative metabolism, and reduced viability. Serum is suitably replaced by serum albumin and amino acids [17,18]. Early cleavage stage embryos have little capacity to metabolize proteins but readily utilize amino acids. One of the toxic byproducts of amino acid metabolism is ammonium that needs to be converted to more useful products such as glutamate or the media renewed every 48—72 h to avoid the accumulating ammonium toxicity [19].

With the background information on embryo metabolic requirements and the need to avoid inhibiting conditions, a culture system involving biphasic media and the growth of embryos to blastocysts has been designed by Jones et al. [3].

This involves a modified human tubal fluid medium (IVF-50; Scandinavian IVF Science AB) for culture of embryos to the eight-cell stage and a specially designed embryo growth medium (EG2). The basic composition for EG2 has been published [20] and we have made some modifications to further improve this medium. We have consistently found that G1 medium [3] fails to provide the support of development from one-cell to eight-cells that is obtained in IVF-50. We grow embryos together in 20–50 µl of medium under paraffin oil to obtain any benefit of autocrine factors [21]. More than 50% of zygotes develop to nascent blastocysts with clearly defined trophoblast and inner cell mass in these culture conditions. Implantation rates of individual embryos is between 23 and 28% so that the transfer of two blastocysts will result in birth rates in excess of 40%. Further improvements in pregnancy success rates will result from patient selection, identification of chromosomally abnormal embryos and optimization of the clinical procedures including embryo transfer technique.

The number of blastocysts produced is significantly associated with the number of oocytes recovered, oocytes inseminated, zygotes and embryos of eight-cell or more, 65–72 h after insemination. Pregnancy rate is significantly influenced by numbers of embryos transferred, the morphology of the leading embryo trans-ferred and mean morphology score of the transferred embryos. Maternal age, etiology of infertility and number of previous IVF cycles did not significantly influence pregnancy rate. These data are discussed in detail by Jones et al. [22]. Some of the interesting observations show, that providing a reasonable ovarian response can be achieved for IVF patients, the past failure of IVF, maternal age up to 40 years and cause of infertility has no apparent influence on pregnancy success rate after transfer of blastocysts. There is also an interesting reduction in tubal pregnancies after blastocyst transfer.

Some important clinical implications of growing embryos to the preimplanta-tion blastocyst stage include:

1. Improved selection of viable embryos. This includes the morphology of blasto-cysts which is already a significant factor in pregnancy success rates [22]. While pregnancy rate can be related to morphology of day 3 embryos, the actual cell numbers of day 3 embryos, but not fragmentation, is significantly related to the further development to blastocysts in vitro. Metabolic activity (utilization of glucose and production of lactate) of the blastocysts does not appear·to be significantly related to the establishment of pregnancy and devel-opment to term.
2. The identification of chromosome aneuploidies in "difficult IVF patients" by fluorescent in situ hybridization (FISH) for chromosomes X, Y, 13, 16, 18 and 21, show that 55–57% of all embryos at day 3 are abnormal [23,24]. Their identification and removal from the cohort of embryos growing to blas-tocysts will further increase the successful implantation and development to term of cleavage stage embryos and blastocysts chosen for transfer.
3. Trophoblast biopsy of blastocysts enables the sampling of a relatively large number of cells [25]. These blastocysts can be DNA fingerprinted to identify

individual embryos and screened for one or several mutations by fluorescent PCR techniques [26]. Genetic diagnosis at the blastocyst stage would involve screening less embryos, increasing the accuracy of diagnosis because of sampling multiple cells, allowing identification of embryos that develop to term, and increasing the success of IVF and diagnosis of genetic disorders in preimplantation embryos for patients. It is likely that preimplantation diagnosis (PGD) will eventually become the first choice for couples who are at risk of transmitting serious genetic disease.

## Maturation of human oocytes in vitro

Oocytes recovered from unstimulated growing follicles in the ovary can be matured in vitro, fertilized and some will develop to term when transferred to patients [27,28]. The maturation conditions are still being optimized for human oocytes because of their reduced embryo developmental competence [29]. It is apparent that primary oocytes cultured in vitro lack a number of the proteins that can be detected by two-dimensional gel electrophoresis in oocytes matured in vivo (C. Anderiesz, A. Trounson, unpublished data). These oocytes are likely to be involved in cell cycle regulation because of the characteristic cleavage arrest observed with in vitro matured oocytes. The protein profile of in vitro matured oocytes can be corrected by exposure of oocytes to ovulating gonadotropin changes within the follicular milieu before culture of the isolated immature oocytes (C. Anderiesz, A. Trounson, unpublished data).

It has been considered that human oocyte maturational and developmental competence is related to follicular diameter and that for successful superovulation the follicles should be of a minimum diameter of 1.6—1.8 cm. To examine this hypothesis, patients having natural cycle IVF or a minimum stimulation with clomiphene citrate have been given an ovulating dose of human chorionic gonadotropin (hCG) when the leading follicle was 0.9—2.5 cm. There was no relationship between developmental competence to the blastocyst stage in vitro and follicle diameter at the time of hCG injection (A. Trounson, G. Jones, unpublished data).

As a consequence of these studies, it is now likely that in vitro maturation systems can be designed to maintain the developmental competence of immature human oocytes from small- to medium-sized antral follicles. These techniques will suit women with polycystic ovaries where large numbers of oocytes can be recovered from follicles of 5—15 mm diameter without any need for FSH treatment to stimulate follicle growth. The successful application of in vitro maturation in this group of patients who are at high risk of ovarian hyperstimulation syndrome, could allow for further applications in nonpolycystic patients who wish to avoid the side effects of large doses of fertility drugs.

**New vitrification methods for cell and tissue cryopreservation**

Despite claims for increasing success rates for cryopreservation of human oocytes and embryos, relatively little new methodology has been applied to human cell cryopreservation. Less than 1–2% of frozen human oocytes will survive present freezing methods and develop to term [30,31] and there is no apparent advantage of freezing immature rather than mature oocytes. Present methods depend on slow cooling of cells in the presence of relatively low concentrations of penetrating and nonpenetrating cryoprotectants. The slow cooling and the need to achieve equilibration conditions by dehydration of the cells during cooling to prevent intracellular ice formation, causes numerous changes in the cell that cannot be reversed. As a consequence, new methods are being explored for both oocyte and embryo cryopreservation.

Increasing the concentration of cryoprotectants and cooling rates will allow solutions to form glass (vitrify) rather than form ice crystals (freeze). Ultrarapid freezing procedures were trialed for cryopreserving oocytes and embryos and while these were very efficient for mouse oocytes and embryos [32], they were less successful for the human [33,34]. It was apparent that both solute concentrations and cooling rate needed to be maximized. Failure to increase cryoprotectant concentrations high enough when rapid cooling can cause irreversible chromosomal damage [35]. Increasing both cryoprotectant and the rate of cooling by using metal grids to cool on [36], or minimum volumes in thin walled plastic straws [37], enables the cryopreservation of the oocytes and embryos of a range of species that have been traditionally susceptible to cryoinjury. The application of these techniques for human oocyte and embryo cryopreservation are likely to revolutionize this aspect of IVF and when combined with oocyte maturation in vitro, will provide a much sought after method for preserving germ cells for patients diagnosed with cancer.

The alternative of cryopreserving ovarian tissue for women with the intention of autotransplantation, culture of primordial follicles or the use of xenotransplantation techniques to recover developmentally competent oocytes has been recently reviewed by Shaw et al. [31]. Concerns about the reseeding of patients with cancer cells may prevent the widespread use of autotransplantation and culture of primordial follicle cells for many months is unlikely to be feasible in the near future. The success of xenotransplantation for recovery of mature oocytes after cryopreservation of ovarian tissue makes this approach the most attractive at the present time for young women diagnosed with cancer, wishing to preserve their germ cells to avoid potential damage by radio- or chemotherapy [38].

**Embryo multiplication**

Embryos can be multiplied by bisection in ruminants to increase the probability of development to term and this is also likely to be the case for human embryos [5]. Embryos may be bisected at any stage of development but bisection of the

blastocyst stage where the inner cell mass (ICM) is duplicated in separate trophoblastic vesicles is the usual technique for twinning in cattle. Implantation
rates increase from around 60—70% to around 110% for each original embryo
[39]. Duplication of the ICM by separation within the same trophectoderm reside
or separate vesicles during hatching from the zona pellucida is one of the likely
mechanisms for monozygotic twinning in the human (Fig. 1).

It is reasonable to consider that patients who are unable to produce many normal embryos because of their age, contraindications for superovulation or their
genetic constitution, could increase their chance of conception and birth by the
mechanical division of the one or the few blastocysts they produce. The problem
for a significant proportion of infertile couples is the production of sufficient
numbers of oocytes and embryos to warrant treatment for the costs of IVF treatment involved. Women who are mosaic for some genetic conditions, for example,
Turner Syndrome, produce few normal embryos during a very restricted time of
ovulatory activity [40]. Identification of the few normal embryos by FISH or
PCR and their bisection could increase implantation rate substantially for such
patients.

Nuclear transfer can also be used to multiply ruminant embryos [41,42] and
these techniques can be used to produce offspring for nonhuman primates [43].
This involves the disaggregation of cleaving embryos and the fusion with mature
enucleated oocytes. A source of donor oocytes is needed to act as surrogate cyto-
plasts for the embryonic nuclei. While this is feasible and the production of a
restricted number of embryos could be considered to help patients who produce
few of their own, ethical concerns are likely to be raised about this approach
because of the close association with somatic cell cloning [5].

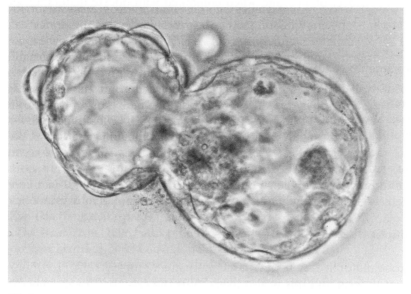

*Fig. 1.*

**Nuclear transfer for correcting genetic and developmental abnormalities**

Nuclear transfer could be used to correct mitochondrial genetic disease. The nucleus of cells of the early developing embryo could be isolated from cytoplasmic mitochondrial elements and introduced into the enucleated cytoplasm of a donor oocyte known to have functionally normal mitochondria. The use of nuclear transfer for this purpose would be arguably ethical and experimental studies are likely to confirm the potential to eradicate the inheritance of mitochondrial defects for women.

Based on some experiments in mice [44], it is believed that zygotes of some patients can be rescued by injection of cytoplasm from mature oocytes [45]. It is rather more difficult to prove the therapeutic benefits of cytoplasmic transfer for human embryos but it remains a technique that may have benefits for the developmental competence of otherwise genetically normal embryos.

Rescue of embryos that begin to show retardation of cleavage or become blocked in development is also possible by nuclear transfer. The nucleus of the failing embryos could be removed from their own cytoplasmic environment and transferred to a developmentally competent donor cytoplast (activated mature enucleated oocyte). This requires the availability of donor oocytes for nuclear transfer. It would be important that oocyte or cytoplast cryopreservation be established to enable the clinical application of this type of embryo rescue technique. Unless the donor embryo can be identified as chromosomally normal, the attempted rescue of a failing embryo may be of little benefit for the patient. This would mean that FISH or fluorescent PCR would be needed to confirm euploidy before or after the reconstruction event.

**Construction of artificial gametes**

Somatic cells can be completely reprogrammed by culture as cell lines and then used for nuclear transfer [46,47]. It is also possible to induce haploidy after nuclear transfer by manipulation of the cytoplast cell cycle [48]. The result is that an oocyte can be formed with a haploid nucleus. A male or female pronucleus can also be formed and also incorporated into the haploid nuclear transfer cytoplast to reconstitute diploidy. These manipulations establish artificial gametes so that in the absence of gametes in one of the partners, they could be formed by nuclear transfer. The unknown and primary difficulty may be a lack of compatibility of maternal and paternal genomic imprinting [49]. The gametes are specifically imprinted for gene expression or inactivation to enable normal development to proceed. The reconstituted nuclear transfer gamete derived from a cultured somatic cell may not be genomically imprinted to be compatible with a sperm- or oocyte-derived nucleus. The use of maternal and paternal somatic cell nuclei may also not be compatible with normal development because chromosomes may be both maternally or paternally derived and hence alleles that are meant to be genomically imprinted may lack this essential requirement for normal development. Experiments are needed in an appropriate animal model to explore this interesting new area to determine the potential for utilization in reproductive medicine [50].

## Embryonic stem cells

Human embryos can be grown in culture to the blastocyst stage and they will attach to the surface of plastic tissue culture dishes to form differentiated outgrowths [51]. When grown under conditions that include fetal fibroblast feeder cells (STO cells), the ICM cells will remain in a primary undifferentiated state and can be passaged to retain this apparent multipotential state (A. Bongso, C. Fong, A. Trounson, unpublished). Similar observations have been made by Pedersen and colleagues [52]. The potential of these putative ES cells needs to be fully established. Similar nonhuman primate ES cells have been derived by Thompson et al. [53,54]. Genuine ES cells in mice will contribute to all the tissue types of the body, including undifferentiated germ cells and hence gametes. The multipotency of human and monkey ES cell lines have yet to be fully characterized.

There is increasing research into the control of lineage differentiation of mouse ES cells in culture. This is determined by molecules that induce specific gene expression patterns, the presence of inhibitors to gene expression and translation, the spatial arrangements of cells to one another and the presence of extracellular matrix molecules. Given the multifactorial influences on lineage formation, it might be considered difficult to control ES cell differentiation into stable somatic cell types that could be multiplied for use in drug evaluation, transplantation and genetic manipulation. However, closely related human embryonal carcinoma (EC) cells have been stably differentiated into neuronal cells that are functional when transplanted [5]. Cloned transgenic bovine embryos have been used to derive dopamine cells that are able to reverse abnormal motor performance in immunosuppressed parkinsonian rats [55]. As a result, there is considerable interest in the derivation of multipotential human ES cells from human embryos for controlled differentiation and potential transplantation, gene therapy and drug evaluation purposes.

Differentiation may also be reversible since somatic cells can be reprogrammed by ooplasm to regenerate all the tissues of the body in ruminants at least [46]. As a consequence, controlled dedifferentiation of somatic cells is also possible. This provides the basis for controlled production of regenerative stem cells for transplantation and gene therapy. This could revolutionize human medicine.

## References

1. Trounson AO, Leeton JF, Wood C, Webb J, Wood J. Pregnancies in humans by fertilization in vitro and embryo transfer in the controlled ovulatory cycle. Science 1981;212:681—682.
2. Trounson AO, Mohr LR, Wood C, Leeton JF. Effect of delayed insemination on in vitro fertilization, culture and transfer of human embryos. J Reprod Fertil 1982;64:285—294.

3. Jones GM, Trounson AO, Gardner DK, Kausche A, Lolatgis N, Wood C. Evolution of a culture protocol for successful blastocyst development and pregnancy. Hum Reprod 1998;13:169—177.

4. Bongso A, Fong CY, Ng SC, Kumar J, Trounson AO, Ratnam S. Delayed embryo transfer: improving IVF and understanding implantation. Hum Reprod 1998;(In press).

5. Trounson A, Pera M. Potential benefits of cell cloning for human medicine. Reprod Fertil Dev 1998;(In press).

6. Bongso A. Oviducted cells and early conception. Reprod Med Rev 1995;4:31—41.

7. Wiemer KE, Cohen J, Amborski GF et al. In vitro development and implantation of human embryos following culture on fetal bovine uterine fibroblast cells. Hum Reprod 1989;4: 595—600.

8. Ménézo YJR, Guerin JF, Czyba JC. Improvement of human early embryo development in vitro by coculture on monolayers of Vero cells. Biol Reprod 1990;42:301—306.

9. Bavister BD. Coculture for embryo development: is it really necessary? Hum Reprod 1992;7: 1339—1341.

10. Van Blerkom J. Development of human embryos to the hatched blastocyst stage in the presence or absence of a monolayer of Vero cells. Hum Reprod 1993;8:1525—1539.

11. Sakkas D, Jaquenoud N, Leppens G et al. Comparison of results after in vitro fertilized human embryos are cultured in routine medium and in coculture on Vero cells: a randomized study. Fertil Steril 1994;61:521—525.

12. Scholtes MCW, Zeilmaker GH. A prospective, randomized study of embryo transfer results after 3 or 5 days of embryo culture in in vitro fertilization. Fertil Steril 1996;65:1245—1248.

13. Gianaroli L, Magli MC, Ferraretti AP et al. Reducing the time of sperm-oocyte interaction in human in vitro fertilization improves the implantation rate. Hum Reprod 1996;11:166—171.

14. Magli MC, Gianaroli L, Fiorentino A, Ferraretti AP, Fortini D, Panzella S. Improved cleavage rate of human embryos cultured in antibiotic-free medium. Hum Reprod 1996;11:1520—1524.

15. Clough JR. Energy metabolism during mammalian embryogenesis. Biochem Soc Trans 1985;13:77—79.

16. Gardner DK, Leese HJ. Noninvasive measurement of nutrient uptake by single cultured preimplantation mouse embryos. Hum Reprod 1986;1:25—27.

17. Bavister BD. Culture of preimplantation embryos: facts and artifacts. Hum Reprod Update 1995;1:91—148.

18. Gardner DK, Lane M. Amino acids and ammonium regulate the development of preimplantation mouse embryos in culture. Biol Reprod 1993;48:377—385.

19. Gardner DK. Mammalian embryo culture in the absence of serum or somatic cell support. Cell Biol Int 1994;18:1163—1179.

20. Barnes FL, Crombie A, Gardner DK et al. Blastocyst development and birth after in vitro maturation of human primary oocytes, intracytoplasmic sperm injection and assisted hatching. Hum Reprod 1995;10:3243—3247.

21. Gardner DK, Lane M, Spitzer A, Batt PA. Enhanced rates of cleavage and development for sheep zygotes cultured to the blastocyst stage in vitro in the absence of serum and somatic cells: amino acids, vitamins, and culturing embryos in groups stimulate development. Biol Reprod 1994;50:390—400.

22. Jones GM, Trounson AO, Lolatgis N, Wood C. The factors affecting the success of human blastocyst development and pregnancy following IVF and embryo transfer. Fertil Steril 1998;(In press).

23. Gianaroli L, Magli MC, Ferraretti AP, Fiorentino A, Garrisi J, Munné S. Preimplantation genetic diagnosis increases the implantation rate in human in vitro fertilization by avoiding the transfer of chromosomally abnormal embryos. Fertil Steril 1997;68:1128—1131.

24. Magli MC, Gianaroli L, Munné S, Ferraretti AP. Incidence of chromosomal abnormalities in a morphologically normal cohort of embryos in poor-prognostic patients. J Assist Reprod Genet 1998;15:296—300.

25. Tarin J, Trounson AO. Embryo biopsy for preimplantation diagnosis. In: Trounson AO, Gardner

48

DK (eds) Handbook of In Vitro Fertilization. Boca Raton: CRC Press, 1993;115–129.

26. Findlay I, Ray P, Rutherford A, Lilford R. Allele dropout and preferential amplification in single cells and human blastomeres: implications for preimplantation diagnosis of sex and cystic fibrosis. Hum Reprod 1995;10:1609–1618.

27. Cha KY, Koo JJ, Ko JJ, Choi DH, Han SY, Yoon TK. Pregnancy after in vitro fertilization of human follicular oocytes collected from nonstimulated cycles, their culture in vitro and their transfer in a donor oocyte program. Fertil Steril 1991;55:109–113.

28. Trounson A, Wood C, Kausche A. In vitro maturation and the fertilization and developmental competence of oocytes recovered from untreated polycystic ovarian patients. Fertil Steril 1994; 62:353–362.

29. Trounson AO, Anderiesz C, Jones GM, Kausche A, Lolatgis N, Wood C. Oocyte maturation. Hum Reprod 1998;13(Suppl 1):101–111.

30. Trounson AO, Bongso A. Fertilization and development in humans. Curr Top Devel Biol 1996;32:59–101.

31. Shaw JM, Dawson KJ, Trounson AO. A critical evaluation of ovarian tissue cryopreservation and grafting as a strategy for preserving the human female germline. Reprod Med Rev 1997;6(In press).

32. Shaw JM, Diotallevi L, Trounson AO. A simple rapid 4.5M dimethyl sulphoxide freezing technique for the cryopreservation of one-cell to blastocyst stage preimplantation mouse embryos. Reprod Fertil Dev 1991;3:621–626.

33. Trounson A, Sjoblom P. Cleavage and development of human embryos in vitro after ultrarapid freezing and thawing. Fertil Steril 1988;50:373–376.

34. Trounson A. Cryopreservation. In: Edwards RG (ed) Assisted Human Conception. Br Med Bull 1990;46:695–708.

35. Shaw JM, Kola I, MacFarlane DR, Trounson AO. An association between chromosomal abnormalities in rapidly frozen two-cell mouse embryos and the ice forming properties of the cryoprotective solution. J Reprod Fertil 1991;91:9–18.

36. Martino A, Songasen N, Leibo SP. Development into blastocysts of bovine oocytes cryopreserved by ultra-rapid cooling. Biol Reprod 1996;54:1059–1069.

37. Vajta G, Kuwayama M, Holm P, Booth PJ, Jacobsen H, Greve T, Callesen H. A new way to avoid cryoinjuries of mammalian ova and embryos: the OPS vitrification. Molec Reprod Devel 1998;(In press).

38. Wood EC, Shaw JM, Trounson AO. Cryopreservation of ovarian tissue: Potential "reproductive insurance" for women at risk of early ovarian failure. Med J Aust 1997;166:366–369.

39. Kippax IS, Christie WB, Rowan TG. Effects of method of splitting, stage of development and presence or absence of zona pellucida on foetal survival in commercial bovine embryo transfer of bisected embryos. Theriogenology 1991;35:25–35.

40. Trounson A, Shaw J, Wood C. Preservation of ovarian function. 4th International Symposium on Turner Syndrome, Sweden. The Netherlands: Elsevier Science B.V., 1995;229–232.

41. Peura TT, Lewis IM, Trounson AO. The effect of recipient oocyte volume on nuclear transfer in cattle. Molec Reprod Devel 1998;50:185–191.

42. Yong Z, Yuqiang L. Nuclear-cytoplasmic interaction and development of goat embryos reconstructed by nuclear transplantation: production of goats by serially cloning embryos. Biol Reprod 1998;58:266–269.

43. Meng L, Ely JJ, Stouffer RL, Wolf DP. Rhesus monkeys produced by nuclear transfer. Biol Reprod 1997;57:454–459.

44. Levron J, Willadsen S, Bertoli M, Cohen J. The development of mouse zygotes after fusion with synchronous and asynchronous cytoplasm. Hum Reprod 1996;11:1287–1292.

45. Cohen J, Scott R, Schimmel T, Levron J, Willadsen S. Birth of infant after transfer of anucleate donor oocyte cytoplasm into recipient eggs. Lancet 1997;350:186–187.

46. Wilmut I, Schnieke AE, McWhir J, Kind AJ, Campbell KH. Viable offspring derived from fetal and adult mammalian cells. Nature 1997;385:810–813.

47. Cibelli JB, Stice SL, Golueke PJ, Kane JJ, Jerry J, Blackwell C, Ponce de León FA, Robl JM. Cloned transgenic calves produced from nonquiescent fetal fibroblasts. Science 1998;280: 1256—1258.

48. Kimura Y, Yanagimachi R. Development of normal mice from oocytes injected with secondary spermatocytes nuclei. Biol Reprod 1995;53:855—862.

49. Obata Y, Kaneko-Ishino T, Koide T, Takai Y, Ueda T, Domeki I, Shiroishi T, Ishino F, Kono T. Disruption of primary imprinting during oocyte growth leads to modified expression of imprinted genes during embryogenesis. Development 1998;125:1553—1560.

50. Trounson A, Wood C. Future developments in IVF and related technologies. In: Trounson AO, Gardner DK (eds) Handbook of In Vitro Fertilization, 2nd edn. Boca Raton: CRC Press, 1998;(In press).

51. Bongso A, Fong C-Y, Ng S-C, Ratnam S. Isolation and culture of inner cell mass cells from human blastocysts. Hum Reprod 1994;9:2110—2117.

52. Lavoir M-C, Conaghan JC, Meneses JJ, Pedersen RA. Studies on the derivation of human pluripotent stem cells. Procceeding The Cloning Symposium: Reprogramming Cell Fate — Transgenesis and Cloning, Melbourne 1998;Abstract.

53. Thomson JA, Kalishman J, Golos TG, Durning M, Harris CP, Becker RA, Hearn JP. Isolation of a primate embryonic stem cell line. Proc Natl Acad Sci USA 1995;92:7844—7848.

54. Thomson JA, Kalishman J, Golos TG, Durning M, Harris CP, Hearn JP. Pluripotent cell lines derived from common marmoset blastocysts. Biol Reprod 1996;55:254—259.

55. Zawada WM, Cibelli JB, Choi PK et al. Somatic cell cloned transgenic bovine neurons for transplantation in parkinsonian rats. Nature Med 1998;4:569—574.

# Surgical management of female infertility

Jean-Bernard Dubuisson and Charles Chapron
*Service de Chirurgie Gynécologique, Clinique Universitaire Baudelocque, C.H.U. Cochin Port-Royal, Paris, France*

**Abstract.** The progress made over the past few years in laparoscopic surgery has brought about considerable changes in the management of women presenting with surgical infertility. It is important to clarify the place of laparoscopic surgery in this indication relative to the other possible treatments.

Combining laparoscopy and microsurgery is the future for reproductive surgery. Laparoscopic tubal microsurgery should be performed by gynaecologists trained in microsurgery and laparoscopic surgery. The techniques of operative laparoscopy may be indicated in selected cases of distal tubal pathology. In these cases, the operative procedures of salpingostomy and fimbrioplasty performed by laparoscopy are similar to the microsurgical ones. Laparoscopic surgery may be indicated for sterilization reversal if the anastomosis is isthmic-isthmic, isthmic-ampullary or ampullary-ampullary. On the contrary, laparoscopic surgery is not recommended for organic proximal occlusion. Microsurgery by laparotomy remains the gold standard. Laparoscopic tubo-cornual anastomosis is still too difficult to perform using laparoscopy, due to the usual bleeding after partial cornual resection and to the depth of the site for the suture. If a salpingectomy is needed, the laparoscopic technique is recommended.

In tubal infertility patients, tubal surgery and IVF should be offered. The choice is governed by several parameters. However, the most important parameter is the severity of the tubal pathology. Patients must be informed of the advantages and disadvantages of each treatment. After tubal surgery, the risk of ectopic pregnancy is higher. In most cases, there is an interval of several months between the operation and the pregnancy. The disadvantages of IVF are the hyperstimulation syndrome associated with ovarian cysts and the multiple pregnancies.

**Keywords:** in vitro fertilization, laparoscopic tubal microsurgery, microsurgery, operative laparoscopy, tubal infertility, tuboplasty.

## Introduction

The progress made over the past few years in laparoscopic surgery has brought about considerable changes in the management of women presenting with surgical infertility. It is important to clarify the place of laparoscopic surgery for this indication relative to the other possible treatments. The most important indication for reconstructive surgery is tubal surgery. Tubal surgery and IVF are complementary options, the goal being to increase the probability of achieving a pregnancy.

The techniques of operative laparoscopy may be indicated in selected cases of

*Address for correspondence:* Prof J.B. Dubuisson, Service de Chirurgie Gynécologique, Clinique Universitaire Baudelocque, C.H.U. Cochin Port-Royal, 123, Bld Port-Royal, 75014 Paris, France. Tel.: +33-1-42-34-12-02. Fax: +33-1-40-51-77-62.

distal tubal pathology. In these cases, the operative procedures performed by laparoscopy are similar to the microsurgical ones. Laparoscopic surgery may be indicated for sterilization reversal if the anastomosis is isthmic-isthmic, isthmic-ampullary or ampullary-ampullary. On the other hand, laparoscopic surgery is not recommended for organic proximal occlusion. Microsurgery by laparotomy remains the gold standard. Laparoscopic tubo-cornual anastomosis is still too difficult to perform using laparoscopy, due to the usual bleeding after partial cornual resection and to the depth of the site for the suture. If a salpingectomy is needed, the laparoscopic technique is recommended.

*Pathology of the fallopian tube related to reconstructive surgery*

There are two degrees of obstruction of the distal tube, partial stenosis or phimosis with some degree of tuboperitoneal patency, and total occlusion with hydrosalpinx and disappearance of the fimbria.

Four main anatomical abnormalities may be observed in phimosis:
1) adhesions encapsulating the infundibulum;
2) a retracted serosal ring strangulating the distal tube at the junction ampulla-infundibulum;
3) severe mucosal adhesions gluing the fimbriae together, and which may even extend into the ampulla (follicular salpingitis); and
4) adhesions affecting only the ostium itself, resulting in ampullar dilatation with apparently normal fimbriae and patency under high-pressure chromotubation.

The anatomical aspects of hydrosalpinges are related to the degree of damage to the mucosa and tube wall [1]:
— Hydrosalpinx simplex with a moderately thin-wall dilated ampulla. At the salpingostomy, the mucosa is normal or atrophic.
— Follicular hydrosalpinx, with fimbrial and intra-ampullar adhesions at salpingostomy forming septa, often associated with a thick wall. This is the most advanced stage of chronic salpingitis.

The most frequent lesions of the proximal tube are fibrosis due to chronic salpingitis and salpingitis isthmica nodosa (SIN).

*Selection of candidates to laparoscopic surgery*

The main counterindications for tubal repair by laparoscopy are as follows [2,3]:
— cohesive pelvic adhesions with a "frozen pelvis";
— past history of extensive tube resection for sterilisation (fimbriectomy);
— thickwall hydrosalpinx, extensive intra-ampullar adhesions and complete destruction of the mucosa suspected at hysterosalpingography and confirmed during the diagnostic phase of laparoscopy and after opening the hydrosalpinx;
— bifocal tube disease (with proximal obstruction or salpingitis isthmica nodosa) [4];

— ongoing genital tuberculosis or sequelae;
— the existence of associated, incurable factors for infertility;
— medical pathology counterindicating surgery or pregnancy; and
— the age of older patients, bearing in mind that each case should be assessed individually.

*Equipment for operative laparoscopy*

Laparoscopic surgical treatment for tubal infertility requires experienced surgeons and theatre staff well-trained in laparoscopic surgery together with suitable and high-performance equipment.

The conventional equipment needed includes automatically controlled electronic insufflator, panoramic 10-mm laparoscopes, video system, electrosurgical unit and basic instrumentation (atraumatic grasping forceps, fine scissors with straight or curved blades, bipolar coagulation forceps with narrow jaws, fine monopolar electrode and an irrigation system). A needle holder and vicryl suture material, 4/0 to 7/0 gauge (Polyglactine 910, Ethicon) are also needed.

More specific equipment may be included according to the surgeon's preference. The sectioning effect of the $CO_2$ laser permits the cutting of the adhesions and the incision of the tube. Its vaporisation effect on fimbrial serosa produces the eversion of the neofimbriae. The $CO_2$ laser can be used either with a bayonet lens via the transumbilical route or with hand forceps by the suprapubic route. The diathermy coagulator (5 mm flat ended probe) enables the tissues to be heated to $100-140°C$ for a few seconds. This effect is obtained at the point where a probe is applied. The thermal effect provokes the retraction of the serosa of the fimbriae and maintains tubal eversion after salpingostomy.

Laparoscopic microinstruments (scissors, forceps, microelectrode, needle holder) are introduced through 3-mm suprapubic trocars. They may be used for tubal anastomosis, fimbrioplasty, fimbriolysis, and tubal adhesiolysis. Two or three suprapubic trocars are inserted under visual control. Their diameter is usually 5 mm. If microinstruments are needed 3-mm trocars are adequate.

*The laparoscopic salpingostomy*

A precise evaluation of the pathology is first required. The peritoneum is inspected, looking for inflammation, adhesions and endometriosis. The morphology of the tubes is evaluated and their patency checked using a methylene blue test [5]. As for the abdomen, particular attention is paid to investigating the regions of the appendix and liver (Fitz-Hugh-Curtis syndrome).

The first phase of the operation must always be devoted to adhesiolysis. Adhesiolysis must be atraumatic and should avoid any injury to the peritoneum, using microsurgical principles. The adhesions are cut and resected under tension. The adhesiolysis is essential to restore normal anatomical relationships and perfect mobility of the tube relative to the ovary. Once this adhesiolysis has been carried out the tubal lesions can be assessed more accurately.

The technique of salpingostomy consists of creating a new ostium in cases when the distal part of the tube is totally occluded (hydrosalpinx). The operation comprises two phases, incision and eversion.

Before opening, the hydrosalpinx is exposed atraumatically. Methylene blue is injected which makes the old ostium show up as a whitish sclerosed area. The ideal is to start opening at this point. The tube is incised using fine laparoscopic scissors or the $CO_2$ laser with a focused shot. Simple laparoscopic inspection of the mucosa in the ampulla and infundibulum provides an excellent means of evaluation of the tubal lesions' severity. Only those patients presenting moderate deterioration of the tube will draw any benefit from salpingostomy, with the others being better referred to IVF. Once the hydrosalpinx has been opened, several incisions of about 1–2 cm are made (between 2 and 4 depending on what is technically feasible). Care should be taken to locate these incisions in between the longitudinal mucosal folds, in an avascular area. Theoretically these incisions should not bleed. If there is any bleeding, immersing the infundibulum in hot normal saline helps to obtain hemostasis. If this fails then elective coagulation of the vessels with the fine monopolar electrode or the bipolar forceps is needed.

Once the hydrosalpinx has been opened, the neo-ostium is kept in the everted position by creating a cuff. The cuff may be maintained using two or three separate stitches of 5 to 7-0 Vicryl. The cuff may also be maintained by distal serosa retraction. Several techniques can be used to provoke the retraction:

— Vaporisation of the tubal serosa with a defocused shot from the $CO_2$ laser. Eversion is maintained thanks to the surface coagulation caused by the laser.
— Bipolar coagulation of the serosa. This enables the same results to be obtained as with the laser. As with the laser method, only the serosa should be coagulated in order to avoid to provoke any lesions in the tubal mucosa.
— Thermocoagulation of the serosa. In this case the 5-mm diathermy probe is applied to the serosa. Once again the serosa whiten and retract creating the required eversion very easily.

Most pregnancies occur within 1 year of the operation. The results of laparoscopic distal tuboplasty are comparable to those for microsurgery [6—9]. Provided that the surgeon has the necessary skill in laparoscopic surgery, operative laparoscopy is now the surgical treatment of choice for distal tubal infertility in view of its undeniable advantages over laparotomy [10].

The fertility results for laparoscopic salpingostomy depend on the severity of the tubal damage. A good correlation exists between the quality of the mucosa and the IUP rate. This classification of Boer-Meisel et al. [11] relies on evaluation of the tubal mucosa alone and enables the patients to be classed into three groups. Patients belonging to group 1 are those whose mucosa is normal with regular folds; patients in group 2 present moderate alterations to the ampullar mucosa, with areas of normal mucosa interspersed with areas where the mucosal folds are rare or inexistent (atrophic mucosa); the patients in group 3 are those whose mucosa is considerably deteriorated with either complete disappearance of the mucosa or the existence of intratubal synechia (follicular salpingitis). Fertility results are about 50% of IUP in group 1, 30% in group 2 and 0% in group 3 [12]. Severely damaged tubes should not be treated by salpingostomy. In vitro fertilization should be selected in these cases.

*Laparoscopic fimbrioplasty*

The principle of fimbrioplasty is to restore the original anatomy of the infundibulum by treating the phimosis. Before the procedure to restore a normal infundibulum is carried out, the first task is to assess the quality of the tubal mucosa and look for any intratubal synechia which are evidence, from the histological point of view, of follicular salpingitis. It adversely affects the prognosis. Salpingoscopy may be required for such evaluation [13–15].

A fine atraumatic forceps inserted via the contralateral trocar to the tube is then cautiously introduced into the phimosis. By gently opening it, the adhesions and bridles in the infundibulum can be observed and exposed. Fimbrioplasty then consists of incising or excising the adhesions using fine scissors, the monopolar electrode or the $CO_2$ laser. When using the latter, a focused shot will enable section-coagulation to be obtained.

After laparoscopic fimbrioplasty the intrauterine pregnancy rate is 40% on average. In cases where the folds are stuck together with extensive synechiae, the rate is extremely low [8].

*Sterilization reversal by laparoscopy*

The first phase in the laparoscopic procedure is diagnostic with the aim of checking to see whether laparoscopic tubal reversal is technically feasible. The distal portion of the tube is visually inspected to assess the quality of the fimbria. Patients with extensive damage (length less than 4 cm) together with those with fimbriectomy are excluded from reconstructive treatment [16]. When the situation is favorable, laparoscopic tubal sterilization reversal is carried out during the same operative procedure.

The position of the three suprapubic trocars is crucial because it directly affects the feasibility of the anastomosis. The trocars must be introduced sufficiently far from the pubis so that movements with the forceps and the needle holders will not be hindered by the uterus when the latter is anteverted. During laparoscopic sterilization reversal, scrupulous attention must be paid to the principles of microsurgery. The most important points are the necessity of dissecting the tubes without trauma, of obtaining meticulous hemostasis by bipolar coagulation without causing any tubal necrosis, and also achieving accurate approximation of the tissues using the suture. The magnification required is obtained by a lens-video camera combination giving excellent definition [17].

Tubal anastomosis consists of two main phases: approximating the ends of the tube and the actual anastomosis itself:

- Approximation is achieved using a stitch placed in the mesosalpinx, level with the tube segments. This enables the two tubal lumina to be perfectly aligned. The suture is made using a single stitch of vicryl 4/0 with an intracorporeal knot.
- Tubal anastomosis may be performed by two techniques: the one-stitch technique [18] and microsurgical anastomosis.
  - The one-stitch technique is carried out in one plane using a single stitch of vicryl 7/0 or 6/0 placed at 12 o' clock position and tied within the corpus. This stitch takes up the serosa and muscularis and tries to avoid the mucosa. The 12 o' clock position suture is adequate to provide a good approximation of the tube segments. A 3 o'clock position or 9 o'clock position single serosal suture may be added if necessary. The mesosalpinx can then be approximated if required using one or two interruptured sutures. Tubal anastomosis via laparoscopy using one stitch has the great advantage of being simple. Catheterization of the tube may be performed. It does not require biological glue. This anastomosis technique ensures perfect tissue healing. Preliminary results are encouraging [19].
  - The microsurgical anastomosis is performed in two layers. The muscle layer is sutured with four separate stitches. The serosal layer is sutured with three separate stitches. The pregnancy rates after laparoscopic anastomosis seem to be similar to those obtained by laparotomy and microsurgery [16,20,21]. Combined laparoscopy and minilaparotomy for reversal of tubal sterilization may be recommended in nonobese patients.

*Microsurgical tubocornual anastomosis*

Proximal obstruction accounts for 10–25% of tubal pathology. Tubal obstruction may be functional (spasm) or organic. The proximal lesions of chronic salpingitis or SIN may progress to complete obstruction. There is a place for fluoroscopic tubal catheterization [22]. However, the response depends mostly on the proximal pathology. It seems better if muscular spasm, luminal plug or polyps are present. In these cases the recanalization of proximally occluded tubes by a transcervical technique could avoid unnecessary microsurgical tubocornual anastomosis. Microsurgery by laparotomy is recommended in patients after failure of the cannulation and if the fimbria are normal. If bipolar lesions are diagnosed, IVF is indicated. Fertility results after microsurgical anastomosis are well-established with an intrauterine pregnancy rate of more 70% after 2 years [23].

In conclusion, combining laparoscopy and microsurgery is the future of reproductive surgery. Laparoscopic tubal microsurgery should be performed by gynaecologists trained in microsurgery and laparoscopic surgery. In tubal infertility patients, tubal surgery and IVF should be offered. The choice is governed by several parameters. The most important parameters are personal considerations and severity of the tubal pathology. Patients must be informed of the advantages and of the disadvantages of each treatment. After tubal surgery, the risk of ectopic pregnancy is more frequent. In most cases, there is an interval of several months between the operation and the pregnancy. The disadvantages of IVF are the hyperstimulation syndrome associated with ovarian cysts and multiple pregnancies.

## References

1. Bateman BG, Nunley WC, Kitchin JD. Surgical management of distal tubal obstruction. Are we making progress? Fertil Steril 1987;48:523−542.
2. Gomel V. Salpingostomy by microsurgery. Fertil Steril 1978;29:380−385.
3. Singhal V, Li TC, Cooke ID. An analysis of factors influencing the outcome of 232 consecutive tubal microsugery cases. Br J Obstet Gynaecol 1991;98:628−636.
4. Dubuisson JB, Aubriot FX, Garnier P et al. Faut-il opérer les lésions tubaires distales bifocales en 1984? A propos de 54 cas. J Gynecol Obstet Biol Reprod 1984;13:925−932.
5. The American Fertility Society. Classifications of adnexal adhesions, distal tubal occlusion, tubal occlusion secondary to tubal ligation, tubal pregnancies, müllerian anomalies and intrauterine adhesions. Fertil Steril 1988;49:944−955.
6. Rock JA, Katayama KP, Martin EJ, Woodruff JD, Jones HW. Factors influencing the success of salpingostomy techniques for distal fimbrial obstruction. Obstet Gynecol 1978;52:591−596.
7. Winston RML, Margara RA. Microsurgical salpingostomy is not an obsolete procedure. Br J Obstet Gynaecol 1991;98:637−642.
8. Canis M, Mage G, Pouly JL et al. Laparoscopic distal tuboplasty: report of 87 cases and a 4-year experience. Fertil Steril 1991;56:616−621.
9. Dubuisson JB, Bouquet de Jolinière J, Aubriot FX et al. Terminal tuboplasties by laparoscopy 65 consecutive cases. Fertil Steril 1990;54:401−403.
10. Chapron C, Dubuisson JB, Chavet X, Morice P. Treatment and causes of female infertility. Lancet 1994;344:333−334.
11. Boer-Meisel ME, Te Velde ER, Habbema JDF, Kardaum JWPF. Predicting the pregnancy outcome in patients treated for hydrosalpinx: a prospective study. Fertil Steril 1986;45:23−29.
12. Dubuisson JB, Chapron C, Morice P et al. Laparoscopic salpingostomy: fertility results according to the tubal mucosal appearance. Hum Reprod 1994;9:334−339.
13. Shapiro BS, Diamond MD, DeCherney AH. Salpingoscopy: an adjunctive technique for evaluation of the fallopian tube. Fertil Steril 1988;49:1076−1079.
14. De Bruyne F, Puttemans P, Boeckx W, Brossens I. The clinical value of salpingoscopy in tubal infertility. Fertil Steril 1989;51:339−340.
15. Herschlag A, Seifer DB, Carcangiu ML et al. Factors influencing the success of salpingostomy techniques for distal fimbrial obstruction. Obstet Gynecol 1978;52:591−599.
16. Gomel V. Tubal reanastomosis by microsurgery. Fertil Steril 1977;28:59−65.
17. Gomel V. Salpingostomy by laparoscopy. J Reprod Med 1977;18:265−267.
18. Dubuisson JB, Swolin K. Laparoscopic tubal anastomosis (the one stitch technique): preliminary results. Hum Reprod 1995;10:2044−2046.
19. Dubuisson JB, Chapron C, Swolin K. A simplified procedure for laparoscopic tubal sterilization reversal: the one tubal stich technique. J Gynecol Surg 1996;12:177−181.
20. Koh CH. Microsurgical laparoscopic tubal resection and anastomosis: techniques and results. Réferences en Gynécologie Obstetrique. No spécial, Congrès Vichy, IFS, 1995;102−104.
21. Yoon TK, Sung HR, Cha SH et al. Fertility outcome after laparoscopic microsurgical tubal anastomosis. Fertil Steril 1997;67:18−22.
22. Thurmond AS, Rosch J. Non-surgical Fallopian tube recanalization for treatment of infertility. Radiology 1990;174:371−374.
23. Dubuisson JB, Chapron C, Ansquer Y, Vacher-Lavenu MC. Proximal tubal occlusion: is there an alternative to microsurgery? Hum Reprod 1997;12:692−698.

# Imaging, infertility and reproductive tract

# Critical evaluation of the fallopian tube

B. Hedon, H. Dechaud, P. Boulot and F. Laffargue

*Faculté de Médecine, Université Montpellier 1, Services de Gynécologie-Obstétrique, Hôpital Arnaud de Villeneuve, Montpellier, France*

**Abstract.** The real clinical benefit of a proper tubal evaluation is questionable since a vast majority of infertility cases end up with in vitro fertilization and embryo transfer (IVF-ET).

*Objectives.* 1) to review the various exploration means in use today to assess tubal function, and 2) to analyse in which clinical situations exploration of the fallopian tube can play a role in the decision making.

*Exploration means.* When exploring the tubes, it is essentially their morphological aspect which is evaluated and hardly, if at all, their functional contribution in the natural procreation process. Hysterosalpingography (HSG) evaluates patency and the internal lining. Ultrasounds, despite recent developments, have not yet proven to be more precise. Laparoscopy gives a direct view on the tubal serosa and its relationships with the ovaries and other reproductive organs. Tubal endoscopy has the theoretical advantage of assessing the tubal mucosa responsible for most of the tubal functions. However, it is still a technically demanding procedure, and the clinical significance of its findings is not yet totally defined.

*Clinical situations.* Despite these limitations, there are a number of clinical situations in which exact knowledge of the tubal status can be helpful to increase the chances of the patient in obtaining a pregnancy:

1) tubal reconstructive surgery in selected cases increases the cumulative probability of pregnancy, adding its results to the results that can be obtained with IVF-ET,

2) if tubal pathology is severe and tubal reconstructive surgery useless or even contraindicated, results of IVF-ET are improved when a salpingectomy is performed, and

3) in failed implantation patients, if the tubes are diseased, salpingectomy increases the probability of obtaining a pregnancy in subsequent IVF-ET attempts.

*Conclusion.* Fallopian tubes should not be the forgotten organs of the infertility work-up. Tubal pathology needs to be diagnosed in order to enable physicians and patients to make the right therapeutic choice between tubal reconstruction and tubal ablation.

**Keywords:** falloposcopy, hydrosalpinx, hysterosalpingography, hystersonography, in vitro fertilization, infertility surgery, infertility work-up, laparoscopic surgery, laparoscopy, salpingectomy, salpingitis isthmica nodosa, tubal pathology, tubal microsurgery, tuboplasty.

Tubal evaluation is part of the basic infertility work-up, at the same level as the other main reproductive parameters such as ovulation and sperm. In fact, the value of tubal explorations needs to be questioned when the treatment of infertility can be assisted procreation (AP) whatever the cause of infertility. Moreover, tubal explorations are more invasive than exploration of other reproductive organs or functions. Adding to that cost and a relative lack of precision, it is

*Address for correspondence:* B. Hedon, Faculté de Médecine, Université Montpellier 1, Services de Gynécologie-Obstétrique, Hôpital Arnaud de Villeneuve, 34295 Montpellier, Cedex 5, France.

understandable why there are voices asking for a revision of the basic infertility work-up, which is oriented more towards the preparation of AP treatments rather than an inefficient search of an explanation to the couple's infertility.

Medical history is often made of brutal shifts in the way patients are managed, these shifts depending on technical breakthroughs, evolving medical knowledge, and also beliefs and fashions. Concerning the revolutionary shifts provoked by the introduction of assisted reproduction into medical practice, it is necessary to remain cautious of the backlash bringing with it even more strength, new reasons and new ways to evaluate tubal reproductive function.

## Evaluation means of the fallopian tubes

### Classical means

### Hysterosalpingography (HSG) [1]

Contrast medium is injected through the cervical os in order to opacify the uterine cavity and the tubal lumen after spilling into the tube via the ostium uterinum. HSG can demonstrate tubal patency when peritoneal spillage is obtained. But, if patency is a required condition, it is far from being enough to be able to conclude on a normal tube. The images obtained need to be analysed more thoroughly in order to detect pathology and to differentiate it from potential artefacts.

A normal salpingography should display:
1) a smooth proximal portion and isthmus, without irregularities,
2) a progressive enlargement of the tubal lumen at the ampullary level with regular parietal coating and presence of mucosal folds, and
3) a peritoneal spillage obtained without accumulation of contrast medium in the tube, with good diffusion in the abdomen outlining intestinal loops and other pelvic structures.

Pathologic findings can be:
1. In the proximal part of the tube:
   — Tubal polyps: pear-shaped enlargement of the tube with a rice-bean-like formation, usually not big enough to obstruct the tube. Although these polyps are usually of endometrial origin, their association with endometriosis is inconstant, and their role in infertility uncertain.
   — Salpingitis isthmica nodosa: the diverticulae and irregularities of the lumen demonstrate destruction of the mucosa by the infectious agent and the related inflammatory reaction.
   — Proximal obstruction with a brutal arrest in the progression of the contrast medium after a normal opacification of the first millimeters or centimeters. This flame-like tubal image differentiates real tubal obstruction from a cornual block possibly related to a functional spasm without pathologic meaning. It is in this case that a selective catheterization of the tubal ostium can overpass the blockage and obtain opacification of the tube.
2. In the distal part:

— Total distal obstruction with no peritoneal spillage despite accumulation of contrast medium in the ampulla outlining a hydrosalpinx.

— Partial distal obstruction (phimosis), where peritoneal spillage is obtained only after accumulation of contrast medium in the ampulla.

— Mucosal pathology appears under the form of parietal irregularities and disorganization or disparition of mucosal folds.

In a meta-analysis using laparoscopy with chromopertubation as gold standard, HSG is found to have a 0.65 sensitivity and a 0.83 specificity for the diagnosis of tubal patency. It is, however, unreliable for the evaluation of peritubal adhesions [1].

HSG is part of the basic infertility work-up and is normally required in every patient whatever her history and possible cause of the couple's infertility. In some patients who are more at risk of sexually transmitted disease or who have a history of pelvic inflammatory disease (PID), antibioprophylaxy should be prescribed in order to avoid an infectious complication.

*Laparoscopy*

Laparoscopy is indicated whenever tubal pathology is suspected because of a patient's history of PID and/or chronic pelvic pain, previous ectopic pregnancy, previous pelvic surgery, or because of abnormal findings on HSG. It is also indicated when there is no clear explanation to the couple's infertility ("unexplained" infertility), because it can reveal pathologies that have not been diagnosed during the basic infertility work-up.

Usually performed under general anesthetic, gynecologic laparoscopy includes the introduction of a 10-mm-wide rigid optic through the umbilicus, and two accessory tools in the pubic region. Although it can be performed as an ambulatory procedure in some clinics, it must be regarded as an invasive procedure requiring specific skills and organisation.

Tubal pathology can be found:

1) in the proximal part: tubal enlargement and rigidity with possible fibrotic nodosities (salpingitis isthmica nodosa);

2) in the distal part: agglutination of fimbrial fringes with serosal covering and tubal distention by fluid (hydrosalpinx). Special attention must be paid to the tubal walls. Thick tubal walls are associated with inflammatory and destroyed mucosa (bad prognosis), whereas thin walled hydrosalpinges can be associated with flattened mucosa (intermediate prognosis); and

3) tubal lesions can be present both in the proximal and the distal parts of the tube. One refers then to bifocal lesions, which, in fact, are a sign of the presence of multifocal lesions spread along the tube. Bifocal (multifocal) lesions are associated with a severe impairment of the tubal potential.

Adhesions can also be diagnosed by laparoscopy. They testify to the inflammatory process that has taken place and might have produced less visible but more significant lesions ion the tubal mucosal surface. Sometimes peritubal adhesions are the only cause of infertility and can easily be divided. When they are associated with tubal lesions, unless they cannot be divided (frozen pelvis), they have no significant prognosis value.

Laparoscopic pelvic examination can be completed with the dye patency test, which offers the advantage over HSG in being performed by the gynecologist under general anesthetic with a direct visual control. But this test is also subject to technical limitations.

Laparoscopy offers the advantage to give access to the possibility of surgery at the same time as the diagnosis. Procedures that can be performed with laparoscopically include: adhesiolysis, salpingoneostomy, fimbrioplasty, and in some circumstances, tubal cannulation.

*Means under development*

*Hysterosonography*

With gynecologic ultrasonographic exploration becoming more precise, especially when using the vaginal probe, attempts to explore fallopian tubes have been made, some authors relying only on ultrasounds to gain knowledge of the tubal status. In fact, tubes are not always clearly visible, even when distally obstructed and distended in the form of hydrosalpinges. Moreover, ultrasonic examination is not yet precise enough to give an idea of the internal tubal lining.

In order to improve the performance of ultrasounds, it has been advocated to use contrast medium as a tool to test tubal patency and possibly to highlight possible mucosal pathology. But, whether isotonic saline or a more specific contrast medium are being utilized, the same limitations are encountered. Because sectorial probes give a plane view, the tube cannot be followed in each of its tortuosities.

Ultrasonographic exploration has potential advantages over HSG: it could easily be performed by the gynecologist as an office procedure; it does not require any special equipment, the same ultrasonic device serving also for all other gynecological and obstetrical purposes; it abolishes the fear generated with the use of radiation in the vicinity of reproductive organs; and during the same ultrasonographic examination, other pelvic organs can be visualized — the uterus and in particular the endometrium and the ovaries. For all these reasons, ultrasonographic examination with a vaginal probe is considered increasingly more as part of the basic infertility work-up, in immediate prolongation of the clinical examination of pelvic organs. However, one must be aware of it's intrinsic limitations, and although it has its own value, it cannot yet replace HSG.

*Falloposcopy*

Rapid advances in the miniaturisation of fiber optics and cannulation devices enable endoscopic examination of small and difficult to reach organs [2]. Falloposcopy is defined as the microendoscopy of the oviductal lumen from the utero-tubal ostium up to the fimbria by a nonincisional transvaginal approach.

It offers the advantage over other conventional means of tubal evaluation in allowing a direct assessment of the tubal epithelium. The staging of the degree of mucosal damage correlates well with pregnancy rates following tubal surgery [3].

The coaxial technique involves hysteroscopic guide-wire cannulation of the tube, passage of a Teflon catheter over the wire, replacement of the guide-wire with the falloposcope and retrograde imaging of the tube. The linear averting catheter technique uses a pressurised tubular polyethylene "balloon" which can unroll itself from within a plastic polymer cannula. The balloon carries the endoscope into and along the tube, protecting the tube and endoscope from damaging one another and negotiating curves and strictures without exerting shear forces on the tubal wall. Imaging of the tubal lumen is carried out during withdrawal of the balloon, keeping the endoscope at the tip of the balloon and flushing sterile isotonic crystalloid around the endoscope. The image obtained is displayed in real time on a video monitor and recorded simultaneously.

The normal appearance of the tube varies depending on the segment being examined. The proximal part has the appearance of a tunnel with a flat and regular wall. The isthmic segment is characterized by the appearance of four or five longitudinal folds. Beyond the isthmo-ampullary junction, the distal segment of the tube becomes too wide for the entire width of the lumen to be visualized. In the distal tube, the epithelium develops into secondary folds.

Pathologic findings include:
1. In the proximal part of the tube: severe narrowing or complete occlusion appearing as a blind-ending tunnel, while a badly damaged but patent proximal tube has an irregular fibrotic appearance with the wall sometimes appearing trabeculated.
2. In the distal part: mobility of the folds may be reduced. If there is a large distention and the folds are flattened, the tubal lumen will appear as a dark cavity. The worst prognostic feature is the presence of intratubal adhesions.

Pregnancy rates are correlated with the aspect of tubal mucosa, demonstrating the predictive value of falloposcopy [4].

In conclusion, falloposcopy is a feasible, reproducible and safe method to investigate the lumen of the fallopian tubes. The accuracy of the diagnosis brought by falloposcopy allows us to think that falloposcopy should be included in the screening of infertile patients. It may be important to consider falloposcopy if treatments requiring tubal function are being considered. Assessment of the tubal epithelium can assist in planning subsequent management and choosing between treatment modalities.

*Transvaginal hydrolaparoscopy* [5]
Recently, a new endoscopic technique has been described as an office procedure to be performed under local anesthetic. Using the posterior vaginal pouch as introduction zone of a 2-mm-wide rigid endoscope, and avoiding abdominal insufflation by simple flotation of pelvic organs in isotonic saline, this technique gives a direct view of the tubes and the ovarian-tubal relationship. This technique is undoubtedly more benign than the usual laparoscopy under general anesthetic

and is accurate enough to allow a precise diagnosis of tubal pathology and adhesions. It cannot be used, though, for just any kind of surgical repair. This theoretical disadvantage becomes an advantage when one considers counseling as an important step in the therapeutic process. Counseling necessitates a dissociation between diagnosis and treatment and this tended to be forgotten due to the fact that the patient was asleep when the surgeon was considering the findings and elaborating the therapeutic strategy.

## Clinical applications

*Decision-making for the therapeutic choice*

*Therapeutic choice in tubal infertility patients*
Many studies compare the performance of tubal reconstructive surgery and IVF-ET, but the most obvious bias is that patients are not the same. In fact, performance of tubal reconstructive surgery is dependent on a number of factors:
1) quality of surgery,
2) intensity of disease,
3) importance of tubal sequelae after surgery,
4) nature and localisation of lesions, and of course
5) age and other fertility factors within the couple.
Among all these factors, residual tubal pathology is probably the most significant that limits the proportion of evolutive intrauterine pregnancies that one can expect. With a better diagnostic accuracy of tubal pathology, one can hypothesise better intrauterine and lower extrauterine pregnancy rates after tubal reconstructive surgery. The fact that no study shows this at present is not a valid argument to say that this hypothesis is wrong, but rather, it is probably related to the limited performances of tubal explorations. A more precise evaluation of tubal capabilities is compulsory if one is to develop tubal reconstructive surgery with better results.

Despite the limitations of tubal reconstructive surgery, it should be the first choice whenever possible (Fig. 1). Cumulative pregnancy rates adding the performances of surgery and of IVF-ET reach a global 80% chance of getting pregnant (Figs. 2 and 3) [6]. The conditions for obtaining such a result are:
1) proper patient selection based on an as accurate as possible assessment of tubal disease, and
2) reasonable delay between surgery and the first IVF-ET attempts in order to allow sufficient time for a natural pregnancy to occur, but also to minimize the age factor.

*Therapeutic choice in unexplained infertility patients*
AP is advocated in unexplained infertility patients because it promotes a number of fertility functions and short cuts a number of others. Despite the fact that the couple's infertility almost certainly has a cause, this is often not diagnosed during

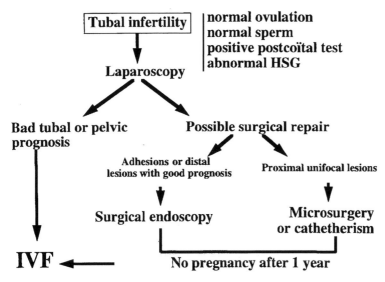

*Fig. 1.* Algorithm of the therapeutic choice in tubal infertility patients, depending on the type of tubal pathology.

the infertility work-up. If the patient is considered as being an "unexplained" infertility patient, the first AP choice would be intrauterine insemination (IUI). If in fact, infertility of the patient were of tubal origin, such inseminations would have a high risk of producing no result at all, or producing an ectopic pregnancy. An accurate diagnosis is the only guarantee that no time and money is being lost.

*The preparation process for IVF-ET*

*Salpingectomy in severe tubal infertility patients undergoing in vitro fertilization*
Tubal pathology, and in particular hydrosalpinges have been proven to impair

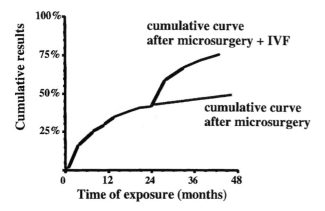

*Fig. 2.* Cumulative rates of intrauterine pregnancies after microsurgery and IVF (after 2 years of pregnancy exposure).

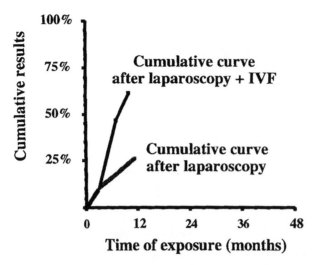

*Fig. 3.* Cumulative rates of intrauterine pregnancies after laparoscopy and IVF (proposed after 6 months of pregnancy exposure).

embryo implantation [7]. In a prospective randomized study we evaluated implantation and pregnancy rates after salpingectomy vs. that without salpingectomy in severe tubal infertility patients undergoing in vitro fertilization [8]. A total of 30 patients with prior salpingectomy were compared to 30 without salpingectomy before IVF treatment. Each of these patients underwent a laparoscopy with or without salpingectomy according to the randomization and subsequently IVF-ET with a long agonist-HMG stimulation protocol. The embryo implantation rate, ongoing pregnancy rates per transfer, per oocyte retrieval and per cycle, cumulative pregnancy rate, and delivery rate of live newborns per transfer were the outcome measures.

There were no significant differences for age, duration of infertility, delay between laparoscopy and IVF, and characteristics of IVF procedures. After the first IVF attempt, the implantation rate was 10.4% in the salpingectomy group and 4.6% in the group without salpingectomy (p = 0.43). Considering all of the IVF attempts, the embryo implantation rates were 13.4 and 8.6%, respectively (p = 0.25). For patients with salpingectomy, the ongoing pregnancy rate per transfer was 34.2% as compared with 18.7% for the group of patients without salpingectomy. Similarly, ongoing pregnancy rates per cycle of IVF were 22 and 12.2%, respectively. After four IVF attempts, the probability of becoming pregnant was greater in the salpingectomy group (75 vs. 63%), but this difference was not statistically significant.

In conclusion, prior salpingectomy in severe tubal infertility patients undergoing in vitro fertilization seems to increase the embryo implantation rate and pregnancy rate per cycle of IVF.

*Table 1.* Results of subsequent IVF-ET attempts after salpingectomy or without salpingectomy in severe tubal infertility patients with implantation failures.

|  | Group A | Group B |
|---|---|---|
| Implantation rate per embryo (first attempt postsalpingectomy or no salpingectomy) | 9.8 (14/143) | 6.25 (p = 0.05) (7/112) |
| Implantation rate per embryo (all attempts postsalpingectomy or no salpingectomy) | 6.8 (18/265) | 4.4 (p = 0.2) (16/361) |
| Clinical pregnancy rate per transfer | 23.5 (16/68) | 9.7 (p = 0.01) (13/134) |
| Evolutive pregnancy rate per transfer | 17.6 (12/68) | 9.7 (p = 0.1) (13/134) |

## *Salpingectomy in implantation failures*

Implantation failure is the most common cause of failure of an IVF-ET attempt. It is recognized as being usually of embryonic origin, but maternal causes are possible.

In a retrospective comparative study (1990–1997) we studied 70 severe infertility patients with a minimum of three previous implantation failures of a minimum nine embryos in total. Of these patients, 35 underwent a bilateral laparoscopic salpingectomy before the fourth attempt. The other 35, serving as control, underwent a fourth attempt without prior salpingectomy, either because this had not been proposed, or because the patient did not give her consent. The results of this study are summarized in Table 1 and demonstrate the importance of performing a good tubal evaluation even when IVF-ET is being considered as therapy.

## References

1. Swart P, Mol BWJ, Van der Veen F, Van Beurden M, Redekop WK, Bossuyt PMM. The accuracy of hysterosalpingography in the diagnosis of tubal pathology: a meta-analysis. Fertil Steril 1995;64:486–491.
2. Kerin JF, Daykhovsky L, Segalowitz J, Surrey ES, Anderson R, Stein A, Wade M, Grundfest WS. Falloposcopy: a microendoscopic technique for visual exploration of the human fallopian tube from the uterotubal ostium to the fimbria using a transvaginal approach. Fertil Steril 1990;54:390–400.
3. De Bruyne F, Puttemans P, Boeckx W, Brosens I. The clinical value of salpingoscopy in tubal infertility. Fertil Steril 1989;51:339–340.
4. Dechaud H, Daures JP, Hedon B. Prospective evaluation of falloposcopy. Hum Reprod 1998;(Submitted).
5. Gordts S, Campo R, Rombauts L, Brosens I. Transvaginal hydrolaparoscopy as an outpatient procedure for infertility investigation. Hum Reprod 1998;13:99–103.
6. Audibert F, Hedon B, Arnal F, Humeau C, Boulot P, Bachelard B, Benos P, Laffargue F, Viala JL. Therapeutic strategies in tubal infertility with distal pathology. Hum Reprod 1991;6: 1439–1442.
7. Wainer R, Camus E, Camier B, Martin C, Vasseur C, Merlet F. Does hydrosalpinx reduce the pregnancy rate after in vitro fertilization? Fertil Steril 1997;68:1022–1026.

8.  Dechaud H, Daurcs J, Arnal F, Humeau C, Hedon B. Does prior salpingectomy improve implantation and pregnancy rates in severe tubal infertility patients undergoing in vitro fertilization? A pilot prospective randomized study. Fertil Steril 1998;69:1020—1025.

Fertility and Reproductive Medicine.
R.D. Kempers, J. Cohen, A.F. Haney and J.B. Younger, editors.

# Microlaparoscopy: indications and applications

Francisco Rísquez
*Centro Médico Docente La Trinidad Caracas, Venezuela*

**Abstract.** Microlaparoscopy refers to a small diameter laparoscope, less than 2 mm in diameter, and made of microfiber optics bundles measured in μm.

Some of the specific advantages of microlaparoscopy are: the patient's safety increases; morbidity decreases, is less aggressive to the patients, sutures and visible scars are avoided; general anesthesia could be eliminated in selected cases, replacing it with simple local anesthesia or analgesia, using local anesthesia allows verbal communication between the patient and the surgeon during and after the surgical procedure, recovery time is shorter, and the technique is performed on an outpatient basis. Microlaparoscopy enables the surgeon to make a diagnosis and in many cases treat the pathology simultaneously. Microlaparoscopy offer cost-benefit advantages and it reduces the complexity of the equipment, because it is easier to handle and transport.

So far, however, clinical experience is limited and only long-term randomized multicenter studies could define the role of microlaparoscopic procedures in gynecology and their obvious transfer towards other surgical areas. We expect that the technique and the instruments can be improved so that it can be implemented preferably with local anesthesia. We also expect improvements in anesthetic techniques which will favorably affect this and other outpatient procedures.

**Keywords:** diagnostic and operative microlaparoscopy, local anesthesia.

## Introduction

Based on the personal clinical experience on microendoscopy as well as experimental work, and preliminary results of an International Multicenter Study on microlaparoscopy inaugurated by the author, the following article discusses technical as well as methodological particularities and controversies of microlaparoscopy including a review of the current literature.

Technological advances in instrumentation as well as video images have accelerated the progress in endoscopy. Laparoscopy has changed the way gynecological pathologies are handled. Previously, the procedures using laparotomy required lengthy surgery and hospitalization times, but now thanks to laparoscopy, they can be performed on an outpatient basis and require only short hospitalizations. Laparoscopy was originally recommended to diagnose female infertility. However, in the past two decades, the scope of laparoscopy has widened so much that today it has become a specialty in itself.

The different diameters achieved with the advent of this new technology has given rise to a confusion in terminology. Microendoscopy is a general term that

*Address for correspondence:* Dr Francisco Rísquez, Av. Luis Roche, Edif Altamira Palace Apt 11-B, Caracas, Venezuela. Fax: +58-2-2844392.

has been used in several medical areas which includes all small diameter endoscopy made of microfiberoptics. In laparoscopy, a small diameter laparoscopy encompasses the different optical technologies such as rod lenses and microfibers and includes the whole spectrum of optical diameters, therefore, the term is too general. Minilaparoscopy is easily confused with minilaparotomy, and refers to small diameter endoscopes, such as the needlescope; whereas microlaparoscopy refers to a small diameter laparoscope, less than 2 mm in diameter, and made of microfiber optics bundles measured in µm. Nowadays, the term microlaparoscopy is widely used and accepted, but for those who still have problems differentiating them we could coin a new term such as "microfiber laparoscopy". However, regardless of the name used, what is important in our new venture is to demonstrate the advantages of this new technology.

**Technical evolution of endoscopes**

Endoscopes are simple cannulas that deliver illuminating light to the operative field, while providing an image to the observer. In the past the image was provided directly through the eyepiece, nowadays is obtained via an attached video camera. The light delivery system was produced via a flexible optical fiber running the length of the cannula, coupling to a distant light source via the proximal end of the endoscope. Until recently, most surgical endoscopes transmitted the image via a system of glass lenses, however, currently laparoscopy is usually performed with conventional rod lens telescopes, the Hopkins being the gold standard design, adapted to the medical field in the early 1960s. The rod lens telescopes used for laparoscopy range from 3.5 to 10 mm, they give a bright an clear image which can be magnified when desired by the use of a zoom on the camera head which is attached to the telescope enabling the surgeon and his assistants to visualize the picture on a monitor. The benefits of the Hopkins rod lens telescopes are the following:

Better light transmission resulting in images of outstanding resolution and contrast. Wider viewing angles offering better visualization of structures and accurate representation of the finest details over the entire field of view. It is possible to design a small diameter Hopkins rod lens telescopes but the narrow rod lens endoscopes are not durable, and break easily when bent, even with minimal flexion. The smaller the diameter of the endoscope, the more fragile it becomes and less light it transmits. The limit between too much flexibility and acceptable rigidity appears at about 3—4 mm in diameter. It is also difficult to design a thin caliber rod lens capable to transmit a bright light, even with the xenon light source.

*Microendoscopy*

The advance in fiber optics and the advent in the 1980s of fused coherent silica bundles has made possible the construction of small coherent image guides made of thousands of picture elements (also known as pixels), each with a diameter as small as 3—4 µm. One of the first applications in medicine of such image guides has been to construct flexible scopes used inside the vessels as an angioscope. Later the increase in the number of pixels and size resulted in an improved picture, and this enabled the manufacturing of small semi rigid telescope. The smallest size commonly in use is around 1 mm over 10,000 pixels.

In a fiber optic telescope each pixel will transit the information at the end of the proximal surface of the image guide which will be magnified by the ocular. The resolution of fiber endoscopes is limited by the diameter of the individual imaging fibers. The more fiber bundles are packed into the endoscope, the better its resolution. Nowadays, fiber design allows up to 50,000 of such fibers to be packed into a 2-mm endoscope, improving the quality of the image and adding an area of visualization, coming close to the quality of optical glass. The increase in fiber number can be accomplished by either augmenting the diameter of the endoscope or reducing the number of light carrying fiber. However, there is still the problem of "pixelation" and illumination that could be partially solved with improvements in the design of light sources and by increasing the sensitivity of video cameras.

**History and evolution**

Parallel to the advances in laparoscopy, smaller diameter endoscopes began to be used in these gynecological areas, sparking an interest in them to replace classic endoscopic techniques. First, the so-called "needlescope" and other small diameter laparoscopes were used [1], mainly for surgical sterilization and diagnostic procedures. This idea remained latent for many years until the recent advances in optic technologies and instruments reduced even further the diameter of these fiber-optics, thus allowing a better view. By the early '90s, small diameter fiber-optics were used in combination with laser beams and under general anesthesia, to coagulate endometriosic areas, myomectomies, adhesiolysis and biopsy evaluation [2,3].

Simultaneously, by the end of the '80s and the beginning of the '90s, the development and evolution of transcervical tubal catheterization and its various applications was on the rise [4]. Pioneers started using microfibers optics in catheterization techniques, introducing them through the operation canal of an hysteroscope into the lumen of the tube, thus describing for the first time the microendoscopy of the tubal lumen, called falloposcopy [5]. After this experience, we started using 0.3—0.5 mm fiber-optics to observe the tubal lumen, replacing the hysteroscope with a simple transcervical tubal catheterization equipment used routinely for procedures such as the removal of tubal obstructions. Therefore, the first step to reach the tubal ostium is to use the introducer with a coaxial catheter and then insert the microendoscope. The 1-mm coaxial catheter used as a guide for the other tubal catheters and metallic guides that will be introduced through the proximal lumen to the distal portion of the tube, has an internal diameter of approximately 0.7—0.8 mm, leaving a residual space of approximately 0.2 mm between the wall of the fiber-optic and the internal wall of the catheter. This space is essential to perform irrigation and create the necessary aqueous interface to see inside the tube with the microendoscope. The key aspect of this procedure is the association of these small microfibers with the techniques of transcervical tubal catheterization. However, we were not satisfied with simple observations, so we used this technique to reach the distal area of a tube which presented an ectopic pregnancy and attempted medical treatment [6]. Unfortunately, in many of these cases blood clots and blood in general hinders the access and several irrigations are needed to obtain a satisfactory view.

With this experience, we started studying the possibility of introducing needles into the abdominal cavity coupled to microendoscopes which varied from 0.3 to 0.5 mm. This allowed the insufflation as well as the visualization of the abdominal cavity. This was done with local anesthesia in order to perform diagnostic procedures on an outpatient basis, eliminating the use of general anesthesia and the scalpel, and enabling the observation of the different tissues as the needles passed through. This procedure was called microlaparoscopy [7], which was very similar to the classic technique and the needlescope, but with the advantage of having a more elaborate and smaller fiber-optic.

Unfortunately, in these first trials there were some difficulties with insufflation because it was slow due to the small caliber of the needles; there was also decreased visibility due to poor illumination, which led us to perform a second comparative study gradually increasing the caliber of the microfiber-optics used.

Evidently, the use of microfiber bundles with a greater diameter yielded better visibility. The execution of the pneumoperitoneum also improved, since it was faster and more effective, and there was better illumination, better field of vision, better resolution and an improvement in technique and instrumentation. The fiber-optics should not exceed 1.8 mm in diameter, so that they could be coupled or introduced in a cannula similar in diameter to the insufflation needle.

Usually, laparoscopy requires neuroleptanalgesia or general anesthesia as well as a surgical incision in the areas were the trocars are placed, but microlaparoscopy eliminates the need for all of these procedures in selected cases. Later, a preliminary report [8] indicated that 30 microlaparoscopies were performed under local anesthesia and sedation, and the view of the pelvic organs was confirmed. There was a marked difference in insufflation speed, visibility and illumination when fibers of approximately 0.5 mm with trocars of 1 mm were used, compared with optics of 1.4 mm and trocars of approximately 2 mm. Evidently, there was a better view and faster insufflation with the latter. Using a 2-mm trocar coupled to the 1.4-mm microendoscope somewhat affected the tolerance levels under local anesthesia, compared to the better acceptance observed with 1-mm trocars. We presented the surgical results of 20 diagnostic microlaparoscopies and 10 surgical microlaparoscopies, among them surgical sterilizations and assisted reproductive procedures like ZIFT. All patients tolerated well the microlaparoscopy under local anesthesia.

In this first stage, half the patients were given preoperative intravenous doses of

5—10 mg of midazolam hydrochloride, and 50—100 mg of fentanyl. The other half received 10 mg of diazepam orally and did not require any sedation, only local anesthesia in the insertion point of the trocars. The technique to introduce the two microlaparoscopy prototypes is very similar to the technique used in classical laparoscopy. First the patient is prepared with proper asepsis and anti-sepsis, a speculum is introduced to view the cervix, and a cannula is inserted which adheres to the cervix in order to manipulate the uterus if necessary. The puncture points where the insufflation needles and the trocars are inserted were infiltrated with 3 mm of 1% xylocaine. A 2-mm incision was made in those patients were the 2-mm needle was used, and a smaller one in those cases where the 0.8-mm needle was used. Before introducing the needle, the abdomen was elevated, and this needle with its envelope coupled to the microendoscope enabled us to see as it entered the abdominal cavity, and immediately after we could perform the pneumoperitoneum. The pelvic area and the abdominal cavity were inspected with the patient in the Trendelenburg position. At the end of the procedure, the patient was transferred to the recovery room and placed under observation for approximately 1 h.

If we compare the images obtained with a microlaparoscope to the images obtained with the classic laparoscope, we see that the focal length, the light inten-sity and the resolution is worse with the microlaparoscope. However, the image obtained with the microlaparoscope allows an adequate inspection of the normal pelvic area and its different pathologies. Occasionally, the patients' respiratory movements made it difficult to obtain a stable image of the organs under obser-vation. Nevertheless, the use of microfiber-optics to perform a microlaparoscopy enabled a full view of the intra-abdominal cavity, including the appendix, liver, bladder, the pelvic area and its annexes, tubes, ovaries, the anterior cul-de-sac, posterior cul-de-sac or Douglas space, and the remainder of the abdominal cav-ity. In the first stages, diagnostic and surgical procedures were performed, such as surgical sterilizations and human reproduction techniques like ZIFT. They were performed in a short time, between 5 and 15 min. These first patients had no complications related to the microendoscopy and the analgesia, whether intraoperative or operative. Some patients reported nausea which resolved spon-taneously within 1 h of the observation period, which is insignificant compared to the effect observed after a general anesthesia in classic laparoscopy proce-dures. Even though the volume of $CO_2$ used was the minimum required and the intraperitoneal pressure was low, one patient had shoulder pain which lasted 2 days, leading us to believe that insufflation is another issue to be solved.

A microlaparoscopy performed with this technique yields the benefits of the widely used insufflation needle or Veress needle, because it is a universally accepted insufflation diameter which causes few complications. These first experiences with microlaparoscopy and local anesthesia proved that small diam-eter endoscopes reduce the size of abdominal incisions, reduce local pain and reduce tissue trauma. It also proved that microlaparoscopy is a procedure where the insertion of the microendoscope and the insufflation needle can be done in a single step. This is comparable to the insertion of a standard insufflation needle, but cannot be compared to the insertion of a trocar without pneumoperitoneum [9,10]. Since the tip of the needle can be easily located through the microlaparoscope, preperitoneal insufflation is reduced as well as the possibility of placing the trocar incorrectly, which happens frequently during classical laparoscopy. In turn, this first puncture allows us to view the abdominal cavity to introduce a second trocar and avoid any possible trauma to the abdominal organs. The fact that these first procedures were performed in an outpatient basis, and not in the regular operation room, allowed us to decrease the cost for the procedure, and therefore, it was better accepted by the patients.

This first work in microlaparoscopy was reviewed in the "Year Book of Infertility and Reproductive Endocrinology", in 1994, by Daniel R. Mishell Jr [11]. According to this author, it makes sense to use this technique in the diagnosis of pelvic pathology in women with normal pelvic exams as well as a normal hysterosalpingography, with no history of pelvic infection or dysmenorrhea. These patients have a slim chance of having a pelvic disease that may cause infertility; therefore the surgical laparoscopy with general anesthesia will be performed only in a small group of women who presented irregularities as detected through the microlaparoscopy. This first work rekindles the old idea of diagnosing and even treating pathologies in the abdominal cavity using small fiber-optics and just local anesthesia. This is how new instruments, with better resolution fiber-optics that are easier to handle, are designed, incorporating anchoring systems for better manipulation and support and an easier penetration through the abdominal wall. Several studies were conducted with different researchers [12–21], in order to confirm the possibility of performing microlaparoscopy with fiber-optics smaller than 2 mm, thus taking advantage of the diameter of the universally accepted Veress needle.

Researchers have used microlaparoscopy for many purposes: to diagnose infertility, to establish a place to access and locate annex trocars, in cases of abdominal pain for pain mapping, using it as a second look instrument, and in patients with ovarian cancer undergoing treatment [22]. The use of these microfiberoptics is emphasized in oncologic cases with tumors given the possibility to use them for biopsies and make differential diagnoses. Nevertheless, to classify ovarian cancer, microlaparoscopy would have the same limitations as conventional laparoscopy.

In the beginning, the diagnosis and treatment made through microendoscopy was not widely accepted; several authors have pointed out some difficulties in making a correct diagnosis due to the limited focal distance, poor lighting and poor resolution, when compared with conventional small diameter endoscopes, like those of approximately 5 mm in diameter [23]. Other authors mention the benefits of reducing the diameter of the fibers so that they can be used in the above-mentioned procedures, and that the use of analgesia or local anesthesia is relatively safe [24,25]. They state that safeguards must be in place, such as resuscitation equipment or the possibility of an immediate transfer to a better equipped center in the event of complications. They add that the use of intravenous sedation must be done with appropriate monitoring equipment, and a general anesthesia support system must be on hand.

Many authors tend to believe that microlaparoscopy can be performed in an office or near an institute with surgical or resuscitation facilities, since these diagnostic procedures seldom have complications. Others have performed comparative studies with independent observers using the microlaparoscope and the classical 10-mm laparoscope, and concluded that the 2-mm microlaparoscope enables a diagnosis comparable to that obtained with the standard 10-mm laparoscope [26], stating that diagnostic microlaparoscopy in the office, using minimum anesthesia is an effective way to make a diagnosis [27].

Taking into account all of the above and the controversy caused by the advent of microlaparoscopy, we decided to carry out a multicenter study, using microlaparoscopy to answer questions such as: is it a procedure that can be performed in the office? Is it easy to perform? What is the level of tolerance? How reproducible is it?, and to define its applications.

To this end, we wrote a questionnaire and sent it to different centers pioneering the new technique, asking them to clearly indicate the equipment used, the diagnostic and surgical indications, the type of anesthesia used, the monitoring procedure used, the feasibility of its applications, the tolerance level, the technique used, the complications, the relationship between initial and final diagnosis, and a brief personal comment about the technique. A series of data were obtained from a group of approximately 408 patients at the different centers; half of them underwent diagnostic microlaparoscopy and the other half underwent surgical microlaparoscopy. The use of different microlaparoscopy equipment was allowed, but the diameters had to be between 1.2 and 2 mm, with a focal distance between 20 and 30 mm.

The patients were divided into three groups: one group received local anesthesia, another analgesia and sedation, and the third group received general anesthesia. The three groups underwent diagnostic and surgical procedures. The abdomen could be viewed successfully in all patients, and the procedure took between 5 and 30 min. It was necessary to monitor all patients with an electrocardiograph, an oxymeter and a sphygmomanometer. Anesthesia was short in those cases where analgesia or general anesthesia was used. There was a significant difference in permanence and postoperative observation between patients receiving local anesthesia, who were under observation approximately 1 h, and patients receiving sedation or general anesthesia, who were under observation between 2 and 4 h. The latter exhibited discrete postoperative after effects from anesthesia, like nausea and in some cases vomiting. This confirms that despite the advances in the different types of microendoscopes used, there are still limitations that must be overcome.

One of these limitations is poor illumination, and in these cases, the situation improved by placing the tip of the microendoscope closer to the target organ. The microendoscopes used in the last series showed improvements over the first one, namely better resolution and color quality. Nevertheless, the size of the image is still small and does not increase when transferred to video as was expected, given the technological advances in that area. Regarding focal distance, even though it is short, it is possible to obtain a good view with proper manipulation. There is still some light reflection when the fiber comes close to smooth and moist surfaces, hindering visibility for short periods of time and forcing the surgeon to retreat and move the microendoscope to solve the problem. The situation worsens with the patient's respiratory movements, but this can be overcome with proper training in the use of these microfiber-optics. After several procedures, the problem of image stability is solved. Pneumoperitoneum is still an issue, even if the amount of gas introduced in the abdominal cavity is reduced: an excess causes discomfort in the patient, and if it goes below levels where the patient does not feel it, the abdominal cavity is not properly distended, thus hindering observation. Therefore, pneumoperitoneum must not exceed 2.5 l and pressure must not exceed 15 mmHg.

In order to study the patients' tolerance level to this procedure, we classified tolerance into three groups: excellent, good, and poor. The following factors make a significant difference in the degree of tolerance: first, the patient's motivation to undergo the procedure; second, the patient's physical conditions; third, the patient's expectations regarding the possibility of pain.

Patients who were highly motivated because the procedure was important for them, i.e., patients requiring surgical sterilization, or diagnostic and even surgical procedures for infertility problems, like the removal of adhesions, tolerated the procedure very well and fell into the "excellent" category. Patients who were less motivated had a lower tolerance to the procedure, and some even required analgesia.

Slim patients who were in good physical condition and who had a thin abdominal wall, tolerated the procedure better than those in poor physical condition, whether due to obesity or other disturbances.

Patients who were properly informed about the procedure and its advantages, for example, that it could be done in an outpatient basis, that it did not require stitches or large incisions, and that it could yield results similar to those obtained with the classic laparoscope, accepted and tolerated the procedure well. The opposite was true for patients without proper conditioning or psychological preparation.

Patients with a high level of anxiety and patients who had intense pelvic pain due to their pathology, i.e., ectopic pregnancies, ruptured cysts and ovarian cyst torsion, required conscious sedation or general anesthesia.

A good evaluation of the procedure was performed and there were no complications, whether intra or perioperative, related to the microlaparoscopy technique with minimal insufflation. A small group of patients had nausea, but it resolved spontaneously in less than 1 h; these patients had undergone the procedure with analgesia or general anesthesia. The length of surgery was approximately $20 \pm 10$ min, which contributed to reduce potential complications from the anesthesia or the surgery itself. Only two minor hemorrhages were reported, one due to a small laceration of the uterus and another due to the laceration of an epigastric vessel. There were no major intra- or perioperative complications related to the microlaparoscopy.

In any surgical procedure there is always a risk of complications, and the rise in the number of endoscopists and of procedures using endoscopic techniques, coupled with poor training in reproductive as well as in gynecological surgery, has increased this risk during classic laparoscopy procedures, both diagnostic and surgical. At present, it is difficult to evaluate the real threat of complications from laparoscopy, since physicians who have a high rate of complications do not report them in the medical literature. In general, most of the problems reported are vascular lesions, which can happen in 0.1 to 0.6% of classic laparoscopy procedures, caused either by the Veress needle, the trocar, or the instruments [28]. These lesions produce immediate hemorrhage. The recent literature on microlaparoscopy describes isolated cases of intestinal perforation with these small needles, but these resolve spontaneously with no need for treatment whatsoever. These reported cases occurred mainly in patients with extensive intracavity alterations, and with extensive adhesions due to neoplasia [29].

On the other hand, we must keep in mind that a reduction in the diameter of the instruments implies a decrease in the force used to introduce it through the abdominal wall, thus decreasing the risk of perforations or trauma.

If we compare universally accepted instruments, like the needles used for intramuscular injections with a diameter of 1 mm (0.039 in.), or the needles used for follicular aspirations, known as follicular puncture needles, with a diameter of approximately 1.67 mm (0.066 in.), we see that with these two needles, the complications reported in the literature are uncommon and infrequent. Therefore, we believe that we must use optic instruments and their accessories with a diameter similar or smaller than the diameter of these needles. Evidently, this could reduce complications due to laparoscopy to a minimum.

Nevertheless, we must take into account that not only diameter is important, but also the instrument's consistency, shape and length. Regarding consistency, it could be flexible; regarding shape and length, it would be ideal if it adapted to the different spaces. Even more so, the length of the fiber-optics or microlaparoscopes should be shortened, to reduce possible complications, and the introduction site will depend on the structure we want to see. In other words, the introduction of an insufflation needle coupled to the fiber-optic can be performed in several points of the abdominal wall, depending on the requirements of the surgeon, and on the surgery or diagnosis to be made. Special care must be taken in those women with previous surgery when introducing the microlaparoscope. It has been already demonstrated that the left upper quadrant (Palmer's point) is the best site to introduce the microlaparoscope avoiding abdominal wall adhesions [30].

**Advantages of microlaparoscopy**

These technological advances and the procedures that can be performed with microlaparoscopy have several advantages. Some of the specific advantages of microlaparoscopy are:

1. The patient's safety increases, because when the insufflation needle is introduced, safety is related to an immediate visualization of the tissues pierced by the needle, thus avoiding an accidental puncture of organs or vascular spaces. Coupling the needle to the microendoscope also avoids the blind introduction of the first trocar, as was done before the advent of this new technology.

2. Morbidity decreases, because the introduction of small caliber instruments produces less tissue trauma. The simple fact of using smaller diameters logically reduces complications during the procedure, like perforating vessels or abdominal organs. Many times, these small punctures only require observation. The smaller caliber also enables us to reach smaller spaces with the microendoscope, something that could not be done with the larger diameter instruments. Also, smaller instruments are easier to transport. This is in tune with the advances in other technological areas, where we see a reduction in the size and caliber of instruments.

3. The use of smaller diameter instruments is less aggressive to the patients, since the introduction of the classic trocar is avoided, as well as sutures and visible scars, and the risk of poor cicatrization or hernia development is reduced.

4. General anesthesia could be eliminated in selected cases, replacing it with simple local anesthesia or analgesia. When microlaparoscopy is performed with local anesthesia for diagnostic and therapeutic purposes, the risk of complications is reduced, as well as the discomfort caused by general anesthesia. In this way, when local anesthesia is used, the discomfort caused by insufflation before the insertion of the trocar is avoided, because introducing the microendoscope coupled to the needle while simultaneously performing the pneumoperitoneum, allows an immediate view during the insufflation process.

5. Using local anesthesia allows verbal communication between the patient and the surgeon during and after the surgical procedure, so if there is pelvic pain, it can be easily located. Recovery time is shorter, and the technique is performed in an outpatient basis; this benefits the patient psychologically and otherwise.

6. Microlaparoscopy enables the surgeon to make a diagnosis and in many cases treat the pathology simultaneously. With the microlaparoscope it is relatively safe to diagnose most gynecological diseases, and it allows to view not only the gynecological area, but also the appendix, liver, bladder and the remainder of the abdominal cavity. It enables the physician to select the treatment modality that can be used during the endoscopy. Introducing the microendo-

scope coupled to the insufflation needle facilitates the introduction of secondary or tertiary trocars. In second-look procedures, the benefits are a short recovery time and less trauma, meaning that it can be performed more frequently. It is also useful in assisted reproductive procedures, such as GIFT, ZIFT and TET, and it has been proven that the pregnancy rate is comparable to other series where classic laparoscope is used. Microlaparoscopy can be used together with other procedures, such as ovarian cystoscopy, where it plays an important role to rule out the possibility of extracystical and peritoneal malignancies [31]. Microlaparoscopy can also be used with tubal cannulation, Falloposcopy and hysteroscopy, among others. It is very valuable for patients with advanced neoplasia which have been previously diagnosed and treated, because this technique enables us to follow up the treatment with minimal aggression. It can also be used in emergencies or in situations where a differential diagnosis is required, for example, in cases of ectopic pregnancies, pelvic infections, and appendicitis, among others [32]. It is a procedure that allows an instant diagnosis and guides us to the definite procedure and treatment [33].

8. Microlaparoscopy offer cost-benefit advantages and it reduces the complexity of the equipment, because it is easier to handle and transport. It can be incorporated to already existing equipment, so its use can be generalized at a minimum additional cost. If it is done in an outpatient basis, the cost of entering an operating room is eliminated. Reducing hospitalization, disability and recovery times, evidently decreases costs and increases benefits, because the patient can reincorporate to her family, society and job in less time.

## Technical improvements

The advances in microendoscopic instruments need to be better developed and tested. Since our first report in 1992 [7], optic instruments and their accessories have improved consistently; however, illumination is still an issue, and a better insufflation technique would allow more freedom during the procedure. The constant technologic development makes it difficult to know all the alternatives, but we know that an era of advances is ahead, where images will be of excellent quality, thus opening the space for microendoscopic instrumentation.

## Questions that need to be addressed

There are still questions that need to be addressed, for example: is this a pro7-cedure that needs local anesthesia or general anesthesia? Is it a procedure that must be performed in the office, in an outpatient basis or in the operating room?

The preferred location for microlaparoscopy is still a controversy [34]. Nevertheless, and referring to the studies done up to date, we see that most diagnostic microlaparoscopy cases and cases where tubal sterilizations are performed, do not require a specialized operating room. Another large variety of operations in patients with intense pelvic pain, ectopic pregnancies, ovarian cysts, pelvic inflammatory disease, torsion of the ovarian pedicle, and combined procedures like tubal catheterization for falloposcopy, hysteroscopic surgery, ovarian cystoscopy and infertility procedures like GIFT, ZIFT and TET have been performed in operating rooms designed for classic laparoscopy. Nevertheless, many of these operating rooms did not meet the requirement of a general operating room, including anesthesia, imaging equipment, laboratory and the support of a blood bank.

We must also remember that unfortunately, not all surgeons are as skilled and prepared in endoscopy. A regulated and lengthy surgical training is required to cope with the speed of technological advances [35]. It is essential to become familiar with the microendoscopic equipment and instruments to avoid intra-operative faults that in many cases can be foreseen [36]. It must be noted that there is a significant difference between handling and manipulating classic laparoscopic instruments and handling microinstruments. This requires specific training, particularly if local anesthesia is used.

## Conclusion

We believe that microlaparoscopy increases the safety and efficiency of endoscopy. This belief is shared by physicians from different countries and for different medical indications [37—46]. So far, however, clinical experience is limited and only long-term randomized multicenter studies could define the role of microlaparoscopic procedures in gynecology and their obvious transfer towards other surgical areas. We expect that the technique and the instruments can be improved so that it can be implemented preferably with local anesthesia. We also expect improvements in anesthetic techniques which will favorably affect this and other outpatient procedures.

In conclusion, we foresee great technological advances in the near future, perhaps based in computer technology, and computer-aided imaging techniques will increase accuracy and therefore safety in the procedure, which in turn will benefit the patient.

## References

1. Dingfelder JR, Brenner WE. The needlescope and other small diameter laparoscopes for sterilization and diagnostic procedures. Int J Gynaecol Obstet 1976;14:53—58.
2. Dorsey JH, Tabb CR. Mini-laparoscopy and fiber optic lasers. Obstet Gynecol Clin North Am 1991;18:613—617.
3. Childers JM, Hatch KD, Surwit EA. Office laparoscopy and biopsy evaluation of patients with intraperitoneal carcinoma using a new optical catheter. Gynecol Oncol 1992;47:337—342.
4. Risquez F, Confino E. Transcervical tubal cannulation, past, present, and future. Fertil Steril 1993;60:211—226.
5. Kerin J, Daykhovsky L, Grundfest W, Surrey E. Falloposcopy: a microendoscopic transvaginal technique for diagnosing and treating endotubal disease incorporating guidewire cannulation and direct balloon tuboplasty. J Reprod Med 1990;1:47—56.

6. Rísquez F, Pennehouat G, Foulot H, Mathieson J, Dubuisson JB, Bonnin A, Madelenat P, Zorn JR. Transcervical tubal cannulation and falloposcopy for the management of tubal pregnancy. Hum Reprod 1992;7:274–275.

7. Rísquez F, Pennehouat G, Kovac's A, Trias A, Briceño P, Bouteville C, Piras M, Madelenat P, Rodriguez O. Microlaparoscopy in Human Reproduction. Presented at the XIV World Congress on Fertility and Sterility. Abstr Book, Abstr 52, pp 49, November, Caracas, Venezuela, 1992.

8. Rísquez F, Penehouat G, Fernandez R, Confino E, Rodriguez O. Microlaparoscopy: a preliminary report. Hum Reprod 1993;8:1701–1702.

9. Dingfelder JR. Direct laparoscope trocar insertion without prior pneumoperitoneum. J Reprod Med 1978;21:45–47.

10. Jarret JC. Laparoscopy: Direct trocar insertion without pneumoperitoneum. Obstet Gynecol 1990;75:725–727.

11. Mishell DR. (Commentary). In: Mishell DR, Lobo RA, Sokol RZ (eds) Year Book of Infertility and Reproductive Endocrinology. Chicago: Mosby-Year Book, 1994;58.

12. Bauer O, Devroey P, Wisanto A, Gerling W, Kaisi M, Diedrich K. Small diameter laparoscopy using a microlaparoscope. Hum Reprod 1995;10:1461–1464.

13. Déchaud H, Hédon B. What is the importance of microlaparoscopy in gynecology? Presented at the 15th World Congress on Fertility and Sterility. Contracept Fertil Sex 1995;23:Abstr OC 315, s69.

14. Molloy D. The diagnostic accuracy of a microlaparoscope. J Am Assoc Gynecol Laparosc 1995;2:203–206.

15. Van Der Wat IJ. Microendoscopy: a new approach in gynecological endoscopy. Presented at the 15th World Congress on Fertility and Sterility. Contracept Fertil Sex 1995;23:Abstr OC 314, s69.

16. Vasquez AR, Partamian JJ, Novelli JE. Minilaparoscopic diagnosis of ectopic pregnancy. Presented at the 15th World Congress on Fertility and Sterility. Contracept Fertil Sex 1995;23:Abstr P109, s100.

17. Barisic D, Ven H, Prieti G, Strelec M. The diagnostic accuracy of a 1.2 mm minilaparoscope. Gynaecol Endosc 1996;5:283–286.

18. Haeusler G, Lehner R, Hanzal E, Kainz C. Diagnostic accuracy of 2 mm microlaparoscopy. Acta Obstet Gynecol Scand 1996;75:672–675.

19. Karabacak O, Bülent TM, Zeki TM, Guner H, Yildiz A, Yildirim M. Small diameter versus conventional laparoscopy: a prospective, self-controlled study. Hum Reprod 1997;12:2399–2401.

20. Connant C, Grochmal SA, Garrat D. In-office laparoscopy with optical catheters: report with initial experience in 413 patients. Presented at the 23rd Annual Meeting of the World Congress of Gynecological Endoscopy, Abstr Book, Oct., New York, USA, 1994.

21. Hibbert ML, Bullert JL, Seymour SD, Poore SE, Davis GD. A microlaparoscopic technique for pomeroy tubal ligation. Obstet Gynecol 1997;90:249–251.

22. Rísquez F, Penehouat G, Audebert A (eds) First International Congress on Microendoscopy in Gynecology and Obstetrics, Abstr. Book, March, Bordeaux, France, 1997.

23. Fuller PN. Microendoscopic surgery: A comparison of microendoscopes and a review of the literature. Am J Obstet Gynecol 1996;174:1757–1762.

24. Love BR, McCorvey R. Low-cost office laparoscopic sterilization. J Am Assoc Gynecol Laparosc 1994;1;379–372.

25. Phipps JH, Hassanien M, Miller R. Microlaparoscopy: diagnostic and sterilization without general anesthesia: a safe practical and cost-effective technique. Gynaecol Endosc 1996;5:223–224.

26. Faber BM, Coddington CC. Microlaparoscopy: a comparative study of diagnostic accuracy. Fertil Steril 1997;67:952–954.

27. Palter S, Olive D. Office microlaparoscopy under local anesthesia for chronic pelvic pain. J Am Assoc Gynecol Laparosc 1996;3:359–364.

84

28. Mintz M. Risks and prophylaxis in laparoscopy: a review of 100,000 cases. J Reprod Med 1977;18:269—272.
29. Bauer O. Micro-access endoscopy: the clinical impact of new technologies. Presented at ESHRE, 12th Annual Meeting. Hum Reprod 1996;11:Abstr 077,36—37.
30. Audebert A. Microlaparoscopy in women with previous surgery. Microendoscopy in gynecology and obstetrics. First International Congress on Microendoscopy in Gynecology and Obstetrics, Abstr, March, Bordeaux, France, 1997.
31. Pennehouat G, Gugliemina JN, Benifla JL, Crequat J. Kystoscopie transvaginale et prise en charge des kystes ovariens uniculaires anechogenes. Jobgyn 1994;2:56—57.
32. Risquez F, Pennehouat G, McCorvey R, Love B, Vazquez A, Partamian J, Rebon P, Lucena E, Audebert A, Confino E. Diagnostic and operative microlaparoscopy: preliminary multicenter report. Hum Reprod 1997;12:1645—1648.
33. Almeida O, Val-Gallas J, Rizk B. Appendicectomy under local anaesthesia following conscious pain mapping with microlaparoscopy. Hum Reprod 1998;13:588—590.
34. Van Der Wat IJ. Microendoscopy in the operating room. Gynaecol Endosc 1997;6:265—268.
35. Rimbach S, Wallwiener D, Bastert G. Falloposcopy: its place in the state-of-the-art spectrum of tubal investigation methods. In: Hedon B, Bringer J, Mares P (eds) Fertility and Sterility a Current Overview, Proceedings of the 15th World Congress on Fertility and Sterility. Montpellier, France. London: Parthenon Publishing, 1995;97—103.
36. Zupi E. Instrumentation for microendoscopy. Presented at the World Congress of Gynaecologic Endoscopy, Abstr Book, June, Rome, Italy, 1997.
37. Curto JM, Buquet RA, Tilli M, Palamas T. Microlaparoscopy in infant and juvenile pathology. Presented at the First International Congress on Microendoscopy in Gynecology and Obstetrics, Abstr Book, March, Bordeaux, France, 1997.
38. Kumar K. Microlaparoscopy under local anesthesia and conscious sedation. Presented at the First International Congress on Microendoscopy in Gynecology and Obstetrics, Abstr Book, March, Bordeaux, France, 1997.
39. Rebón P, Partamian JJ, Vazquez A, Novelli J. Microlaparoscopic management of ectopic pregnancy. Presented at the First International Congress on Microendoscopy in Gynecology and Obstetrics, Abstr Book, March, Bordeaux, France, 1997.
40. Gordts S, Brosens I (eds) Second International Congress on microendoscopy in gynecology and obstetrics, Abstr Book, May, Leuven, Belgium, 1998.
41. Benifla JL, Massoud E, Kadoch O, Tardif D, Goncalves O, Meneux E, Batallan A, Darai E, Madelenat P. Microlaparoscopy under local anesthesia and intravenous sedation: technique and tolerance. Report of 100 patients. Presented at the Second International Congress on Microendoscopy in Gynecology and Obstetrics, Abstr Book, May, Leuven, Belgium, 1998;62.
42. Déchaud H, Zayat A, Astruc M, Boulot P, Hédon B. Microlaparoscopy during the third trimester of pregnancy. Presented at the Second International Congress on Microendoscopy in Gynecology and Obstetrics, Abstr Book, May, Leuven, Belgium, 1998;40.
43. Edén E. The patients experience and tolerance of microlaparoscopy under local anaesthesia: a randomized study comparing the new technique with conventional laparoscopy. Presented at the Second International Congress on microendoscopy in gynecology and obstetrics, Abstr Book, May, Leuven, Belgium, 1998;42.
44. Hutchon DJR. Safe creation of the pneumoperitoneum: a computer simulation of verres needle vs direct trochar entry. Presented at the Second International Congress on Microendoscopy in Gynecology and Obstetrics, Abstr Book, May, Leuven, Belgium, 1998;64.
45. Mage G, Wattiez A, Canis M, Goldchmit R, Bruhat MA. Office microendoscopy: Definitions and terminology. Presented at the Second International Congress on Microendoscopy in Gynecology and Obstetrics, Abstr Book, May, Leuven, Belgium, 1998;13.
46. O'Donovan PJ. Out patient microhysteroscopy, set up, personnel and equipment. Presented at the Second International Congress on Microendoscopy in Gynecology and Obstetrics, Abstr Book, May, Leuven, Belgium, 1998;40.

# Ovarian imaging

Roger A. Pierson

*Womens' Health Imaging Research Laboratory, Department of Obstetrics, Gynaecology and Reproductive Sciences, College of Medicine, University of Saskatchewan, Saskatoon, Saskatchewan, Canada*

**Abstract.** There is much physiologic information available in the exquisite detail of ovarian images generated by high-resolution imaging instruments. Ultrasonography and magnetic resonance imaging are being used in clinical and research settings to increase our understanding of ovarian biology and its relationship to the events of conception. Physiologically dominant ovarian follicles are identifiable by ultrasonography at approximately day 7 postmenstruation. Computer-assisted image analyses of the attributes of normal preovulatory follicles include thick, low-amplitude walls and a gradual transformation zone at the fluid-follicle interface. We are actively evaluating the acoustic characteristics indicative of viability and atresia of ovarian follicles. The walls of preovulatory follicles were characterized by increased heterogeneity, increased wall breadth and a more gradual transformation at the fluid-follicle wall interface. Atresia is characterized by thin walls, high numerical pixel value (bright) signals and highly variable signals from the follicular fluid. The physiologic status of follicles as small as 6 mm may be determined. No differences in image attributes have been detected in 4- to 5-mm follicles. Image attributes of physiologically selected small follicles (< 6 mm) include higher amplitude walls and smooth echotexture of follicle fluid compared to subordinate follicles of the cohort. Similarly, time series analyses combining image attributes of the follicles and their individual growth profiles show marked differences in the characteristics of ovulatory and atretic follicles in both natural ovarian cycles and under ovulation induction conditions. The implications for the timing oocyte retrieval from small follicles for in vitro maturation are profound. If acoustic markers for oocyte competence are determined, oocyte retrieval and in vitro maturation from 4- to 6-mm follicles may become a routine clinical procedure. Computer-assisted image analysis and ultrasonographic assessment of ovarian follicular development also are natural extensions of the technologic advances in ovulation induction therapy. Similarly, magnetic resonance images of the ovaries are being used to assess physiologic attributes of ovarian follicles and corpora lutea. A combined approach of imaging, image analysis and mathematical modelling to describe the patterns of follicular development will elucidate many previously unanswered questions in the fundamental biology of ovarian function.

**Keywords:** image analysis, imaging, MRI, ovary, ultrasonography.

Noninvasive imaging of the ovaries is transforming the way that we think about normal and abnormal ovarian function. We now have the unprecedented opportunity to observe ovarian function in the same women over time, to determine what happens to individual follicles and to apply many new techniques to age old puzzles. It is important to remember that changes in the anatomy and physiology of the ovarian follicles and luteal glands form the basis for the images that

---

*Address for correspondence:* Roger A. Pierson PhD, Reproductive Biological Unit, Department of Obstetrics/Gynaecology, Royal University, 103 Hospital Drive, Saskatoon, Saskatchewan S7N OW8, Canada. Tel.: +1-306-966-4458. Fax: +1-306-966-8796. E-mail: Pierson@erato.usask.ca

we see, therefore, reminders of the biology underlying the images are placed where marriage of concept and visualization are critical.

Transvaginal high-resolution diagnostic ultrasonography has become the most important development in infertility investigation since the widespread application of radioimmunoassay techniques for the measurement of reproductively active hormones. Relatively high frequency (e.g., 5.0 and 7.5 MHz) or broadband (4–9 MHz) intravaginal transducers and color-flow Doppler techniques have dramatically increased image resolution facilitating detailed examination of the ovaries and other female reproductive organs. There is a great deal of physiologically important information not readily appreciated by the human eye available in the exquisite detail of the images created by the current generation of ultrasonographic instruments. These image data may be evaluated in many forms. We believe that the physiologic events underlying ovarian follicular growth and development may be evaluated in minute detail using computer-enhanced ultrasonography. Similarly, magnetic resonance imaging is beginning to emerge as a research tool in ovarian imaging. Future developments in equipment may make MRI as user friendly as ultrasonography is now. Combinations of the information available in ultrasonography, magnetic resonance imaging, computer-assisted image analysis and mathematical modelling foreshadow a new era in our understanding of the basic biology of ovarian follicular development, ovulation and luteogenesis.

The purpose of this manuscript is to identify some of the important issues in ovarian biology and to describe the contributions of ovarian imaging technology to our understanding of these problems. Finally, we will speculate on the applications of emerging imaging technologies to our future understanding of ovarian function, conception and contraception.

## Ovaries

The role of the ovary as the master gland of the female reproductive tract necessitates a dynamic morphology. The structure of the ovary changes every day of the menstrual cycle as follicles grow, regress or ovulate. Because ovarian follicles have both endocrine (production of estrogens and nonsteroidal hormones) and exocrine (nurture and release of oocytes) functions, seemingly minute changes in the follicles or luteal glands may have profound physiologic implications.

The primary functions of a preovulatory follicle are the nurture and release of an oocyte capable of being fertilized and subsequent structural and functional transformation into a luteal gland capable of adequate progesterone production. It is also important to remember that follicular development is a concomitant, concerted development of all of the components of the follicle. The follicular phase of the ovarian cycle has been divided into functional divisions describing the events which occur during folliculogenesis. They are:

1) the recruitment phase, during which many receptive follicles are recruited and develop;

2) the selection and dominance phases, during which one follicle undergoes favoured growth and development while other follicles in the recruited cohort are committed to atresia; and

3) the ovulation phase, during which the dominant follicle ruptures and expels the oocyte/cumulus complex. Images of the follicles generated during each phase will reflect their physiologic status.

Transvaginal color Doppler imaging has been used to identify the ovarian arteries. In most cases, the ovarian vessels may be identified as they enter the ovarian hilus, removing all doubt about the identity of the ovarian vasculature. Resistance to blood flow in the ovarian vasculature has been studied at various times during the ovarian cycle using spectral Doppler techniques; the ovary bearing the preovulatory follicle or corpus luteum exhibits lower resistance to blood flow than the vessels of the contralateral ovary. The lowest impedance to blood flow during the ovarian cycle occurs on the day of the luteinizing hormone (LH) peak while highest resistance to blood flow was observed on day 1 of menses [1]. The temporal relationships of blood flow and ovarian status in regard to development of the preovulatory follicle, development and regression of the corpus luteum apparently have not been fully investigated.

**Assessment of ovarian follicular development**

The ovarian follicular population may be evaluated at any time during the menstrual cycle. However, the period of greatest interest usually is the late follicular phase when the development of the follicle physiologically selected to ovulate may be identified and monitored. The dominant follicle appears to be identifiable on the basis of size at approximately day 7 postmenstruation and grows at a rate of approximately 2 mm per day [2–8]. Serial ultrasound examinations may be performed during the follicular phases of one or more menstrual cycles to ascertain that the processes of follicular selection and growth are occurring within clinically normal limits [8,9]. If subtle abnormalities in follicular growth are detected, corrective measures may be taken. These types of studies appear to be most useful in the elucidation of problems associated with idiopathic infertility.

The profiles for serum estradiol concentrations and ultrasonographically determined diameters of preovulatory follicles normally run parallel courses [10]. Therefore, serial ultrasonography and evaluation of systemic estrogen levels have great potential in the isolation and identification of the causes of follicular phase defects. For example, patients may present with estradiol concentrations that appear to be within clinically normal limits for the preovulatory phase of the menstrual cycle, however, ultrasound examination may reveal the presence of six to 20 follicles of 5- to 10-mm diameter and the absence of a dominant follicle of preovulatory diameter. Alternatively, ultrasound examination during the late follicular phase may reveal a follicle of ostensibly preovulatory diameter (e.g., 22 mm) and the patient may exhibit clinically low estradiol concentrations. Follicles with this particular pattern of growth and regression have an atypical morphology, appear flaccid, fail to ovulate and regress over the ensuing week.

Using serial ultrasonography and assessment of circulation hormone levels, it appears possible to identify subtle defects in the processes of follicular recruitment, development, physiologic selection for the preovulatory follicle, final follicular maturation and ovulation. Seemingly minor disturbances in the continuum of folliculogenesis may be responsible for much infertility previously classified as idiopathic. Assessment of follicular dynamics and mapping the fates of individual follicles in normative and infertile patients is the subject of ongoing research in our laboratory.

**Preovulatory follicles**

The follicle destined to ovulate is physiologically selected for preferential development and eventual ovulation, while other follicles in its cohort are condemned to atresia. The processes by which the selection mechanism occurs have not been determined and remain among the great mysteries in reproductive biology. The current concepts regarding physiological selection of the dominant follicle in women and nonhuman primates have been critically evaluated and it has been determined that the selection process is completed only during the ovarian cycle in which the individual ovulation occurs [3–5]. In this regard, it has been postulated that selection, final growth and maturation of the ovulatory follicle may be due simply to chance development of a follicle within the recruited cohort coincident with luteal regression and increased preovulatory FSH levels.

Preovulatory follicles differ from the other follicles in their cohort in that they have a more extensive and permeable capillary network [6,7,11]. The considerable vascularity which exists around the dominant follicle may allow it to accumulate more of the circulating gonadotropins and thus survive while the other members of its cohort undergo atresia. However, enhanced vascularity may be either a cause or reflection of selection.

Studies using transvaginal color flow mapping to assess blood flow to the follicle and the vascular perfusion of the follicular wall during the dominance phase are ongoing. Although data have not yet been critically evaluated, it appears that there is a very gradual decrease in impedance to blood flow in the vessels immediately surrounding the follicle as the interval to ovulation decreases. Immediately prior to ovulation, the perifollicular vessels are easily identified and spectral Doppler flow wave forms may be generated. However, it is rare to visualize the perifollicular vessels in one image plane due to their tortuous path around the periphery of the follicle [1,12].

Research is just beginning into the assessment of echotextural characteristics and vascular patterns of individual preovulatory follicles to evaluate the probability of ovulation. It appears that ultrasonographic confirmation of ovulation may be important for many patients undergoing clinical evaluation for ovulatory dysfunction.

# Ovulation

Ovulation is the culmination of a complex series of events which is set into motion with a sudden, very brief rise in peripheral LH concentrations and results in the evacuation of the follicular fluid, collapse of the preovulatory follicle and expulsion of the oocyte from the follicle [13—15]. Disintegration of the apex of the follicle, final maturation of the oocyte, and evacuation of the follicular fluid must be closely coordinated for successful ovulation. Subsequent functional and morphologic changes in the cells which formerly comprised the follicular epithelium and theca interna also must be completed to form the luteal gland. Direct observation of ovulation by laparoscopy or ultrasonography is quite dramatic, however, it must be remembered that the event of ovulation is the result of a long series of biochemical, physiologic and morphologic changes in the tissues of the follicle [15].

Ovulation occurs on approximately day 14 postmenstruation in a classic "textbook" 28-day menstrual cycle [2—4]. Transabdominal ultrasound scanning has been used for many years to detect the occurrence of ovulation in women [16]. However, rupture of the follicle and evacuation of the follicular fluid and cumulus/oocyte complex has only recently been demonstrated by real-time ultrasonography [17,18]. On average, ovulation appeared to take approximately 10 min from initiation to complete follicular evacuation. However, the time required for ovulation varied from less than 1 min to more than 20 min. The site of follicular evacuation was immediately detectable. The point of follicular rupture from the surface of the ovary may be recognised for up to a week and the luteal gland typically remains ultrasonographically detectable until the subsequent ovulatory cycle [19,20].

The first noticeable micromorphologic alterations following the LH surge are that the capillaries which surround the preovulatory follicle become increasingly fenestrated and the theca interna becomes edematous due to plasma effusion from the newly fenestrated vasculature [6,7,11]. The collagen networks comprising the theca externa and tunica albuginea dissociate due to increased plasmin released by granulosa cells and increased collagenase activity originating from the fibroblasts of the albuginea [21]. Weakening of the follicle wall occurs over the entire wall, however, rupture is localized to the apex. The cells comprising the wall of the follicle are not destroyed, but reorganized, facilitating transformation to the corpus luteum [15].

Color flow mapping studies of the follicular vasculature have only recently begun. There is a single report of a single ovulation in the literature [22]. Studies regarding vasculature changes during ovulation are ongoing [12]. In our series of color flow studies, volumetric estimations of the follicular fluid are made from follicular measurements at defined times before and during ovulation. Color flow maps and spectral Doppler wave forms also are generated at defined times during follicular evacuation. The patterns of blood flow during collapse of the follicle have not yet been critically evaluated. However, variation in resistance to blood flow appears to be quite dramatically decreased between preovulatory measurements and those taken following initiation of follicular rupture. Variation in flow characteristics appear very slight once follicular evacuation has begun.

**Ovulation failure**

Evaluation of ovulation and the period of early luteogenesis in control patients and patients referred for idiopathic infertility is revealing previously undescribed flaws in the ovulatory process. It appears that failure of ovulation probably occurs by one of two mechanisms. The luteinized, unruptured follicle syndrome (LUF) has been debated, however, transvaginal ultrasound has been used to provide detailed descriptions of the process [23,24]. The physiologically selected follicle attains preovulatory diameter and fails to rupture and release the oocyte/cumulus complex. The oocyte/cumulus complex apparently remains trapped within the lumen of the follicular structure. The walls of the follicle appear to thicken and acquire echotexture similar to that displayed by luteinized tissue following normal ovulations. The follicular fluid/follicle interface acquires hazy, indistinct borders. The LUF remains identifiable for the duration of the menstrual cycle and apparently regresses following a time course similar to that of clinically normal corpora lutea [12]. Basal body temperature charts and midcycle progesterone concentrations remain within clinically normal limits. Menstrual periods may be reported to be normal or somewhat lighter than normal for individual patients. A variation of the LUF syndrome is the hemorrhagic anovulatory follicle, in which the same series of event occurs, however, there is capillary leakage into the lumen of the follicle and the same level of peripheral luteinization does not develop.

A second proposed mechanism for failure of ovulation appears to involve the growth of the physiologically selected follicle beyond normal preovulatory diameter without ovulation. The dysfunctional dominant follicle appears to remain static for 1 to several days and then regresses. The rate of follicular regression appears to be highly variable, although in several instances in our laboratory, the rate of regression has been the same as the rate of follicular growth. There apparently is no luteinization of the follicular wall. The walls of the follicle appear thin and highly echoic. The follicular fluid/follicle interface appears sharp and distinct. Menstrual periods following this type of ovulatory failure typically occur within a normal cycle length although the amount of flow appears quite variable.

As diagnostic techniques are developed, we believe that transvaginal ultrasonography will assist in the diagnosis and treatment of subtle ovulatory dysfunction by the practicing clinician.

**Corpus luteum**

The corpus luteum is the forgotten gland in reproductive endocrinology. The corpus luteum undergoes profound neoangiogenesis during its development, is dependent on vascular flow for normal function, and exhibits degradation of the vascular supply during regression. This cyclicity in vascularization and the role of the corpus luteum in regulating ovarian function from ovarian cycle to ovarian cycle, in addition to its role in the establishment and maintenance of pregnancy make the luteal gland a primary target for research based upon color-flow Doppler ultrasonography.

The walls of the follicle are in close opposition immediately following evacuation of the follicular fluid. The cells of the former follicular wall begin the structural and functional transformation to the cells which will comprise the corpus luteum and the walls of the evacuated follicle become profoundly vascularized during the 48- to 72-h period following ovulation. Blood and lymphatic vessels colonize the developing corpus luteum. It appears that following approximately 60% of ovulations in women, there is a slight haemorrhage into the evacuated follicle. The degree of haemorrhage is extremely variable, however, there does not appear to be any effect of luteal morphology on progesterone production during the luteal phase of the menstrual cycle [12,20].

Color Doppler imaging combined with high-resolution grey scale ultrasonography allows evaluation of the functional development of luteal glands, as well as other reproductive organs of interest and provides the ability to locate blood flow in very small vessels that cannot be visualized with conventional gray-scale imaging and the flow velocity waveforms resulting from spectral Doppler interrogation may be analysed to assess functional integrity. More recently, the addition of power-flow color Doppler provides a technique with which we may study the perfusion of the corpus luteum.

A pronounced ring of vascularity, which appears to follow the path of the vascular supply surrounding the former preovulatory follicle and becomes even more apparent as the corpus luteum matures, is typically observed upon color flow Doppler interrogation of the luteal gland. During the period of active progesterone secretion during the estrous cycle and during early pregnancy, resistance to vascular flow is usually low as would be expected of an active endocrine tissue. As luteal regression ensues, the vascular flow characteristics change profoundly. The color flow mapping patterns become much less pronounced and increased resistance to flow is observed within the vessels. Definitive studies of the vascular dynamics within the corpus luteum have apparently not yet been performed, however, this is expected to develop into a promising research area with profound ramifications to infertility assessments, maternal recognition of pregnancy and etiology of early embryonic loss. The role of Doppler ultrasonography in studies of corpora lutea associated with early embryonic loss, either impending or demonstrated remains to be elucidated, however, it is highly probable that vascular changes in the corpus luteum may be indicative of impending early embryonic death.

A precise role for color flow Doppler assessment of luteal vascularity has yet to be defined, it seems probable that there is a profound role for this imaging modality in the study of luteal angiogenesis. Transvaginal color flow ultrasonography evaluation of luteal blood flow in pregnant and nonpregnant women has shown low rates of luteal flow were observed in nonpregnant women while highest rates of blood flow were observed in the luteal glands of women with intrauterine pregnancies [25].

## Polycystic ovarian syndrome

Polycystic ovarian syndrome (PCOS) resulting in anovulation also is a common cause of infertility. The patterns of follicular turnover, initiation of follicular growth and physiological selection of a dominant follicle are poorly understood in PCOS patients. It is hoped that new research will elucidate the specific defects in processes of follicular growth and development and allow targeted therapies to ameliorate the infertility associated with the condition. Although the diagnosis of PCOS is traditionally made on clinical history and endocrine assessment, the ultrasonographic appearance of the ovaries of a PCOS patient strongly supports the clinical diagnosis and in many cases PCOS may be identified solely on the ultrasonographic morphology of the ovaries. The ultrasonographic morphology of PCOS has been described as ovaries containing from 15 to 40 follicles of 4- to 10-mm diameter. The typical distribution of follicles is like that of a string-of-pearls around the cortex of the ovary, although some women have follicles evenly distributed throughout the parenchyma [26]. The attributes of PCOS morphology are being constantly updated as subtle differences in endocrine profiles are elucidated [27]. Many PCOS patients present a difficult problem during ovulation induction with mild or more potent ovulation inducing agents. Serial transvaginal ultrasonography is an extremely important adjunct in assessment of the ovarian response to the pharmaceutical agents used in the ovulation induction protocol.

## Ovulation induction

Ovulation induction therapy may be performed for a variety of reasons varying from simply providing adequate stimulation to achieve a single ovulation in women who are anovulatory to the production of many well developed oocytes for fertilization in the assisted reproductive technologies. In many instances, the goal of ovarian superstimulation is to stave off atresia in a recruited cohort of follicles, sustain the development of the recruited follicles to a preovulatory state and to obtain a number of properly matured oocytes for fertilization.

In some of the assisted reproductive technologies, the objective of ovarian stimulation is to facilitate the development of three or four follicles which will provide oocytes capable of being fertilized. In in vitro fertilization (IVF) protocols, the stimulation of many more follicles may be desired. In centers where IVF is performed in concert with an embryo cryopreservation program, up to three fresh embryos may be transferred at the time of the procedure and additional embryos frozen for future use. Induction of ovulation in women with ostensibly normal ovarian function combined with intrauterine insemination also is increasingly being used as a therapy for idiopathic infertility and in cases where the male partner has a mild to medium level of oligospermia.

Ultrasonography is essential in determining the numbers and fates of individual follicles induced to grow with the exogenous gonadotrophins. It is also important to note that the linear relationship between circulating estradiol 17β concentrations and follicular diameter we expect based upon unstimulated cycles may not exist during ovulation induction [28]. Thus the role of ultrasonography is extremely important in this area. The timing of the hCG administration is critical in all ovulation induction protocols. In monitoring the course of an ovulation induction, the responses of individual follicles to the ovulatory dose of hCG may be as important as monitoring the number and rates of growth of the follicles. The number of follicles which ovulate may be discerned and unruptured follicles remaining in the ovaries assessed. If conception does not occur, appropriate actions may be taken for subsequent therapies.

## Clomiphene citrate

Clomiphene citrate is a weak estrogen agonist with a long half-life which exerts its effect by binding to hypothalamic estrogen receptors and thus facilitates increased gonadotrophin secretion. The additional FSH released by the effects of clomiphene citrate binding at this level recruits follicles and sustains their continued development [29]. The normal physiological mechanism for selection and dominance of preovulatory follicles may be overwhelmed and more than one preovulatory follicle may develop. The incidence of multiple follicular development reportedly ranges from 20 to 60% per cycle. Follicles stimulated to grow with clomiphene citrate appear to follow the normal course of preovulatory development, estrogen levels are consistent with those observed in spontaneous cycles and the diameter of preovulatory follicles is reportedly 22—23 mm [30—32].

However, in many cases it may be observed that the follicles do not ovulate until they attain a diameter of 30—35 mm, or alternatively, do not ovulate and regress [33]. The administration of human chorionic gonadotrophin (hCG) to initiate the changes associated with ovulation may then be necessary. It is important to appreciate that hCG should not be administered as an empiric therapy or according to a specific menstrual cycle date. The hCG injection is best administered following serial ultrasonographic examinations to ascertain progressive growth of the dominant follicles. Clinically, it has traditionally been assumed that initiation of menstrual bleeding following clomiphene citrate administration in amenorrheic women indicates that ovulation has occurred. However, it is increasingly important to verify this notion with follow-up ultrasonographic examinations and assessment of circulating midluteal phase progesterone concentrations.

Follicles induced to grow with clomiphene citrate may be slightly different from those recruited during spontaneous cycles [12]. Follicles may grow to a larger diameter than typically observed in natural cycles, e.g., 25—30 mm, and the walls exhibit a characteristically brighter echotexture depending on the dose, number of days of clomiphene citrate therapy and the number of cycles previously stimulated. The walls also do not appear to become as thick as those seen in uninduced preovulatory follicles [34]. Many of the follicles exhibit morphologies consistent with luteinized unruptured follicle syndrome on follow-up examinations. The appropriate follow-up studies for these preliminary observations are ongoing.

**Exogenous gonadotrophins**

Ovulation induction with exogenous human menopausal gonadotrophins (hMG) or recombinant FSH (rFSH) typically follows a complex regimen which involves the injection of a supraphysiologic dose of FSH and LH on a daily basis. The relative purity of the FSH component varies with the manufacturer of the drug. Some of the gonadotrophins contain approximately equal quantities of FSH and LH while others contain an FSH to LH ratio of approximately nine to one. FSH derived from recombinant sources is now available for clinical use and has no LH contamination. One of the remaining controversies in ovulation induction is the role of LH in follicle and oocyte maturation.

Programs of ovulation induction with hMG may be carried out in many iterations. In some centers the initial follicle recruitment is stimulated with clomiphene citrate or GnRH analogues and then completed with human menopausal gonadotropins. The menstrual cycles for groups of women may be synchronized using GnRH analogues or oral contraceptives to suppress ovarian activity. There are many variations of ovulation induction protocols and each center has protocols which work best in their hands. Ovulation induction with exogenous gonadotrophins is commenced on cycle day 3 in our program and intensive ultrasonographic surveillance is initiated after 5 days of unmonitored ovarian stimulation. Alternatively, rFSH or hMG therapy may be initiated between day 2 and day 5 of a natural menstrual cycle depending on the ovarian response desired. Depending on the ultrasonographic assessment of follicular development of the individual response for each woman, the daily dose of gonadotrophins may be increased or decreased to either stimulate more follicles or to prevent ovarian hyperstimulation, respectively.

The ovarian response to induction with exogenous gonadotrophins is typically assessed by daily measurement of serum estradiol using standard radioimmunoassay techniques and serial ultrasonographic examinations. Both methods play a complementary role in controlled ovarian hyperstimulation, however, the importance of intensive ultrasonographic monitoring during the stimulation cycle cannot be overemphasized. When the diameter of the largest follicle first attains a predetermined diameter (18—20 mm in our center), hCG 5,000 to 10,000 IU is administered to trigger the final phases of follicular maturation leading to ovulation. Oocyte retrieval for the assisted reproductive technologies is typically scheduled for 30–34 h following hCG. Ovulation is expected to occur 34–48 h following the hCG in women who are undergoing intrauterine insemination. In our center, ultrasonographic examinations are continued until all follicles have either ovulated or showed ultrasonographically detectable signs of atresia.

Numerous reports on naturally cycling women have stated that the wide range of values reported for the maximal diameter of preovulatory follicles precludes its use as a single index for the prediction of ovulation [8,16,19]. However, follicular diameter was a more accurate predictor of impending ovulation than plasma measurements of FSH, LH or estradiol-17β [35]. Some of the disparity in measurements of preovulatory follicular diameter may, in part, be attributed to different scanning protocols. In most cases, scans were performed daily and measurements were made as much as 24 h prior to ovulation [8,16,19,35], while other measurements were taken just prior to ovulation [17,34].

The relationship between follicle size and oocyte maturity has yet to be resolved. In most ovulation induction protocols, hCG is administered when the leading preovulatory follicle attains 18–20 mm. It has been postulated that oocyte maturity may be achieved at a mean follicular diameter of 15–16 mm in hMG-stimulated cycles [36]. However, it is possible that follicle diameter does not correlate well with the stage of maturity and quality of the oocyte. The results of a recent study have been interpreted to demonstrate that there were no differences in the fertilization rate of oocytes aspirated from follicles in the following size categories: 10–14 mm, 15–19 mm and 20 mm, although the lack of differences may also be due to in vitro maturation of the oocytes [37]. The characteristics and appropriate sizes of follicles which will produced oocytes in states of maturity appropriate for fertilization remains the subject of much controversy and research. These observations support the necessity of monitoring the development of individual follicles; any follicle attaining a diameter of > 14 mm has the potential to ovulate viable oocytes which can maximize the benefit of the ovulation induction cycle. Previous reports have suggested that reduced oocyte quality and fertilization rates result from ova from smaller follicles [38].

## New imaging techniques

### Magnetic resonance imaging in the bovine model

MRI observations from bovine ovaries in vitro have revealed that the nuclear magnetic resonance (NMR) relaxation properties of ovarian follicular fluid appear to depend upon the physiologic status of the follicle [39]. We have developed the hypothesis that the follicle physiologic status of the follicle will be reflected in the image attributes of T1 and T2 NMR relaxation rates of follicular fluid. Nonendocrinologically active (prephysiologic selection or atretic) ovarian follicles contain fluid that has long T1 and T2 relaxation times at resting values of approximately 6,500 and 500 ms, respectively. As the time of physiologic selection approaches, both the T1 and T2 times of the fluid decrease as the follicle becomes more endocrinologically active. If the follicle is physiologically selected to ovulate, the T1 time will continue to decrease while the T2 time rapidly recovers to the resting value. If the follicle is committed to atresia, both T1 and T2 times will recover to the resting value with the T2 recovery being slower than the T2 recovery for the preovulatory follicle.

We have developed the hypothesis that the T1 value is inversely related to estradiol-17β levels in the follicular fluid while the T2 value reflects an unknown factor associated with the event of physiologic selection. Conventional MRI relaxometry may be useful for identifying the physiologic status of ovarian follicles and we expect that improvements in MRI speed and resolution combined with the use of intravaginal coils will soon allow relaxometric observations of ovarian follicles in vivo in women.

*Computer-assisted ultrasonographic imaging of follicular development in unstimulated and stimulated ovarian cycles*

Physiologically dominant ovarian follicles are identifiable by ultrasonography at approximately day 7 postmenstruation in unstimulated cycles. The image attributes of ultrasonographic images of normal preovulatory follicles include thick, low-amplitude walls and a gradual transformation zone at the fluid-follicle interface. We are actively evaluating the acoustic characteristics indicative of viability and atresia of ovarian follicles in unstimulated cycles and under ovarian stimulation protocols. The walls of preovulatory follicles are characterized by increased heterogeneity, increased wall breadth and a more gradual transformation at the fluid-follicle wall interface. Atresia is characterized by thin walls, high numerical pixel value (bright) signals and highly variable signals from the follicular fluid [40].

Follicular dynamics in women undergoing ovarian superstimulation are extremely variable. Follicle growth profiles are determined and images of the follicles are analyzed using linear time-series techniques. Three-dimensional surface maps of the image are then made to assess the textures of the follicular fluid and the follicle wall using the regional pixel intensity mapping technique at physiologically important time points (e.g., day of hCG administration, day before ovulation. The physiologic status of follicles as small as 6 mm may be determined. No differences in image attributes have yet been detected in 4- to 5-mm follicles. Image attributes of physiologically selected small follicles ($<6$ mm) include higher amplitude walls and smooth echotexture of follicle fluid compared to subordinate follicles of the cohort. Similarly, time series analyses combining image attributes of the follicles and their individual growth profiles show marked differences in the characteristics of ovulatory and atretic follicles. Follicles which eventually ovulate, or provide superior grades of oocytes exhibit walls which are thicker and of quantitatively lower peak values throughout their development than do the walls of follicles which are destined to atresia. In addition, follicles which ovulate typically have smooth, even textures in the areas corresponding to follicular fluid whereas images of follicles which do not ovulate exhibit rough surfaces in the fluid areas and higher (brighter) walls. The correlations among the computer-assisted analyses, follicular fluid hormonal analyses, histological appearances appear to be very high [40].

The implications for timing oocyte retrieval from small follicles for in vitro maturation are profound. If acoustic markers for follicle and/or oocyte competence are determined, oocyte retrieval and in vitro maturation from 4- to 6-mm follicles may become a routine clinical procedure.

Computer-assisted image analysis and ultrasonographic assessment of ovarian follicular development are natural extensions of the technologic advances in ovulation induction therapy. The overall ovarian response, growth profiles and ultrasonographically detectable characteristics of individual follicles, doses and types of stimulatory agents may be interactively evaluated as therapeutic manipulation of the ovaries unfolds. The response of the individual follicles to the ovulation inducing dose of hCG may be as important as the number and rates of growth of the follicles. Follicles may be as individual as patients in their response to stimulation. Thus, assessment of the development and fates of individual follicles is critical in tailoring ovarian stimulation to individual patients in order to increase the probability of conception.

*Mathematical modeling of ovarian follicular development*

One of the newest methods of investigating ovarian function is mathematical modeling of follicular development. The hypothesis that imaging attributes derived from ultrasonography or MR imaging may be integrated into a comprehensive model of ovarian folliculogenesis which includes mathematical description of growth of ovarian follicles in a competitive environment under the influence of estradiol-17β and other hormones such as FSH and LH is under active investigation in our laboratory [41]. Image attributes from MRI or ultrasonography integrated into the mathematical model appear to allow inference of hormone levels from noninvasive image data and obviate the need for routine hormonal analyses. In the models simplest form, the growth of every follicle is governed by a first order nonlinear differential equation where the follicles maturity as measured by the intrafollicular estradiol-17β content, blood serum estradiol level, serum FSH levels, and imaging characteristics as determined by ultrasonography and MRI.

**Concluding remarks**

Many of the difficulties in understanding ovarian biology may be overcome with the application of imaging technology to what were previously thought to be purely endocrine problems. The door is open to enhanced comprehension of basic ovarian biology, clinical enhancement of follicular growth and development, suppression of follicular function when desired and control of ovarian cyclicity if we have the vision to wander down what is now a somewhat hazy path.

## Acknowledgements

Original research in Dr Piersons laboratory is supported by the Medical Research Council of Canada.

## References

1. Collins W, Jurkovic D, Bourne T, Kurjak A, Campbell S. Ovarian morphology, endocrine function and intrafollicular blood flow during the periovulatory period. Hum Reprod 1991;6:319—324.
2. Hodgen GD. The dominant ovarian follicle. Fertil Steril 1982;38:281—300.
3. Gougeon A. Dynamics of follicular growth in the human: a model from preliminary results. Hum Reprod 1986;1:81—87.
4. Baird DT. A model for follicular selection and ovulation: lessons from superovulation. J Steroid Biochem 1987;27:15—23.
5. Greenwald GS, Terranova PF. Follicular selection and its control. In: Knobil E, Neill J (eds) The Physiology of Reproduction. New York: Raven Press, 1988;387—446.
6. Moor RM, Seamark RF. Cell signalling, permeability, and microvascular changes during follicle development in mammals. J Dairy Sci 1986;69:927—943.
7. Guraya SS. Biology of Ovarian Follicles in Mammals. New York: Springer-Verlag, 1985;320.
8. Bomsel-Helmreich O. Ultrasound and the preovulatory human follicle. Oxford Rev Reprod Biol 1985;7:1—72.
9. Renaud RL, Macler J, Dervain I, Ehret MC, Aron C, Plas-Roser S, Spira A, Pollack H. Echographic study of follicular maturation and ovulation during the normal menstrual cycle. Fertil Steril 1980;33:272—279.
10. Hackelöer BJ, Fleming R, Robinson HP, Adam AH, Coutts JRT. Correlation of ultrasonic and endocrinologic assessment of human follicular development. Am J Obstet Gynecol 1979;135: 122.
11. Carson R, Findlay J, Mattner P, Brown B. Relative levels of thecal blood flow in atretic and non-atretic ovarian follicles of the conscious sheep. Austr J Exp Biol Med Sci 1986;64:381—387.
12. Pierson RA. 1998. Unpublished data.
13. Balboni GC. Structural changes: ovulation and luteal phase. In: Serra GB (ed) The Ovary: Comprehensive Endocrinology. New York: Raven Press, 1983;123—142.
14. Morioka N et al. Mechanisms of mammalian ovulation. In: Development of Preimplantation Embryos and Their Environment. New York: Alan R Liss, Inc., 1989;65—85.
15. Espey LL, Lipner H. Ovulation. In: The Physiology of Reproduction, 2nd edn. New York, NY: Raven Press, 1994;725—780.
16. Queenan JT, O'Brien GD, Bains LM, Simpson J, Collins WP, Campbell S. Ultrasound scanning of ovaries to detect ovulation in women. Fertil Steril 1980;34:99—105.
17. Pierson RA, Martinuk SD, Chizen DR, Simpson CW. Ultrasonographic visualization of human ovulation. In: Evers JCL, Heineman MJ (eds) From Ovulation to Implantation. Proceedings of the VIIth Reinier de Graaf Symposium, Maastricht, the Netherlands, 1990;73—79.
18. Hanna MD, Chizen DR, Pierson RA. Characteristics of follicular evacuation during human ovulation. J Ultrasound Obstet Gynaecol 1994;4:488—493.17.
19. Lenz S. Ultrasonic study of follicular maturation, ovulation and development of corpus luteum during normal menstrual cycles. Acta Obstet Gynecol Scand 1985;64:15.

20. Bächström T, Nakata M, Pierson RA. Ultrasonography of normal and abnormal luteogenesis. In: Jaffe R, Pierson RA, Abramowicz JS (eds) Imaging in Infertility and Reproductive Endocrinology. Philadelphia USA: Lippencott, 1994;143−154.

21. Woessner JF et al. Connective tissue breakdown in ovulation. Steroids 1989;54:491−499.

22. Bourne TH, Jurkovic J, Waterstone J, Campbell S, Collins WP. Intrafollicular blood flow during human ovulation. J Ultrasound Obstet Gynecol 1991;1:53−59.

23. Haines CJ. Luteinized unruptured follicle syndrome. Clin Reprod Fertil 1987;5:321−332.7.

24. Katz E. The luteinized unruptured follicle and other ovulatory dysfunctions. Fertil Steril 1988;50:839-845.

25. Zalud I, Kurjak A. The assessment of luteal blood flow in pregnanat and nonpregnant woman by transvaginal color Doppler. J Perinat Med 1990;18:215−219.

26. Hann LE, Hall DA, McArdle CR, Seibel M. Polycystic ovarian disease: Sonographic spectrum. J Radiol 1984;150:531.

27. Falcone T, Bourque J, Granger L, Hemmings R, Miron P. Polycystic ovary syndrome. Curr Prob Obstet Gynecol Fertil 1993;16:65−72.

28. Marrs R, Vargyas D, March C. Correlation of ultrasonic and endocrinologic measurements in human menopausal gonadotropin therapy. Am J Obstet Gynecol 1983;145:4−11.

29. Blankenstein J. Use of clomiphone citrate for ovulation induction. In: Collins RL (ed) Ovulation Induction. 1991;62−68.

30. O'Herlihy C, Robinson H. Ultrasound timing of human chorionic gonadotrophin administration in clomiphene citrate stimulated cycles. Obstet Gynecol 1982;59:40−45.

31. Vargyas J, Marrs R, Kletsky O et al. Correlation of ultrasonic measurement of ovarian follicular size and serum estradiol levels in ovulatory patients following clomiphene citrate for in vitro fertilization. Am J Obstet Gynecol 1982;144:569−575.

32. Leerentveld RA, VanGent I, DerStoep M, Wladimiroff JW. Ultrasonographic assessment of Graafian follicle growth under monofollicular and multifollicular conditions in clomiphene citrate stimulated cycles. Fertil Steril 1985;40:461−465.

33. Pierson RA, Hanna MD, Chizen DR, Olatunbosun OA. Ovulation induction, ultrasonographic imaging and computer assisted image analysis. In: An Emphasis on Outcomes, Proceedings of the Serono Symposium. Alberta: Kananaskis, 1992;19−25.

34. Martinuk SD, Chizen DR, Pierson RA. Ultrasonographic morphology of the human preovulatory follicle wall prior to ovulation. Clin Anat 1992;5:1−14.

35. Bryce RL, Shuter B, Sinosich MJ, Stiel JN, Picker RH, Saunders DM. The value of ultrasound, gonadotropin, and estradiol measurements for precise ovulation prediction. Fertil Steril 1982;37:42.

36. Silverberg KM, Olive DL, Burns WN, Johnson JV, Groff TR, Schenken RS. Follicular size at the time of human chorionic gonadotropin administration predicts ovulation outcome in human menopausal gonadotropin stimulated cycles. Fertil Steril 1991;56:296−303.

37. Haines CJ, Emes AL. The relationship between follicle diameter, fertilization rate and microscopic embryo quality. Fertil Steril 1991;55:205.

38. Veek LL, Wortham JWE, Witmyer J, Sandow BA, Acosta AA, Garcia JE, Jones GS, Jones HW. Maturation and fertilization of morphologically immature human oocytes in a program of in vitro fertilization. Fertil Steril 1983;39:594−599.

39. Sarty GE, Kendall EJ, Pierson RA. Magnetic resonance imaging of bovine ovaries in vitro. Magnetic resonance materials in physics, biology and medicine. (MAG*MA) 1996;4:205-211.

40. Pierson RA, Adams GP. Computer-assisted image analysis, diagnostic ultrasonography and ovulation induction: strange bedfellows. Theriogenology 1995;43:105−112.

41. Sarty GE, Pierson RA. Analysis of ovarian follicular response to superstimulation in a three dimensional parametric space. Proceedings of the 16th World Congress on Fertility and Sterility 1998;(In press).

# Ovarian stimulation in ART

Fertility and Reproductive Medicine.
R.D. Kempers, J. Cohen, A.F. Haney and J.B. Younger, editors.

# Impact of the use of recombinant follicle stimulating hormone

Basil C. Tarlatzis and Helen Bili
*1st Department of Obstetrics and Gynaecology, Aristotle University of Thessaloniki, Greece*

**Abstract.** The inherent disadvantages of the existing gonadotropins and the availability of molecular biology techniques led to the synthesis of human recombinant gonadotropins. Recently, FSH was manufactured by means of recombinant DNA technology using a Chinese hamster ovary cell line, transfected with the genes encoding FSH (recombinant FSH; recFSH). The efficacy and safety of GnRH-a/recFSH treatment in ovarian stimulation for IVF/ET, were tested in two large randomized prospective studies. In the first one, the use of Puregon (Organon) was compared with pFSH (Metrodin), after pituitary down regulation with buserelin, in 981 women undergoing IVF/ET. Significantly more oocytes and high-quality embryos were obtained in the group receiving recFSH, as compared to pFSH. Moreover, fewer ampules of recFSH were needed to stimulate the ovaries compared to pFSH and in a significantly shorter treatment period, indicating that this FSH preparation is possibly more potent than urinary FSH. However, the pregnancy rates, were similar in the two groups, although the ongoing pregnancy rates were significantly higher after Puregon treatment when the pregnancies resulting from frozen-thawed embryo replacements were also included (25.7 vs. 20.4%, p = 0.05). In addition, the comparison of the IM with the SC administration of recFSH showed that both routes were equally effective, and no allergic reactions were observed, whereas no anti-recFSH antibodies were detected. In the other study involving Gonal-F (Serono Labs), 235 patients undergoing IVF/ET and ICSI (119 treated with recFSH and 114 with pFSH (Metrodin) after pituitary desensitization with buserelin) were analyzed. More oocytes and embryos were obtained in the recFSH group, indicating that the availability of gonadotropins with less batch to batch variability would be of benefit. In conclusion, recFSH represents a significant improvement in ovarian stimulation, as it is pure, potent, consistent from batch to batch and can be produced in unlimited amounts. Moreover, it allows the individualization of ovarian stimulation regimens according to the specific needs of the patients treated. However, new protocols are needed in order to address the effectiveness vis-a-vis the cost of these new preparations.

**Keywords:** in vitro fertilization, ovarian stimulation, recombinant FSH.

## Introduction

Exogenous human gonadotropin preparations have been widely used over the last 30 years for the induction of ovulation in anovulatory patients suffering from infertility. Ovarian stimulation has an important role in infertility management and is applied either to induce ovulation in anovulatory women or to increase follicle recruitment for assisted reproduction techniques (ART). The first gonadotropins obtained from pituitary extracts were an equal mixture of follicle stimulating hormone (FSH) and luteinizing hormone (LH). Human pituitary gonadotro-

*Address for correspondence:* Basil C. Tarlatzis MD, Infertility and IVF Center, Geniki Kliniki, 2 Gravias Street, Thessaloniki 546 45, Greece. Tel.: +30-31-821-681 and 265-273. Fax: +30-31-821-420. E-mail: tarlatzis@hol.gr.

pins are no longer used in view of the potential risk for Jakob Creutzfeldt disease, observed in some patients treated by pituitary extracts for growth hormone supplementation [1].

The next step in ovulation induction was the development of gonadotropins extracted from urine of postmenopausal women (HMG; Humegon, Organon; Pergonal, Serono Labs). These preparations contain an equal amount of FSH and LH activity (approximately 75 IU of each per ampule). It soon became evident that HMG was very effective and was, hence, established as the standard treatment for ovarian stimulation.

In addition, over the last decade, a new formulation was developed consisting mainly of FSH (75 IU) and to a lesser extent of LH activity ($< 0.7$ IU), with a specific activity of about 150 IU FSH/mg protein (pFSH; Metrodin, Serono Labs). Metrodin has been successfully used alone or in combination with HMG, in the treatment of women with polycystic ovarian syndrome as well as to induce multiple follicular development for ART, such as in vitro fertilization/embryo transfer (IVF/ET). Recently, another highly purified FSH preparation (Metrodin HP, Serono Labs) became available which is devoid of any significant LH activity and has a specific activity of approximately 9,000 IU FSH/mg protein.

Gonadotropins are currently administered in combination with gonadotropin releasing hormone analogues (GnRHa) in order to suppress the endogenous LH or to avoid the premature LH surges, frequently observed in stimulated cycles. On the other hand, several comparative clinical studies have shown that in GnRHa-suppressed cycles, pFSH is as effective as HMG in ovulation induction [2,3]. This suggests that the residual endogenous LH levels or the LH content of the existing preparations are adequate to support follicular development.

### Human menopausal gonadotropin preparations

Until recently, the only available preparations of HMG and pFSH were crude urinary extracts, with a purity of only 1−2% and heavy protein contamination which could cause local tissue reactions and pain necessitating deep intramuscular (IM) injection. These preparations have decreased specific biological activity and contain variable isoforms of the gonadotropins with different pharmacokinetic properties which are responsible for the great interindividual variations in the half-life of these hormones. In general, the half-life for pFSH after IM administration ranges from 30 to 40 h [4], whereas LH has a much shorter half-life [4], and this is the reason for the administration of long-acting HCG as a therapeutic substitute for the LH surge. On the other hand, because of their origin, the existing preparations present a great degree of variation in their activity from batch to batch. These problems have made it very difficult to prepare consistent formulation regimens for ovulation induction, enabling to tailor the protocol to the individual patients' needs. Moreover, the wide application of new ART, like ICSI, increased the demands for gonadotropins and created during the last 3 years a worldwide shortage of human menopausal gonadotropin preparations.

**Human recombinant FSH (recFSH)**

The main clinical disadvantages of the existing preparations and the availability of recombinant DNA technology have recently led to the production of human recFSH (Puregon, Organon; Gonal-F, Seroño Labs).

Recombinant FSH, is obtained from chinese hamster ovary cells which are known to be suitable host cells for the production of glycosylated recombinant proteins. For this purpose, a genomic clone containing the entire coding sequence for the FSH β-subunit, either alone or together with the α-subunit gene, was transfected into chinese hamster ovarian cells [5]. The polypeptide backbone of recFSH is identical to that of natural FSH, whereas recombinant and natural carbohydrate structures are either identical or closely related [6]. Like natural FSH preparations, recFSH exhibits considerable charge heterogeneity while its bioactivity was confirmed by in vitro bioassays and in vivo clinical studies [7,8]. Moreover, chimeric molecules with extended half-life by modifying the carboxyterminal peptide (CTP) has been synthesized and is available for phase I clinical trials [9]. The potential clinical benefits of this new molecule may include less frequent administration and more fixed ovulation induction protocols [9]. The specific bioactivity of recFSH is > 10,000 IU of FSH/mg of protein. Thus, the high degree of purity allows the subcutaneous (SC) administration of recFSH. The advantages of recFSH over the urinary product can be summarized as follows:

1) an improved batch to batch consistency;
2) High purity allowing convenient, SC self-administration and chemical characterization for quality control;
3) Complete absence of LH which will enable studies on the control of ovarian follicular function; and
4) Production of short- or long-acting recFSH molecules enabling more efficient ovulation induction.

**Clinical applications of recFSH**

During the last few years, extensive clinical research was conducted aiming to establish the long-term safety and efficacy of recFSH vis-à-vis the disadvantages of current urinary gonadotropin preparations.

The availability of highly specific recombinant FSH has benefitted research and clinical practice. Thus, in preliminary studies on human exposure to recFSH performed in hypogonadotropic hypogonadal women [10,11] it was evident that in spite of the multiple follicular development after recFSH administration, the estradiol (E2) concentrations in follicular fluid and in serum were extremely low. Therefore, LH even in very small amounts is required to induce adequate androgen production by theca cells, which in turn will be converted to estrogens under the influence of FSH. Moreover, it is plausible that human follicle maturation may not require estrogens, in contrast to the evidence in rodents, and E2 seems to be necessary for the preparation of the genital tract to accept embryos for implantation.

The first pregnancies [12—14] obtained after treatment with recFSH in ovulatory women for IVF/ET were concomitantly reported by two separate groups of investigators, using the two available preparations (Gonal-F and Puregon). These reports, indicate that recFSH can successfully stimulate multiple follicular development and steroidogenesis in ovulatory women pretreated with a GnRHa for IVF/ET.

Clinical trials in World Health Organization (WHO) group II patients were subsequently designed [15,16] and a pregnancy was reported [17] after induction of ovulation with IM administration of recFSH in a patient with polycystic ovary syndrome. Moreover, Homburg [16] used pFSH or recFSH to induce ovulation in WHO group II patients without finding any significant difference in the efficacy of these regimes. The results of these studies [15—17] suggest that exposure to endogenous LH is sufficient to support the FSH-induced follicular development in WHO group II women. Thus, all the aforementioned data fully support the hypothesis of gonadotropin synergism in estrogen production (two-cell theory).

On the other hand, Devroey et al. [18] in a pilot study examined the ability of five different GnRHa/recFSH regimens to induce follicular and oocyte development for IVF/ET. The stimulation protocols were: recFSH alone (group I), recFSH together with buserelin, intranasally in the short (group II) or in the long protocol (group III), and recFSH in association with triptorelin depot (group IV) or daily SC injections (group V). In all patients treatment with recFSH resulted in multiple follicular growth and increased E2 and inhibin levels without any significant difference between the five groups in the parameters assessed, except for the LH levels that were significantly lower in women treated with triptorelin (groups IV and V). Overall, 10 clinical pregnancies were achieved in the five groups, from which eight were ongoing, and thus, the clinical and ongoing pregnancy rate per transfer was 18.6 and 23.2%, respectively [19]. These data demonstrate that GnRHa/recFSH treatment is effective and that, even after profound LH suppression, the residual LH levels are adequate to induce normal steroidogenesis.

The efficacy and safety of GnRHa/recFSH treatment in ovarian stimulation for IVF/ET were further tested in two large multicenter prospective studies. In the first one involving Gonal-F [20], 123 patients undergoing IVF/ET (60 treated with recFSH and 63 with pFSH after pituitary desensitization with leuprolide acetate) were analyzed. No significant differences were found between the two groups, demonstrating that recFSH is as effective as pFSH in ovulation induction for IVF/ET.

In the other multicenter prospective study [21], the use of recFSH (Puregon) was compared with pFSH (Metrodin) after pituitary downregulation with buserelin intranasally, in 981 women undergoing IVF/ET (585 subjects received recFSH and 396 urinary FSH). Significantly more oocytes and high-quality embryos were obtained in the group receiving recFSH as compared to pFSH (Table 1).

*Table 1.* Patients characteristics and IVF/ET results in 981 women treated by recFSH (Puregon) or pFSH (Metrodin) after pituitary desensitization with buserelin.

|  | recFSH | pFSH | p |
|---|---|---|---|
| Patients (n) | 585 | 396 |  |
| Age (years) | 32.2 | 32.3 | n.s |
| Number (%) of subjects with cause of infertility |  |  |  |
|     Tubal disease | 377 (64.4) | 254 (64.1) |  |
|     Endometriosis | 45 (7.7) | 30 (70.6) |  |
|     Tubal disease + Endometriosis | 23 (3.9) | 15 (3.8) |  |
|     Unknown | 117 (20.0) | 79 (19.9) |  |
|     Other | 23 (3.9) | 18 (4.5) |  |
| Treatment length (days) | 10.7 | 11.3 | < 0.0001 |
| Total FSH ampules (n) | 28.5 | 31.8 | < 0.0001 |
| $E_2$ on HCG day (pmol/l) | 6084 | 5179 | < 0.0001 |
| Follicles $\geq$ 15 mm on HCG day (n) | 7.49 | 6.67 | < 0.0002 |
| Oocytes recovered (n) | 10.84 | 8.95 | < 0.0001 |
| Mature oocytes (n) | 8.55 | 6.76 | < 0.0001 |
| High quality embryos (n) | 3.11 | 2.61 | = 0.0003 |
| Ongoing pregnancy rate per cycle (%) | 22.17 | 18.22 | n.s |
| Ongoing pregnancy rate per transfer (%) | 25.97 | 22.02 | n.s |
| Ongoing pregnancy rate (plus frozen-thawed embryo cycles | 25.70 | 20.40 | = 0.05 |

n.s = Not significant. (Adapted from [21].)

Furthermore, significantly fewer ampules of recFSH were needed to stimulate the ovaries compared to pFSH and in a significantly shorter treatment period, indicating that this recFSH preparation seems to be more potent than urinary FSH. Ongoing pregnancy rates per attempt and transfer in the recFSH group were 22.17 and 25.97%, respectively, and in the urinary FSH group, 18.22 and 22.02%, respectively (p = NS). The ongoing pregnancy rates including pregnancies resulting from frozen-thawed embryo transfers were 25.7% for recFSH and 20.4% for urinary FSH (p = 0.05) (Table 1). Despite the higher number of follicles recruited and the increased serum estradiol concentration on the day of HCG administration the incidence of ovarian hyperstimulation syndrome (OHSS) although higher after recFSH treatment was not statistically significant. Therefore, given the higher potency of this recFSH preparation, careful monitoring to prevent the occurence of this syndrome is essential. The results of this study showed that recFSH is more effective than urinary FSH in inducing multiple follicular development and in achieving an ongoing pregnancy.

It is important to note that no anti-recFSH antibodies were detected in any of the women treated by the two recFSH preparations [18,19,21].

In a recent prospective randomized trial done by Bergh et al. [22], which was carried out in two centers, it was also found that recFSH is more effective than urinary FSH in inducing multiple follicular development in couples undergoing

108

ICSI (Table 2). The authors also found an unexpected rate of low ovarian response in the urinary FSH group and they concluded that there is a need for gonadotropins with less batch-to-batch variability.

In another very recent prospective randomized multicentre trial [23], the efficacy of fixed doses of recFSH (Puregon, Organon) (100 vs. 200 IU/day) was examined in women downregulated with a GnRH agonist. In the 100 IU fixed dose group, significantly less oocytes and embryos were obtained in comparison with the 200 IU fixed dose group. Clinical pregnancy rates per cycle were similar in both groups, despite the increased cancellation rate in the low-dose group. On the other hand, less ampules of recFSH were used in the 100 IU group compared to the 200 IU group (Table 3).

**The impact of recFSH use**

It is generally accepted that the introduction of recFSH represents an improvement in ovarian stimulation. However, it is equally important to assess the impact of the wide use of recFSH in daily clinical practice.

As shown in the initial studies [10,11] in hypogonadotropic hypogonadal patients (WHO I), the complete absence of LH in recFSH preparations, led to extremely low estrogen production in response to recFSH administration. Therefore, in this category of patients with very low endogenous LH levels, it may be necessary to coadminister exogenous LH. Confirming this assumption, Hull et al. [24] treated a 28-year-old woman with Kallman's syndrome with a combination of recFSH (Gonal-F) 150 IU and recLH (LHadi, Serono Labs) 75 IU subcutaneously. As shown in Table 4, stimulation with pFSH (Metrodin) resulted in high number of large follicles but with relatively low E2 levels. On the other hand, the administration of recFSH together with recLH was associated with higher E2 levels and normal oocyte development, as testified by the achievement of pregnancy.

These findings were corroborated by Loumaye et al. [25] who treated 28 hypogonadotropic hypogonadal women by 150 IU/day recFSH (Gonal-F) and different doses (0, 25, 75 or 225 IU/day) of recLH (LHadi). Their preliminary results

*Table 2.* Stimulation characteristics of patients receiving human chorionic gonadotrophin (HCG; values are means ± SD).

| | Gonal-F | Metrodin HP | p Value |
|---|---|---|---|
| Patients (n) | 119 | 102 | |
| Days of FSH[a] treatment (n) | 11.0 ± 5.1 | 13.5 ± 3.7 | <0.0001 |
| Ampoules FSH (75 IU equivalent) (n) | 21.9 ± 5.1 | 31.9 ± 13.4 | <0.0001 |
| Follicles >10 mm on HCG day (n) | 12.7 ± 4.9 | 8.4 ± 4.2 | <0.002 |
| E$_2$ on the day of HCG (nmol/l) | 6.55 ± 5.75 | 3.95 ± 3.90 | <0.0001 |
| Oocytes retrieved (n) | 12.2 ± 5.5 | 7.6 ± 4.4 | <0.0001 |

[a]FSH: Follicle-stimulating hormone. (Adapted from [22].)

*Table 3.* Data concerning the 100 IU vs. the 200 IU group.

| | 100 IU | 200 IU | p Value |
|---|---|---|---|
| Patients per stated cycle (n) | 101 | 98 | na |
| Age (years) | 32.7 | 32.4 | na |
| Cancellation rate (%) | 31 | 15 | na |
| Follicles $\geqslant$ 15 mm (n) | 7.1 | 9.1 | < 0.001 |
| Follicles $\geqslant$ 17 mm (n) | 5.1 | 5.6 | ns |
| Oocytes retrieved (n) | 6.2 | 10.6 | < 0.001 |
| Total dose (IU) | 1114 | 1931 | < 0.001 |
| Treatment length (days) | 11.2 | 9.3 | < 0.001 |
| Transferable embryos after ICSI (n) | 3.67 | 4.39 | ns |
| Transferable embryos after IVF (n) | 4.14 | 6.38 | < 0.001 |
| Embryo-development rate in ICSI (%) | 46 | 52 | ns |
| Embryo-development rate in IVF (%) | 5 | 60 | ns |
| Embryos transferred (n) | 2.1 | 2.6 | < 0.01 |
| Clinical pregnancy rate per ET (%) | 36 | 28 | ns |
| Miscarriage rate (%) | 36 | 4 | < 0.01 |
| Implantation rate (%) | 17 | 13 | ns |
| Ongoing pregnancy rate per ET (%) | 23 | 28 | ns |
| Patients with abdominal pain/OHSS (n) | 5 | 14 | 0.02 |

na: not applicable, ns: not significant. (Adapted from [23].)

indicate that in these patients, LH is necessary to support follicular steroidogenesis (Table 5).

Furthermore, 75 IU/day of recLH seem to be an effective dose for most patients, since with this dose, high E2 levels and maximal endometrial growth were observed. Finally, the pregnancies obtained with 75 and 225 IU/day of recLH confirm that normal oogenesis and endometrial priming was achieved using these regimes.

Similarly, it has been observed that the administration of high doses of GnRH

*Table 4.* Results of ovarian stimulation in a patient with Kallman's syndrome using preparations of FSH with or without LH.

| | HMG | pFSH | | | recFSH + recLH |
|---|---|---|---|---|---|
| | | Cycle 1 | Cycle 2 | Cycle 3 | |
| Total FSH ampules (n) | 35 | 32 | 72 | 68 | 30 |
| Treatment length (days) | 21 | 16 | 33 | 25 | 15 |
| Follicles $\geqslant$ 10 mm on HCG day (n) | 7 | 9 | 25 | 17 | 7 |
| E$_2$ on HCG day (pmol/l) | 2947 | 550 | 1125 | 884 | 1200 |
| E$_2$ ratio to total follicles | 421 | 61 | 45 | 59 | 171 |
| Midluteal progesterone (nmol/l) | 194 | 100 | 100 | 100 | 150 |

Adapted from [24].

*Table 5.* Results of ovarian stimulation in 28 hypogonadotropic hypogonadal women treated by 150 IU/day recFSH (Gonal-F) and different doses (0, 25, 75 or 225 IU/day) of recLH (LHadi).

| | recLH (IU/day) | | | |
| --- | --- | --- | --- | --- |
| | 0 | 25 | 75 | 225 |
| Patients (n) | 8 | 5 | 7 | 8 |
| Preovulatory $E_2$ (pmol/l) | $250 \pm 150$ | $505 \pm 235$ | $961 \pm 198$ | $1491 \pm 423$ |
| Endometrial thickness (mm) | $4.3 \pm 1.2$ | $7.0 \pm 2.5$ | $9.2 \pm 0.6$ | $8.6 \pm 0.9$ |
| Preovulatory progesterone (nmol/l) | $< 3$ | $< 3$ | $< 3$ | $< 3$ |
| Midluteal progesterone (nmol/l) | $50 \pm 49$ | $62 \pm 44$ | $63 \pm 31$ | $98 \pm 24$ |
| Pregnancies | – | – | 2 | 1 |

Adapted from [25].

antagonists in combination with recFSH may be associated with cessation of follicular growth and drop of E2 levels, probably due to profound suppression of endogenous LH levels, further supporting the "two-cell and two-gonadotropin" theory.

Data from the existing studies [20,22] show that recFSH is associated with more follicles, oocytes and good quality embryos as compared to urinary FSH administration. On the other hand, during the last years the combination of rapidly developing medical technology, patients' expectations and the overutilization of medications and procedures, have contributed to a sharp rise in health care costs. Thus, it has become important to assess health care quality and the true economic impact of new preparations and procedures. However, as indicated in the large multicenter trials [21,22] their use is associated with a higher number of embryos that can be transferred or frozen, supporting a higher efficacy of recFSH. On the other hand, two recent studies [23,26] showed that the administration of low doses of recFSH results in a satisfactory pregnancy rate with lower consumption of medication. It seems, therefore, that there is a need to re-evaluate the ovarian stimulation protocols, especially in the GnRH antagonists era, taking into account the optimal number of oocytes needed to acheive satisfactory pregnacy rates. Furthermore, the use of long- or short-acting molecules of recFSH may enable the individualization of treatment protocols and thus reduce the cost of treatment. Finally, the cost of treatment with recombinant gonadotropins is expected to be balanced by the more efficient and reproducible production of this preparation.

**Conclusion**

Recombinant FSH provides a new tool for gaining a better insight into the role of gonadotropins in human folliculogenesis. The first data suggest that FSH alone can induce growth of preovulatory follicles. Follicle growth does occur in the presence of subnormal E2 levels but LH is necessary for adequate biosynthesis of E2. Furthermore, the initial clinical trials using the two available recFSH preparations indicate that both can successfully and safely stimulate follicle and oocyte development leading to pregnancy without any serious side effects. This encouraging experience with recFSH paves the way for its wider use both in research and in routine clinical practice. However, new protocols are needed in order to address the effectiveness vis-a-vis the cost of these new preparations.

## References

1. Yovich J, Grudzinskas G. Ovarian stimulation. In: Yovich J, Grudzinskas G (eds) The Management of Infertility. Avon, UK: Heinemann Medical Books, 1990;21–36.
2. Bentick B, Shaw RW, Iffland CA, Burford G, Bernard A. A randomized comparative study of purified FSH and HMG after pituitary desensitization with buserelin for superovulation and IVF. Fertil Steril 1988;50:79–84.
3. Edelstein MC, Brzyski RG, Jones GS, Simonetti S, Muasher SJ. Equivalency of human menopausal gonadotropin and follicle stimulating hormone stimulation after gonadotropin-releasing hormone agonist suppression. Fertil Steril 1990;53:103–106.
4. Mizunuma H, Takagi T, Honjyo S, Ibuki Y, Igarashi M. Clinical pharmacodynamics of urinary follicle-stimulating hormone and its application for pharmacokinetic stimulation program. Fertil Steril 1990;53:440–445.
5. Keene JL, Matzuk MM, Otani T, Fauser BC, Galway AB, Hsueh AJ. Expression of biologically active human follitropin in chinese hamster ovary cells. J Biol Chem 1989;246:4769–4775.
6. Hard K, Mekking A, Damm JBL, Kamerling JP, de Boer W, Wijnands RA, Vliegenthart JFG. Isolation and structure determination of the intact sialylated N-linked carbohydrate chains of recombinant human follitropin (hFSH) expressed in Chinese hamster ovary cells. Eur J Biochem 1990;193:263–271.
7. Mannaerts B, De Leeuw R, Geelen J, Van Ravestein A, Van Wezenbeek P, Schuurs A, Kloosterboer H. Comparative in vitro and in vivo studies on the biological characteristics of recombinant human follicle-stimulating hormone. Endocrinology 1991;129:2623–2630.
8. Le Cotonnec JV, Porchet HC, Beltrami V, Khan A, Toon S, Rowland M. Clinical pharmacology of recombinant human follicle-stimulating hormone (FSH). I. Comparative pharmacokinetics with urinary human FSH. Fertil Steril 1994;61:669–678.
9. Fauser BCJM. Recombinant human FSH: future prospects for clinical use. In: Fauser BCJM (ed) FSH Action and Intraovarian Regulation. Proceedings of the IX Reinier e Graaf Symposium, Noordwijk, The Netherlands, vol 6. The Parthenon Publishing Group, UK, September 1996.
10. Shoot DC, Coelingh-Bennink HJT, Mannaerts BM, Lamberts SW, Bouchard P, Fauser BC. Human recombinant follicle-stimulating hormone induces growth of preovulatory follicles without concomitant increase in androgen and estrogen biosynthesis in a woman with isolated gonadotropin deficiency. J Clin Endocrinol Metab 1992;74:1471–1473.
11. Shoham Z, Mannaerts B, Insler V, Coelingh-Bennink HJT. Induction of follicular growth using recombinant human follicle-stimulating hormone in two volunteer women with hypogonadotropic hypogonadism. Fertil Steril 1993;59:738–742.
12. Germond M, Dessole S, Senn A, Loumaye E, Howles C, Beltrami V. Successful in vitro fertilization and embryo transfer after treatment with recombinant human FSH. Lancet 1992;339: 1170–1171.
13. Devroey P, Van Steirteghem A, Mannaerts B, Coelingh-Bennink HJT. Successful in vitro fertilization and embryo transfer after treatment with recombinant human FSH. Lancet 1992;339: 1170–1171.
14. Devroey P, Mannaerts B, Smitz J, Van Steirteghem A. First established pregnancy and birth after

ovarian stimulation with recombinant follicle-stimulating hormone (Org 31489). Hum Reprod 1993;8:863–865.

15. Homnes P, Giroud D, Howles C, Loumaye E. Recombinant human follicle-stimulating hormone treatment leads to normal follicular growth, estradiol secretion, and pregnancy in a World Health Organization group II anovulatory woman. Fertil Steril 1993;60:724–726.

16. Homburg R. Efficacy of recFSH (Gonal-F) for inducing ovulation in WHO II an-ovulatory patients. Preliminary results of a comparative multicentre study. In: Mori T, Aono T, Tominaga T, Hiroi M (eds) Proceedings of the VIIIth World Congress on in Vitro Fertilization and Alternate Assisted Reproduction, Kyoto, Japan, Sept 1993. Serono Symposia. New York: Raven Press, 1994.

17. Donderwinkel PFJ, Schoot D, Coelingh-Bennink HTJ, Fauser BC. Pregnancy after induction of ovulation with recombinant FSH in polycystic ovary syndrome. Lancet 1992;340:983–984.

18. Devroey P, Mannaerts B, Smitz J, Coelingh-Bennink H, Van Steirteghem A. Clinical outcome of a pilot efficacy study on recombinant human follicle-stimulating hormone (Org 32489) combined with various gonadotrophin-releasing hormone agonist regimens. Hum Reprod 1994; 9:1064–1069.

19. Devroey P, Ubaldi F, Smitz J, Van Steirteghem A. Recombinant follicle stimulating hormone. Ass Reprod Rev 1994;4:2–9.

20 Loumaye E, Alvarez S, Barlow D et al. Efficacy of recombinant human follicle stimulating hormone (Gonal-F) for stimulating multiple follicular development in assisted reproduction technologies. In: Mori T, Aono T, Tominaga T, Hiroi M (eds) Proceedings of the VIIIth World Congress on in Vitro Fertilization and Alternate Assisted Reproduction, Kyoto, Japan, Sept 1993. Serono Symposia. New York: Raven Press, 1994.

21. Out HJ, Mannaerts BMJL, Driessen SGAJ, Coelingh-Bennink HJT. A prospective, randomized, assessor-blind, multicentre study comparing recombinant and urinary follicle-stimulating hormone (Puregon vs. Metrodin) in in vitro fertilization. Hum Reprod 1995;10:2534–2540.

22. Bergh C, Howles CM, Borg K, Hamberger L, Josefsson B, Nilsson L, Wikland M. Recombinant human follicle stimulating hormone (r-hFSH; Gonal-F) vs. highly purified urinary FSH (Metrodin HP): results of a randomized comparative study in women undergoing assisted reproductive techniques. Hum Reprod 1997;12(10):2133–2139.

23. Healy D, Out HJ. Stimulataion regimens: the use of fixed dosages of recombinant FSH. Abstract Book. 14th Annual Meeting of the ESHRE. Organon Sponsored Symposia. Goteborg, Sweden, June 23–24, 1998.

24. Hull M, Corrigan E, Piazzi A, Loumaye E. Recombinant human luteinizing hormone: an effective new gonadotropin preparation. Lancet 1994;344:334–335.

25. Loumaye E, Piazzi A, Baird D et al. A prospective, randomized, parallel group study to determine the effective dose of recombinant human luteinizing hormone to support FSH-induced follicular development in hypogonadotrophic hypogonadal (HH) women. Abstracts of the 11th Annual Meeting of ESHRE, Hamburg. June 28–July 1, 1995.

26. Devroey P, Tournaye H, Van Steirteghem A, Hendrix P, Out HJ. The use of a 100 IU starting dose of recombinant follicle stimulating hormone (Puregon) in in vitro fertilization. Hum Reprod 1998;13:565–566.

# Ovarian stimulation in ART: use of GnRH-antagonists

R. Felberbaum and K. Diedrich

*Department of Obstetrics and Gynecology, Medical University of Lübeck, Germany*

**Abstract.** Due to their different pharmacological mode of action GnRH-antagonists are able to suppress serum-concentrations of LH within hours. Instead of "down regulation" and "desensitization", a classic competitive blockage of the GnRH-receptors on the cell membrane of the gonadotrophic cells seems to take place. During the last few years the GnRH-antagonists Cetrorelix and Ganirelix have been used in clinical studies to prove that these compounds reliably prevent the premature LH-surge within controlled ovarian hyperstimulation (COH). Cetrorelix has been applied in single- and multiple-dose protocols, while Ganirelix was used until now only according to the multiple-dose "Lübeck" protocol. In the multiple-dose protocol COH is started on day 2 or 3 of the cycle with HMG (human menopausal gonadotropin) or recombinant FSH. Daily administration of the GnRH-antagonist with its minimal effective dose (0.25 mg/day s.c.) occurs from the 6th day of stimulation onward until ovulation induction. In the single-dose protocol 3 mg of the GnRH-antagonist Cetrorelix is injected on day 8 of the stimulation cycle. Until now more than 1,000 patients have been treated with these protocols. Both protocols have been proven to be safe and effective. Fertilization rates of $> 50\%$ in IVF and $> 60\%$ in ICSI (intracytoplasmic sperm injection), as well as clinical pregnancy rates of about 30% per transfer sound most promising. Estradiol secretion is not compromised by the GnRH-antagonist in its minimal effective dose using rec. FSH for COH. The incidence of a premature LH-surge is far below 2%, while the pituitary response remains preserved under this regime in a dose-dependent manner, allowing the induction of ovulation by GnRH or GnRH-agonists. However, luteal phase support remains mandatory. The incidence of severe OHSS (ovarian hyperstimulation syndrome) seems to be lower than in the long agonistic protocol. Treatment time is shortened as well as the patient's burden being lowered. The combination of softer stimulation regimes like clomiphene citrate (CC) and low-dose HMG with midcyclic administration of GnRH-antagonists may be the way to cheap, safe and efficient ovarian stimulation.

**Keywords:** ART, Cetrorelix, controlled ovarian hyperstimulation, Ganirelix, GnRH-agonists, OHSS, premature LH-surge.

## Introduction

The use of GnRH-agonists for the purpose of ovarian stimulation marks in some way the beginning of a modern management within assisted reproduction. Premature LH-surges had been responsible for a reduced effectiveness of ovarian stimulation by human menopausal gonadotropin (HMG) in an in vitro fertilization (IVF) program. At the same time, they negatively affected oocyte and embryo quality, and due to this, the obtained pregnancy rates [1,2]. The introduction of agonist treatment has remedied most of these difficulties and drawbacks,

*Address for correspondence:* Prof K. Diedrich, Medizinische Universität zu Lübeck, Klinik für Frauenhellkunde und Geburtshilfe, Ratzeburger Allee 160, D-23538 Lübeck, Germany.

and the rate of stimulated cycles which must be terminated has been reduced to about only 2%. Ovulation induction has become plannable so that the psychological pressure on patients and physicians has been eased to some extent. Suppression of endogenous hormone production by GnRH analogues followed by HMG stimulation has developed from second-line into first-line therapy [3]. Different treatment schedules are presently applied, including the so-called "long protocol", which aims at a complete pituitary suppression, and the "short" and "ultrashort" protocol, in which the initial "flare-up" of gonadotropins is attempted to be harvested for ovarian stimulation [4,5]. Among these protocols the "long protocol" is generally the most effective and is most often used at present. In Germany, for instance, more than 70% of all performed stimulated cycles for ART (assisted reproduction techniques) are realized according to the "long protocol" [6]. It can be taken for granted that controlled ovarian hyperstimulation (COH) using human urinary or recombinant gonadotrophins in combination with GnRH-analogues has been proven to be highly efficient for ART [5,7]. However, the "long protocol" has the disadvantages of a long treatment period until desensitization occurs, as well as relatively high costs due to an increased requirement for HMG. On the other hand, excessive ovarian stimulation with rescue rates of more than 30 oocytes is not seldomly seen, as large numbers of follicles and aspirated oocytes are almost regarded as criteria of success [8]. It seems to be at least debatable if this is still acceptable in the presence of ICSI (intracytoplasmic sperm injection), with its high fertilization outcome independent of sperm morphology [9]. The question arises whether we can avoid the complexities and costs of prolonged pharmaceutically driven treatments [10]. A reduction in the amount of gonadotropins used and a reduced number of mature oocytes (metaphase II) could be the goal to aim for, reducing the burden and risk for the patient, as well as the financial costs. For this, the introduction of GnRH-antagonists into protocols for COH seems to open new pathways.

**GnRH-antagonists**

In parallel with the development of GnRH-agonists, other analogues were synthesized which also bind to the pituitary GnRH-receptors but that are not functional in inducing the release of gonadotrophins. These compounds are far more complex than GnRH-agonists with modifications in the molecular structure not only at positions 6 and 10, but also at positions 1, 2, 3 and 8. In comparison to the GnRH-agonists the pharmacological mechanism by which GnRH-antagonists suppress the liberation of gonadotrophins is completely different. While the agonists act on chronic administration through the down regulation of receptors and desensitization of the gonadotrophic cells, the antagonists bind competitively to the receptors and thereby prevent the endogenous GnRH from exerting its stimulatory effects on the pituitary cells avoiding any "flare-up" effect. Within hours, the secretion of gonadotrophines is reduced. This mechanism of action is dependent on the equilibrium between endogenous GnRH and the applied antagonist. Due to this, the effect of the antagonist is highly dose-dependent, in contrast to the agonists [11].

While in the first generation of GnRH-antagonists allergic side effects due to an induced histamine release hampered the clinical development of these compounds, modern GnRH-antagonists like the Ganirelix (Organon, Oss, The Netherlands) or Cetrorelix (ASTA-Medica, Frankfurt/M, Germany) seem to have solved these problems, and thus may become available medically in the near future, both of them having been used at our department [12].

## GnRH-antagonists within COH

In 1991 Dittkoff et al. showed that a GnRH-antagonist that is applied for a short period is capable of suppressing the ovulation-inducing midcycle LH-peak [13]. They administered 50 μg of Nal-Glu per kg body weight per day for 4 days in the midcycle phase. The LH peak failed to occur, estradiol production came to a halt, and follicular growth was interrupted. After discontinuing the antagonists, gonadal function normalized within days. Apparently, antagonists neither deplete the FSH and LH stores of gonadotrophic cells nor inhibit gonadotropin synthesis.

Trying to transfer these results into a clinical stimulation protocol for the routine use within an IVF-unit the so-called "multiple-dose Lübeck protocol" was designed [14,15]. Starting on cycle day 2 patients are treated with two ampoules of gonadotrophins — urinary or recombinant preparations — per day. From cycle day 7, when a premature LH surge may be imminent until ovulation induction the GnRH-antagonist is administered daily. On day 5 the dosages of gonadotrophins has to be adjusted to the individual ovarian response of the patient to the stimulation, as assessed by estradiol values and measurement of follicles. This treatment was continued until induction of ovulation with 10,000 IU HCG i.m., given when the leading follicle reached a diameter of 18–20 mm, measured by transvaginal ultrasound, and when estradiol values indicated a satisfactory follicular response.

Figure 1 shows the hormone profiles for LH of the first 47 patients treated with the GnRH-antagonist Cetrorelix at the Department of Obstetrics and Gynecology at the Medical University of Lübeck for the purpose of COH with the different dosages of 3, 1, 0.5 and 0.25 mg/day. In all four groups on day 7 of the cycle, when Cetrorelix administration was started, a significant decrease in LH concentrations could be observed. Afterwards, LH levels could be maintained at a low level and not a single patient's stimulation had to be cancelled due to a premature rise in the LH level. In the case of FSH the hormone profiles were quite different. Almost no suppression over the time of stimulation could be observed until the day of HCG administration. This may be mainly due to the fact, that exogenous FSH had been constantly administered during COH with the distinct longer half-life time of FSH in comparison to LH. Pharmacokinetic studies have shown that without FSH supplementation under Cetrorelix treatment FSH secretion is

116

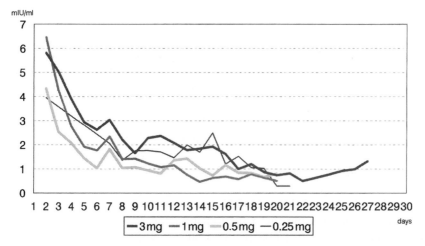

*Fig. 1.* Mean courses of LH-serum concentration (mIU/ml) during COH with HMG and concomitant midcyclic GnRH-antagonist treatment (Cetrorelix) in different dosages (3 mg/day, 1 mg/day, 0.5 mg/day and 0.25 mg/day) according to the multiple dose protocol.

as well suppressed as LH in a dose-dependent manner, although to a lesser extent than LH values [16].

Estradiol serum concentrations showed constantly increasing values under GnRH-antagonist treatment, reflecting ovarian follicle maturation (Fig. 2). The fact that in the 0.5-mg group a more pronounced increase in estradiol values from day 7 onwards was observed caused severe discussions about the possibility of direct effects of the GnRH-antagonist on gonadal sexual steroid production. However, stepping down to 0.25 mg per day this observation could not be

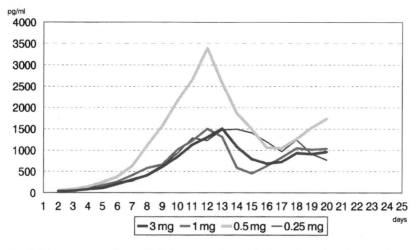

*Fig. 2.* Mean courses of estradiol-serum concentration (pg/ml) during COH with HMG and concomitant midcyclic GnRH-antagonist treatment (Cetrorelix) in different dosages (3 mg/day, 1 mg/day, 0.5 mg/day and 0.25 mg/day) according to the multiple dose protocol.

repeated. On the other hand, all of the in vitro studies that have been performed in our department for a period of longer than 1 year, examining the possible interference of the GnRH-antagonist with sexual steroid secretion of the granulosa lutein cells, have not shown any evidence for a direct effect of the GnRH-antagonist, at least with a dosage of 0.25 mg per day according to the "Lübeck" protocol [17].

Subsequent dose-finding studies using 0.5 mg Cetrorelix/die as well as 0.25 mg Cetrorelix/die and 0.1 mg Cetrorelix/die proved the efficacy and safety of 0.25 mg Cetrorelix/die in avoiding premature LH-surges, while under 0.1 mg Cetrorelix/die premature LH-surges could be observed [18,19]. In these studies ICSI for treatment of male subfertility of the husband was allowed, leading to fertilization rates within the range to be expected after normal oocyte maturation. It is really essential to emphasize that stepping down with the dosage of Cetrorelix did not have a negative impact on the outcome of the treatment. There were no significant differences regarding two-pronuclei fertilization rates, increase in estradiol values, cleavage rate, clinical pregnancy rate per ET and implantation rate between the group treated with 0.5 mg Cetrorelix per day and those patients treated with only 0.25 mg per day (Table 1). The clinical pregnancy rates per transfer were 30.7% in the 0.5 mg group and 29.6% in the 0.25 mg group. Interestingly, about 16% of the patients treated in this study with 0.5 mg Cetrorelix per day and 10% of those treated with only 0.25 mg per day showed a significant rise in LH concentrations during the follicular phase, while progesterone concentrations remained low. These patients showed a significantly lower cleavage rate and no pregnancy occurred in this subgroup of patients. As these patients showed higher estradiol concentrations than patients who did not have a rise of LH, these findings may suggest, that an earlier administration of the antagonist may be necessary in high responders to avoid the LH rise, which may compromise the quality and maturity of the recovered oocytes [19].

*The "French protocol": single-shot injection*

In parallel to the multiple-dose administration a different protocol for adminis-

*Table 1.* Stimulation and ICSI outcome in patients treated with HMG and concomitant midcyclic GnRh antagonist (Cetrorelix) administration at 0.5 and 0.25 mg/day [19].

|  | 0.5 mg/day | 0.25 mg/day |
| --- | --- | --- |
| No. of patients | 32 | 30 |
| No. of HMG ampoules | 35 | 33 |
| Duration of HMG treatment (days) | 11 | 10 |
| No. of follicles > 15 mm the day of HCG | 10 | 10 |
| Estradiol the day of HCG (pg/ml) | 2122 | 2491 |
| Fertilization rate (%) | 55 | 59 |
| Cleavage rate (%) | 78 | 76 |
| Clinical pregnancy rate (%) | 31 | 30 |

tration of GnRH-antagonists within COH was developed by the French investigators Bouchard, Frydman and Olivennes, in which the compound was used with a dosage of 2 or 3 mg as single or dual administration around day 9. In this protocol the antagonist was injected at the time when estradiol reached 150–200 pg/ml and the follicle size was > 14 mm, which is usually the case on day 8 or 9 of the cycle [20,21]. They could not observe premature LH rises in any of the cycles that have been studied and published until now. Because it could be demonstrated that 3 mg of Cetrorelix are able to suppress LH values for as long as 96 h, acting like an intermediate depot preparation, the protocol was modified; 3 mg of Cetrorelix was then injected on cycle day 8 as a "jour fixe". If within these 96 h the criteria for ovulation induction were not met, 0.25 mg of Cetrorelix was administered as daily injections. The injection of 3 mg Cetrorelix was capable of preventing LH surges in the patients treated, introducing a very simple treatment protocol. Clinical pregnancy rates of over 30% per transfer were reported, which sound very promising.

## Results of phase III studies

Both of the protocols described have been used in prospective, randomised open label phase III studies, comparing the results obtained in the GnRH-antagonist groups with those after treatment according to the long agonistic protocol.

In total, 188 patients treated with Cetrorelix with its minimal effective dose of 0.25 mg/day according to the multiple-dose protocol were compared with 85 patients treated according to the long protocol, using Buserelin as nasal spray for desensitization of the pituitary gland. While in 84% of the patients from the antagonist group an embryo transfer could be performed, this was only possible in 79% of the cases in the agonist group, reflecting a lower cancellation rate using Cetrorelix. The clinical pregnancy rate (intrauterine pregnancies with documented heart activity of the embryo) in the antagonist group was 27% per transfer and 33% in the agonist group. However, this difference was not statistically significant. Also, no differences were to be found in the implantation rates, which were 15.3% after having used the antagonist and 16.7% after COH according to the long protocol. Concerning those patients treated with ICSI due to male infertility of the couple there were no differences to be observed regarding oocytes in the metaphase II or fertilization rates after ICSI. It may be difficult to attribute to the use of a GnRH-antagonist the higher percentage of excellent embryos to be transferred in the Cetrorelix group (45%) in comparison to the agonist group (27%) (Table 2). The distribution of follicles on the day of HCG-injection for ovulation induction was quite similar in the two groups with a certain tendency towards fewer small follicles in the group of patients having been treated by Cetrorelix. Although this tendency did not reach statistical significance it became very clear that the synchronization of follicular recruitment is not impaired by the use of a GnRH-antagonist according to the multiple-dose protocol. Also, the estradiol profiles throughout the treatment time showed no significant differ-

*Table 2.* COH for ICSI with HMG and Cetrorelix (multiple dose protocol; 0.25 mg/day) vs. long protocol (HMG/Buserelin; nasal spray).

|  | Cetrorelix | Buserelin |
|---|---|---|
| ICSI (n) | 46 | 27 |
| COC | 465 | 316 |
| Metaphase II (ICSI) (%) | 80 | 82 |
| ICSI Fertilisation rate (%) | 63 | 64 |
| Embryos (ICSI) | 92 | 55 |
| Excellent embryos (ICSI) (%) | 45 | 27 |

ences between the two groups. Only a certain tendency towards higher estradiol levels on the day of HCG was to be observed on the day of HCG (Fig. 3). However, the incidence of ovarian hyperstimulation syndrome (OHSS) II—III was significantly different in the two groups. While in the Cetrorelix group only three cases (1.7%) were observed, all of them grade II, the incidence in the Buserelin group was 6.5% with one case of severe OHSS that required hospitalization. The tendency is towards higher estradiol levels in the late stimulatory phase in the agonist group, because fewer amounts of small follicles on the day of HCG in the Cetrorelix group may be of causal importance for this lower incidence after having used the antagonist.

A total of 115 patients have been treated according to the French single-shot protocol using 3 mg of Cetrorelix injected on day 8 of the cycle. Their results

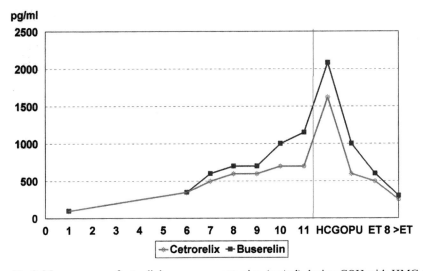

*Fig. 3.* Mean courses of estradiol-serum concentration (pg/ml) during COH with HMG and concomitant midcyclic GnRH-antagonist treatment (Cetrorelix) in its minimal effective dose (0.25 mg/day) according to the multiple dose protocol in comparison to estradiol serum concentrations during COH according to the long protocol (HMG/Buserelin).

were compared to 36 patients treated with Triptorelin as a depot preparation according to the long protocol. No significant statistical differences were observed between the two groups regarding stimulation length (9.4 and 10.7 days), estradiol levels on the day of HCG (1,786 pg/ml in the Cetrorelix group and 2,549 pg/ml in the Triptorelin group), fertilization rate (56% in the Cetrorelix group and 17.8% in the Triptorelin group), and implantation rate (13.8% in the Cetrorelix group and 17.8% in the Triptorelin group). As in the case of the multiple-dose protocol the pregnancy rate showed to be a little more favourable in the agonist group (25% per oocyte pick up (OPU)) than in the Cetrorelix group (18.6% per OPU). However, these differences were again not statistically significant. Again the incidence of OHSS (II−III) was remarkably lower within these patients, who had been treated with Cetrorelix (3.5%) than in those, who had been stimulated according to the long protocol using Triptorelin (11.1%) (Table 3). Interestingly, in all of the patients who had started to show a rise in the LH level on day 8, when Cetrorelix was to be administered, the LH rise could be cut down by the administration of the antagonist (Fig. 4). None of these cycles had to be cancelled and pregnancies also occurred.

In a prospective, open nonrandomised study, also using 0.25 mg of Cetrorelix according to the multiple-dose "Lübeck" protocol, 346 patients were treated in several European centres. By replacing a mean of 2.66 embryos per cycle a clinical ongoing pregnancy rate of 25% per transfer could be obtained. The abortion rate was of 14%. The median exposure time to Cetrorelix was 5 days, the mean time of stimulation with gonadotrophins was 10.4 days per cycle, and the median number of ampoules of HMG used per cycle was 23. The incidence of premature luteinization in this presently largest study using Cetrorelix for COH was as low as 0.89% after having started antagonist administration.

**Preserved pituitary response**

Based on the mechanism of competitive binding, it is possible to modulate the degree of hormone suppression by the dose of antagonist to be administered. This preservation of the pituitary response due to competitive mechanisms could be clearly demonstrated using a GnRH test during GnRH-antagonist treatment. A period of 3 h before injecting the hCG for ovulation induction, 25 mg of

Table 3. COH for IVF/ICSI with HMG and Cetrorelix single shot administration (3 mg at day 8) vs. long protocol (HMG/Triptorelin depot).

|  | Cetrorelix | Triptorelin |
| --- | --- | --- |
| Fertilisation rate (%) | 56 | 59 |
| Embryos obtained | 5.4 | 7.6 |
| Implantation rate (%) | 13.8 | 17.8 |
| Clinical pregnancy rate/OPU | 18.6 | 25 |
| OHSS (%) | 3.5 | 11.1 |

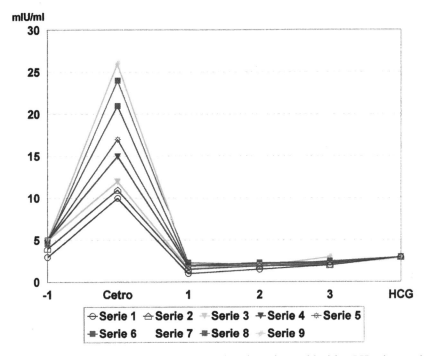

*Fig. 4.* Courses of estradiol-serum concentrations in patients with rising LH values at day 8. Single dose injection of 3 mg Cetrorelix s.c.

GnRH were administered in patients treated with 1 or 3 mg Cetrorelix per day. Blood samples for LH measurement were taken before and 30 min after GnRH treatment. The mean increase was 10 mIU/ml for the 3-mg group, while the average maximum concentration of serum LH in the 1-mg group was about 32.5 mIU/ml. These results were highly significant [11]. They could open new paths in the treatment of patients at higher risk for developing OHSS, as it would allow the avoidance of, in some cases, deleterious effects of HCG administration. Ovulation induction is possible using GnRH-agonists or native GnRH itself under antagonistic treatment. This could help to lower the incidence rate of an early onset OHSS [22].

### COH with rec. FSH and concomitant midcyclic GnRH antagonist treatment

Cetrorelix and Ganirelix are presently tested within the frame of clinical phase II studies in combination with recombinant FSH. In contrast to urinary compounds these preparations are free of LH activity. Their effectiveness within COH according to the long protocol has been proven. Even after down regulation of the pituitary gland endogenous LH secretion seems to be sufficient for normal ovarian sexual steroids biosynthesis. However, extreme suppression of LH secretion by high doses of GnRH-antagonists could cause problems according to the two cells/two gonadotrophin hypothesis of follicular estrogen production [23]. It could cause a situation very similar to WHO-I infertile patients having ovarian stimulation with pure FSH, depletion of any LH-activity could induce follicular growth in the absence of any estrogen secretion, as has been described for these patients [24]. It is the merit of the prospective, multicentric double-blinded dose-finding phase II study with Ganirelix to have elucidated this question and demonstrated the correctness of the two cell/two gonadotrophin theory. In this study Ganirelix was administered according to the multiple-dose "Lübeck protocol" with six different dosages (0.0625, 0.125, 0.25, 0.5, 1 and 2 mg/day). While in the lower dosages estradiol secretion was normal and sufficient, injecting 2 mg Ganirelix s.c. per day almost no increase in the estradiol secretion could be seen. In some cases even the follicles did not grow, an observation that still awaits a scientific explanation. The treatment outcome in the 0.25 mg group was an overwhelming success, showing a clinical pregnancy rate of 40.3% per transfer. By increasing the dosage of Ganirelix the pregnancy rates decreased and the abortion rates increased. Thus, 0.25 mg was defined as the minimal effective dose to be administered according to the multiple-dose protocol. However, we must wait and see whether this obvious great success can be repeated in the ongoing phase III study, using 0.25 mg Ganirelix per day (Table 4).

## Future aspects on GnRH-antagonists in COH

Since 1992, we have experienced a veritable revolution in infertility treatment of the male as a consequence of the inauguration of ICSI with its excellent fertilization outcome irrespective of sperm morphology [25,26]. However, it seems as if our therapeutic approach has been overdone in the meantime. The burden and risks to our patients, as well as the costs have skyrocketed. Excessive ovarian stimulation with rescue rates of more than 30 oocytes is not uncommon. On the other hand, the incidence of moderate and severe OHSSs has increased from

Table 4. COH for IVF/ICSI with rec. FSH and concomitant mid-cyclic GnRH antagonist (Ganirelix) administration in six different dosages (multiple-dose protocol).

| Daily dose of Ganirelix (mg/day) | 0.625 | 0.125 | 0.25 | 0.5 | 1 | 2 |
|---|---|---|---|---|---|---|
| Patients (n) | 31 | 65 | 69 | 69 | 65 | 30 |
| COC[a] | 9 | 9.5 | 10 | 8.8 | 9.3 | 8.6 |
| Embryos[a] | | | | | | |
| Total[a] | 5.4 | 5.9 | 5.4 | 4.6 | 5.3 | 4.9 |
| Good quality[a] | 3.8 | 3.3 | 3.3 | 2.5 | 3.3 | 3.5 |
| Implantation rate (%) | 14.2 | 16.6 | 21.9 | 9 | 8.8 | 1.5 |
| Clinical pregnancies | 7 | 17 | 25 | 8 | 9 | 1 |
| Clinical pregnancy/ET (%) | 25.9 | 28.3 | 40.3 | 14.8 | 15.3 | 4.3 |
| Abortion rate (%) | 0 | 12 | 4 | 25 | 56 | — |

[a]Mean.

< 1 to about 7%, while our therapeutic possibilities still remain poor [27—29]. If a healthy single-fetus pregnancy is the goal to aim for, a multiple pregnancy rate of over 20% demonstrates how often we fail in our attempt. The development of recombinant gonadotropins and their introduction onto the market entailed an important scientific advance, while treatment costs increased tremendously [30]. Because of the lowering in price of these compounds, they were expected to replace the urinary ones almost completely, however, recombinant gonadotropins remain extremely expensive. After years of intensive clinical trials, GnRH-antagonists are now to be introduced onto the market. They will probably replace GnRH-agonists within COH for ARTs, due to the advantages of their mode of action as compared to agonistic analogues. A reduction in gonadotrophins used for COH seems to be feasible using GnRH-antagonists. Although our knowledge regarding oocyte and embryo quality after COH with concomitant GnRH-antagonist treatment may still be limited, the rates of excellent embryos transferred seem to be satisfactory. The long agonist protocol was regarded as advantageous since recruitment of a larger follicle cohort could be stimulated by gonadotropins at a very early point of folliculogenesis. As for the short agonistic protocol, this is not the case in protocols for COH using antagonists, where stimulation starts almost immediately after having completing the recruitment of follicles in the spontaneous cycle. From a theoretical point of view, this could lead to a larger number of small and intermediate follicles at the time for ovulation induction by HCG. This would actually enhance the risk of onset of OHSS. In spite of this very reasonable hypothesis, all data available up to now seem to indicate a remarkably lower incidence of moderate and severe OHSS after COH with gonadotropins and concomitant GnRH antagonist treatment, which may be below 2%. Overall, the most promising aspect of introducing GnRH antagonists into COH may be the possibility of making this treatment less aggressive and much softer than an agonistic long-protocol, using old-fashioned schemes of stimulation such as clomiphene citrate (CC) in combination with HMG.

## Conclusions

Due to the different pharmacological method of action GnRH-antagonist allowed us to significantly reduce the length of a stimulation cycle. The flare-up phenomenon is completely avoided. Premature LH surges are a rare event under this treatment modality, that also uses Cetrorelix in a daily fashion (multiple-dose "Lübeck" protocol), as in the single-shot protocol (single-shot "French" protocol). In fact, Cetrorelix and Ganirelix, used with their minimal effective dose of 0.25 mg/day according to the multiple-dose protocol, allow sufficient LH to be secreted from the pituitary gland for a normal estradiol secretion under stimulation with preparations of rec. FSH, avoiding any LH-activity. As the pituitary responsiveness is maintained under GnRH-antagonist treatment it seems to be possible to induce ovulation by native GnRH or a GnRH-agonist, avoiding the necessity of HCG with its, in some cases, deleterious effects on OHSS. Combin-

124

ing GnRH-antagonist treatment with softer stimulation regimes like clomiphene citrate/HMG may be the way to a cheap, safe and efficient ovarian stimulation for ART.

## References

1. Loumaye E. The control of endogenous secretion of LH by gonadotrophin-releasing hormone agonists during ovarian hyperstimulation for in vitro fertilization and embryo transfer. Hum Reprod 1990;5:357-376.
2. Stanger JD, Yovich JL. Reduced in vitro fertilization of human oocytes from patients with raised basal luteinizing hormone levels during the follicular phase. Br J Obstet Gynecol 1985;92: 385—393.
3. Macnamee MC, Howles CM, Edwards RG, Taylor PJ, Elder KT. Short-term luteinizing hormone-releasing hormone agonist treatment: prospective trial of a novel ovarian stimulation regimen for in vitro fertilization. Fertil Steril 1989;52:264—269.
4. Loumaye E, de Cooman S, Anoma M, Psalti I, Depreester S, Schmit M, Thomas K. Short-term utilization of a gonadotropin releasing hormone agonist (Buserelin) for induction of ovulation in an in vitro fertilization program. Ann NY Acad Sci 1988;541:96—102.
5. Smitz J, Ron-El R, Tarlatzis BC. The use of gonadotrophin releasing hormone agonists for in vitro fertilization and other assisted procreation techniques: experience from three centres. Hum Reprod 1992;7(Suppl 1):49—66.
6. Deutsches IVF Register. Jahrbuch 1997. DIR Bundesgeschäftsstelle Ärztekammer Schleswig Holstein, Bismarckallee 8-12, 23795 Bad Segeberg, Germany.
7. Loumaye E, Porchet HC, Beltrami V, Giroud D, Le Cotonnec JY, O'Dea L, Piazzi A, Howles CM, Galazka A. Ovulation induction with recombinant human follicle-stimulating hormone and luteinizing hormone. In: Filicori M, Flamigni C (eds) Ovulation Induction. Basic Science and Clinical Advances. Amsterdam: Elsevier Science B.V. 1994;227—236.
8. Balen A. The effects of ovulation induction with gonadotrophins on the ovary and uterus and implications for assisted reproduction. Hum Reprod 1995;10:2233—2237.
9. Küpker W, Al-Hasani S, Schulze W, Kühnel W, Schill T, Felberbaum R, Diedrich K. Morphology in intracytoplasmic sperm injection: preliminary results. J Assist Reprod Genet 1995;12: 620—626.
10. Edwards RG, Lobo R, Bouchard P. Time to revolutionize ovarian stimulation. Hum Reprod 1996;11:917—919.
11. Felberbaum RE, Reissmann T, Küpker W, Bauer O, Al-Hasani S, Diedrich C, Diedrich K. Preserved pituitary response under ovarian stimulation with HMG and GnRH-antagonists (Cetrorelix) in women with tubal infertility. Eur J Obstet Gynecol Reprod Biol 1995;61:151—155.
12. Reissmann T, Felberbaum R, Diedrich K, Engel J, Comaru-Schally AM, Schally AV. Development and applications of luteinizing hormone-releasing hormone antagonists in the treatment of infertility: an overview. Hum Reprod 1995;10:1974—1981.
13. Dittkoff EC, Cassidenti DL, Paulson RJ, Sauer MV, Wellington LP, Rivier J, Yen SSC, Lobo RA. The gonadotrophin-releasing hormone antagonist (Nal-Glu) acutely blocks the luteinizing hormone surge but allows for resumption of folliculogenesis in normal women. Am J Obstet Gynecol 1991;165:1811—1817.
14. Diedrich K, Diedrich C, Santos E et al. Suppression of the endogenous luteinizing hormone surge by the gonadotrophin releasing hormone antagonist Cetrorelix during ovarian stimulation. Hum Reprod 1994;9:788—791.
15. Felberbaum R, Reissmann T, Küpker W, Al-Hasani S, Bauer O, Schill T, Zoll C, Diedrich C, Diedrich K. Hormone profiles under ovarian stimulation with human menopausal gonadotrophin (HMG) and concomitant administration of the gonadotropin releasing hormone (GnRH)-antagonist Cetrorelix at different dosages. J Assist Reprod Genet 1996;13:216—222.

16. Duijkers IJM, Klipping C, Willemsen WNP, Krone D, Schneider E, Niebch G, Romeis P, Hermann R. Single and multiple dose pharmacokinetics and pharmacodynamics of the gonadotrophin-releasing hormone antagonist Cetrorelix in healthy female volunteers. Hum Reprod 1998;13(Abstract book 1):123.

17. Ortmann O, Oltmanns K, Weiss JM, Felberbaum R, Polack S, Diedrich K. Effects of the GnRH antagonist Cetrorelix on steroidogenesis inhuman granulosa lutein cells. Hum Reprod 1998;13(Abstract book 1):254.

18. Albano C, Smitz J, Camus M, Riethmüller-Winzen H, Siebert-Weigel M, Diedrich K, Van Steirteghem AC, Devroey P. Hormonal profile during the follicular phase in cycles stimulated with a combination of human menopausal gonadotrophin and gonadotrophin-releasing hormone antagonist (Cetrorelix). Hum Reprod 1996;11:2114—2118.

19. Albano C, Smitz J, Camus M, Riethmüller-Winzen H, Van Steirteghem A, Devroey P. Comparison of different doses of gonadotropin-releasing hormone antagonist Cetrorelix during controlled ovarian hyperstimulation. Fertil Steril 1997;67:917—922.

20. Olivennes F, Fanchin R, Bouchard P, De Ziegler D, Taieb J, Selva j, Frydman R. The single or dual administration of the gonadotrophin-releasing hormone antagonist Cetrorelix in an in vitro fertilization — embryo transfer programme. Fertil Steril 1994;62:468—476.

21. Olivennes F, Fanchin R, Bouchard P, Taieb J, Selva J, Frydman R. Scheduled administration of a gonadotrophin-releasing hormone antagonist (Cetrorelix) on day 8 of in vitro fertilization cycles: a pilot study. Hum Reprod 1995;10:1382—1386.

22. Olivennes F, Fanchin R, Bouchard P, Taieb J, Frydman R. Triggering of ovulation by a gonadotropin-releasing hormone (GnRH) agonist in patients pretreated with a GnRH antagonist. Fertil Steril 1996;66:151—153.

23. Adashi EY. Endocrinology of the ovary. Hum Reprod 1994;9(Suppl 2):36—51.

24. Schoot DC, Harlin J, Shoham Z, Manaerts BMJL, Lalou N, Bouchard P, Coelingh Bennink HJT, Fauser BCJM. Recombinant human follicle-stimulating hormone and ovarian response in gonadotrophin-deficient women. Hum Reprod 1994;9:1237—1242.

25. Palermo G, Joris H, Devroey P, Van Steirteghem AC. Pregnancies after intracytoplasmic injection of single spermatozoon into an oocyte. Lancet 1992;340:17—18.

26. Van Steirteghem AC. IVF and micromanipulation techniques for male-factor infertility. Curr Opin Obstet Gynecol 1994;6:173—177.

27. Golan A, Ron-El R, Herman A, Weintraub Z, Soffer Y, Caspi E. Ovarian hyperstimulation syndrome following D-Trp-6-luteinizing hormone-releasing hormone microcapsules and menotropins for in vitro fertilization. Fertil Steril 1988;50:912—916.

28. Ron-El R, Herman A, Golan A, Nachum H, Soffer Y, Caspi E. Gonadotropins and combined gonadotropin-releasing hormone agonist-gonadotropins protocols in a randomized prospective study. Fertil Steril 1991;55:574—578.

29. Bauer O, Diedrich K. Komplikationen der assistierten Reproduktion. Gynäkologe 1996;29:464—473.

30. Recombinant Human FSH Study Group. Clinical assessment of recombinant human follicle-stimulating hormone in stimulating ovarian follicular development for in vitro fertilization. Fertil Steril 1995;63:77—86.

# Managing nonresponders

P.N. Barri, F. Martínez, B. Coroleu, N. Parera and A. Veiga
*Service of Reproductive Medicine, Department of Obstetrics and Gynecology, Institut Universitari Dexeus, Barcelona, Spain*

**Abstract.** Patients with a poor response to classical ovarian stimulation protocols have lower pregnancy rates. Although oocyte and embryo quality are not impaired in these patients the lower chances of achieving a pregnancy are commonly related to the reduced number of oocytes and embryos.

We have carried out a prospective study in a group of 80 poor responders comparing the standard long protocol of GnRH analog with the short protocol, the mini- or low-dose analogue protocol, a repeated long protocol and a combination of clomiphene and gonadotropins. Although we have seen some differences the final goal, the pregnancy rates, were not improved.

It is still too early to evaluate the potential of the new recombinant gonadotropins to be used in these cases. So far, natural cycles and oocyte donation are the last hope for these patients.

**Keywords:** bad response, IVF, ovarian stimulation.

## Introduction

One aspect which all IVF teams agree on is the usefulness of using follicular stimulation protocols to obtain more oocytes, thus increasing the yield of an IVF cycle. In our experience, the number of embryos available for transfer is a determining factor for the success of the process. In 1997 we obtained eight pregnancies in the 130 IVF cycles with transfer of a single embryo (6% pregnancies/ET), whereas in the 844 IVF cycles with transfer of more than two embryos we obtained 324 pregnancies (38% pregnancies/ET) ($p < 0.0001$).

Given the importance of a suitable ovarian response to stimulation in attaining the final objective of a high number of good quality oocytes and embryos, it seems obvious that those cycles in which response is very poor should be cancelled. We defined bad-response cycles as those in which plasmatic estradiol on the day of HCG administration was less than 1,000 pg/ml and in which no more than three oocytes had been obtained [1].

### What is a bad responder?

Sometimes a bad response may be sporadic or accidental, depending on the par-

*Address for correspondence:* P.N. Barri, Service of Reproductive Medicine, Department of Obstetrics and Gynecology, Institut Universitari Dexeus, Paseo Bonanova 67, 08017 Barcelona, Spain. Tel.: +34-93-227-4700/227-4710. Fax: +34-93-205-7966.

ticular menstrual cycle. For this reason, we think that a patient should be considered as a "bad responder" when she has repeated an inadequate response in at least two IVF cycles.

It is important for us to study the factors of age, previous history, and endocrinological characteristics which may cause a patient to respond badly to stimulation.

## Physiopathological bases of ovarian ageing

The events that occur with ovarian ageing were described several years ago with the concept of the "pre-eminent follicle" [2]. In the majority of cases, the ageing ovary progressively loses its follicle pool and reduces its level of inhibin [3], and the pituitary reacts by increasing FSH secretion; this translates into an increase in basal estradiol levels [4,5]. This situation brings with it a greater risk of an excessively premature LH peak and ovulation, and in other cases of early luteinization. On these occasions there is an accelerated rate of follicular growth which shortens the follicular phase and consequently the cycle.

The reason for this perimenopausal transition beginning in the mid or late thirties seems to be related to a granulosa cell compromise. Ovaries of women with a poor functional reserve have fewer follicles, and the follicles have a hypoxic environment [6] and contain fewer granulosa cells [7]. Granulosa cells may also have a decreased function indicated by reduced steroid and glycoprotein production in vitro, decreased mitosis and increased apoptosis [8].

Recent publications speak of the functional antagonism between gonadotropin liberating factors (GnRH) and the inhibiting or attenuating factors (GnSIF) as being responsible for certain imbalances in ovarian-pituitary-hypothalamus relationships, leading eventually to a bad ovulatory response in apparently normal patients [9,10].

Based on this knowledge, three types of bad responders should be differentiated:
1) elderly patients with an abnormal endocrinological profile, which suggests a poor ovarian reserve;
2) young patients with an altered endocrinological profile; and
3) young patients with an absolutely normal basal hormonal profile.

The last category of young patients who respond badly to stimulation despite having an apparently normal ovarian reserve present a real challenge to our possibilities of diagnosis and treatment [11].

## Evaluation of the functional reserve of the ovary

There is a series of parameters to analyse in order to discover a patient's ovarian functional reserve.

*Age*

The patient's age plays a crucial role in the prognosis of an IVF cycle. Numerous studies show that as age rises cancellation rates increase, the number of oocytes and embryos falls, and although fertilisation rates are unchanged the pregnancy rate worsens significantly [12,13]. However, if an elderly patient has a good functional reserve and her ovaries respond well, her chances of becoming pregnant if she receives three embryos are similar to those of younger patients [14]. The negative influence of age affects not only the number of oocytes but also their quality. There is evidence that the incidence of oocyte chromosome degeneration and meiotic nondisjunction increase notably with age [15,16].

*Basal FSH*

As well as the patient's chronological age, it is essential to know her basal plasmatic FSH level measured in the early follicular phase (days 3—5). According to our data, basal FSH levels greater than 15 mIU/ml are associated with a worse response to stimulation [17]. Some authors accept that more importance should be given to FSH levels than to the patient's age [18,19]. Another advantage of measuring basal FSH levels is their high predictive value for later values of this hormone during 1 year, since they do not vary significantly during this period [20].

*Estradiol*

Data have recently been published stating that patients with $E_2$ levels greater than 80 pg/ml in the early follicular phase have a worse response and higher cancellation rates [21—23].

In our experience basal estradiol has a discriminatory value only in the identification of those patients who, despite having normal FSH levels, will respond

*Table 1.* The clomiphene test.

| | Basal FSH level | | | |
|---|---|---|---|---|
| | Normal $FSH_1 < 10.5$ (n = 98) | | Abnormal $FSH_1 > 10.5$ (n = 81) | |
| | Normal responders (n = 84) | Bad responders (n = 14) | Normal responders (n = 56) | Bad responders (n = 25) |
| Age (years) | 36.46 | 39.7 | 37.20 | 39.20 |
| $FSH_1 + FSH_2$ (mIU/ml) | 17.80[a] | 24.8[a] | 34.40 | 42.50 |
| $Estradiol_1$ (pg/ml) | 58.30[b] | 118.0[b] | 39.81 | 39.28 |

[a,b] $p < 0.01$.

badly to stimulation. However, we have found no significant differences in basal estradiol levels among patients who already had abnormal levels of FSH (Table 1).

## Clomiphene test

The clomiphene test measures the ovary's ability to control secretion of FSH [24–26]. A possible explanation of the sensitivity of FSH to clomiphene is the lower level of inhibin secretion of ovarian follicles with functional deficits [3].

We consider it useful to ask for a clomiphene test in patients who are over 37 years of age, who have undergone ovarian surgery or suffered from endometriosis. This test has allowed us to find great differences between patients who respond well to stimulation and those who respond badly. We have observed differences not only in the sum of both FSH values, but also in the second estradiol measurement, which was significantly lower in the group of bad responders (Table 2).

## Basal LH

Recently, importance has been given to plasmatic LH levels, both measured in isolation, with day 3 LH levels $< 3$ mIU/ml being a bad prognosis for good response [27], and by studying the FSH/LH quotient. It seems that high values for this quotient ($> 3$) are associated with high cancellation rates [28].

## Inhibin

As the functional pool of follicles reduces, the ovary loses its ability to restrain the pituitary, which becomes evident with the increase in FSH levels. There is some recent evidence of significantly lower plasmatic inhibin levels in patients who respond badly to stimulation [29,30].

## Dynamic tests

There are several dynamic tests which may be useful when basal determinations

Table 2. The clomiphene test: comparison of normal/bad response.

| | Normal responders (n = 134) | Bad responders (n = 45) |
|---|---|---|
| Age (years) | 36.70[a] | 39.40[a] |
| $FSH_1$ (mIU/ml) | 10.40[b] | 13.80[b] |
| $FSH_1 + FSH_2$ (mIU/ml) | 24.10[c] | 35.47[c] |
| $Estradiol_1$ (pg/ml) | 51.29 | 69.14 |
| $Estradiol_2$ (pg/ml) | 372.60[d] | 256.00[d] |

[a,b,c,d]$p < 0.001$.

are not informative.

However, neither the leuprolide test [31] nor the EFORT test [32] is necessary as screening since the best information that they can provide is given by basal hormone levels.

*Ultrasound scanning*

The development of high-frequency transvaginal transducers has made possible a notable improvement in resolution power of current ultrasound equipment. Some authors have recently published an age-related decrease in antral follicles ($\geqslant 2$ mm), and based on this we recommend measurement of the number of antral follicles to find a patient's response ability [33].

New three-dimensional echography systems already allow it to be shown that the pool of selectable (2—5 mm) follicles in young low responders with normal basal serum FSH is low when compared to controls [34].

**Risk factors for bad response to ovarian stimulation**

In summary we consider the following risk factors to be relevant for the prediction of a poor response:
1) patient's age,
2) family history of premature ovarian failure,
3) history of pelvic surgery on the adnexa,
4) endometriosis,
5) obesity
6) idiopathic infertility, and
7) smoking.

**Alternative protocols for use in patients with a history of bad response**

Currently, most IVF cycles are carried out under a long protocol of GnRH analogues which were started in the luteal phase of the cycle before stimulation with gonadotropins. However, when a patient responds badly to a conventional protocol, other protocols must be presented which allow the treatment to be individualised, adapting it to the characteristics of each case.

Various therapeutic strategies have been used to improve the response of these patients.

*Reducing the dose of GnRH analogue*

With the aim of reducing the intensity of pituitary suppression several schemes have been proposed with lower analogue doses [35] or even interrupting their administration [36].

Retrospective analysis of the wide-ranging series carried out under one of these mini-protocols or low-dose analogue protocols shows that lower cancellation rates and better responses can be obtained [37].

### Changing the GnRH analogue

It is well known that in addition to their pituitary action GnRH analogues also have a direct gonadal action that varies depending on the analogues [38].

We retrospectively compared buserelin and leuprolide in a group of 50 patients (each patient did two cycles, one with each analogue). Our results showed that with leuprolide we consumed less gonadotropins, and obtained a higher estradiol level and more oocytes and embryos [1].

### Changing the timing of GnRH analogue administration

In a patient with a history of bad response there are several studies which recommend following a short protocol with simultaneous administration of the analogue and the gonadotropins, taking advantage of the "flare-up" produced by the analogues [39,40].

### Other alternative protocols

Until now, neither the use of growth hormone combined with GnRH analogues and gonadotropins [41–43] nor increase in the dose of gonadotropins [45] has been shown to be more effective in obtaining an adequate response in these patients.

The classic combination of clomiphene citrate and gonadotropins was also tried in these patients, but with variable results [45,46]. Recently a bromocriptine rebound protocol has been proposed in which 2.5 mg/day of bromocriptine is added to the conventional scheme of a long protocol. Preliminary protocols seem to suggest a better response in both quantity and quality of oocytes and embryos [47,48].

In view of the lack of prospective studies we decided to carry out a prospective study in 80 patients with bad response to a conventional long protocol. These patients were randomized, assigning them four different protocols (Fig. 1):
1) 20 patients repeated a long protocol,
2) 20 patients changed to a short protocol,
3) 20 patients followed a mini-protocol with low doses of analogue, and
4) 20 patients were stimulated without analogues under a combination of clomiphene citrate and gonadotropins.

As Table 3 shows, we observed some differences in comparing long protocol cycles with mini-protocol or clomiphene cycles. However, as far as final yield is concerned, that is to say pregnancy rates, neither protocol was more efficient than the previous long protocol.

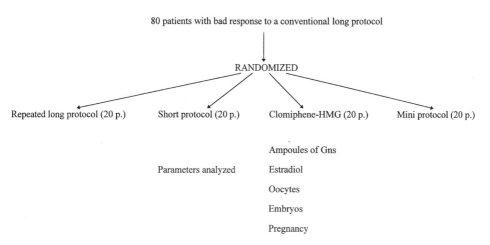

*Fig. 1.* Alternative protocols: prospective randomized study.

## Are gamete and embryo quality affected in bad responders?

According to our experience, oocyte quality is not impaired in young low responders because normal fertilization rates are observed [11]. Embryo quality seems also to be adequate in these patients because the normal rates were obtained in cleavage, implantation, blastocyst formation and miscarriage. In most cases the low pregnancy rate is related to the reduced number of oocytes and embryos common in low responders [49].

## What can the future offer in the treatment of low responders?

### Recombinant gonadotropins

In the last year, two new preparations containing recombinant FSH have come to the market (Follitropin-$\alpha$ and Follitropin-$\beta$). The phase III clinical studies published to date have shown that recombinant gonadotropins were more powerful

*Table 3.* Alternative protocols.

| Prospective randomized study |
| --- |
| 1. Long protocol vs. repeated long protocol and long protocol vs. short protocol<br>    No differences in the parameters analyzed |
| 2. Long protocol vs. mini- or low-dose GnRH protocol<br>    ↑ Number of oocytes $2.8 \pm 0.8$ vs. $5.4 \pm 1.1$ ($p = 0.033$) |
| 3. Long protocol vs. clomiphene-HMG<br>    ↓ Number of oocytes $3 \pm 0$ vs. $1.8 \pm 0.6$ ($p = 0.05$)<br>    ↓ Ampoules of HMG $45 \pm 14.6$ vs. $20.1 \pm 5.2$ ($p = 0.005$) |

than gonadotropins of urinary extraction and in normal patients produced more oocytes and embryos, so that pregnancy rates tended to improve [50–52].

The challenge is to show that these drugs can also achieve better responses in bad responders. Although it seems that the basic character of recombinant FSH would make it more powerful, there is no study which refers to the specific application of recombinant gonadotropins in bad responders. The only trial in these patients has been stimulation with recombinant FSH before the menstrual period. Preliminary results of this protocol have shown no additional benefit either from the use of recombinant preparations or from beginning them before menstruation [53].

*Natural cycle*

Some years ago an evaluation was made of the cost-benefit relationship of a possible return to the natural cycle without stimulation for IVF [54]. Although pregnancy rates were low this was perhaps the only therapeutic alternative to be considered in patients with repeated failure to respond to stimulation [55,56].

Recent publications [57–59] have specifically referred to the usefulness of trying spontaneous IVF cycles in bad responders.

*Oocyte donation*

Oocyte donation is a valid alternative which must be proposed to patients in whom all protocols, including the natural cycle, have failed.

These patients have excellent implantation and pregnancy rates when they receive anonymously donated oocytes from women under the age of 35 years [1,60,61].

## Conclusions

In the case of a patient who responds badly to stimulation, it is essential to establish an appropriate diagnosis. In this way it is possible to differentiate patients who respond badly occasionally from those who will always respond badly, whichever protocol is used.

Although the therapeutic options are limited, the alternative protocols and natural cycle can be attempted before resorting to oocyte donation.

## References

1. Barri PN. Respuesta anómala a la estimulación de la maduración folicular en fecundación in vitro. Tesis doctoral. Barcelona: Universidad de Barcelona, 1993.
2. Thatcher SS, Naftolin F. The aging and aged ovary. Sem Reprod Endocrinol 1991;9(3): 189–199.
3. Seifer DB, Gardiner AC, Lambert-Messerlian G, Schweyer AL. Differential secretion of dimeric inhibin in cultured luteinized granulosa cells as a function of ovarian reserve. J Clin Endocrinol Metab 1996;81:736–739.

4. Klein NA, Battaglia DE, Fujimoto VY, Davis GS, Bremner WJ, Soules MR. Reproductive aging: accelerated ovarian follicular development associated with a monotropic FSH rise in normal older women. J Clin Endocrinol Metab 1996;81:1038–1045.

5. Christin-Maitre S, Bouchard P. Physiopatologie des anomalies de la receptivité ovarienne. Contr Fertil Sex 1996;24(2):105–110.

6. Friedman CI, Danforth DR, Herbosa-Encarnación C, Arbogast L, Alak BM, Seifer DB. Follicular fluid vascular endothelial growth concentrations are elevated in women of advanced reproductive age undergoing ovulation induction. Fertil Steril 1997;68:607–612.

7. Seifer DB, Naftolin F. Moving toward and earlier and better understanding of perimenopause. Fertil Steril 1996;69(3):387–388.

8. Seifer DB, Gardiner AC, Ferreira KA, Peluso JJ. Apoptosis as a function of ovarian reserve in women undergoing in vitro fertilization. Fertil Steril 1996;66:593–598.

9. Koning de J. Gonadotropin surge-inhibiting potentiating factors governs LH secretion during the ovarian cycle: physiology and pathology. Hum Reprod 1995;10(11):2854–2861.

10. Mroueh JM, Arbogast LK, Fowler P, Templeton AA, Friedman CI, Danforth DR. Identification of gonadotropin surge-inhibiting factor/attenuin in human follicular fluid. Hum Reprod 1996;11(3):490–496.

11. Barri PN, Gallinerlli A, Coroleu B, Parera N, Gallostra I, Calderón G, Veiga A. Management of poor responders. In: Gomel V, Leung P (eds) Proceedings of the 10th World Congress of IVF and Assisted Reproduction. Vancouver, May 1997. Vancouver: Monduzzi Editore, 1997; 265–276.

12. Hull MGR, Fleming CF, Hughes AO, McDermott A. The age-related decline in female fecundity: a quantitative controlled study of implanting capacity and survival of individual embryos after IVF. Fertil Steril 1996;65(4):783–790.

13. Templeton A, Morris JK, Parslow W. Factors that affect outcome of IVF treatment. Lancet 1996;348(November 23):1402–1406.

14. Alrayves S, Fakih H, Khan I. Effect of age and cycle responsiveness patients undergoing ICSI. Fertil Steril 1997;68:123–127.

15. Tim AST, Tsakok MFM. Age-related decline in fertility: a link to degenerative oocytes. Fertil Steril 1997;68:265–271.

16. Volaricik K, Sheean L, Goldfarb J, Woods L, Abdul-Karim FW, Hunt P. The meiotic competence of in vitro matured human oocytes is influenced by donor age: evidence that folliculogenesis is compromised in the reproductively age ovary. Hum Reprod 1998;13(1):150–160.

17. Martinez F, Coroleu B, Llueca A, Aran B, Barri PN. Valor predictivo de los niveles de FSH en día 3 del ciclo para la respuesta a la estimulación ovárica en ciclos de FIV. Prog Obstet Ginecol 1992;35:502–506.

18. Roest J, Van Heusden AM, Mous H, Zeilmaker GH, Verhoeff A. The ovarian response as a predictor for successful IVF treatment after the age of 40 years. Fertil Steril 1996;66:969–973.

19. Magarelli PC, Pearlstone AC, Buyalos RP. Discrimination between chronological and ovarian age in infertile women aged 35 years and older: predicting pregnancy using basal FSH, age and number of AIH cycles. Hum Reprod 1996;11(6):1214–1219.

20. Brown JR, Liu HC, Sewitch KF, Rosenwaks Z, Berkeley AS. Variability of day 3 FSH levels in eumenorrheic women. J Reprod Med 1995;40(9):620–624.

21. Smotrich BB, Widra EA, Gindoff PR, Levy MJ, Hall JL, Stillman RJ. Prognostic value of day 3 estradiol on in vitro fertilization outcome. Fertil Steril 1995;64(6):1136–1140.

22. Hansen LM, Batzer FR, Gutmann JN, Corson SL, Kelly MP, Gocial B. Evaluation ovarian reserve: FSH and $E_2$ variability during cycle days 2–5. Hum Reprod 1996;11(3):486–489.

23. Buyalos R, Daneshmand S, Brzechffa PR. Basal estradiol and FSH predict fecundity in women of advanced reproductive age undergoing ovulation induction therapy. Fertil Steril 1997;68: 272–277.

24. Navot P, Rosenwaks Z, Margalioth J. Prognostic assessment of female fecundity. Lancet 1987;2: 645–647.

136

25. Loumaye E, Billion JM, Mine JM, Psalti I, Pensis M, Thomas K. Prediction of individual response to COH by means of a clomiphene challenge test. Fertil Steril 1990;53:295—301.
26. Hoffman GE, Sosnowski J, Scott RT, Thie J. Efficacy of selection criteria for ovarian reserve screening using the clomiphene citrate challenge test in a tertiary center population. Fertil Steril 1996;66(1):49—53.
27. Noci I, Biagiotti R, Maggi M, Ricci F, Cinotti A, Scarselli GF. Low day 3 LH values are predictive of reduced response to ovarian stimulation. Hum Reprod 1998;13(3):531—534.
28. Mukherjee T, Copperman AB, Lapinski R, Sandler B, Bustillo M, Grunfeld L. An elevated day 3 FSH/LH ratio in the presence of a normal day 3 FSH predicts a poor response to controlled ovarian stimulation. Fertil Steril 1996;65—3:588—593.
29. Balasch J, Creus M, Fabregues F, Carmona F, Casamitjana R, Ascaso C, Vanrell JA. Inhibin, follicle-stimulating hormone, and age as predictors of ovarian response in in vitro fertilization cycles stimulated with gonadotropin-releasing hormone agonist-gonadotropin treatment. Am J Obstet Gynecol 1996;175(5):1226—1230.
30. Seifer DB, Lambert-Messercian G, Hogan JW, Gardiner AC, Blazar AS, Berk CA. Day 3 serum inhibin-B is predictive of assisted reproductive technologies outcome. Fertil Steril 1997;67: 110—114.
31. Padilla SL, Smith RD, Garcia J. The leupron screening test. Tailoring the use of leuprolide acetate in ovarian stimulation for IVF. Fertil Steril 1991;56(1):79—83.
32. Fanchin R, de Ziegler D, Olivennes F, Taieb J, Dzik A, Frydman R. EFORT test: a simple and reliable screening test for detecting poor responders in IVF. Hum Reprod 1994;9(9): 1607—1611.
33. Chang MY, Chiang CH, Chiu TH, Hsieh TT, Soong YK. The antral follicle count predicts the outcome of pregnancy in a COH/IUI programme. J Assist Reprod Genet 1998;15(1):12—17.
34. Pellicer A, Ardiles G, Neuspiller F, Remohi J, Simon C, Bonilla-Musoles F. Three dimensional ultrasound in low responders. Fertil Steril (In press).
35. Feldeberg D, Farmi J, Ashkenazi J, Dicker D, Shalev J, Ben-Rafael Z. Minidose GnRH agonist is the treatment of choice in poor responders with high FSH levels. Fertil Steril 1994;62(2): 343—346.
36. Fujii S, Sagara M, Kudo H, Kagiya A, Sato S, Saito Y. A prospective randomized comparison between long and discontinuous-long protocols of gonadotropin releasing hormone agonist for in vitro fertilization. Fertil Steril 1997;67:1166—1168.
37. Olivennes F, Righini C, Fanchin R, Torrisi C, Hazout A, Glissant M, Hernandez H, Frydman R. A protocol using a low dose of GnRH agonist might be the best protocol for patients with high FSH concentration on day 3. Hum Reprod 1996;11(6):1169—1172.
38. Balasch J, Jove I, Moreno V, Civico S, Puerto B, Vanrell JA. The comparison of two Gn-RH agonists in an IVF program. Fertil Steril 1992;58(5):991—994.
39. Padilla SL, Dugan K, Maruschak V, Shalika S, Smith RO. Use of the flare-up protocol with high dose of FSH and HMG for IVF in poor responders. Fertil Steril 1996;65(4):796—799.
40. Toth TL, Awwad JT, Veeck LL, Jones HW, Muasmer S. Suppression and flare regimens of GnRH agonist. Use in women with different basal gonadotropin values in an IVF program. J Reprod Med 1996;41:321—326.
41. Dor J, Seidman DS, Amudai E, Bider D, Levran D, Mashiach S. Adjuvant GH therapy in poor responders to IVF: a prospective randomized placebo controlled double blind study. Hum Reprod 1995;10(1):40—43.
42. Suikkari AM, Maclachlan V, Koistinen R, Seppala M, Healy D. Double blind placebo controlled study: human biosynthetic GH for ART. Fertil Steril 1996;65(4):800—805.
43. Homburg R, Ben-Rafael Z. The place of cotreatment with GH and hMG in ovarian stimulation. J Assist Reprod Genet 1996;13(5):371—373.
44. Land JA, Yarmolinskaya MI, Dumoulin J, Evers JH. High-dose hMG stimulation in poor responders does not improve IVF outcome. Fertil Steril 1996;65(5):961—965.
45. Benadiva CA, Davis O, Kligman I, Liu HC, Rosenwaks Z. Clomiphene citrate and hMG: an

alternative stimulation protocol for selected failed IVF patients. J Assist Reprod Genet 1995; 12(1):8—12.

46. Awonuga AO, Nabi A. In vitro fertilization with low-dose clomiphene citrate stimulation in women who respond poorly to superovulation. J Assist Reprod Genet 1997;14(9):503—507.

47. Jinno M, Yoshimura Y, Ubukata Y, Nakamura Y. A novel method of ovarian stimulation for in vitro fertilization: bromocriptine rebound method. Fertil Steril 1996;66:271—274.

48. Jinno M, Katsumata Y, Hoshiai T, Nakamura Y, Matsumoto K, Yoshimura Y. A therapeutic role of protactine supplementation in ovarian stimulation for in vitro fertilization: the bromocriptine rebound method. J Clin Endocrinol Metab 1997;82:3603—3611.

49. Scholtes MC, Zeilmaker GH. Blastocyst transfer in day-5 embryo transfer depends primarily on the number of oocytes retrieved and not on age. Fertil Steril 1998;69:78—83.

50. Recombinant human FSH study group. Clinical assessment of recombinant human FSH in stimulation ovarian follicular development before in vitro fertilization. Fertil Steril 1995;63:77—86.

51. Out HJ, Driessen SGA, Mannaerts BHJL, Coelingh Bennink HJT. Recombinant follicle stimulating hormone (follitropin beta, Puregon) yields higher pregnancy rates in in vitro fertilization than urinary gonadotropins. Fertil Steril 1997;68:138—142.

52. Berg C, Howles C, Borg K. Recombinant human FSH (gonal-F) vs. highly purified urinary FSH (metrodin-HP). Results of a randomized comparative study in women undergoing ART. Hum Reprod 1997;12:52—56.

53. Rombauts L, Suikkari AM, Maclahlan AM, Trounson AO, Healy DL. Recruitment of follicles by recombinant human follicle-stimulating hormone commencing in the luteal phase of the ovarian cycle. Fertil Steril 1998;69:665—669.

54. Daya S, Gunby J, Hugues EG, Collins JA, Sagle MA, Younglai EV. Natural cycles for in vitro fertilization: cost-effectiveness analysis and factors influencing outcome. Hum Reprod 1995; 10(7):1719—1724.

55. Kumar A, Benny P, Lenton EA, Cooke ID. Retrograde tubal embryo transfer in natural cycle in in vitro fertilization. Hum Reprod 1997;12(3):484—486.

56. Fabregues F, Peñarrubia J, Creus M, Moreno V, Civico S, Puerto B, Balasch J, Vanrell JA. Caracteristicas del desarrollo folicular y resultados de la FIV en ciclo no estimulado en pacientes con FSH basal elevada. Prog Obstet Ginecol 1997;40(3):2—6.

57. Lindheim SR, Vidali A, Ditkoff E, Sauer MV, Zinger M. Poor responders to ovarian hyperstimulation may benefit from an attempt at natural cycle oocyte retrieval. J Assist Reprod Genet 1997;14:174—176.

58. Heilebaut S, De Sutter P, Dhont M. Management of transient ovarian failure: pregnancy after in vitro fertilization and ICSI. A case report. J Assist Reprod Genet 1998;15(2):76—78.

59. Olivennes F, Frydman R. Friendly IVF: the way of the future? Hum Reprod 1998;13(5): 1121—1124.

60. Borini A, Bianchi L, Violini F, Maccolini A, Cattoli M, Flamigni C. Oocyte donation program: pregnancy and implantation rates in women of different ages sharing oocytes from single donor. Fertil Steril 1996;65(1):94—97.

61. Remohí J, Gartner B, Gallardo E, Yalil S, Simon C, Pellicer A. Pregnancy and birth rates after oocyte donation. Fertil Steril 1997;67(4):717—723.

# Aging and reproduction hazards

Fertility and Reproductive Medicine.
R.D. Kempers, J. Cohen, A.F. Haney and J.B. Younger, editors.

# Changes in male reproductive health?

D. Stewart Irvine

*Clinical Consultant, MRC Reproductive Biology Unit, Centre for Reproductive Biology, Edinburgh, Scotland, UK*

**Abstract.** A substantial body of evidence has accumulated in recent years suggesting that human semen quality may be deteriorating. Unfortunately the evidence remains inconclusive, with a number of publications showing clear evidence of a fall in sperm counts, and an almost equal number showing clear evidence of no change. Most of the evidence is retrospective, based on analyses of data sets collected for other purposes and there is little data from outside Europe and North America. There is as yet no evidence for any adverse change in male fertility as such. This apparent fall in sperm counts has been associated with evidence of other changes in male reproductive health, including possible increases in congenital malformations and testis cancer in man, and associated problems in wildlife. The latter evidence, particularly that relating to a birth-cohort associated increase in testis cancer is more convincing. It has been suggested that these changes may be due to environmental xenoestrogens acting during development. There is certainly good evidence of the environmental burden of potential hormone disrupting chemicals, but little evidence of the extent, if any, of human exposure. Although there is now a large quantity of data indicating that xenoestrogen exposure is a plausible hypothesis, evidence of causality, rather than association, remains to be provided. The potential importance of these changes for human health is considerable, and urgent research is required to clarify the situation.

**Keywords:** male infertility, semen analysis, sperm count, testicular cancer.

## Introduction

During the past two decades, a number of reports have appeared which have raised serious concerns about the development of reproductive problems in animals and man [1,2]. There have been reports of alligators with abnormal male genital development [3], of reproductive changes in fish and birds [4, 5], and at the same time, there have been controversial reports of changes in human semen quality [6—8], alongside reports of an increasing incidence of congenital malformations of the male genital tract, such as cryptorchidism and hypospadias [9,10], and of an increasing incidence of testicular cancer [11, 12]. However, there is controversy over whether or not these reported changes in male reproductive health are genuine [13], and if so, what the causes and implications are, in particular, the implications for clinicians caring for couples with infertility.

*Address for correspondence:* Dr D. Stewart Irvine BSc MD MRCOG, Clinical Consultant, MRC Reproductive Biology Unit, Centre for Reproductive Biology, 37 Chalmers Street, Edinburgh EH3 9EW, Scotland, UK. Tel.: +44-131-229-2575. Fax:+44-131-228-5571. E-mail: d.s.irvine@ed.ac.uk

**Testicular cancer**

Although many of the changes seen in male reproductive health are controversial, there is little argument that testis cancer is increasing in frequency, with unexplained increases in the age standardised incidence being observed in Europe [11,14,15] and in the USA [16,17]. In the west of Scotland, the number of testicular germ cell tumours registered has more than doubled between 1960 and 1990 [18], while a recent study from Norway reported an increase in the age standardised incidence for testis cancer from 2.7 to 8.5 per 100,000 from 1955 to 1992 [12]. A similar study reported a 61% increase in testis cancer in southern Norway from 1986–1987 to 1991–1992 [15]. In parts of the USA, the overall age-adjusted incidence rate of testis cancer has increased 3.5-fold during the past 60 years [17]. There is substantial geographical variation in both the incidence of testis cancer and in the observed rate of increase [11], a variation which mirrors that seen in semen quality.

The observed increases, both in Europe and the USA appear to be a birth cohort effect [14,17]. Bergstrom and colleagues [14] evaluated data from Denmark, Norway, Sweden, East Germany, Finland and Poland, including data on over 30,000 cases of testis cancer from 1945 to 1989 in men aged 20–84. They found considerable regional variation in both the incidence of testis cancer and in the observed rate of increase, ranging from a 2.3% increase annually in Sweden to 5.2% annually in East Germany. Notably, in all six countries, birth cohort was a stronger determinant for testis cancer risk than calendar time, such that men born in 1965 had a risk of testis cancer that was 3.9 times (95% CI 2.7–5.6; Sweden) to 11.4 times (95% CI 8.3–15.5; East Germany) higher than for men born in 1905. Similarly, Zheng and colleagues [17] working in the USA, concluded that the increase in testis cancer seen in men born after 1910 was mainly explained by a strong birth-cohort effect.

It is clear that men with a history of cryptorchidism have a significantly increased risk of testis cancer, estimated to be about 3.6-fold (95% CI 1.8–6.9) in one study [19] and 5.2-fold (2.1–13.0) in another [20]. The risk of testis cancer has also been found to be elevated in association with other congenital malformations including inguinal hernia, hypospadias and hydrocele [20], and it has been suggested that paternal (but not maternal) occupation before conception may alter the subsequent testis cancer risk of offspring [21], as may the parental use of agricultural fertilizers [22] or childhood residence in areas with a high nitrate concentration in ground water [23]. Whilst fathers of testis cancer sufferers have been found to have a slight increase in their own risk of the disease (about 2-fold, 95% CI 1.01–3.43) a much more significant risk attaches to the brothers of men with testis cancer, who have been estimated to have a 12-fold increase in their own risk (95% CI 3.3–31.5) [24]. These latter observations support the possible involvement of a genetic component in the aetiology of testis cancer, but also leave room for a role for factors acting during intrauterine or early neonatal life, and which might be shared by brothers. For example, in a case control study in the UK, Davies et al. [25] found that while cryptorchidism was a major risk factor for testis cancer (7.19, 95% CI 2.36–21.9) each extra quarter pint of milk consumed increased the risk by 1.39 (95% CI 1.19–1.63).

## Cryptorchidism and congenital malformations

The incidence of congenital malformation of the male genital tract may also be changing, with increases observed in the prevalence of cryptorchidism and hypospadias [26]. Cryptorchidism, for example, has increased by as much as 65–77% over recent decades in the UK [9]. In contrast, data from the USA suggested that rates of cryptorchidism have not changed [27], although one recent large study from the USA reported that rates of hypospadias have doubled from the 1970s to 1980s [28]. Here too, regional differences have been observed, although the data are less robust than is the case with testicular cancer. In one multicentre study of 8,122 boys from seven malformation surveillance systems around the world, Kallen et al. concluded that, even when differences in ascertainment were taken into account, true geographical differences exist in the prevalence of hypospadias at birth [10]. Intriguingly, this study also concluded that there seemed to be an inverse correlation between the fertility of a population (estimated from mean parity in control women) and the prevalence of isolated hypospadias at birth.

## Changing semen quality: historical data on normal men

In 1974, Nelson and Bunge [29] reported data on men presenting for vasectomy in Iowa, USA, finding a mean sperm concentration for this group of $48 \times 10^6/$ml. They compared their data with previously published data in studies of semen quality in fertile men which had reported average values for sperm concentration between 100 and $145 \times 10^6/$ml [30–32]. In 1951, MacLeod and Gold published their landmark study of semen quality in 1,000 male partners in infertile relationships, and a similar number of men of proven fertility [33], finding in the latter group an average sperm concentration of $107 \times 10^6/$ml. Nelson and Bunge thus interpreted their data as suggesting that the earlier studies were broadly consistent with each other, implying that semen quality had fallen, and speculated that their data "would tend to incriminate an environmental factor to which the entire population has been exposed" [29].

This study was followed by several reports of semen quality in fertile men which found intermediate values for average sperm concentration of $70–81 \times 10^6/$ml [34–36]. These data were reviewed by MacLeod and Wang [37] drawing together much of the available data on semen quality in fertile and infertile men, and relying heavily on their extensive data on semen quality in the male partners of infertile marriages. They concluded, that there was no evidence of a general fall in semen quality. Leto and Frensilli [38] later reported a decline in semen quality amongst potential semen donors, 77% of volunteer donors having acceptable semen quality (by AATB standards) in 1973, compared to only 37%, by the same standards, in 1980. In addition, they observed a significant overall decline in the donors' sperm concentration over the same time. In 1980, James [39] reported the first (admittedly nonsystematic) review of published data on semen quality in men of proven fertility, and in unselected normal men. Using the simple technique of unweighted rank correlation (recognising its short-comings), he noted significant negative correlations between year of publication and average sperm concentration amongst 17 papers containing data on 7,639 fertile men, and amongst 12 papers containing data on 354 unselected men.

**Changing semen quality: historical data on infertile men**

Whilst MacLeod and Wang had not seen any change in the semen quality of the male partners of infertile couples presenting in New York, two European studies reached different conclusions. In Denmark, Bostofte et al. [40] compared 1,077 men presenting for assessment of infertility in 1952 with 1,000 similar men presenting 20 years later in 1972. They observed a significant fall in sperm concentration, a decrease in qualitative motility and an increase in the proportion of sperm with abnormal morphology. Unfortunately, the two populations were not directly comparable, the men examined in 1972 being younger and of slightly higher social class. Notwithstanding this, the median sperm concentration appeared to fall from $73.4 \times 10^6$/ml in 1952 to $54.5 \times 10^6$/ml 20 years later, whilst no change was noted in ejaculate volume. Similar findings were reported in a Swedish study, the median sperm concentration amongst 185 men being investigated for infertility in 1960–1961 being $109 \times 10^6$/ml, falling to $65 \times 10^6$/ml in 1980–1981 [41].

Although controversial in their own way, these early publications failed to raise major public health concerns, perhaps because the data came from selected groups of men, unrepresentative of the general population, including men attending infertility clinics [40–42], semen donors [38] or candidates for vasectomy [29]. Perhaps also because the matter was debated in "the peaceful obscurity of the specialist journals" [43].

**Changing semen quality: the Carlsen meta analysis**

In 1992, Carlsen et al. [8] reawakened concern over the possibility of secular trends in semen quality, publishing a meta analysis of data on semen quality in normal men. The authors undertook a systematic review of available data on semen quality in normal men, published since 1930. Standard techniques applicable to meta-analysis were used to identify relevant papers, and care was taken to exclude data on infertile couples, men selected on the basis of their semen quality, and data generated using nonclassical approaches to semen analysis. Data was obtained on 14,947 men, published in 61 papers between 1938 and 1990. Unfortunately, most of the data published related to mean values for sperm concentration, with only 19/61 studies reporting the median value. Using weighted linear regression, the authors observed a decline in average ejaculate volume from 3.40 ml in 1940 to 2.75 ml in 1990. A similar analysis for sperm concentration suggested an apparent decline from $113 \times 10^6$/ml in 1940 to $66 \times 10^6$/ml in 1990. A similar significant decline in mean sperm concentration was seen when the 39 papers reporting data on men of proven fertility were analysed separately. There was no change in the average age of the men studied, and no apparent influence of age on the observed secular trend in semen quality. Given that a high proportion of the reported studies emanated from the USA (28 studies, including data on 8,329 men), this subgroup was analysed separately, and a similar trend observed. In discussing the implications of this review, the authors considered the possibilities that racial, geographical or other aspects of the populations studied could be important, together with the obvious difficulties of methodological and selection bias inherent in meta-analysis.

Predictably, the central message of this meta-analysis, that sperm counts had declined by about 50% over the past 50 years, attracted enormous attention, and generated much controversy [43—46]. Several workers published reanalyses and reinterpretations of the data presented. Bromwich and colleagues [45] noted that sperm concentration data tend not to be normally distributed, that mean sperm concentration is thus not an ideal measure of central tendency, and went on to speculate that much of the apparent change in semen quality could be accounted for by a change in the "accepted" definition of the lower limits of "normal" semen quality from around $60 \times 10^6$/ml in the 1940s [47] to the figure of $20 \times 10^6$/ml commonly accepted today [48]. This change might have led to the exclusion of men with sperm concentrations between 20 and $60 \times 10^6$/ml in the earlier studies, however, it has been pointed out that at least some of the earlier papers did include men with semen quality in this range [49].

Others presented different statistical approaches to the data suggesting that alternative models including the quadratic, spline fit and stair-step provided a better fit than the linear regression used by Carlsen et al. and might lead to different interpretation. For example, the use of linear or quadratic models tends to suggest that any change in semen quality is gradual and may be continuing, whereas the stair-step model tends to suggest that "something happened" which is not continuing. A sudden apparent fall in semen quality may be due to substantial changes in analytical methodology, subject selection criteria, study selection criteria or to the widespread introduction of a global environmental factor. Yet as Keiding and Skakkebaek point out, all of the statistical models agree on one qualitative message — a decline in semen quality over time [50]. It is very clear that the numerous epidemiological pitfalls of work in this area mean that "answering even simple questions is difficult" [43].

**Changing semen quality: contemporary data in favour**

Most of the papers that appeared immediately following the meta-analysis of

Carlsen et al. [8] provided alternative interpretations of the data — new data has since begun to emerge. This data has been able to address some of the inherent problems in a meta-analysis which used data that had been collected in different countries, at different times, on different populations and with different methods of semen analysis. Unfortunately, the available data still fail to reach a conclusion on whether or not there is any secular trend in semen quality.

Auger and colleagues published data on semen quality in fertile Parisian men [7]. They examined data on 1,750 men in a single geographical area, with consistent methods of subject recruitment and laboratory technique during a 20-year period. All their study subjects were men of proven fertility, those presenting for vasectomy and the siblings of infertile men being specifically excluded. They observed a fall in all of the classical measures of semen quality over time. Due to the size of their data set, and the length of the data collection period, these workers were able to examine the independent effects of age at donation, and year of birth, taking into account any effect of the duration of abstinence. Sperm concentration was found to be affected by age with each year of advancing age being associated with a 3.3% fall in sperm concentration. Importantly, men born later were found to have poorer semen quality, with each later year of birth being associated with a 2.6% fall in sperm concentration. Similar, although less dramatic, falls were noted in the other parameters of semen quality.

A number of other groups have published data suggesting a secular trend in semen quality amongst normal men. In a study of 577 unselected candidate semen donors in Scotland, born between 1951 and 1973, Irvine et al. [6] noted that the median sperm concentration fell from $98 \times 10^6$/ml amongst donors born before 1959 to $78 \times 10^6$/ml amongst donors born after 1970, while the median total sperm number/ejaculate fell from $301 \times 10^6$ to $214 \times 10^6$. In a similar study of 416 consecutive candidate semen donors in Belgium, Van Waeleghem et al. [51] observed declines in sperm concentration, motility and morphology. They observed a fall in sperm concentration from a mean of $71 \times 10^6$/ml to $58.6 \times 10^6$/ml when donors assessed between 1977 and 1980 were compared with those assessed between 1990 and 1995. Corresponding figures for grade-a motility were 52.7 vs. 31.7%, and for normal morphology 39.2 vs. 26.6%.

**Changing semen quality: contemporary data against**

In contrast, a number of reports have failed to find any evidence of a secular trend in semen quality. In Finland, Vierula and colleagues [52] studied 238 normal men and 5,481 men from infertile couples. They found a mean sperm concentration of $133.9 \times 10^6$/ml, a median of $90 \times 10^6$/ml, with the comparable figures for total sperm number/ejaculate being 396.6 and $309 \times 10^6$, respectively, amongst the normal men. Interestingly, these figures are significantly higher than other recent European data, being comparable to the data published by MacLeod and Gold in the USA in the 1950s [33]. Unfortunately no analysis of secular trends was presented in the group of normal men. In a similar way, a study of 302 volunteer semen donors in Toulouse, France, between 1977 and 1992 found no evidence of changes in semen quality with time [53]. Handelsman [54] examined the semen quality of 509 volunteer semen donors with a mean age of 33, presenting to one Australian unit between 1980 and 1995, and observed a median sperm concentration of $69 \times 10^6$/ml, but found no evidence of any effect of year of observation or year of birth on sperm concentration, total sperm number or ejaculate volume. In the same report, they included data on 180 men contributing semen samples in the course of clinical studies, and found that men who volunteered for studies conducted in 1987–1989 had higher sperm counts ($103–142 \times 10^6$/ml) than men volunteering for similar studies in 1990–1994 ($63–84 \times 10^6$/ml). They concluded that significant biases are introduced by subject self-selection in this area, and advocated caution in generalising from such data to the population when the sample cannot be shown to be representative of that population. This leaves open the question of whether such a representative sample can ever be obtained.

Two significant papers from the USA have provided evidence of unchanging semen quality in the populations studied. Fisch and colleagues [55] conducted a retrospective review of data on 1,283 men electing to store sperm with a commercial semen banking service prior to vasectomy between 1970 and 1974. This study involved data collection in three locations within the USA: Minnesota in the north (n = 600), New York in the east (n = 400) and Los Angeles in the west (n = 221). Unfortunately, the data was complicated by the fact that some subjects were represented by data from one semen sample, whilst others were represented by the arithmetic mean of several samples. In addition, different techniques for semen analysis were used in the different locations, at different times. Overall, this group of workers found a small but significant increase in sperm concentration with time, equivalent to about 0.65% per year. Sperm concentration rose from $77 \times 10^6$/ml in 1970 to $89 \times 10^6$/ml in 1994, whilst there were no significant changes in ejaculate volume or sperm motility. Interestingly, there was no apparent effect of age on sperm concentration, although they did observe a (positive) effect of abstinence on sperm count and ejaculate volume. The duration of abstinence did not appear to change during the period of data collection, and, notably, was not affected by age. What was particularly interesting, however, were the very marked regional variations in semen quality apparent between the three geographical locations contributing subjects to the study. For example, sperm concentrations were highest in New York (mean = $131.5 \times 10^6$/ml), intermediate in Minnesota ($100.8 \times 10^6$/ml), and lowest in California ($72.7 \times 10^6$/ml). Unfortunately, interpretation of these striking regional differences is complicated by the fact that there were differences between the centres in respect of the mean age of the subjects, in their reported duration of abstinence, and in the techniques of semen analysis.

In a study published at the same time, Paulsen and co-workers presented data on multiple semen samples from 510 normal men participating in research studies in Seattle, northwestern USA, between 1972 and 1993 [56]. These men were highly selected on the basis of normal blood chemistry, endocrine profiles and physical examination. Between 4 and 30 samples per subject were analysed and in contrast to all previous studies discussed above, sperm concentrations were determined by Coulter counter. The (geometric) mean sperm concentration in 1972 was $46.5 \times 10^6$/ml, and regression analysis showed a weak increase with time, which was statistically significant, but regarded by the authors as clinically insignificant.

In addition to the Finnish data mentioned above [52], two substantial reports have addressed the question of semen quality in the male partners of infertile couples. De Mouzon and colleagues have published what is (to date) the largest retrospective review of semen quality data [57]. Based upon the French national IVF register, they reviewed the results of 19,848 semen analyses from 7,714 men undergoing IVF for tubal disease, and having a normal semen analysis prior to IVF. They found a significant decrease in semen quality with later year of birth, the average sperm concentration in men born before 1939 being $92.5 \times 10^6$/ml, falling to $77.1 \times 10^6$/ml for men born after 1965. In a smaller study, Berling and Wölner-Hanssen [58] reported on semen quality in 718 semen samples submitted by infertile men from 1985 to 1995 in one Swedish centre, and found no relationships with age or date of birth.

## Changing semen quality?

Most recently, a very careful reanalysis of the historical data [8] on semen quality in normal men has been published [59]. These workers used multiple linear regression models, controlling for abstinence time, age, the proportion of the sample with proven fertility, specimen collection method, study goal and geographical location to examine regional differences and the interaction between region and year of publication. Using a linear model, they found that sperm concentrations and the rate of decline in sperm concentration differed significantly across regions. They concluded that there was evidence of a decline in sperm concentrations in the USA of $-1.5 \times 10^6$/ml/year (95% CI $-1.9$ to $-1.1$), and in Europe of $3.13 \times 10^6$/ml/year (95% CI $-4.96$ to $-1.30$), but not in nonwestern countries. Results were similar when other (nonlinear) models were used, and these workers concluded that their results were unlikely to be due to either confounding or selection bias [59].

Thus the available literature on secular changes in semen quality is at best inconclusive. To a greater or lesser extent, all of the available data suffer from the problems of being retrospective, collected in different countries, at different times, using different methods of subject selection and recruitment, and different laboratory methodology. The retrospective nature of the data means that control of important confounding variables is often imperfect, weakening the conclusions reached. More evidence is clearly needed, yet one is tempted to wonder whether the inherent difficulties in laboratory methodology, subject selection and the large number of potential confounding variables involved mean that it may never be possible to resolve the issue of secular trends in human semen quality with certainty.

## Regional variations: a possible clue?

Whilst the position with regard to secular changes in semen quality remains unresolved, an important observation to emerge from this work is the striking regional differences that are apparent. For example, the study by Fisch et al. [55] has already been alluded to, in which sperm concentrations were highest in New York (mean = $131.5 \times 10^6$/ml), intermediate in Minnesota ($100.8 \times 10^6$/ml), and lowest in California ($72.7 \times 10^6$/ml). Within Europe, similar patterns can be observed. Semen quality in normal Finnish men would appear to be high, with a mean sperm concentration of $133.9 \times 10^6$/ml reported [52], whilst in Paris and Edinburgh lower mean values of $98.8 \times 10^6$/ml and $104.5 \times 10^6$/ml have been reported [6,7]. In contrast, semen quality in normal men in Belgium has been reported at $66.8 \times 10^6$/ml, and in Denmark at $69.2 \times 10^6$/ml [51,60]. Whether or not there are also regional differences in the occurrence or otherwise of secular changes in semen quality is unknown [53], but it is clear that geography is an important confounding variable which requires to be taken into account when examining such data [61,62]. An example of how local this effect might be was provided by one study which found evidence of deteriorating semen quality in a group of patients resident within the area of one water supply company, but no change in the semen of similar patients living nearby [63]. Data from the French CECOS [64] has provided strong support for the existence of regional differences within France, and the recent meta-analysis by Swan et al. [59] noted that intraregional differences were at least as large as the mean decline in sperm concentration.

It is possible that these regional differences, which might be due to ethnic, environmental or lifestyle factors, could provide a valuable tool in addressing the hypothetical causes of changes in semen quality [65]. Why, for example, is the quality of semen in Finland and Denmark so apparently different? The "Finnish exception" has already provided the first evidence that these differences in semen quality may be reflected in real changes in the biological fertility of the population. Using time to pregnancy in fertile couples as a measure of fertility [66] Joffe [67] has examined antenatal population and cross-sectional studies in Finland and the UK. In both comparisons, fertility was significantly greater in Finland, than in the UK. The author therefore concluded that "the previously reported difference in sperm counts between Finland and elsewhere in northwest Europe (including Britain) is probably not artefactual, suggesting that the reported worldwide decline in semen quality is also real".

## The cause of changes in male reproductive health?

The cause of any observed changes in male reproductive health remains unknown. It is clear that lifestyle factors such as occupation [68], smoking [69], dress habits [70] and even time spent commuting [68,71] may be relevant. However, the hypothesis which has attracted most attention concerns exposure to environmental xenoestrogens during development [72].

Sertoli cells play an important role in regulating the environment within the seminiferous tubules, each Sertoli cell supporting the development of a limited number of germ cells [73]. Any perturbation in the development of the reproductive system which leads to a reduction of the Sertoli cell number will reduce the individual's ultimate capacity for sperm production in adult life. In most mammals, Sertoli cell replication occurs during fetal and postnatal life, Sertoli cell number becoming fixed at some stage of development. In the rat, Sertoli cell multiplication commences around 19—20 days of gestation and ceases at around 15 days of postnatal life [74]. In some primates, there is a rapid and substantial proliferation of Sertoli cells at the onset of puberty [75]. In man the total number of Sertoli cells increases significantly between late foetal and prepubertal life, with a further increase during puberty [76]. Hence any "window" for adverse effects on Sertoli cell multiplication may be longer in man than in other species.

The idea that exposure to "oestrogens" may affect male reproductive development is founded on the observation that FSH is involved in determining the Sertoli cell number [77], and that oestrogens produced by Sertoli cells may keep FSH levels in check by negative feedback whilst the Sertoli cell number is being determined. Hence, short-term exposure of neonatal rats to estradiol results in a suppression of FSH levels, and in consequent reductions of testicular weight and spermatogenesis in adult life, whilst exposure of rodents in utero to the synthetic oestrogen diethylstilboestrol (DES) results not only in reductions of testis size and spermatogenesis in adult life, but also in an increased incidence of cryptorchidism and hypospadias [78]. In a similar way, the male offspring of women exposed to DES during pregnancy have an increased incidence of cryptorchidism and hypospadias at birth, and of abnormal spermatogenesis in adult life [79]. It is not clear, however, whether they are any less fertile as a result [80]. The effect on testicular descent, and perhaps also on increase in testis cancer risk, would presumably be mediated through interference with the secretion of Müllerian inhibiting substance (MIS) [81,82] — testis cancer may also be a congenital condition which becomes manifest at or after puberty [83].

Thus, our understanding of the development of the male reproductive system leads to the conclusion that exposure to exogenous oestrogens may perturb this in such a way as to give rise to the changes which appear to be emerging in human health. This raises two important questions: are we exposed to more exogenous oestrogens than hitherto, and can exposure to exogenous oestrogens cause these changes in animal models?

There is certainly concern over the growing number of chemicals that may be viewed as "endocrine disrupters". The Danish Environmental Protection Agency has recently released a report raising concern over environmental chemicals with oestrogenic effects [84], whilst recent commentaries in the Lancet [85] and

BMJ [86] have highlighted the need for further research in this complex area. It is clear that there are chemicals in the environment which are "oestrogenic", and which can perturb sexual development in exposed animals [87—89]. In mammals, it has been shown that exposure of pregnant mice to ethinyl estradiol increases the frequency of gonadal dysgenesis, cryptorchidism and testicular cancer, in association with impaired Leydig cell development and reduced Sertoli cell numbers [90—92]. Gestational exposure of rats to xenoestrogens has been shown to result in reduced testicular size and sperm production [93], and we now know that exposure of pregnant sheep to xenoestrogens suppresses fetal FSH. In an attempt to estimate the familial and genetic contributions to variation in human testicular function, Handelsman [94] has studied 11 pairs of monozygotic and six pairs of dizygotic twins, and observed that sperm concentration, testicular size and SHBG all had a strong familial effect, but was unable to confirm any genetic component.

## Conclusions

Although the "environmental oestrogen" hypothesis has attracted much attention, and there exists some biological data to confirm its plausibility, evidence that it is causally related to changes in human male reproductive health remains circumstantial. The evidence for secular changes in semen quality and other changes in male reproductive health is inconclusive, with the exception of testicular cancer, although evidence for regional differences in reproductive health would appear to be stronger. In both cases, association does not imply causality, and several other possible explanations require consideration. As far as semen quality is concerned, sperm count is a poor index of fertility, and there is as yet no data on secular changes or regional differences in sperm function, although there may be some evidence of regional differences in fertility.

Whilst the available evidence is inconclusive and circumstantial its weight is considerable, and at the very least it should raise concerns that deserve to be addressed by properly designed, coordinated and funded research. Delay may compromise the fertility and reproductive health of future generations [65,86].

## References

1. Colborn T, Dumanoski D, Myers JP. Our Stolen Future. London: Penguin Group, 1996.
2. Cadbury D. The Feminization of Nature: Our Future at Risk. London: Hamish Hamilton Ltd., 1997.
3. Guillette LJ Jr, Gross TS, Masson GR, Matter JM, Percival HF, Woodward AR. Developmental abnormalities of the gonad and abnormal sex hormone concentrations in juvenile alligators from contaminated and control lakes in Florida. Environ Health Perspect 1994;102:680—688.
4. Giesy JP, Ludwig JP, Tillit DE. Deformities in birds of the great lakes region. Environ Sci and Technol 1994;28:128A,130A—135A.
5. Sumpter JP, Jobling S. Vitellogenesis as a biomarker for estrogenic contamination of the aquatic environment. Environ Health Perspect 1995;103:173—178.

6. Irvine DS, Cawood EHH, Richardson DW, MacDonald E, Aitken RJ. Evidence of deteriorating semen quality in the UK: birth cohort study in 577 men in Scotland over 11 years. Br Med J 1996;312:476–471.

7. Auger J, Kunstmann JM, Czyglik F, Jouannet P. Decline in semen quality among fertile men in Paris during the past 20 years. N Engl J Med 1995;332:281–285.

8. Carlsen E, Giwercman A, Keiding N, Skakkebæk NE. Evidence for decreasing quality of semen during past 50 years. Br Med J 1992;305:609–613.

9. Ansell PE, Bennet V, Bull D et al. Cryptorchidism: a prospective study of 7,500 consecutive male births, 1984–88. Arch Dis Child 1992;67:892–899.

10. Kallen B, Bertollini R, Castilla E et al. A joint international study on the epidemiology of hypospadias. Acta Paediatr Scand 1986;324(Suppl):1–52.

11. Adami HO, Bergstrom R, Mohner M et al. Testicular cancer in nine Northern European countries. Int J Cancer 1994;59:33–38.

12. Hoff Wanderas E, Tretli S, Fossa SD. Trends in incidence of testicular cancer in Norway 1955–1992. Eur J Cancer Part A 1995;31:2044–2048.

13. Setchell BP. Sperm counts in semen of farm animals 1932–1995. Int J Androl 1997;20(4):209–214.

14. Bergstrom R, Adami HO, Mohner M et al. Increase in testicular cancer incidence in six European countries: a birth cohort phenomenon. J Natl Cancer Inst 1996;88(11):727–733.

15. Hernes EH, Harstad K, Fossa SD. Changing incidence and delay of testicular cancer in southern Norway (1981–1992). Eur Urol 1996;30(3):349–357.

16. Devesa SS, Blot WJ, Stone BJ, Miller BA, Tarone RE, Fraumeni JF Jr. Recent cancer trends in the United States. J Natl Cancer Inst 1995;87:175–182.

17. Zheng T, Holford TR, Ma Z, Ward BA, Flannery J, Boyle P. Continuing increase in incidence of germ-cell testis cancer in young adults: experience from Connecticut, USA, 1935–1992. Int J Cancer 1996;65(6):723–729.

18. Hatton MQF, Paul J, Harding M, MacFarlane G, Robertson AG, Kaye SB. Changes in the incidence and mortality of testicular cancer in Scotland with particular reference to the outcome of older patients treated for non-seminonmatous germ cell tumours. Eur J Cancer Part A: General Topics 1995;31:1487–1491.

19. Moller H, Prener A, Skakkebaek NE. Testicular cancer, cryptorchidism, inguinal hernia, testicular atrophy, and genital malformations: case-control studies in Denmark. Cancer Cause Control 1996;7(2):264–274.

20. Prener A, Engholm G, Jensen OM. Genital anomalies and risk for testicular cancer in Danish men. Epidemiology 1996;7:14–19.

21. Knight JA, Marrett LD. Parental occupational exposure and the risk of testicular cancer in Ontario. J Occ Env Med 1997;39(4):333–338.

22. Kristensen P, Andersen A, Irgens LM, Bye AS, Vagstad N. Testicular cancer and parental use of fertilizers in agriculture. Cancer Epidem Biomark Prev 1996;5(1):3–9.

23. Moller H. Work in agriculture, childhood residence, nitrate exposure, and testicular cancer risk: a case-control study in Denmark. Cancer Epidem Biomark Prev 1997;6(2):141–144.

24. Westergaard T, Olsen JH, Frisch M, Kroman N, Nielsen JW, Melbye M. Cancer risk in fathers and brothers of testicular cancer patients in Denmark. A population-based study. Int J Cancer 1996;66(5):627–631.

25. Davies TW, Palmer CR, Ruja E, Lipscombe JM. Adolescent milk, dairy product and fruit consumption and testicular cancer. Br J Cancer 1996;74(4):657–660.

26. Editorial. An increasing incidence of cryptorchidism and hypospadias. Lancet 1985;i:1311.

27. Berkowitz GS, Lapinski RH, Dolgin SE, Gazella JG, Bodian CA, Holzman IR. Prevalence and natural history of cryptorchidism. Pediatrics 1993;92(1):44–49.

28. Paulozzi LJ, Erickson JD, Jackson RJ. Hypospadias trends in two US surveillance systems. Pediatrics 1997;100(5):831–834.

29. Nelson CMK, Bunge RG. Semen analysis: evidence for changing parameters of male fertility

potential. Fertil Steril 1974;25:503—507.

30. Hotchkiss RS. Semen analysis of 200 fertile men. Am J Med Sci 1938;196:362.

31. Farris EJ. The number of motile spermatozoa as an index of fertility in man: a study of 406 semen specimens. J Urol 1949;61:1099—1104.

32. Falk HC, Kaufman SA. What constitutes a normal semen? Fertil Steril 1950;1:489—503.

33. MacLeod J, Gold RZ. The male factor in fertility and infertility. II. Spermatozoon counts in 1,000 men of known fertility and in 1,000 cases of infertile marriage. J Urol 1951;66:436—449.

34. Sobrero AJ, Rehan N-E. The semen of fertile men. II. Semen characteristics of 100 fertile men. Fertil Steril 1975;26:1048.

35. Rehan NE, Sobrero AJ, Fertig JW. The semen of fertile men: statistical analysis of 1,300 men. Fertil Steril 1975;26:492—502.

36. Smith KD, Steinberger E. What is oligospermia? In: Troen P, Nankin HR (eds) The Testis in Normal and Infertile Men. New York: Raven Press, 1977;489—503.

37. MacLeod J, Wang Y. Male fertility potential in terms of semen quality: a review of the past, a study of the present. Fertil Steril 1979;31:103—116.

38. Leto S, Frensilli FJ. Changing parameters of donor semen. Fertil Steril 1981;36:766—770.

39. James WH. Secular trend in reported sperm counts. Andrologia 1980;12:381—388.

40. Bostofte E, Serup J, Rebbe H. Has the fertility of Danish men declined through the years in terms of semen quality? A comparison of semen qualities between 1952 and 1972. Int J Fertil 1983;28:91—95.

41. Osser S, Liedholm P, Ranstam J. Depressed semen quality: a study over two decades. Arch Androl 1984;12:113—116.

42. Menkveld R, Van Zyl JA, Kotze TJW, Joubert G. Possible changes in male fertility over a 15-year period. Arch Androl 1986;17:143—144.

43. Farrow S. Falling sperm quality: fact or fiction? Br Med J 1994;309:1—2.

44. Olsen GW, Bodner KM, Ramlow JM, Ross CE, Lipshultz LI. Have sperm counts been reduced 50 percent in 50 years? A statistical model revisited. Fertil Steril 1995;63:887—893.

45. Bromwich P, Cohen J, Stewart I, Walker A. Decline in sperm counts: an artefact of changed reference range of "normal"? Br Med J 1994;309:19—22.

46. Brake A, Krause W. Decreasing quality of semen (letter). Br Med J 1992;305:1498.

47. Macomber D, Sanders MB. The spermatozoa count. Its value in the diagnosis, prognosis and treatment of sterility. N Engl J Med. 1929;200:981—984.

48. World Health Organization. WHO Laboratory Manual for the Examination of Human Semen and Sperm-Cervical Mucus Interaction. Cambridge: University Press, 1992.

49. Keiding N, Giwercman A, Carlsen E, Skakkebaek NE. Commentary: importance of empirical evidence. Br Med J 1994;309:22.

50. Keiding N, Skakkebaek NE. Sperm decline — real or artefact? (letter). Fertil Steril 1996;65:450—451.

51. Van Waeleghem K, De Clercq N, Vermeulen L, Schoonjans F, Comhaire F. Deterioration of sperm quality in young healthy Belgian men. Hum Reprod 1996;11:325—329.

52. Vierula M, Niemi M, Keiski A, Saaranen M, Saarikoski S, Suominen J. High and unchanged sperm counts of Finnish men. Int J Androl 1996;19:11—17.

53. Bujan L, Mansat A, Pontonnier F, Mieusset R. Time series analysis of sperm concentration in fertile men in Toulouse, France between 1977 and 1992. Br Med J 1996;312:471—472.

54. Handelsman DJ. Sperm output of healthy men in Australia: magnitude of bias due to self-selected volunteers. Hum Reprod 1997;12(12):2701—2705.

55. Fisch H, Goluboff ET, Olson JH, Feldshuh J, Broder SJ, Barad DH. Semen analyses in 1,283 men from the United States over a 25-year period: no decline in quality. Fertil Steril 1996;65:1009—1014.

56. Paulsen CA, Berman NG, Wang C. Data from men in greater Seattle area reveals no downward trend in semen quality: further evidence that deterioration of semen quality is not geographically uniform. Fertil Steril 1996;65:1015—1020.

57. De Mouzon J, Thonneau P, Spira A, Multigner L. Semen quality has declined among men born in France since 1950. Br Med J 1996;313:43.
58. Berling S, Wölner-Hanssen P. No evidence of deteriorating semen quality among men in infertile relationships during the last decade: a study of males from Southern Sweden. Hum Reprod 1997;12(5):1002–1005.
59. Swan SH, Elkin EP, Fenster L. Have sperm densities declined? A reanalysis of global trend data. Environ Health Perspect 1997;105(11):1228–1232.
60. Jensen TK, Giwercnam A, Carlsen E, Scheike T, Skakkebaek NE. Semen quality among members of organic food associations in Zealand, Denmark. Lancet 1996;347:1844.
61. Lipshultz LI. "The debate continues" — the continuing debate over the possible decline in semen quality. Fertil Steril 1996;65:909–911.
62. Fisch H, Goluboff ET. Geographic variations in sperm counts: a potential cause of bias in studies of semen quality. Fertil Steril 1996;65:1044–1046.
63. Ginsburg J, Okolo S, Prelevic G, Hardiman P. Residence in the London area and sperm density (letter). Lancet 1994;343:230.
64. CECOS FFd, Auger J, Jouannet P. Evidence for regional differences of semen quality among fertile French men. Hum Reprod 1997;12(4):740–745.
65. Irvine S. Is the human testis still an organ at risk? Br Med J 1996;312:1557–1558.
66. Joffe M, Villard L, Li Z, Plowman R, Vessey M. A time to pregnancy questionnaire designed for long-term recall: validity in Oxford, England. J Epidemiol Commun Health 1995;49:314–319.
67. Joffe M. Decreased fertility in Britain compared with Finland. Lancet 1996;347:1519–1522.
68. Thonneau P, Ducot B, Bujan L, Mieusset R, Spira A. Effect of male occupational heat exposure on time to pregnancy. Int J Androl 1997;20:274–278.
69. Vine MF, Margolin BH, Morrison HI. Cigarette smoking and sperm density: a meta analysis. Fertil Steril 1994;61:35–43.
70. Tiemessen CHJ, Evers JLH, Bots RSGM. Tight-fitting underwear and sperm quality. Lancet 1996;347:1844–1845.
71. Thonneau P, Ducot B, Bujan L, Mieusset R, Spira A. Heat exposure as a hazard to male fertility. Lancet 1996;347:204–205.
72. Sharpe RM, Skakkebaeck NE. Are oestrogens involved in falling sperm counts and disorders of the male reproductive tract. Lancet 1993;341:1392–1395.
73. Orth JM, Gunsalus GL, Lamperti AA. Evidence from Sertoli cell-depleted rats indicates that spermatid number in adults depends on numbers of Sertoli cells produced during perinatal development. Endocrinology 1988;122:787–794.
74. Orth JM. Proliferation of Sertoli cells in fetal and postnatal rats: a quantitative autoradiographic study. Anat Rec 1982;203:485–492.
75. Marshall GR, Plant TM. Puberty occurring either spontaneously or induced precociously in rhesus monkey (Macaca mulatta) is associated with a marked proliferation of Sertoli cells. Biol Reprod 1996;54:1192–1199.
76. Cortes D, Muller J, Skakkebaek NE. Proliferation of Sertoli cells during development of the human testis assessed by stereological methods. Int J Androl 1987;10:589–596.
77. Orth JM. The role of follicle-stimulating hormone in controlling Sertoli cell proliferation in testes of fetal rats. Endocrinology 1984;115:1248–1255.
78. Sharpe RM. Declining sperm counts in men — is there an endocrine cause? J Endocrinology 1993;136:357–360.
79. Stillman RJ. In utero exposure to diethylstilbestrol: adverse effects on the reproductive tract and reproductive performance in male and female offspring. Am J Obstet Gynecol 1982;142:905–921.
80. Wilcox AJ, Baird DD, Weinberg CR, Hornsby PP, Herbst AL. Fertility in men exposed prenatally to diethyl stilbestrol. N Engl J Med 1995;332:1411–1416.
81. Kuroda T, Lee MM, Haqq CM, Powell DM, Manganaro TF, Donahoe PK. Mullerian inhibiting substance ontogeny and its modulation by follicle-stimulation hormone in rat testes. Endocri-

nology 1990;127:1825—1832.

82. Hirobe S, He WW, Lee MM, Donahoe PK. Mullerian inhibiting substance messenger ribonucleic acid expression in granulosa and sertoli cells coincides with their mitotic activity. Endocrinology 1992;131:854—862.

83. Skakkebaek NE, Berthelsen JG, Giwercman A, Muller J. Carcinoma-in-situ of the testis: possible origin from gonocytes and precursor of all types of germ cell tumours except spermatocytoma. Int J Androl 1987;10:19—28.

84. Danish Environmental Protection Agency. Male Reproductive Health and Environmental Chemicals with Estrogenic Effects. Copenhagen: Ministry of Environment and Energy, 1995.

85. Ginsburg J. Tackling environmental endocrine disrupters. Lancet 1996;347:1501—1502.

86. de Kretser DM. Declining sperm counts. Environmental chemicals may be to blame. Br Med J 1996;312:457—458.

87. Jobling S, Sheahan D, Osborne JA, Matthiessen P, Sumpter JP. Inhibition of testicular growth in rainbow trout (Oncorhynchus mykiss) exposed to estrogenic alkylphenolic chemicals. Environ Tox Chem 1996;15:194—202.

88. White R, Jobling S, Hoare SA, Sumpter JP, Parker MG. Environmentally persistent alkylphenolic compounds are estrogenic. Endocrinology 1994;135:175—182.

89. Jobling S, Reynolds T, White R, Parker MG, Sumpter JP. A variety of environmentally persistent chemicals, including some phthalate plasticizers, are weakly estrogenic. Environ Health Perspect 1995;103:582—587.

90. Yasuda Y, Kihara T, Tanimura T. Effects of ethinyl estradiol on the differentiation of mouse fetal testis. Teratology 1985;32:113—118.

91. Yasuda Y, Kihara T, Tanimura T, Nishimura H. Gonadal dysgenesis induced by prenatal exposure to ethinyl estradiol in mice. Teratology 1985;32:219—227.

92. Walker AH, Bernstein L, Warren DW, Warner NE, Zheng X, Henderson BE. The effect of in utero ethinyl oestradiol exposure on the risk of cryptorchid testis and testicular teratoma in mice. Br J Cancer 1990;62:599—602.

93. Sharpe RM, Fisher JS, Millar MM, Jobling S, Sumpter JP. Gestational exposure of rats to xenoestrogens results in reduced testicular size and sperm production. Environ Health Perspect 1995;103:2—9.

94. Handelsman DJ. Estimating familial and genetic contributions to variability in human testicular function: a pilot twin study. Int J Androl 1997;20(4):215—221.

# Age and fertility (a review of relevant gynaecological issues)

Allan Templeton
*Department of Obstetrics and Gynaecology, University of Aberdeen, Foresterhill, Aberdeen, UK*

**Abstract.** In this chapter the effects of aging during the reproductive life span are reviewed with particular respect to the outcome of fertility treatment. In women over the age of 35 years there is a steep decline in the success of IVF treatment such that the predicted live birth per cycle in a women aged 40 is almost half that seen in a women aged 35 years. Similar effects are seen with COH and IUI treatment, where it is doubtful that the life birth rates seen in women over 40 can justify the use of treatment in this age group. Live birth rates with donor insemination may be enhanced where intrauterine insemination is used and comparative studies are urgently needed, particularly in the older age groups. Attempts to reverse the effects of age on fertility treatment are invariably ineffective, the one exception being the use of donor eggs, where success is correlated to the age of the donor. Besides age, a number of other factors including basal FSH and E2 levels, as well as ovarian stimulation tests, can be used as predictors of outcome. Finally the acquisition with age of uterine problems may be expected to affect implantation, but these are confined to intracavity fibroids and postradiation or chemotherapy damage.

**Keywords:** age, donor insemination, fertility treatment, intrauterine insemination, IVF, treatment outcome.

## Introduction

In stark contrast to men, it has been projected that the life expectancy at birth for women will increase in the developed world to about 90 years by the year 2020 [1]. This will, however, make no difference to the length of the reproductive life span, which will remain essentially unaltered, and will make up only one-third of the total life span for many women. This chapter is concerned with ageing during the reproductive years and is primarily concerned with the effects of age on the ovary and the acquisition of pelvic and particularly uterine disorders. The focus of the chapter is the effect of these factors on the outcome of fertility treatment.

## Fecundity

Leridon's research on age-specific fertility in selected populations not using contraception indicated a decline in fertility throughout the reproductive years, and certainly after the age of 20 [2]. This decline is gradual until the age of 35, after

*Address for correspondence:* Prof Allan Templeton MD, Department of Obstetrics and Gynaecology, University of Aberdeen, Foresterhill, Aberdeen, AB25 2ZD, UK. Tel.: +44-1224-840590. Fax: +44-1224-648440. E-mail: allan.templeton@abdn.ac.uk

which it steepens considerably. Similarly, the French "Federation des Centres d'Etude et de Conservation du Sperme Humain" (CECOS) study of the results of artificial insemination in over 2,000 nulliparous women with azoospermic husbands indicates a significant decrease in the cumulative success rate for women over the age of 30 years [3]. Assessing all pregnancies, this study showed a mean rate per cycle of 10.5% at 26—30 years, 9.1% at 31—35 years and 6.5% over the age of 35. Similarly, the cumulative success rates after 12 cycles of treatment were 74, 61 and 54%, respectively.

If both these studies are accepted as reasonable estimates of natural fecundity, it is clear that this is lower in women in their 30s and particularly in women in their late 30s. This will have relevance for the timing of infertility investigations, and particularly surgical interventions such as laparoscopy. Older women who are not sterile will require longer to conceive than younger women and should therefore be given longer, in the absence of a history suggestive of disease, prior to considering laparoscopy. In practice the reverse is often true with younger women given longer with the result that laparoscopy is more likely to reveal pelvic pathology than in older women.

Fertility treatment cannot reverse the process of aging (except of course by egg donation). The effects of age are particularly important on single cycle interventions such as IVF and gamete intrafallopian transfer (GIFT). Interventions such as tubal surgery can be expected to provide enhanced fertility over a longer period of time in successive cycles. It might be expected that the replacement of several embryos in IVF treatment or the stimulation of several follicles, as is frequently done with intrauterine insemination, would diminish the effects of age. However, it seems that this is not necessarily the case, as outlined below.

**Fertility treatment**

*In vitro fertilisation*

It is well-established that age is the major factor determining the outcome of in vitro fertilisation [4]. Using the database established by the Human Fertilisation and Embryology Authority (HFEA) of all IVF cycles carried out in the UK, during 1991—94 (over 50,000 cycles) the relationship between age and live birth rate was modelled by the method of fractional polynomials. A logistic regression was used to predict the probability of a live birth for individual women [4]. Live birth rates were maximal in women aged 30 years and were less in both younger and older women. For a woman aged 30, the predicted live birth rate (95% confidence limits) was 16.1 (15.0—17.3). For older women the predicted live birth rates were 13.9 (13.4—14.3) for age 35, 7.3 (6.7—7.8) for age 40, and 1.9 (1.4—2.5) for age 45. There were no pregnancies through IVF in women over the age of 46 years. Of these cycles, 59% involved the transfer of three embryos, 31% two embryos, and 10% one embryo. (The transfer of more than three embryos is prohibited in the UK). The equivalent figures for live births using oocyte recovery as the denominator were 17.7, 18.5, 15.5, 8.6 and 2.5 and for embryo transfer, 21.1, 21.6, 17.9, 10.0 and 3.0%, respectively.

Similarly, the effects of age were apparent in the recently published 1995 Assisted Reproduction Technology Success Rates from the USA and Canada, where 77% of women having assisted reproduction (IVF and GIFT) are between 30 and 40 years of age [5,6]. Success rates are fairly constant, at around 25% live birth rate per cycle, until the age of 34 years when there is a steep decline. Again no pregnancies were recorded among women over the age of 46 years.

Analysis of the UK data showed that previous pregnancy, and particularly previous live birth, enhanced the likelihood of a successful outcome to IVF treatment. In fact, the chance of pregnancy was almost doubled if this previous live birth was a result of IVF treatment [4]. Analysis of the American database indicates the same effect and confirms that the enhancement is evident in all age groups.

Furthermore, the American results indicate that in women under the age of 35, the replacement of more than three embryos does not enhance the outcome of IVF treatment, all that is achieved is an increase in the multiple birth rate. Similarly, in all age groups studied in the UK database, the number of eggs fertilised and available for transfer appears to be more important in predicting outcome than the number of embryos actually transferred.

There is of course a dramatic reversal of the effects of age when donor eggs are used. Here it is evident that the outcome is related to the age of the egg donor rather than the egg recipient. In the UK all egg donors must be aged 35 or younger. Live birth rates per embryo transfer in women who received donated eggs were 22% for women under the age of 30, 28% for women aged 30—34, 26% for women aged 35—39, and 19% for women aged 40—44. Thus, although the results are dependent mainly on the age of the egg donor, there was a significant downward trend in the birth rates above the age of 30 indicating a small but significant uterine effect on the outcome. Whether this is an effect of age per se, or the acquisition of pathology as part of the aging process is unclear at this stage. It has been suggested that the effect of ageing on uterine receptivity can be reversed by the use of high doses of progesterone, and that where approximately physiological levels have been used, a decline in implantation with increasing age is evident [7]. However, this is yet to be confirmed in randomised studies. Similarly, the suggestion that amenorrhoeic women may have improved implantation after sex steroid replacement, compared to cycling women, needs to be confirmed [8,9]. It appears that the endometrium fails to respond to steroid replacement only in exceptional cases, including after radiotherapy or chemotherapy, although there may also be an impaired responsiveness in Turner syndrome [10].

In summary, none of the ways of reversing the effects of age on the outcome of IVF treatment have been proven to be effective. These attempts have included varied stimulation protocols, oocyte manipulation, coculture and embryo hatching [11].

*Controlled ovarian hyperstimulation and intrauterine insemination*

Two meta-analyses have confirmed the effectiveness of controlled ovarian hyperstimulation and intrauterine insemination in the treatment of unexplained infertility, endometriosis and male factor infertility, although the treatment appears to be less effective in the case of endometriosis and male factor infertility [12,13]. Furthermore, these analyses have indicated that separately both controlled ovarian hyperstimulation (COH) and intrauterine insemination (IUI) enhance conception rates per cycle, although in the case of IUI alone for male factor infertility, it is unlikely that this would ever be clinically useful as the conception rate per cycle is so low. Neither of the meta-analyses have addressed specifically the separate effects of age on the outcome of treatment, although other studies have. Pearlstone et al. [14] analysed over 400 cycles in 85 women over the age of 40 and demonstrated a pregnancy rate of 3.5% per cycle, although the live birth rate was only 1.2% per cycle (confidence limits 0.2–2.3%). No woman over the age of 43 became pregnant and no woman aged 40–43 where the FSH was elevated above 25 IU/l became pregnant. Frederick et al. [15] confirmed in a smaller retrospective study the very poor success rates in women over the age of 40 compared to women less than 40 where rates of 10% per cycle were generally achieved. In the older women the pregnancy rate per cycle was 5.2% but because of the concomitant high abortion rate, the live birth rate per cycle was only 1.4%. The cumulative pregnancy rate per patient was at best 3.9%. Agarwal and Buyalos [16] reported a series of 664 cycles involving 290 women, aged 22–48 years. Stimulation was with clomiphene and intrauterine insemination was carried out. The clinical pregnancy rate in those under 30 was 19% per cycle and in those over 40, 5% per cycle. Almost all of the pregnancies had occurred by the fourth cycle of treatment, regardless of the age. Finally, Brzechffa and Buyalos [17] analysed retrospectively 363 cycles in which ovarian stimulation with human menopausal gonadotrophin and intrauterine insemination was carried out. They found that age was the main determinant of outcome and furthermore that the use of high doses of hMG was also indicative of a poor outcome.

Thus, it is doubtful that controlled ovarian stimulation and intrauterine insemination is useful in women over 40. Assessment of background spontaneous pregnancy rates should be carried out and data are now available from a number of studies in this respect [18]. Also, comparisons with the likely outcome of IVF treatment should be considered before embarking on treatment in this age group. Women over 40 years should be aware that their chance of a birth per treatment cycle is unlikely to be better than 1–2%.

*Donor insemination*

The above-mentioned CECOS study indicated the progressive fall with age in the success rates of donor insemination used to treat the wives of azoospermic men [3]. Similarly, the HFEA database has indicated a progressive fall in success rates in women over the age of 25 treated with donor insemination [19]. Live birth rates per treatment cycle under the age of 25 were 10.7% and in the age group 25–29, 11.4%. For each subsequent 5-year age group, the live birth rates were 9.8, 6.8 and 2.7%, respectively, and over the age of 45, 2.2%, although only 93 cycles were recorded in this age group. The effects of ovarian stimulation and also intrauterine insemination are not yet available for analysis, using this database. However, Kang and Wu [20] report the effects of age in this respect. Using IUI with frozen donor sperm they report cycle conception rates of 20% for women aged 35 and less, 12% aged 35–40 years and 6% over the age of 40 years. However, they also reported cumulative pregnancy rates of 42% over the age of 40 after seven cycles of treatment. Thus it appears that treatment in older age groups may be justified, particularly where IUI is used. However, further prospective comparative studies are needed in this area, particularly as the alternative treatment is IVF and intracytoplasmic sperm injection (ICSI) with either husband's sperm or with frozen donor sperm.

## Other factors predicting a reduction in fertility

Although menstrual irregularity and anovulation precede the menopause, normal women over the age of 40 experience a decrease in fertility despite regular, apparently ovulatory, cycles. It is well-established that the follicular phase in older women is significantly shorter [21], although the preovulatory follicles may be the same size [22] and the luteal phase is, if anything, longer [23]. Furthermore, there may be both an elevation of FSH and serum or intrafollicular oestradiol levels in the older woman [22,24], but with other follicular fluid steroids indicative of healthy follicles [22]. Thus it appears that there are changes in follicular response in older women, but that generally the follicles appear healthy. Whether this response is a result of intrinsic ovarian aging or changes in the hypothalamic-pituitary axis associated with age, is unclear, although further studies indicate the problem is follicular recruitment [25], suggesting there may be a numerical problem in the availability of follicles.

Higher FSH levels and ovarian reserve screening using a variety of challenges including clomiphene and GnRH agonist, may be predictive of outcome, although age remains the major influence [26]. Toner et al. [27] indicated that age and FSH were independent predictors of IVF response, although others have indicated that the interaction is more important [26,28].

Despite these observations, the major problem associated with age relates to the oocyte, which shows both reduced ability to fertilise and reduced implantation potential in the older woman. Furthermore, even if implantation occurs, there is an increased risk of aneuploidy, early pregnancy loss, and also miscarriage. Even after the detection of fetal cardiac activity, there is a profound impact of age on pregnancy outcome. In one study among infertile women, a 5-fold increase in the spontaneous abortion rate was observed in women over 40 years (20%) compared to 31–35 years (4%) [29]. It has previously been observed that infertile women have a higher rate of both clinical [30] and subclinical pregnancy loss [31]. However, in IVF treatment it has been clearly demonstrated that miscarriage rates are related to the age of the egg (donor) rather than the age of the uterus (recipient) [32].

Thus, it is unlikely that clinical or embryological manipulations, whether aimed at the follicle or the egg, can alter the intrinsic-age-related changes within the oocyte. However, besides age, it appears that elevated FSH and E2 levels, as well as the response to ovarian stimulation, may be helpful in predicting the outcome of fertility treatment.

## Other gynaecological problems affecting fertility

Besides the effects of age on the hypothalamic pituitary ovarian axis described above, the major age-related factors likely to affect fertility are uterine fibroids, endometriosis and pelvic infection. It is well-established that the likelihood of acquiring one of these pathologies increases with age.

Uterine leiomyomas are thought to occur in 30% of women over the age of 30, although surprisingly little is known about the pathophysiology [33]. A number of factors are associated with the risk of developing uterine leiomyoma, but adjusting for these and allowing for age, the major factor is black race [34]. Perhaps surprisingly the protective effect of smoking has been confirmed in several observational studies [35,36].

In general it can be stated that the effect of fibroids on fertility in any individual patient remains uncertain [37]. It appears that fibroids that are not distorting the cavity of the uterus will not impair fertility. This conclusion is most secure in the context of IVF treatment [38—40]. However, fibroids that have been shown to distort the uterine cavity will significantly reduce the chance of successful implantation [38].

In the USA, endometriosis is the third most common gynaecological disorder necessitating hospital admission [41]. It is more commonly diagnosed in older women and highest rates are among white women age 40—44 years. The association of endometriosis with infertility is well-documented although a causal relationship with minimal or mild endometriosis remains uncertain. The findings of the recent Canadian surgical treatment study [42], may lend support to the concept that certain cases of mild endometriosis cause subfertility. On the other hand, drug treatment of mild endometriosis appears to have no effect on fertility [43]. However, it is well-established that regardless of age, the presence of endometriosis does not have an adverse effect on the outcome of IVF treatment. Fertilisation and implantation rates appear to be the same or better than other diagnostic groups [4].

Turning to pelvic inflammatory disease (PID), age-specific rates for acute episodes of PID are highest for women under the age of 25. Teenagers have the highest relative risk. The consequences of PID, namely chronic pelvic infection, infertility and ectopic pregnancy, are seen more frequently in older age groups [44].

It is now recognised in the Western world that chlamydia is the main organism causing PID and is particularly prevalent in men and women under the age of 30 years and particularly teenagers. Pelvic inflammatory disease was the most common gynaecological reason for admission to hospital in the USA during 1998—90. The highest rates were in age groups less than 40 years. Tubal disease remains a major cause of infertility, particularly secondary infertility, and in the UK accounted for 40% of all IVF cycles carried out in 1995—96. Overall, there appears to be no detrimental effect of tubal infertility on the outcome of IVF treatment, although there is evidence of a slightly reduced implantation rate (birthrate per embryo transfer) compared to unexplained infertility [4]. The contribution of hydrosalpinges to this reduction in birth rate has recently been reviewed [45], but it is less clear that removal of hydrosalpinges prior to IVF has proven beneficial. Such a recommendation will require the completion of a randomised controlled study.

## Conclusion

Age is the main determinant of the outcome of fertility treatment and the effect is almost entirely ovarian in origin. The acquisition of gynaecological disease may affect fertility, but is much less likely to affect the outcome of treatment except in specific circumstances.

## References

1. Murray CJ, Lopez AD. Alternative projections of mortality and disability by cause 1990—2020: global burden of disease study. Lancet 1997;349:1498—1504.
2. Leridon H. Human Fertility: The Basic Components. Chicago: University of Chicago Press, 1977;107.
3. CECOS, Schwartz D, Mayaux MJ. Female fecundity as a function of age. N Engl J Med 1982; 306:404—406.
4. Templeton A, Morris JK, Parslow W. Factors that affect outcome of in vitro fertilisation treatment. Lancet 1996;348:1402—1406.
5. Centers for Disease Control and Prevention. US Dept. of Health and Human Services. 1995 Assisted Reproductive Technology Success Rates. National Summary and Fertility Clinic Reports 1997;3:1—23.
6. Society for Assisted Reproductive Technology and the American Society for Reproductive Medicine. Assisted reproductive technology in the United States and Canada: 1995 results generated from the American Society for Reproductive Medicine/Society for Assisted Reproductive Technology Registry. Fertil Steril 1998;69:389—398.
7. Meldrum DR. Female reproductive aging — ovarian and uterine factors. Fertil Steril 1993; 49:1—5.
8. Edwards RG, Matcos S, Macnamel M, Balmaceda JP, Walters DE, Asch R. High fecundity of amenorrhoeic women in embryo-transfer programmes. Lancet 1991;338:292—294.
9. Remohi J, Yalil S, Gartner B, Simon C, Gallardo E, Pellicer A. Pregnancy and birth rates after oocyte donation. Fertil Steril 1997;67:717—723.
10. Khastgir G, Abdalla H, Thomas A, Korea L, Latarche L, Studd J. Oocyte donation in Turner syndrome: an analysis of the factors affecting the outcome. Hum Reprod 1997;12:279—285.

164

11. Marcus SF, Brinsden PR. In vitro fertilization and embryo transfer in women aged 40 years and over (review). Hum Reprod Update 1996;2:459—468.
12. Hughes EG. The effectiveness of ovulation induction and intrauterine insemination in the treatment of persistent infertility: a meta-analysis. Hum Reprod 1997;12:1865—1872.
13. Cohlen BJ, Vanderkerckhove P, Te Velde ER, Habbema JDF. Intrauterine insemination for treating male subfertility. In: Templeton A, O'Brien S, Cooke I (eds) Evidence-Based Fertility Treatment. London: RCOG Press (In press).
14. Pearlstone AC, Fournet N, Gambone JC, Pang SC, Buyaloss RP. Ovulation induction in women age 40 and older: the importance of basal follicle-stimulating hormone level and chronological age. Fertil Steril 1992;58:674—679.
15. Frederick JL, Denker MS, Rojas A, Horta I, Stone SC, Asch RH, Balmaceda JP. Is there a role for ovarian stimulation and intrauterine insemination after age 40? Hum Reprod 1994;9: 2284—2286.
16. Agarwal SK, Buyalos RP. Clomiphene citrate with intrauterine insemination: is it effective therapy in women above the age of 35 years? Fertil Steril 1996;65:759—763.
17. Brzechffa PR, Buyalos RP. Female and male partner age and menotrophin requirements influence pregnancy rates with human menopausal gonadotrophin therapy in combination with intrauterine insemination. Hum Reprod 1997;12(1):29—33.
18. Collins JA, Burrows EA, Willan AR. The prognosis for live birth among untreated infertile couples. Fertil Steril 1995;64:22—28.
19. HFEA. Human Fertilisation and Embryology Authority. Sixth Annual Report, 1997;11—45.
20. Kang BM, Wu T-CJ. Effect of age on intrauterine insemination with frozen donor sperm. Obstet Gynecol 1996;88:93—98.
21. Sherman B, Wallace R, Treloar A. The menopausal transition: endocrinologic and epidemiologic considerations. J Biol Sci 1979;6:19.
22. Klein NA, Battaglia DE, Miller PB, Branigan EF, Giudice LC, Soules MR. Ovarian follicular development and the follicular fluid hormones and growth factors in normal women of advanced reproductive age. J Clin Endocrinol Metab 1996;81:1946—1951.
23. Gindoff PR, Jewelewicz R. Reproductive potential in the older woman. Fertil Steril 1986; 46:989—1001.
24. Buyalos RP, Daneshmand S, Brzechffa PR. Basal estradiol and follicle-stimulating hormone predict fecundity in women of advanced reproductive age undergoing ovulation induction therapy. Fertil Steril 1997;68:272—277.
25. Batista MC, Cartledge TP, Zellmer AW, Merino MJ, Axiotis C, Bremner WJ, Nieman LK. Effects of aging on menstrual cycle hormones and endometrial maturation. Fertil Steril 1995; 64:492—499.
26. Scott RT Jr, Hofmann GE. Prognostic assessment of ovarian reserve (Review). Fertil Steril 1995;63:1—11.
27. Toner JP, Philput CB, Jones GS, Muasher SJ. Basal follicle-stimulating hormone level is a better predictor of in vitro fertilization performance than age. Fertil Steril 1991;55:784—791.
28. Magarelli PC, Pearlstone AC, Buyalos RP. Discrimination between chronological and ovarian age in infertile women aged 35 years and older; predicting pregnancy using basal follicle stimulating hormone, age and number of ovulation induction/intrauterine insemination cycles. Hum Reprod 1996;11:1214—1219.
29. Smith KE, Buyalos RP. The profound impact of patient age on pregnancy outcome after early detection of fetal cardiac activity. Fertil Steril 1996;65:35—40.
30. Templeton A, Fraser C, Thompson B. The epidemiology of infertility in Aberdeen. Br J Med 1990;301:148—152.
31. Hakim RB, Gray RH, Zacur H. Infertility and early pregnancy loss. Am J Obstet Gynecol 1995;172:1510—1517.
32. Abdalla HI, Burton G, Kirkland A, Johnson MR, Leonard T, Brooks AA, Studd JW. Age, pregnancy and miscarriage: uterine versus ovarian factors. Hum Reprod 1993;8:1512—1517.

33. Andersen J, Barbieri RL. Abnormal gene expression in uterine leiomyomas (Review). J Soc Gynecol Invest 1995;2:663–672.
34. Marshall LM, Spiegelman D, Barbieri RL, Goldman MB, Manson JE, Colditz GA, Willett WC, Hunter DJ. Variation in the incidence of uterine leiomyoma among premenopausal women by age and race. Obstet Gynecol 1997;90:967–973.
35. Parazzini F, Negri E, La Vecchia C, Rabaiotti M, Luchini L, Villa A, Fedele L. Uterine myomas and smoking. Results from an Italian study. J Reprod Med 1996;41:316–320.
36. Samadi AR, Lee NC, Flanders WD, Boring JR 3rd, Parris EB. Risk factors for self-reported uterine fibroids: a case control study. Am J Pub Health 1996;86:858–862.
37. Miller CE. Are fibroids a cause of infertility? Infertil Reprod Med Clin N Am 1997;4:639–647.
38. Farhi J, Ashkenazi J, Feldberg D, Dicker D, Orvieto R, Ben Rafael Z. Effect of uterine leiomyomata on the results of in vitro fertilization treatment. Hum Reprod 1995;10:2576–2578.
39. Ramzy AM, Sattar M, Amin Y, Mansour RT, Serour GI, Aboulghar MA. Uterine myomata and outcome of assisted reproduction. Hum Reprod 1998;13:198–202.
40. Stovall DW, Parrish SB, Van Voorhis BJ, Hahn SJ, Sparks AET, Syrop CH. Uterine leiomyomas reduce the efficacy of assisted reproduction cycles: results of a matched follow-up study. Hum Reprod 1998;13:192–197.
41. Velebil P, Wingo PA, Zia Z, Wilcox LS, Peterson HB. Rate of hospitalization for gynecologic disorders among reproductive-age women in the United States. Obstet Gynecol 1995;86:764–769.
42. Marcoux S, Maheux R, Berube S. Canadian collaborate group on endometriosis. Laparoscopic surgery in infertile women with minimal or mild endometriosis. N Engl J Med 1997;337:217–222.
43. Hughes EG, Fedorkow DM, Collins JA. A quantitative overview of controlled trials in endometriosis-associated infertility. Fertil Steril 1993;59:973–970.
44. Washington AE. Pelvic inflammatory disease: linking epidemiological trends, determinants and prevention. In: Templeton A (ed) The Prevention of Pelvic Infection. RCOG Press, 1996;3–13.
45. Nackley AC, Muasher SJ. The significance of hydrosalpinx in in vitro fertilization. Fertil Steril 1998;69:373–384.

© 1998 Elsevier Science B.V. All rights reserved.
Fertility and Reproductive Medicine.
R.D. Kempers, J. Cohen, A.F. Haney and J.B. Younger, editors.

# Oocyte donation

José Remohí, Manuel Muñoz, Gerardo Ardiles and Fernando Neuspiller
*Instituto Valenciano de Infertilidad, Valencia, Spain*

**Abstract.** Oocyte donation is an increasingly popular method that is used to reach the target of having a healthy child at home, in couples with irreversible infertility. The indications of this technique have increased from early egg donation because of premature ovarian failure (POF), heritable maternal genetic abnormalities, physiologic menopause, low responders to ovarian stimulation and women who have previously undergone multiple unsuccessful in vitro fertilization attempts. In the following years, perhaps we will be able to establish new indications for oocyte donation.

This article concerns the protocol that recipients underwent at the Instituto Valenciano de Infertilidad and our general results obtained with this technique.

We also review the lessons learned from oocyte donation, like the handling of ovarian suppression, the long-term effects of oestradiol administration, several aspects about the age of the recipients, aspects about the endometrial thickness and serum oestradiol levels as predictors of outcome, the handling of low responders and aspects about donors with endometriosis and polycystic ovary syndrome.

**Keywords:** age, endometrial thickness, endometriosis, low responders, oestradiol levels, ovarian suppression.

Oocyte donation is an increasingly popular method for establishing pregnancies in irreversibly infertile women. It was in the mid-1980s that the first descriptions were reported [1,2] of pregnancies resulting from donated oocytes fertilized in the laboratory and transferred into women deprived of ovarian function.

## Indications

These early egg donations were all achieved in women suffering from premature ovarian failure (POF) and who had received hormonal replacement regimens designed to duplicate the endocrine environment of the menstrual cycle [3]. Subsequently, the indications for ovum donation were expanded to cases with heritable, maternal genetic abnormalities [4], physiologic menopause [5], low responders to ovarian stimulation [4], and women who had previously undergone multiple unsuccessful IVF attempts [6]. Perhaps the future will bring new indications for this technique of assisted reproduction.

*Address for correspondence:* José Remohí MD, Instituto Valenciano de Infertilidad, C/ Guardia Civil 23, 46020 Valencia, Spain.

## Protocol for recipients

The protocol of steroid replacement for recipients is briefly described. Patients with ovarian function were desensitized with daily SC administration of 1 mg leuprolide acetate (LA, Procrin; Abbott S.A., Madrid, Spain) or 3.75 mg of LA depot beginning in the secretory phase of the previous cycle. Hormonal replacement started on day 1 of the cycle with administration of 2 mg/day E2 valerate (Progynova; Schering Spain, Madrid, Spain) from days 1 to 8; 4 mg/day from days 9 to 11; and 6 mg/day from day 12 onwards. After 13 days of E2 valerate administration, recipients were ready to receive oocytes and they waited until a donation became available. In case of spotting during E2 valerate administration, the patient was cycled with 10 mg medroxyprogesterone acetate (Progevera; Schering Spain) for 10 days, and a new cycle was started.

At the day of recovery of the donated oocytes, 100 mg/day of natural P in oil IM was administered, or 800 mg/day of intravaginal micronized progesterone (Progeffik: Effik Spain). Embryo transfer was performed 48 h after oocyte recovery using the vaginal route. The regimen of 6 mg/day E2 valerate and P was maintained for 15 days, after which a urinary $\beta$-hCG analysis was performed. In the case of positive results, E2 valerate and P were maintained at the same dosage until day 100 of the pregnancy.

## Results

Our general results of the ovum donation program were published and are shown in Table 1 [7]. A total of 627 ETs was performed in 397 women during the study period. A mean of 4.1 ± 1.0 (mean ± SEM) embryos were replaced per transfer. A total of 2,340 embryos were replaced into the uterus and 430 were implanted (implantation rate, 18.3%). This resulted in 325 clinical pregnancies, 66 of which were early miscarriages (20.3%), five tubal pregnancies (1.5%), and 33 preterm deliveries (10.2%). The total number of term deliveries was 221. Because all 33 preterm gestations ended in at least a live birth, the number of term pregnancies plus the number of preterm deliveries has been considered as the total number of live birth deliveries. The pregnancy rate (PR), after one cycle was 53.4% (CI

*Table 1.* Cumulative pregnancy and live birth rates in 627 cycles of oocyte donation.

| No. of attempts | Total cycles | Pregnancies[a] | Cumulative pregnancy rate | 95% Confidence interval | Live births[a] | Cumulative live birth rate | 95% Confidence interval |
|---|---|---|---|---|---|---|---|
| 1 | 397 | 212 (53.4) | 53.4 | 59.9−55.9 | 169 (42.6) | 42.6 | 40.1−45.1 |
| 2 | 149 | 70 (47.0) | 75.3 | 71.8−78.8 | 52 (34.9) | 62.6 | 58.6−66.6 |
| 3 | 53 | 26 (46.4) | 86.8 | 82.1−91.4 | 21 (39.6) | 77.4 | 71.6−83.1 |
| ⩾4 | 28 | 17 (60.7) | 94.8 | 90.6−99.0 | 12 (42.8) | 88.7 | 88.1−89.3 |

[a]Values in parentheses are percentages.

50.9—55.9%), with a delivery rate of 42.6% (CI 40.1—45.1%). Accumulated PR increased up to 94.8% (CI 90.6—99.0%) after four transfers. Similarly, live birth rates reached 88.7% (CI 88.1—89.3%) after four attempts of ET by ovum donation.

As mentioned above, 71 of the 325 clinical pregnancies were miscarriages or ectopic pregnancies, whereas the remaining 33 were the result of spontaneous (n = 12) or induced (n = 21) embryo reduction. From the 430 initially implanted embryos, a total of 326 newborn infants were the result. Table 2 also shows the mean weights at birth as well as the number of perinatal deaths and major congenital malformations in the population studied. Mental retardation due to immaturity is included in this list as well as Poland syndrome, spina bifida, myelomeningocele, and phocomelia.

Complications during pregnancy included 29 cases of pregnancy-induced hypertension, two cases of gestational diabetes, four cases of premature rupture of membranes, and one case of placenta previa.

The results have been analyzed further, taking into account several interesting parameters such as age of the recipient, ovarian function, and indication for entering the ovum donation program. There were no statistical differences among the life tables calculated for each age group. Women in the age group < 30 years showed the highest cumulative live birth rate with the lowest number of attempts.

**Lessons learned from oocyte donation**

*Ovarian suppression*

Initial reports of ovum donation in normally ovulatory women were based on the measurements of LH surge in recipients and donors and synchronization within 24 h of each other [8,9]. However, Serhal and Craft [10] simplified the technique by administering exogenous steroids to women undergoing oocyte donation regardless of their ovarian function and demonstrated that pregnancy can be achieved by simple administration of E2 valerate and P in regularly cycling women and that the advocated pituitary suppression with GnRH-a before steroid therapy [11] was unnecessary. In this preliminary report, neither the actual per-

*Table 2.* Outcome of newborns obtained from ovum donation.

| Pregnancy | Delivered | Weight[a] (g) | Live births | Perinatal death | Malformations |
|-----------|-----------|---------------|-------------|-----------------|---------------|
| Single | 188 | 3058 ± 316 | 183 | 5 | 2 |
| Twins | 122 | 2450 ± 730 | 1117 | 5 | 2 |
| Triplets | 12 | 2139 ± 548 | 12 | 0 | 0 |
| Quadruplets | 4 | 1540 ± 189 | 4 | 0 | 1 |
| Total | 326 | | 316 | 10 | 5 |

[a]Values are means ± SEM.

formance of oocyte donation in low responders nor the ovarian function during the artificial cycle were properly analyzed [10].

In a second paper, the performance of low responders in oocyte donation was reported to be similar to women with POF. The authors observed ovulation especially in young women and employed sublingual E2 valerate or GnRH-a [12] to override this problem. A recent report using transdermal E2 has shown that women with regular menses employing exogenous steroids in the absence of pituitary suppression have an LH surge, but neither follicular development nor a rise in serum P were observed, suggesting ovarian quiescence [13].

We published our results comparing cycles with or without the use of aGnRH [14]. A total of 69 women undergoing oocyte donation because of either POF (n = 10) or low response in IVF (LR, n = 59) were included in our study. There was no difference between groups I (POF) and II (LR) regarding age and cause of infertility of the donors (polycystic ovaries: 13 and 15 cases; tubal infertility: six and seven; idiopathic infertility: six and four; endometriosis: three and five; male infertility: six and four; and fertile women: three and two, respectively). The percentage of subnormal semen samples was also no different between groups (37.8 and 35.1%, respectively). Similarly, some of the characteristics of the stimulation, such as the number of days a patient was treated with GnRHa before ovarian stimulation began, the total number of days under GnRH treatment, the number of ampoules of gonadotrophins, as well as days of stimulation, were considered. There was no difference between groups I and II regarding these parameters.

Analyzing the results of embryo transfer after oocyte donation, there was no difference between groups 1 and II in the numbers of donated oocytes and embryos replaced (3.8 ± 0.2 and 4.2 ± 0.1, respectively). A total of 37 embryo transfers were performed in each group, resulting in a 48.6% clinical pregnancy rate in the group treated with GnRHa, while women without analogues displayed a 56.8% clinical pregnancy rate per transfer; these rates were not significantly different. Implantation rates, defined as the number of embryonic sacs visualized, were also the same, being 17.8 and 17.4% respectively. Three sets of twins and two sets of triplets were obtained in group I, while group II displayed two sets each of twins and triplets.

Spontaneous luteinization, as recognized by elevated serum progesterone values (> 1 ng/ml) was followed in women not treated with GnRHa, i.e., those included in group II who had ovarian function. A total of seven out of the 32 (21.9%) low responders had elevated serum progesterone values.

Our data confirmed previous observations in which the presence or absence of ovarian function, and subsequently the use of GnRH analogues, does not influence the outcome of ovum donation [14].

*Oestradiol administration*

The clinical experience of maintaining recipients on oestrogens for 2—4 weeks before starting on progesterone demonstrated that even after 35 days of unopposed oestrogen administration, endometrial receptivity was adequate [10,15]. Using the "long follicular phase protocol", a 48.5% pregnancy rate was reported [15]. In our report, the unopposed administration of oestrogens was extended beyond these limits.

Data from our center with oocytes donated by 182 women undergoing IVF were distributed among 186 women treated by ovum donation. Five groups of recipients were established according to the duration of oestradiol valerate (EV) administration, in a "prolonged follicular phase" protocol, before embryo replacement, employing EV at increasing doses up to 6 mg/day. Several groups of recipients were established according to the duration of EV administration in order to evaluate the clinical results of oocyte donation. Group 1 was made up of 18 women who underwent 23 cycles of oocyte donation in which EV was administered for 13—16 days before progesterone injection; group 2 was composed of 68 patients (85 cycles) who were treated for 17—35 days; group 3, 53 women (63 cycles) in whom EV was administered for 36—50 days; group 4 consisted 25 patients (32 cycles) in whom EV was given for 51—65 days; and group 5 was composed of 22 women (27 cycles) who received EV for $> 65$ days before progesterone administration. There was no difference among groups in fertilization rates or the number of embryos transferred per cycle of donation. Similarly, the pregnancy, implantation and abortion rates were similar among groups regardless of the prolongation of the follicular phase with EV. Of the patients two were treated with EV for $> 100$ days; one patient was transferred after 108 days of unopposed EV administration but she did not get pregnant. A single pregnancy reached term after 100 days of EV administration in another woman. In addition, a twin pregnancy also successfully finished after 8 days of continued EV ingestion.

After these encouraging results, we decided to continue with a long protocol of EV administration in our anonymous program. Our updated results are consistent with our first report [16] and show that the follicular phase can be prolonged $> 65$ days without impairing the results of ovum donation. We believe that there is actually no doubt, however, that EV administration can be prolonged as long as necessary before progesterone administration, with no detrimental effects on pregnancy, implantation or abortion rate. This is of enormous help in the synchronization of donors and recipients in anonymous program.

*Age of recipients*

There is an evident decline in fecundity with age, clearly observed in populations in which contraception has not been used [17]. In such circumstances, fecundity decreases and infertility increases with age. There is a clear cutoff for poor reproductive potential $> 40$ years [17]. The fundamental physiological question is whether the uterus, the egg, or both are responsible for this impairment of fertility with age. There is little doubt that the quality of the egg is affected by age.

However, aging of the uterus is a more controversial subject. Chetkowski et al. [18], using a mathematical model, were able to demonstrate a significant age-related drop in both embryo quality and uterine receptivity.

Several reports have analyzed the impact of age on the reproductive performance of women > 40 years of age and even > 50 years of age [19—23] undergoing oocyte donation. Although some authors have observed decreased pregnancy rates in women > 40 years of age as compared with younger patients [19,24,25], others have not found such differences [23,26—29]. Thus, although the model seems to be valid, some controversy still exists as to whether the uterus ages with the ovary.

Recipients of different ages should receive oocytes from the same source and quality so as to test the receptivity of their uteri because we know that implantation in ovum donation is influenced by the source of the oocytes [30,31]. The quality of the oocytes can be corrected when oocytes from the same cohort of follicles are distributed randomly between women < 40 and > 40 years of age undergoing ovum donation. This approach has been used recently by Navot et al. [29], who found similar PRs between younger and older patients, concluding that uterine aging is not an important factor in determining the success of oocyte donation. From this study it can be inferred that waning oocyte quality rather than reduced uterine receptivity is responsible for the age-related decline in female fertility potential in natural life and assisted reproduction.

Further evidence, however, reveals that the uterus may be affected by age. Meldrum [27] showed that a decrease in ongoing and delivered PRs in older patients may be corrected by increasing the dose of exogenous P administered to the recipient. From this study it can be concluded that the uterus may be affected by age, although P may correct the defect. In keeping with this concept, it is of enormous interest to assure an adequate action of P on the endometrium in women entering an ovum donation program.

Our data was drawn up using live birth rates as the end point. It shows the overall results as compared by age. There were no statistical differences among the life tables calculated for each age group. Women in the age group < 30 showed the highest cumulative live birth rate with the lowest number of attempts.

*Serum oestradiol levels and endometrial thickness*

Adequate endometrial preparation with exogenous steroids is mandatory in ovum donation for a successful outcome. Several markers of sufficient endometrial priming are currently employed, including endometrial thickness by ultrasound and serum oestradiol (E2). Our data [32] was analyzed and published to assess the value of these parameters as predictors of ovum donation outcome and to analyze the correlation between serum E2 levels and the endometrial thickness. A total of 465 ovum donation cycles were included in the study. Endometrial thickness and serum E2 levels the day of oocyte donation were recorded and compared to several IVF parameters. The cycles were classified according to serum E2 values and endometrial thickness. Comparison among the groups established showed that endometrial thickness was significantly (p = 0.002) higher when serum E2 >400 pg/ml as compared to <100 pg/ml. Pregnancy and implantation rates were no different among groups, women with serum E2 <50 pg/ml having similar outcomes to the remaining cases. Endometrial thickness showed a similar picture in terms of pregnancy and implantation. Also, women with an endometrium <4 mm in size had normal pregnancy and implantation rates. There was a positive correlation (p = 0.0044) between endometrial thickness and implantation, as well as between endometrial thickness and serum E2 (p = 0.0184). None of the parameters tested was able to predict the ovum donation outcome. It was concluded that endometrial thickness is preferred to serum E2 for the monitoring of endometrial development, although none of them is able to predict success in oocyte donation.

*Low responders*

To analyze endometrial response (endometrial dating and implantation) to exogenous administration of E2 valerate and P in women with low response to gonadotropins undergoing oocyte donation, a cycle in which endometrial specimens were obtained and subsequent cycles with ET were evaluated. The control group was made up of patients with POF undergoing the same procedure.

A total of 37 women with low response to gonadotropins in previous cycles and 33 women with POF took part.

First, the artificial cycle with E2 valerate and P in the absence of previous pituitary suppression was used to determine endometrial adequacy. Followed by successive artificial cycles in which ET was performed on cycle day 17. Oocytes were donated from infertile patients undergoing IVF.

Serum steroid levels were measured during the artificial cycle. Histologic dating of the endometrium was carried out on cycle days 15 and 26. IVF/ET pregnancies were ultrasonographically documented.

Our results showed that postovulatory changes on cycle day 15 were observed in 36.4% of low responders treated with E2 valerate and P in the absence of simultaneous pituitary suppression. Pregnancy rates were higher in women with previous sufficiently (77.8%) or insufficiently (80%) estrogen-primed endometrium than in the cases showing postovulatory changes (37.5%). PRs per transfer were significantly higher in low responders (63.8%) than in patients with POF (37.2%). Patients with endometriosis had a 71.4% PR per transfer. Embryos derived from oocytes from polycystic ovaries had a 48.3% PR.

With this evidence we concluded that oocyte donation is a reliable alternative for women with low response to gonadotropins, including those with severe endometriosis. The efficacy of the steroid replacement regimen in controlling ovarian function may influence outcome. Thus, women with functional ovaries despite exogenous steroid replacement might be treated differently [4].

*Patients with endometriosis and PCO as donors*

It is also worth noting the positive results observed in women with stage III—IV endometriosis who usually enter the program because of a low response to gonadotropins or repeated IVF failure. We have previously shown that women with endometriosis perform similar to other low responders in ovum donation, providing the rational for an effect of endometriosis on the oocyte and resulting embryo, rather than on the uterine environment at implantation [32]. Our recent data confirms the good prognosis of endometriosis patients with this technology.

## References

1. Lutjen P, Trounson A, Leeton J, Findlay J, Wood C, Renow P. The establishment and maintenance of pregnancy using in vitro fertilization and embryo donation in a patient with primary ovarian failure. Nature 1984;307:174—175.
2. Navot D, Laufer N, Kopolovic J, Rabinowitz R, Birkenfield A, Lewin A et al. Artificially induced endometrial cycles and establishment of pregnancies in the absence of ovaries. N Engl J Med 1984;314:806—811.
3. Rosenwaks Z. Donor eggs: their application in modern reproductive technologies. Fertil Steril 1987;47:895—909.
4. Remohí J, Vidal A, Pellicer A. Oocyte donation in low responders to a conventional ovarian stimulation for in vitro fertilization. Fertil Steril 1993;59:1208—1215.
5. Sauer MV, Paulson PJ, Lobo RA. Pregnancy after age 50: applying oocyte donation to women following natural menopause. Lancet 1993;341:321—323.
6. Burton G, Abdalla HI, Kirkland A, Studd JW. The role of oocyte donation in women who are unsuccessful with in vitro fertilization. Hum Reprod 1993;7:1103—1105.
7. Remohí J, Gartner B, Gallardo E, Yalil S, Simón C, Pellicer A. Pregnancy and birth rates after oocyte donation. Fertil Steril 1997;67:717—723.
8. Trounson A, Leeton J, Besanko M, Wood C, Conti A. Pregnancy established in an infertile patient after transfer of a donated embryo fertilized in vitro. Br Med J 1983;286:835—838.
9. Rosenwaks Z, Veeck LL, Liu H-C. Pregnancy following transfer of in vitro fertilized donated oocytes. Fertil Steril 1986;45:417—420.
10. Serhal PF, Craft IL. Ovum donation — a simplified approach. Fertil Steril 1987;48:265—269.
11. Meldrurn DR, Wisot A, Hamilton F, Gutlay-Yeo AL, Marr B, Huynh D. Artificial agonadism and hormone replacement for ooeyie donation. Fertil Steril 1989;52:509—511.
12. Serhal PF, Craft IL. Oocyte donation in 61 patients. Lancet 1989;2:1185—1187.
13. de Ziegler D, Cornel C, Bergeron C, Hazout A, Bouchard P, Frydman R. Controlled preparation of the endometrium with exogenous estradiol and progesterone in women having functioning ovaries. Fertil Steril 1991;56:851—855.
14. Remohí J, Gutiérrez A, Vidal A, Tarín JJ, Pellicer A. The use of gonadotrophin-releasing hormone analogues in women receiving oocyte donation does not affect implantation rates. Hum Reprod 1994;9:1761—1764.
15. Navot D et al. An insight into early reproductive processes through the in vivo model of ovum donation. J Clin Endocrinol Metab 1991;72:408—414.
16. Remohí J, Gutierrez A, Cano F. Long oestradiol replacement in an oocyte donation programme. Hum Reprod 1995;6:1387—1391.
17. Menken J, Trussell J, Larsen U. Age and infertility. Science 1986;233:1389—1394.
18. Chetkowski RJ, Rode RA, Burruel V, Nass TE. The effect of pituitary suppression and the women's age on embryo viability and uterine receptivity. Fertil Steril 1991;56:1095—1103.
19. Flamigni C, Borini A, Iolini F, Bianchi L, Serrao L. Oocyte donation: comparison between

recipients from different age groups. Hum Reprod 1993;8:2088−2092.

20. Antinori S, Versaci C, Ghólami GH, Panci C, Caffa B. Oocyte donation in menopausal women. Hum Reprod 1993;8:1487−1490.

21. Pantos K, Meimeti-Damianaki T, Vaxevanoglou T, Kapetanakis E. Oocyte donation in menopausal women aged over 40 years. Hum Reprod 1993;8:488−491.

22. Borini A. Oocyte donation and pregnancy in women over 50. Assist Reprod Rev 1994;4:60−63.

23. Balmaceda JP, Bernardini L, Ciuffardi I, Felix C, Ord T, Sueldo CE et al. Oocyte donation in humans: a model to study the effect of age on embryo implantation rate. Hum Reprod 1994;9:2160−2163.

24. Abdalla HI, Baber R, Kirkland A, Leonard T, Power M, Studd JWW. A report on 100 cycles of oocyte donation; factors affecting the outcome. Hum Reprod 1990;5:1018−1022.

25. Yaron Y, Botehan A, Amit A, Kogosowski A, Yovel I, Lessing JB. Endometrial receptivity: the age-related decline in pregnancy rates and the effect of ovarian function. Fertil Steril 1993;60: 314−318.

26. Check J, Askari HA, Fisher C, Vanaman L. The use of a shared donor oocyte program to evaluate the effect of uterine senescence. Fertil Steril 1994;61:252−256.

27. Meldrum DR. Female reproductive aging — ovarian and uterine factors. Fertil Steril 1993;59: 1−5.

28. Rotsztejn DA, Asch RH. Effect of aging on assisted reproductive technologies (ART): experience from egg donation. Sem Reprod Endocrinol 1991;9:272−279.

29. Navot D, Drews MR, Bergh PA, Guzman I, Karstaedt A, Scott RT et al. Age-related decline in female fertility is not due to diminished capacity of the uterus to sustain embryo implantation. Fertil Steril 1994;61:97−101.

30. Remohí J, Vidal A, Pellicer A. Oocyte donation in low responders to conventional ovarian stimulation for in vitro fertilization. Fertil Steril 1993;59:1208−1215.

31. Simón C, Gutiérrez A, Vidal A, De los Santos MJ, Tarín JJ, Remohí J et al. Outcome of patients with endometriosis in assisted reproduction: results from in vitro fertilization and oocyte donation. Hum Reprod 1994;9:725−729.

32. Remohí J, Ardiles G, García Velasco JA, Gaitán P, Simón C, Pellicer A. Endometrial thickness and serum oestradiol concentrations as predictors of outcome in oocyte donation. Hum Reprod 1997;12(10):2271−2276.

# Obstetrical and pediatric outcome
# of ART procedures

Fertility and Reproductive Medicine.
R.D. Kempers, J. Cohen, A.F. Haney and J.B. Younger, editors.

# Long-term follow up of ART children including psychological aspects

Francois Olivennes and Sylvie Tine-Brissaud

*Department of Obstetrics and Gynecology, Hospital A. Beclere, Clamart, France*

**Abstract.** The first child conceived through the use of IVF is now 20 years of age. During this time, major progress has been made in various aspects of IVF and the number of children that are conceived with its help is growing.

Very few reports have been published on the long-term follow up of IVF children. Most of these present reassuring data, however, lack the methodology that would lead to an undoubtable conclusion that IVF has no detrimental effect on the growth, and the motor and psychological development of the children conceived with this technique.

Pediatric follow-up studies are very difficult to organise, especially when choosing a control group which takes into consideration the differences that exist between fertile and infertile couples. The number of children to be included, the type of evaluation and its extent, the length of the follow up, and the risk of a high rate of loss for follow up also constitute difficulties. There is also a clear ethical problem in singularising these children by enrolling them in specific medical and psychological studies. However, the evaluation of assisted reproductive technologies (ART) is mandatory, and the wellbeing of the children has to be evaluated especially since new techniques involve the use of gametes and embryos.

**Keywords:** children, follow up, IVF.

The first child conceived with in vitro fertilization and embryo transfer (IVF-ET) will be 20 years old this year. Since then, thousands of scientific papers have been published on various aspects of IVF-ET, but very few address perinatal complications and child follow up. This lack of data is a clear drawback for the evaluation of new technology that helps to treat infertile couples.

IVF-ET is now part of the infertility treatment. The number of children born worldwide after IVF is estimated to be over 300,000. In the last world meeting concerning IVF, the collaborative study group reported a total of 19,000 IVF children for the year 1995 [1].

If child follow-up studies are difficult to organize they are, however, mandatory to confirm the safety of IVF-ET. The follow up should include, of course, the assessment of the perinatal outcome which can affect the development of the children born prematurely or small for gestational age. This subject will be addressed in a specific chapter of this book.

**Address for correspondence:** Dr Francois Olivennes, Department of Obstetrics and Hynecology, Hospital A. Beclere, 157 rue de la Porte Trivaux, 92140 Clamart, France. Tel.: +33-1-45-37-40-53. Fax: +33-1-45-37-49-81.

The observation of the wellbeing of the children should take place at birth where, for example, malformations are recorded. However, evaluation is needed on further characteristics, and long-term follow-up studies are also necessary to evaluate the motor and intellectual development of the children as well as his (or her) growth. The potential effects of in vitro fertilization on the child development should not be underestimated. If there are no worrying data published on long-term assessment of IVF children, we will know that very few studies have addressed this issue, and if no data support the potential adverse effect on the long-term development, no data confirm the total safety.

This is of course the case for the large amount of children born after classical IVF, but the introduction of new techniques applied to gametes and embryos reinforce the necessity of a scientific evaluation of their safety. The follow up of children born after ICSI will not be part of this paper since it will be treated in a specific chapter, but represent an illustration of the importance of the follow up when using a technique which bypasses the normal fertilization process, and is indicated for the majority of the cases in couples with severe male infertility where a higher proportion of genetic abnormalities are observed.

However, it is clear that child follow-up studies are extremely difficult to organise which could explain the reason for this lack of available.literature. We will give a summary on the studies on long-term follow up of IVF children.

The first report on IVF-ET children was made by Mushin et al. [2]. They reported the follow up of 33 of their 52 children (lost for follow up: 36.5%). The children aged 12—37 months were assessed by a semistructured interview and development tests were performed (Bayley scale and Denver development screening test). The authors concluded that no particular abnormalities were observed.

In 1986, Yovich et al. [3] reported the evolution of their 20 first IVF children. Development tests were made at 1 year of age and no abnormalities was observed.

In 1989, the group from Norfolk reported the follow up of 110 IVF children compared to a control group of spontaneously conceived children [4]. The rate of loss for follow up was 24.5%. The children were aged 13—30 months. No difference was found between the two groups of children for the malformations, neurological and psychomotor evaluation made with the Bayley scale.

In 1992, Brandes et al. [5] compared a group of 116 IVF children aged 12—14 months to a matched control group (birthweight, term, rank of the pregnancy, mode of delivery, sex, age and socioeconomic status of the parents) of non-IVF children. No difference was found between the groups, but a correlation was found between the multiple births and a lower developmental index (Bayley and Stanford-Binet).

In 1994, Ron-el et al. [6] did not find a significant difference in the development of a group of 30 IVF children aged 28 months as compared to 30 spontaneously conceived ones.

More recently, Saunders et al. [7] followed up a group of 314 children aged 22.5—25.5 months. These children were compared to a control group matched for the number of children, the term and the date of birth. However, the families of the selected control group had differences with the general population. They were of higher socioeconomic class and the unemployment rate was 2 times lower. The parents of the control group were also significantly younger than those of the IVF group (34.9 vs. 31.9 for the mother and 37.6 vs. 34.5 for the fathers, representing a drawback of the study). The authors did not find any difference between the two groups of children for the malformations, growth and neurological development.

Also in 1996, Cederblad et al. [8] published the results of a study in which a group of 99 IVF children aged 33−85 months were studied. The loss for follow up was 21.5%. The parents differed from the general population by being of a higher socioeconomic class. Children were assessed with a Griffith test. No difference was observed between the results, which were available, of the IVF children and the general population, the IVF children having globally a slightly higher developmental index. Logistic regression showed a link between the birthweight and the tests results.

A study carried out by Epelboin et al. in Paris (1995, unpublished data) interviewed the parents with a questionnaire. Information was obtained for a total of 285 children out of the 300 conceived in their center (lost for follow up: 5%). No particularities were observed for the medical and surgical medical history, as well as for the scholastic performance. A correlation of 98% was found between a medical examination and the administered questionnaire for a subgroup of 126 children seen by a pediatrician after the questionnaire.

We have published the results of a study on the cohort of 422 children conceived in our center between 1982 and 1989 [9]. We managed to obtain information on 375 children (lost for follow up: 11.2%). A telephone interview with a standardized questionnaire, established by a group of three pediatricians, was carried out. No particularity was observed for the medical and surgical history, the malformation rate, the growth (weight and height) and the scholastic performances. We were surprised by the high rate of parents who kept the origin of the conception secret to their child (or children) (58.7% of the parents of children < 10 years old and 34% for the children > 10 years old).

As mentioned above, for the children conceived with special techniques, the follow up of those conceived with ICSI is addressed in a specific chapter. Only three studies present the long-term follow up of children born after frozen/thawed embryos.

Sutcliffe et al. [10] reported the follow up of 91 IVF children to 83 spontaneously conceived children. The children were assessed at 2 years of age. The results of the tests were slightly lower for the IVF children coming from frozen/thawed embryos but the two groups were not matched. The prematurity was not taken into account and was twice as high in the IVF group. Moreover, there was a 4-month difference in the mean age of the two groups of children at the time of the evaluation. The authors conclude that no excess of abnormalities can be demonstrated between these groups of children.

Salat-Baroux et al. [11] presented the results of a survey on 84 children (mean age: 5.2 ± 1.0 years), though with a high rate of loss for follow up (44%). A total of four malformations were found (4.7%). We have studied the total cohort of the children conceived in our center between 1986 and 1994 and representing 93 children. We obtained information on 89 of them (lost for follow up: 4.3%). We did not observe adverse outcome concerning the growth, medical and surgical history. Only one malformation (short uretere) was observed. The scholastic performance evaluated by the parents were within normal range [12].

The studies on the psychological aspects in IVF children are also rare [13]. With IVF, for the first time in human history, fertilization takes place outside the mother's body. This has raised many questions about the psychological consequences for the children (in western societies about 1% of first born babies are conceived by IVF). This subject brings much speculation, most of which is negative. For example, an unnatural (cold) conception might not engender a good (warm) relationship between parents and children [14]; the medical specialist is a "third" parent and might interfere with the parent-child relationship [15]; the "real" child of these infertile parents may have difficulties meeting expectations created by the "fantasy" child [16], and the Freudian psychoanalysts are simply wondering how one now deals with such a "primitive scene"? However, other assumptions are: IVF infants are seen as very precious, which may create, subsequently, overprotective parents with highly elevated expectations [17]. After a long period of infertility, parents can have problems in the process of child rearing, or the IVF child might be seen as different within the family environment.

In reality, very few studies are actually focused on the psychological development of IVF children, they are more about parent-children relationships or psychosocial outcomes.

Some researchers [2,3,8] found that IVF children exhibit a high level of psychomotor development, which is apparently due to the elevated social status and high motivation of IVF parents.

Regarding the psychomotor development, no deviations were found with other children, according to Raoul-Duval et al. [18] and Ron-El et al. [6].

The most extensive study was carried out by Golombok et al. [17,19,20]. The study compared families with IVF child, families with a child conceived after donor insemination (DI), adoptive families and normally fertile families. The children were assessed between 4 and 8 years of age. The assessment of the psychological development has been done from different perspectives: mother, child's teacher and child itself. The various measures on the child's psychological development yielded no significant differences. Nevertheless, IVF families scores higher on open expression of affection by the mother, and quality of parent-child interaction. The above study, like the one from Colpin et al. [15], is based on a theoretical framework to underpin the influence of the parents' contribution to the development of the IVF child. Parental warmth and sensibility promote a positive development for the child, and no significant differences were found between IVF and DI parents. Children in all type of families were functioning well. However, only 62% of DI families have accepted to take part in this study, and according to telephone conversations, they were not experiencing problems, though they have decided to keep the child's origin secret. Like Weaver et al. [21], Golombok and associates report a high degree of protectivness among IVF parents, and they point out that overprotectivness and a high degree of warmth do not result in a better wellbeing for the child when a certain threshold is passed. Another consequence of IVF technique on children is the multiple birth which may occur. Twins and triplets are very often preterm babies and we know that prematurity may lead to developmental problems. In case of triplets, the social and psychological consequences for the parents may lead as well to psychological problems for the children [22,23]. Multiple birth is a serious complication of the IVF treatment, and it is a concern for many teams who choose to transfer less embryos.

It can be concluded that the parent-child relationship in IVF families seems to be better than in "spontaneous child families", however, the psychological consequences on children are not really established yet.

Studies which follow up IVF children on a long-term basis are rare as well as studies on the psychological impact of the IVF technique on the child and on the parent/child relationship. Moreover, the methodology of the published studies cannot scientifically eliminate any fine adverse effects of IVF on the development of the children. The studies, most of the time, have a high rate of loss for follow up. They are often done on a group of children chosen on unknown criteria, the children are young and their overall small number do not allow for the detection of rare abnormalities, control groups are absent in the majority of the studies and the evaluation is not always standardized.

The follow-up studies are extremely difficult to organize [24]. The major problems are:

1) the evaluation of the size of the population. Should we include the whole cohort or a sample of it;
2) the choice of a control group;
3) the definition of the evaluation criteria. What tests, at which age and for how long [25,26]; and
5) the loss for follow up rate is a major drawback of any long-term studies [27]. There is a clear ethical problem of singularizing the children in a long-term study. The effect of such a study by itself on the development of the children should be evaluated.

Finally the financial cost of such studies are important and source of financing on this topics are rare.

If most of the studies published on the follow up of IVF children are reassuring, it is clear that these studies are clearly not sufficient to undoubtedly eliminate any fine adverse effects on the wellbeing of IVF children. The main problem of IVF remains the high rate of multiple pregnancies leading to pediatric complications related to their high rate of perinatal adverse outcome.

184

## References

1. World Collaborative Report on IVF: preliminary data for 1995. J Assist Reprod Genet 1997; 14(Suppl):251—265.
2. Mushin DN, Spensley J, Barreda Hanson M. Children of IVF 1985. J Clin Obstet 1985;12: 865—876.
3. Yovich JL, Parry TS, French NP, Granaug AA. Development assessment of 20 IVF infants at their first birthday. J In Vitro Fertil Embryo Transfer 1986;4:253—257.
4. Morin N, Wirth F, Johnson DH, Frank LM, Presburg H, Van De Water V. Congenital malformations and psychological development in children conceived by IVF. J Pediatr 1989;115: 222—227.
5. Brandes JM, Scher A, Itzkovits J, Thaler L, Sarid M, Ghershoni Baruch R. Growth and development of children conceived by IVF. Pediatrics 1992;90:424—429.
6. Ron-El PR, Lahat E, Golan A, Lerman M, Bukowski I, Herman A. Development of children born after superovulation induced by long acting GnRH agonist and menotropins and by IVF. J Pediatr 1994;125:734—737.
7. Saunders K, Spensley J, Munro J, Halasz G. Growth and physical outcome of children conceived by in vitro fertilization. Pediatrics 1996;97(5):688—692.
8. Cederblad M, Friberg B, Ploman F, Sjöberg NO, Stjernqvist K, Zackrisson E. Intelligence and behaviour in children born after in vitro fertilization treatment. Hum Reprod 1996;11: 2052—2057.
9. Olivennes F, Kerbrat V, Rufat P, Blanchet V, Fanchin R, Frydman R. Follow up of a cohort of 422 children aged 6 to 13 years conceived by in vitro fertilization. Fertil Steril 1997;67(2): 284—289.
10. Sutcliffe A, D'souza S, Cadman J, Richards B, Mckinlay I, Lieberman B. Outcome in children from cryopreserved embryos. Arch Dis Child 1995;72:290—293.
11. Salat-Baroux J, Mandelbaum J, Junca AM, Plachot M, Alvarez S, Alnot MO, Antoine JM. Congélation des embryons humains après FIV: résultats immédiats et à long terme. Bull Acad Natl Méd 1996;180(1):83—93.
12. Olivennes F, Schneider Z, Remy V, Blanchet V, Kerbrat V, Fanchin R, Hazout A, Glissant A, Fernandez H, Dehan M, Frydman R. Perinatal outcome and follow up of 82 children aged 1 to 9 years old conceived from cryopreserved embryos. Hum Reprod 1996;11:1565—1568.
13. McMahon CA, Ungerer JA, Beaurepaire J. Psychosocial outcomes for parents and children after in vitro fertilization: a review. J Reprod Infant Psychol 1995;13:1—16.
14. Gross P, Honer A. Multiple parenthoods, new reproductive techniques, individualization and family change. Soziale Welt 1990;41:97—116.
15. Colpin H, Demyttenaere K, Vandemeulebroecke L. New reproduction technology and the family: the parent—child relationship after IVF. J Child Psychol Psychiat 1995;36:1429—1441.
16. Hammer-Burns L. Infertility as a boundary ambiguity: one theoretical perspective. Fam Process 1987;26:359—372.
17. Golombok S, Brewaeys A, Cook R, Giavazzi MT, Guerra D, Mantovani A, Van Hall E, Crosignani PG, Dexeus S. The European study of assisted reproduction families: family functioning and child development. Hum Reprod 1996;11(10):2324—2331.
18. Raoul-Duval A, Bertrand-Servais M, Frydman R. Comparative prospective study of the psychological development of children born by IVF and their mother. J Psychosom Obstet Gynaecol 1993;14:117—126.
19. Golombok S, Cook R, Bish A. Families created by the new reproduction technologies: quality of parenting and social and emotional development of the children. Child Devel 1995;66:285—298.
20. Golombok S. Parenting and secrecy issues related to children of assisted reproduction. J Assist Reprod Genet 1997;14:375—378.
21. Weaver SM, Clifford E et al. A follow up study of "successful" IVF/GIFT couples: social-emotional wellbeing and adjustment to parenthood. J Psychosom Obstet Gynaecol 1993;14:s5—

s16 special issue.

22. Garel M, Blondel B. Assessment at 1 year of psychological consequences of having triplets. Hum Reprod 1992;7:729—732.

23. Garel M, Salobir C, Blondel B. Psychological consequences of having triplets: a 4-year follow-up study. Fertil Steril 1997;67(6):1162—1165.

24. Mutch LM, Johnson MA, Morley R. Follow-up studies: design, organisation and analysis. Arch Dis Child 1989;64(10):1394—1402.

25. Aylward GP. Developmental assessment: caveats and a cry for quality control. J Pediatr 1987; February:253—254.

26. Dworkin PH. British and American recommendations for developmental monitoring: the role of surveillance. Pediatrics 1989;84(6):1000—1010.

27. Aylward GP, Hatcher RP, Stripp B, Gustafson NF, Leavitt LA. Who goes and who stays: subject loss in a multicenter, longitudinal follow-up study. Devel Behav Pediatr 1985;6(1):3—8.

# Obstetrical complications of ART and selective reduction

Pierre Boulot, Jacques Vignal, Hervé Dechaud, Jean-Michel Faure and
Bernard Hedon
*Fetal Medicine Unit, Department of Obstetrics and Gynecology, Hopital Arnaud de Villeneuve, Montpellier, France*

**Abstract.** Multifetal pregnancy reduction (MFPR) is performed in cases of high-order multiple fetal gestations, including triplets, quadruplets, quintuplets or more in order to decrease the chance of complications (early or late miscarriages, prematurity, low birth weights, in utero fetal death, major permanent handicaps such as cerebral palsy, necrotizing enterocolitis and chronic seizure disorders) generally resulting in the birth of twins and more rarely singeltons.

MFPR is an invasive procedure which carries some intrinsic risk of pregnancy loss. MFPR can be performed transcervically, transvaginally or transabdominally. Reported fetal loss rates following MFPR range from 8% up to to 16%. To date, data from large monocentric studies and data from the most recent cases in recently expanded studies suggest that the fetal loss rate following MFPR is plateauing at 8%. Transabdominal and transvaginal procedures yield better short-term results than the transcervical procedure.

Series comparing outcome obstetrical data from quintuplets of quadruplets reduced to twins and nonreduced multiples suggest that the obstetric outcome of pregnancies (essentially twins) following reduction is improved when compared to the data from nonreduced pregnancies.

A reduction from triplet to twin decreases the chance of very early prematurity and short-term morbidity. Although MFPR decreases the number of babies going home per couple, it increases the proportion of surviving infants without complications. However, data fails to demonstrate an improvement in the long-term outcome of the survivors as no information from a prolonged follow-up is available in any study.

First-trimester selective reduction improves the prognosis of high-order multiple pregnancies. The benefits to the remaining fetuses with regards to the length of gestation, birth weight and perinatal morbidity are well-established for mutliple pregnancies with more than three embryos. Information on the risks (miscarriage) and advantages of reduction (gain in fetal growth and prematurity, decrease in maternal complications) should be supplied to all couples with multiple pregnancies by an experienced obstetrician. Reducing multifetal pregnancy to twins appears to be the more appropriate medical attitude for the majority of both medical teams and couples. Reduction seems necessary for triplet pregnancies when there are poor prognosis factors such as structural uterine anomalie or severe maternal disease. It remains unclear whether the long-term outcome of triplets is improved by the procedure.

**Keywords:** assisted reproductive technique, ethics, multifetal pregnancy reduction, perinatal mortality, triplet gestation, twins.

---

*Address for correspondence:* Dr Pierre Boulet, Hopital Arnaud de Villeneuve, Service Gyn/Obs, 371, Avenue Doyen G. Giraud, 34295 Montpellier Cedex, France. Tel.: +33-4-67-33-6486. Fax: +33-4-67-33-6468. E-mail: gyneco-bm@ chu-momtpellier.fr

Over the past 10 years, the number of women carrying three or more fetuses has increased dramatically as a result of infertility treatments including the use of ovulation-inducing agents and assisted reproductive technology (ART). First-trimester selective terminations of multiple pregnancies were first carried out in twin pregnancies when one of the twins showed a genetic or chromosomal anomaly or malformation. Reduction is now performed in most cases on high-order multiple fetal gestations, including quadruplets, quintuplets or more in order to decrease the chance of complications (early or late miscarriages, prematurity, low birth weights, in utero fetal death, major permanent handicaps such as cerebral palsy, necrotizing enterocolitis and chronic seizure disorders, etc.) generally resulting in the birth of twins and more rarely singletons. The deliberate sacrifice of the number of apparently healthy embryos in a wanted high-multiple pregnancy is an alternative to the abortion of all the fetuses or to the acceptance of the risk of extremely premature delivery. Although the procedure poses no problems when dealing with high-order multiple fetal gestations (quadruplets, quintuplets or more), the same is not true concerning triplets where the indications have not been clearly established. Numerous terms have been used to describe the procedure. By consensus, "selective termination" signifies a procedure done on a multiple pregnancy in which an embryo is affected by a severe disease. This procedure is also called selective fetocide or selective abortion. The term selective reduction signifies that the procedure is performed only because of the excessive number of apparently normal embryos. The term "multifetal pregnancy reduction" (MFPR) seems to be the more accurate and was adopted by the American College of Obstetricians and Gynecologists in 1991 [1,2].

**Incidence of multiple gestations**

In the last 10 years, there has been a progressive increase in the incidence of high-order multiple pregnancies principally due to the increased use of ovulation induction, ovulation stimulation and assisted reproduction techniques. The rates in France in 1972 were 8.9/1,000 and 0.9/10,000, respectively, and rose to 13/1,000 and 4.2/10,000 in 1993. Such incidences were similar in european countries and in the USA [3].

The 1993 ART World Report representing 27 countries indicated that out of 16,629 pregnancies, 23.7% were twins, 4.3% were triplets and 0.3% were quadruplets or more [4]. The 1994 report of the Society of Assisted Reproductive Technologies Registry, representing 249 programs in North America performing 27,000 cycles, indicated that in 98.5% of cycles, ovarian stimulation was used, producing 6,114 pregnancies, of which 35% were multiples (28.3% twins, 5.9% triplets, 0.6% high-order [5]). Data from the French national database FIVNAT recording pregnancies obtained after ART, indicate that the triplet pregnancy rate over 10 years remains stable at the level of 4% [6]. Over a 9-year period (1986–1994), there was an incidence of 23.5% for twins, 3.3% for triplets and 0.1% for high-order pregnancies in France, resulting from IVF programs and

16,987 pregnancies. This was accompanied by 2.4% of MFPR (404 selective reductions in the registered pregnancies).

## Technical considerations

Three echoguided techniques have been used since the first attempts at the beginning of the 1980s. MFPR can be performed transcervically, transvaginally or transabdominally. In an evaluation of technical aspects and risks from 2,756 cases of the literature [7], we found the distribution of each technique to be as follows: transabdominal procedure 2,145 cases (83.3%), transcervical approach 363 cases (14.1%) and transvaginal approach 248 cases (9.6%).

Before performing the procedure, a careful ultrasonic assessment of the pregnancy is highly recommended, preferably using transvaginal examination. Attention should be paid to placentation. Although the majority of multiple pregnancies obtained after superovulation or multiple embryo transfer are polychorionic gestations, the risk of monochorionic twinning associated with ART is increased. Indeed, some series have reported triplet gestations that include one singleton and an adjacent monoamniotic twin gestation [8]. Only a multichorial placentation allows a safe procedure for the remaining embryos as monochorionic placentae almost always have some vascular anastomoses between the two fetal circulations. Attention should be given to the actual number of living fetuses as a spontaneous partial embryo loss may occur (natural phenomenon known as vanishing twin syndrome). Lastly, a careful search for fetal anomalies and discordancy in crown–rump length should be performed.

The transabdominal technique is by far the most commonly used [1,2,7,9,10]. Under local anesthesia, a 18–21 gauge needle is transabdominally inserted through the uterine wall, then into the amniotic cavity, and finally pushed into the fetal thorax at a level above the diaphragm. Then potassium chloride solution (amount ranging from 0.5 to 5 cc) is injected, leading to the cessation of the heartbeat. The procedure is repeated for the adjacent sac(s) if requested. There are multiple reasons for choosing the interval between 10 and 12 weeks gestation (WG) to perform a transabdominal procedure; before this time, a spontaneous loss of an embryo may occur, which could cancel the need to perform a MFPR. Therefore, waiting until 10 to 12 WG allows for the ultrasonography search of morphologic abnormalities. Chances of diagnosing anomalies increase with each advancing week of gestation. The nuchal fold measurement of each embryo is obtainable, as well as the crown–rump length. As a poor obstetrical outcome is associated with an increase in nuchal translucency or with a significant lag in crown–rump length between embryos, these fetuses would be selected for reduction [1,12]. Beyond 12 WG, the chance of spontaneous loss is diminished and may rarely occur. Lastly, by waiting until 12 WG, the couple will have time to reflect and make an informed decision [13].

The transvaginal technique is carried out in an earlier stage of pregnancy. This technique is analogous in many respects to oocyte aspiration for in vitro fertilization and may be very useful when the attempt is made very early in gestation. Indeed, this procedure permits transvaginal aspiration or transvaginal embryo-puncture of the early embryo using potassium chloride. This procedure is performed at approximately 6–7 weeks by means of a 17–21 gauge needle affixed to a vaginal ultrasound probe [9,8,14]. However, delaying the procedure to at least 9–10 weeks is desirable to permit at least a rudimentary fetal visualization and the search for worrisome signs such as an increased nuchal fold, inappropriate crown–rump length or cystic hygroma. It is probably preferable to wait until 8 weeks or later in the event that a "vanishing twin" may occur, thus leading to the risk of losing the only remaining embryo(s) if selective termination is carried out very early.

A third technique, the first to be introduced, is the transcervical minisuction to remove embryos at 8–11 weeks using a Karmann cannula No. 6 to 10 inserted through the cervix under echoguidage [15]. Because of the dilation of the cervix combined with the removal of the gestational sac which may alter intrauterine volume, loss of the entire pregnancy reaches higher levels than with others techniques [1,7,9,12,16]. The major concern about using the transvaginal and transcervical procedures remains the risk of ascending infection that could lead to the entire loss of the pregnancy. However, no controlled data to evaluate this risk or to assess the need of antibiotic prophylaxis is available to date.

The decision of which embryos(s) to choose is mainly based on the technical issue of which embryo is easiest to reach. However, malformed embryos or embryos recognized as having worrisome signs should preferably be suppressed. It is reported that it is better to target the embryo in the fundal area of the uterus, and not to choose the embryo closest to the cervix because devitalization of tissue near the cervix might predispose it to ascending infection and would result in an increased risk of fetal loss.

## Subsequent outcome

Data dealing with embryo losses related to the procedure are helpful when counseling patients faced with multiple pregnancies. MFPR is an invasive procedure which carries some intrinsic risk of pregnancy loss. Reported fetal loss rates following MFPR range from 8 to 16%. The report by Evans et al. [9] covering data from 1988 to early 1991 including cases all performed by the transabdominal potassium chloride injection, indicate an overall 16.4% pregnancy loss rate up through 24 WG [1,7,14,17]. A second collaborative paper [10] shows that the risks diminish with increased experience, suggesting that the procedure should be performed by trained operators in experienced centers (learning curve). The overall pregnancy loss rate has decreased to 11.7%. For example, in the case of transabdominal procedures, the rate declined from 16 to 8% while transcervical and transvaginal cases were associated with a loss rate of approximately 13%. To date, data from large monocentric studies and data from the most recent cases in the recently expanded Evans' study [1] suggest that the fetal loss rate following

MFPR is plateauing at 8%. Reducing multifetal pregnancy leads to fetal loss rates which vary with the starting number of embryos. Pregnancy loss rates before 24 WG were 20.9% for patients starting with sextuplets, 17.1% for quintuplets, 13% for quadruplets and decreased to 7.6% for triplets reduced to twins. Other results suggest that the overall loss rates were related to the finishing number of embryos. The study revealed that the lowest pregnancy loss rates were for cases reduced to twins, also there were increased loss rates when reducing to singletons. However, this latter finding might reflect a tendency to perform multifetal pregnancy reduction to singletons for medical reasons (fetal anomalies, structural uterine anomalies or poor maternal conditions). In our survey of 2,576 cases of the literature [7], we found a fetal loss rate before 24 WG that reached 12, 20 and 10%, respectively, for the transabdominal approach, the trancervical approach and the transvaginal approach. Other results from this survey indicated total fetal loss rates (miscarriage plus in utero fetal death) that were significantly different, namely 16.7% when dealing with transabdominal procedures, 24.8% with transcervical cases and 10.9% with transvaginal cases. This strongly suggests that the transcervical approach should be abandoned. Maymon et al. [18] reviewed 804 cases of the literature in order to analyze the relationship between procedures and subsequent perinatal risks. When evaluating the miscarriage rate, no significant difference was found between the transvaginal, transabdominal and transcervical techniques (11, 13 and 15% respectively). They found that the transabdominal option yields better short-term results, such as the lowest infant mortality rate and a significant lower infection rate. The transvaginal approach has a significant lower preterm delivery rate. The preterm delivery rate before 36 WG with the transcervical procedure is higher than for those of the transabdominal and transvaginal. In Berkowitz's largest monocentric series including 400 patients, 368 patients delivered after 24 weeks gestation whereas 32 (8%) lost their entire pregnancies [2]. More interestingly, fetal losses were related to the starting number of embryos. The loss rates were 7.3 and 8.4% for women having three and four fetuses at the time of the procedure, 6.1% for those with five fetuses, and 17.6% for those with six or more fetuses.

It remains difficult to know whether fetal loss is directly related to the procedure itself or would have occurred as natural miscarriages of a multifetal pregnancy. The natural course of early multifetal pregnancy is being clarified with both the use of transvaginal sonography and the prospective observation of expectantly managed multiple pregnancies, essentially triplets. All series of post in vitro fertilization pregnancies indicate that the rate of miscarriage, even on singletons remains superior to the average [5,6,7,20]. Kol reports that spontaneous fetal death occurred in 5% of multiple pregnancies [19]. Lipitz [21] reports a spontaneous fetal loss rate among expectantly managed triplets of nearly 21% before 24 WG. Our data show this rate to be 7.5% before 24 WG among triplets [17]. These data suggest that the spontaneous loss rate in women carrying three or more fetuses may be similar to or even higher than the fetal loss rate observed following MFPR.

**Performing multifetal pregnancy reduction on multifetal gestations with more than three embryos**

The review of the literature about the natural history of quadruplets clearly indicates that extreme premature delivery remains the main risk. It has also been shown that as the number of fetuses rises, the risk of maternal and fetal complications during labour and delivery will also increase [22,28]. The preterm delivery rate varies from 96 to 100%, whereas births before 28 WG reach 14.6% and those before 32 WG reach 48%. The possibility of reducing quaduplets to twins dramatically decreases the risk of prematurity. In a large monocentric series of 142 quadruplets mostly reduced to twins, Berkowitz et al. reported that the mean gestational age at delivery time was 34.9 WG; 49% were delivered after 36 WG, 35% between 32 and 36 WG, 11% between 28 and 32 WG and 5% between 24 and 28 WG [2]. In Evans' study, among 653 quadruplets mostly reduced to twins, there were 37.1% of the births after 37 WG, 33.8% between 33 and 36WG, 10.4% between 29 and 32 WG and 4.9% before 25 and 28 WG [1]. Two series comparing outcome obstetrical data from multiples reduced to twins and nonreduced multiples suggest that the obstetric outcome of twins following reduction is not equivalent to that of twin gestations in which selective embryo reduction has not been performed. Groutz et al. [29] compared the outcome of twins obtained by means of MFPR with that of spontaneously conceived twins; patients who initially had carried quadruplets delivered significantly earlier than those who had originally carried triplets or nonreduced twin gestation (33.2 vs. 35.9 and 36.9 WG). In Alexander's study [30], twins following reduction from high-order multiples were delivered at a lower gestational age than the nonreduced group and the mean fetal birth weights differed significantly (reduced 2,038 g, nonreduced 2,512 g), suggesting that MFPR does not reverse completely the decreased gestational age and impaired fetal growth associated with high-order multiples. However, it is unclear whether these results concerning birth weights are due to earlier delivery, to an effect of the procedure or to the initial placentation of more than two embryos.

There are few data available on the natural history of quintuplet pregnancies, as series are limited and anecdotal. To date, the majority of quintuplets undergo MFPR, leading to a better obstetrical outcome. Among a series of 21 quintuplet pregnancies mostly reduced to twins, Berkowitz et al. [2] reported a mean gestational age at delivery of 35 WG, whereas 3% of births occurred between 24 and 28 WG, 13% between 28 and 32 WG and 36% between 32 and 36 WG. In Evans' study, among the 170 quintuplets mostly reduced to twins, there were 32.9% of births after 37 WG, 32.4% between 33 and 36WG, 12.4% between 29 and 32 WG and 5.3% before 25 and 28 WG [1]. Concerning indications, selective terminations are currently performed in high-order multiple fetal pregnancies (quadruplets, quintuplets or more). The ability to carry four or more fetuses to viability is not assured. Without any intervention, it is quite likely that women would lose all fetuses or deliver four or five infants with major risks of permanent handicaps.

These rare obstetric circumstances are generally accepted for reduction because prematurity rates, fetal growth retardation rates and perinatal mortality rates are very high (13,17).

**Performing multifetal pregnancy reduction on triplets**

One important challenge in triplet pregnancies is the high rate of premature delivery, ranging from 87.5 to 91.6%, while the mean age at delivery is 33.9 WG [17]. Analyzing the natural history of triplet gestation provides information about the risk of very early prematurity. The prematurity rate before 32 WG ranges from to 6.6% for Newmann [22] to 26.5% in the French national collecting data (FIVNAT) [6]. The proportion of births occurring between 32 WG reaches approximately 25% according to the series of the literature, while the rate of premature deliveries occurring between 24 and 28 weeks is nearly 7% [22–28]. We reviewed three series that compare the outcome of reduced triplets vs. nonreduced triplets [13,17,21]. The mean gestational age at delivery for the gestations resulting from reduced triplets was nearly 36.5 WG, while the mean gestational age at delivery (34.4 WG) in expectantly managed groups is comparable to that reported in the literature. There is a significant decrease in prematurity among reduced groups compared to triplets since pregnancies of the reduced populations continue for 2 weeks longer on average. However, reduction does not seem to be effective for avoiding extreme premature births, although they occur less frequently in reduced groups than in expectantly managed groups. In the 1996 collaborative Evans' study, the prematurity rate observed in the interval between 25 and 28 WG was 3.3 and 7.5% between 29 and 32 WG among triplets managed with MFPR [1].

As for the fetal growth, there was a significant and important weight gain among reduced pregnancies, since the birth weights of infants in reduced group were nearly 450 g higher in all series. Furthermore, the proportion of fetal weights < 1,500 g was lower among the reduced groups. In our study, we showed that the proportion of infants whose weights were under the third centile, was lower in the reduced group when compared to the nonreduced group. In Lipitz's study [21], the incidence of infants weighing less than 1,000 g and infants whose weights were between 1,000 and 1,500 g were 1.7 vs. 6.7% and 5.1 vs 19.7%, respectively, in comparison to the nonreduced group. It would thus appear that MFPR does improve fetal growth. This weight gain reveals the absence of any detrimental effects of selective reduction on the growth of the surviving twins. However, we think that the increase in birth weight may be partially explained by the avoidance of placental functional insuffiency in triplet cases. The increase in gestational age at delivery, since birth weight and gestational age are linked, might play a role. Our series and the Lipitz's study reported a decrease in the incidence of perinatal mortality and neonatal respiratory complications and reported a decrease in the incidence of intraventricular hemorrhaging among the patients undergoing MFPR [17,21]. Bollen reported that 8% of surviving triplets suffer from neurological sequelae and this percentage may rise because many of these children were too young to permit full evaluation [13]. All these data suggest that a reduction from triplet to twin decreases the chance of very early prematurity and short-term morbidity. Although MFPR decreases the number of babies going home per couple, it increases the proportion of surviving infants without complications. However, data fails to demonstrate an improvement in the long-term outcome of the survivors as no information from a prolonged follow up is available in any study.

MFPR on triplets is usually performed within centers experienced in the management of high-order gestations. In Evans' study [9], 42% of the 1,084 procedures performed were for reducing triplets. This rate is similar for the expanded series including 1,789 gestations out of which 759 were triplets. In the French national study [31], 41% of 262 cases of reductions performed were on triplets. Similar data are reported from monocentric series, with a mean rate of 40%, (44% for Wapner [32], 43% for Salat-Baroux [15], 26% for Dommergues [32], 57.5% for Tabsh [34], 24% for Lipitz [20], 50% for Trimor-Trisch [14], 60% in our experience [17], 44% for Berkowitz [11], and 49% in his expanded series [2]). However, reducing triplets remains controversial. Although data shows an improvement in preterm deliveries and fetal growth, the advantages of the procedure remain uncertain because assessment in the long term is unavailable. With regard to triplets, there is no consensus among specialists concerning the use of MFPR. Some authors consider that the procedure, when applied to triplets, can be criticized because the medical risks related to these gestations do not systematically justify reduction. MFPR in triplets (resulting in twins and less often in singletons) should be considered in pregnancies with serious maternal disease (i.e., heart disease, diabetes), poor uterine conditions (bicornuate uterus, previous cesarean section, history of early preterm delivery of a prior singleton infant, exposure to distilbene) or in cases where an embryo is affected by a severe disease. In the absence of worrisome factors, one might consider that the decision belongs to the well-informed couple. The results shown above indicate that the reduction of triplets improves some obstetrical parameters and avoids serious maternal complications [9,10,13,17,21,35]. Consequently, the couples with triplets should be informed of the possibility of performing reduction and their related risks as well as the risks of naturally managed triplet gestation. Additional reasons for requesting MFPR include financial and social concerns, the obligation of the mother to stop her professional activities and the anticipation of a poor quality of life after the birth of triplets [36]. Like others, our opinions on the subject have evolved during the past decade [1,16] and we consider that the ultimate decision should be made by the woman and her spouse thus allowing greater patient autonomy and choice.

### How many embryos should be left?

The number of fetuses which should be left after the procedure is a further topic for discussion. Although reducing multifetal pregnancy to twins appears to be the more appropriate medical attitude for the majority of both medical teams and couples, some argue for reducing a multifetal gestation to a singleton in the hope of lowering the obstetrical risks related with the course of a twin gestation. Since twin gestations are at a higher risk for obstetric complications compared to singletons, selective reduction to a singleton may be justified. From 5 to 7% of twin deliveries occur before 32 WG leading to an incidence of long-term sequelae higher than that observed in singleton pregnancies. This risk might be sufficient to perform a reduction on triplets to obtain a singleton. Brambati et al. [12] reported the results of 100 postreduction pregnancies, 32 of which were reduced to singletons and the remainder to twins. As the outcome of pregnancies reduced to singletons was significantly better than those reduced to twins, the authors concluded that these results make a woman's request ethically justified. When couples ask for the reduction of triplets to singletons, their requests should be carefully assessed. Some couples argue that abortion on demand justifies the procedure when considering the womens' right to decide what to do with her pregnancies within the legal period. Consequently, fetal reduction in high-order or even twin pregnancies may be performed to reduce the number of fetuses according to the patients' convenience. In our opinion, such a request involves risks for the surviving singleton as data indicate that the loss rate of pregnancies reduced to singletons is greater than those reduced to twins [1]. Twins are at a greater risk than singletons but these risks can be managed, and the children can benefit from the recent advances in neonatal care leading to a successful outcome for the majority.

In conclusion, first-trimester selective reduction improves the prognosis of high-order multiple pregnancies. The benefits to the remaining fetuses with regards to the length of gestation, birth weight and perinatal morbidity are well established for multiple pregnancies with more than three embryos. Information on the risks (miscarriage) and advantages of reduction (gain in fetal growth and prematurity, decrease of maternal complications) should be supplied to all couples with multiple pregnancies by an experienced obstetrician. Reduction seems necessary for triplet pregnancies when there are poor prognosis factors such as structural uterine anomaly or severe maternal disease. It remains unclear whether the long-term outcome of triplets is improved by the procedure.

Practitioners involved in ART must have a complete and accurate understanding of the medical consequences of iatrogenic multifetal pregnancy, as well as the social, financial and psychological aspects. For ethical reasons, efforts should be made to prevent these high-risk situations which are side effects of infertility treatments. Although it is a relatively safe and effective technique, MFPR should never be considered as a routine procedure, and should never be thought of as a routine part of fertility treatment. However, an unanticipated multiple pregnancy may occur when more than two embryos are transferred. Therefore, we consider the MFPR to be the best tool under theses exceptional circumstances.

196

## Acknowledgements

We would like to thank Mrs Childress for her precious help in editing the manuscript.

## References

1. Evans MI, Kramer RL, Yaron Y, Drugan A, Johnson MP. What are the ethical and technical problems associated with multifetal pregnancy gestation? Clin Obstet Gynecol 1998;41:47—54.
2. Berkowitz RL, Lynch Lauren, Stone J, Alvarez M. The current status of multifetal pregnancy reduction. Am J Obstet Gynecol 1996;174:1265—1272.
3. Influence des grossesses multiples. In Grande prématurité: dépistage et prévention du risque. Expertise collective. INSERM 1997. 7—21 Ed INSERM.
4. ART World collaborative report 1993. 15th World Congress on Fertility and Sterility. Montpellier, 1995.
5. Assisted reproductive technology in the United States and Canada: 1994 results generated from the American Society for Reproductive Medicine/Society for Assisted Reproductive Technology Registry. Fertil Steril 1996;66:697—705.
6. Dossier FIVNAT 1996. 10 ans d'évolution de la FIV en France. Analyse des résultats 1986—1994.
7. Dechaud H, Picot MC, Hedon B, Boulot P. First-trimester multifetal pregnancy reduction: evaluation of technical aspects and risks from 2,756 cases of the literature. Fetal Therapy (In press).
8. Wenstrom KD, Syrop CH, Hammit DG, Van Voorhis BJ. Increased risk of monochorionic twinning associated with assisted reproduction. Fertil Steril 1993;60:510—513.
9. Evans MI, Dommergues M, Wapner RJ, Lynch L, Dumez Y, Goldberg JD, Zador IE, Nicolaides KH, Johnson MP, Golbus MS, Boulot P, Berkowitz RL. Efficacy of transabdominal multifetal pregnancy reduction: collaborative experience among the worlds largest centers. Obstet Gynecol 1993;82:61—66.
10. Evans MI, Dommergues M, Wapner RJ, Lynch L, Dumez Y, Goldberg JD, Nicolaides KH, Johnson MP, Golbus MS, Boulot P, Aknin AJ, Monteagudo A, Berkowitz RL. Transabdominal versus transcervical and transvaginal multifetal pregnancy reduction: international collaborative experience of more than thousand cases. Am J Obstet 1994;170:902—909.
11. Berkowitz RL, Lynch l, Lapinski R, Bergh P. First-trimester transabdominal multifetal pregnancy reduction: a report of 200 completed cases. Am J Obstet Gynecol 1993;169:17—21.
12. Brambati B, Tului L. First-trimester fetal reduction: its role in the management of twin and higher order multiple pregnancies. Hum Reprod Update 1995;1:397—408.
13. Bollen N, Camus M, Tournaye H, Wisanto A, Van Steirteghem A, Devroey P. Embryo reduction in triplet pregnancies after assisted procreation: a comparative study. Fertil Steril 1993;60:504—509.
14. Timor-Tritsch IE, Peisner BD, Monteagudo A, Lerner JP, Sharma S. Multifetal pregnancy reduction by transvaginal puncture: evaluation of the technique used in 134 cases. Am J Obstet Gynecol 1993;168:799—804.
15. Salat-Baroux J, Aknin J, Antoine JM, Alamowitch R. The management of multiple pregnancies after induction for superovulation. Hum Reprod 1988;3:399—401.
16. Boulot P, Hedon B, Pelliccia G, Lefort G, Deschamps F, Arnal F, Humeau C, Laffargue F, Viala JL. Multifetal pregnancy reduction: a consecutive series of 61 cases. Br J Obstet Gynecol 1993;100:63—68.
17. Boulot P, Hedon B, Pelliccia G, Peray P, Laffargue F, Viala JL. The effects of selective reduction in triplet gestations: a comparative study on 80 cases managed with or without this procedure. Fertil Steril 1993;60:497—503.

18. Maymon R, Herman A, Shulman A, Halperin R, Arieli S, Bukovsky I, Weinraub Z. First-trimester embryo reduction: a medical solution to an iatrogenic problem. Human Reprod 1995; 10:668–673.
19. Kol S, Levron J, Lewit N, Drugan A, Itskovitz-Elder J. The natural history of multiple pregnancies after assisted reproduction: is spontaneous demise a clinically significant phenomenon? Fertil Steril 1993;60:127–130.
20. Hecht BR, Magoon MW. Can the epidemic of iatrogenic multiples be conquered? Clin Obstet Gynecol 1998;41:127–137.
21. Lipitz S, Reichman B, Uval J, Shalev J, Achiron R, Barkai G, Maschiach S. A prospective comparison of the outcome of triplet pregnancies managed expectantly or by multifetal reduction to twins. Am J Obstet Gynecol 1994;170:874–879.
22. Newman R, Hamer C, Miller M. Outpatient triplet management: a contemporary review. Am J Obstet Gynecol 1989;161:547–553.
23. Seoud MA, Kruithoff C, Muasher SJ. Outcome of triplet and quadruplet pregnancies resulting from in vitro fertilization. Eur J Obstet Gynecol Reprod Biol 1991;41:79–84.
24. Vervliet J, De Cleyn K, Renier et al. Management and outcome of 21 triplet and quadruplet pregnancies. Eur J Obstet Gynecol Reprod Biol 1989;33:61–69.
25. Gonen Y, Blankier J, Casper RF. The outcome of triplet, quadruplet and quintuplet pregnancies managed in a perinatal unit: obstetric, neonatal and follow-up data. Am J Obstet Gynecol 1990;162:454–459.
26. Elliott JP, Radin TG. Quadruplet pregnancy: contemporary management and outcome. Obstet Gynecol 1992;80:421–424.
27. Collins MS, Bleyl J. Seventy-one quadruplet pregnancies: management and outcome. Am J Obstet Gynecol 1990;162:1384–1392.
28. Lipitz S, Reichman B, Paret G, Modan M, Shalev J, Serr D, Mashiach S, Frenkel Y. The improving outcome of triplet pregnancies. Am J Obstet Gynecol 1989;161:1279–1284.
29. Groutz A, Yovel I, Amit A, Yaron Y, Azem F, Lessing JB. Pregnancy outcome after multifetal pregnancy reduction to twins compared with spontaneously conceived twins. Hum Reprod 1996;11:1334–1336.
30. Alexander JM, Hammond KR, Steinkampf MP. Multifetal reduction of high-order multiple pregnancy: comparison of obstetrical outcome with nonreduced twin gestations. Fertil Steril 1995;64:1201–1203.
31. Dommergues M, Aknin J, Boulot P, Nisand I, Lewin F, Oury JF, Herlicoviez M, Dumez Y, Evans M. Pour le Club Francophone de Médecine Foetale. Réductions embryonnaires dans les grossesses multiples. Une enquête multicentrique française. J Gynecol Obstet Biol Reprod 1994;23:415–418.
32. Wapner RJ, Davis GH, Johnson A, Weinblatt VJ, Fischer RL, Jackson LG, Chervenak FA, MC Cullough LB. Selective reduction of multifetal pregnancies. Lancet 1990;335:90–94.
33. Dommergues M, Nisand I, Mandelbrot L, Isfer E, Radunovic N, Dumez Y. Embryo reduction in multifetal pregnancies following infertility therapy: obstetrical risks and perinatal benefits are related to operative strategy. Fertil Steril 1991;55:801–811.
34. Tabsh KA. Transabdominal multifetal pregnancy reduction: report of 40 cases. Obstet Gynecol 1990;75:739–741.
35. Smith-Levitin M, Kowlaik A, Birnholz J, Skupski DW, Hutson JM, Chervenak FA, Rosenwaks Z. Selective reduction of multifetal pregnancies to twins improves outcome over nonreduced triplet gestations. Am J Obstet Gynecol 1996;175:878–882.
36. Vauthier-Brouzes D, Lefebvre G. Selective reduction n multifetal pregnancies: technical and psychological aspects. Fertil Steril 1992;57:1012–1016.

# Are anomalies increased after ART and ICSI?

Joe Leigh Simpson

*Department of Obstetrics and Gynecology, Baylor College of Medicine, Houston, Texas, USA*

**Abstract.** Various pitfalls preclude facile analysis of ART pregnancies, but available data provide no indication that congenital anomalies are increased in ART pregnancies. Offspring resulting from IVF or ICSI show the same 2–3% anomaly rate as the general population. The sole adverse finding has been the nearly 1% prevalence of sex choromosomal aberrations following ICSI. Guidelines for minimizing surveillance biases in generating data are offered.

**Keywords:** assisted reproductive technologies, congenital anomalies, intracytoplasmic sperm injection, in vitro fertilization.

## Introduction

Offspring conceived by assisted reproductive technologies (ART) could plausibly be at increased risk for congenital anomalies. Fortunately, patients and ART teams alike can be comforted by extant data [1]. Nonetheless, reports of increased sex chromosomal polysomy after intracytoplasmic sperm injection (ICSI) highlight potential concerns. Given that the media will surely place a spot light on even poorly substantiated claims, it behoves the ART community to generate data validating ART safety.

The purpose of this communication is: 1) to summarize current information on congenital anomalies in standard IVF and ICSI pregnancies, 2) to examine pitfalls that impede determining whether the anomaly rate after ART is comparable to the 2–3% in the general population, and 3) to summarize recommendations for assessing anomalies while concomitantly taking into account potential confounding variables [1].

### Is the ART population comparable to the general population?

In assessing both pregnancy losses and congenital anomalies, a major underlying concern is that the ART population is not necessarily comparable to the general population.

First, the underlying infertility that necessitated ART may be associated with factors that persist and increase the rate of pregnancy loss or anomalies in offspring. Frequency and severity of past illnesses are not necessarily comparable in the ART and the general population. Infection producing tubal occlusion

*Address for correspondence:* Joe Leigh Simpson, Chairman and Professor, Department of Obstetrics and Gynecology, Baylor College of Medicine, 6550 Fannin, Suite 729A, Houston, TX 77030, USA.

could persist in a chronic state. Women undergoing ART are usually older (mean age about 33 or 34 years) than women conceiving naturally (mean age about 27 or 28 years); paternal age is also increased. Advanced maternal age is associated with increased risk of pregnancy loss and liveborn aneuploidy, whereas advanced paternal age is associated with fresh Mendelian mutations. Women undergoing ART and women in the general population also differ with respect to potential confounding variables like maternal toxin exposure and nutrition. The overall effect of the above confounders is uncertain. The higher maternal age in women undergoing ART places these women at increased risk compared to women in the general population, but lower exposures to toxins like alcohol and cigarettes place these same women at decreased risk. The aggregate effect of these contradictory trends is uncertain.

Pregnancies utilizing ICSI for oligospermic men having Y-deletions involving DAZ illustrate that the ART population differs from the general population on the basis of likelihood of anomalies in offspring. Azoospermic men with Y-deletions of DAZ obligatorily transmit the deleted Y to all male offspring, who will also be azoospermic or oligospermic. Thus, underlying genetic problems not only can explain the infertility that necessitates a couple to seek ART, but place offspring at increased risk irrespective of the manner by which pregnancy is achieved — natural or ART. Another example is men infertile due to congenital absence of the vas deferens (CAVD). Because a relationship exists between CAVS and mutations in the cystic fibrosis gene, a male with CAVD usually has two mutant CF alleles. If the female is heterozygous for ΔF508, offspring could show ΔF508 CF homozygosity or compound heterozygosity.

**Pregnancy losses associated with conventional IVF**

Spontaneous abortions are considered to be increased following in vitro fertilization (IVF). Although usually assumed to be the result of hormonal perturbations adversely affecting implantation, an increased abortion rate is of potential concern given that 50–60% of clinically recognized spontaneous abortions show chromosomal abnormalities. The increased pregnancy loss in ART could well reflect hormonal perturbations, but cytogenetic abnormalities have not been excluded as an explanation for the increased abortion rate. If chromosomal abnormalities are the explanation for the increased abortion rate, a corollary is that an increased risk would also exist for ART liveborns being cytogenetically abnormal.

For an early international meeting, Seppala et al. [2] collected data on 1,084 IVF pregnancies from multiple centers, finding the abortion rate to be 29.9%. In a 1988 international survey, Cohen et al. [3] collected IVF pregnancies from 55 centers worldwide. Of 2,329 pregnancies, 577 (24.8%) resulted in "early abortion", 36 "late abortion", three therapeutic abortion, and 120 ectopic pregnancy. Data collected from Australia and New Zealand between 1979 and 1987 showed 24.3% (641/2,634) spontaneous abortions [4]. In the UK the 430 IVF pregnancies reported from Bourne-Hallam Medical Centre showed 93 (23%) resulted in spontaneous abortion [5]. In the latest (1995) US cohort reported by the American Society of Reproductive Medicine and Society for Assisted Reproductive Technology [6] the spontaneous abortion rate was 18.6% in standard IVF, 18.9 and 21.6% with cryopreserved embryos. Data from the French national IVF registry consistently show abortion rates of 16—20% (1986—93) [7—9].

The 20—25% rate of spontaneous abortion in ART is generally considered to be elevated, but in fact this rate is barely increased over background [1,7]. Weeks of observations may be greater in women undergoing ART than in the general population because in ART pregnancy surveillance begins earlier. Surveillance is often more rigorous than in spontaneously conceived pregnancies. A better comparison might involve life table analysis that takes into account the differing number of weeks of observations.

**Anomalies associated with conventional IVF**

The fact that congenital anomalies could be increased in ART pregnancies is plausible for several reasons:
1) Selective mechanisms operating in vivo against morphologically abnormal sperm might not be comparably operative in vitro.
2) Altered hormonal milieu in vitro may predispose to perturbations of meiosis or mitosis and, hence, chromosomal aneuploidy.
3) Point mutations could result from the various chemical exposures inherent during extracorporeal fertilization. To assess whether any of these theoretical concerns have validity, various surveys and registries have generated data on ART anomaly rates. Although the vigilance of ART workers in initiating surveillance is salutary, an unassailable problem is that comparisons must be made to outcomes of birth defect registries, not necessarily the best comparison group.

Fortunately, data have since the onset been reassuring. In the 1988 survey of Cohen et al. [3] involving 55 centers worldwide there were 1,454 ART births, anomalies occurred in 23 of 938 singleton births (2.5%) and in eight of 22 (36%) multiple births. A problem is the disparate rates among centers, suggesting lack of consistent criteria. For example, some anomalies recorded would not necessarily have been detected in birth defects registries: small umbilical hernias, nonpigmented skin, "hip click" that may or may not actually indicate congenital hip dislocations, and an extra digit. The ART surveillance by Cohen et al. [3] thus could have recorded as anomalies variants not ordinarily included in birth defect registries. It follows that the ART anomaly rate could have been spuriously overestimated.

In Australia and New Zealand, ART units recorded in the late 1980s that the incidence of major congenital anomalies was 2.2% (37/1697 infants) [10]. Six of the 37 infants had spina bifida and four had transposition of the great vessels. This survey led Lancaster [11] to claim a possible relationship between neural tube defects (NTD) and ovulation-induction agents. We and others later showed in case control studies that no such association existed nor have any other IVF registries shown this [12]. Still, Lancaster and Shafir find the high incidence to persist in Australia/New Zealand [13]. The anomaly rate estimate for all malformation in Australia/New Zealand ART is now 2.9%, based on 185 malformations among 6,388 singleton births (1979—93) [14].

The UK Medical Research Council Working Party on Children Conceived through IVF surveyed 1,267 pregnancies conceived by IVF and GIFT [15] between 1978 and 1987. Data covered all UK clinics registered with a voluntary licensing authority. One or more congenital anomalies were detected in the 1st week of life in 35 of 1,581 IVF infants (2.2%). A slight increase in central nervous system anomalies did not reach statistical significance. Overall, 2.2% of individuals had one or more malformations diagnosed within the 1st year of life, comparable to the general UK population.

The UK Bourne-Hallam cases [15] were reported separately from the larger MRC survey [14]. Of 961 babies born between 1978 and 1987, 763 still lived in the UK. In these 763, the malformation rate was 2.7% in multiple births and 2.4% in singletons. Individual anomalies were also considered comparable to those expected on the basis of maternal age-adjusted rates derived from a Liverpool Congenital Malformation Register. Again, some anomalies listed would not have been detected in neonatal surveys: mild hypospadias, undescended testes, hydronephrosis, polycystic kidney disease and laryngeal cleft. Four cases of patent ductus arteriosis might have reflected simply prematurity.

Another European registry of interest is FIVNAT (French In Vitro National Registry) [8,9]. The anomaly rate as observed yearly (malformations per newborns) was 3.4, 3.0, 2.5, 3.8 and 3.5, respectively, between 1986 and 1990.

In the USA a registry maintained by the American Society Reproductive Medicine/Society and its Society for Assisted Reproductive Technologies (ASRM/SART) have provided valuable information. As an example of data comparable in time to most of the studies previously cited, the 1990 cohort recorded 38 congenital anomalies in 28 infants among 3,110 total liveborns [17]. This reports unconventionally recorded data as total anomalies per total infants, rather than the more conventional method of infants with anomalies per total number of infants. Using the latter approach, the anomaly rate would be 28/3,110, or 0.9%. As in other studies, certain anomalies would not have been detected on neonatal examination: periventricular cyst, hydronephrosis, pyloric stenosis, retinopathy, and pulmonary hypoplasia. Anomalies detected in pregnancy termination cases were also pooled with anomalies in liveborns, an inappropriate practice because some abnormal pregnancies that were terminated might have been lost spontaneously had not iatrogenic intervention occurred. If the pregnancy loss had been spontaneous rather than iatrogenic, the anomaly might have passed unrecognized.

Given biases toward overestimating anomaly rates, the US data are surprising in only showing an anomaly rate of 1%. Lower than expected anomaly rates in

US figures continue to be reported in the ASRM/SART registry, notwithstanding report of the 1993 cohort in which 5,103 deliveries resulted in 6,870 babies [18] having 2.3 "birth defects per neonates delivered". In the latest (1995) cohort there were 0.7 "birth defects per neonate" with standard IVF and 1.0 per neonate with IVF/ICSI.

Of particular interest, given the lower than expected reported rate in the USA, was experience in a single large US center. Palermo et al. [19] analyzed IVF pregnancies from The New York Hospital/Cornell Medical College, finding 23 of 653 (3.5%) to have major anomalies; and 20 of 653 (3.1%) had minor anomalies. These rates were considered comparable to rates in the general New York population [20].

In conclusion, anomaly rates in ART seem comparable to that in the general populations, notwithstanding difficulties in defining a proper comparison (control) group.

## Anomalies associated with ICSI

Concern has been raised that increased rates of certain abnormalities could occur following intracytoplasmic sperm injection (ICSI). This concern is distinct from transmission of a Y-deletion involving DAZ from men who require ICSI as result of oligospermia or azoospermia. The latter is of minimal clinical concern because DAZ deletions are not pleiotropic, seeming only to affect spermatogenesis. A greater concern would exist if risk for other anomalies is increased.

To this end the Centre for Reproductive Medicine of the Brussels Free University has long monitored their ICSI pregnancies. Anomalies have been systematically assessed in neonates, antenatal cytogenetic studies offered routinely and selected case control studies performed [21,22]. In the latest tabulations, Bonduelle et al. [22] reported 46 major malformations among 1,987 children. The 2.3% rate is comparable to background levels. Among their early follow-up studies, Bonduelle et al. [23] reported a study of 163 couples undergoing subzonal insemination (SUZI), intracytoplasmic sperm injection (ICSI), or both. Couples were followed prospectively, including a systematic neonatal exam by a geneticist. Follow-up exams were conducted at 12 months and again at 2 years of age. In the cohort, 21 children were born after SUZI, 24 after ICSI, and 10 after combining the two techniques. Only two of the 55 infants showed major malformations; none of the 55 infants had chromosomal abnormalities. In another study [24], 130 children born after ICSI were matched with 130 children born after IVF. Surveillance consisted of prenatal chromosomal studies, prenatal ultrasound examination, and physical examinations at birth, 2 months, and 1 year of age. Five major anomalies were detected in the ICSI group, compared to six in the matched IVF group.

Other groups have reported comparable anomaly rates. Reporting the New York Hospital/Cornell Medical College experience, Palermo et al. [25] reported the frequency of major anomalies to be 1.6%, even lower than the rate in their standard IVF cases [19]. Tarlatzis [26] tabulated a 22% rate with ejaculated sperm in the ESHRE Task Force data, a group that included cases from Brussels. Overall, the consensus is that major structural or functional in abnormalities following ICSI are not increased over general population expectations of 2—3%.

In contrast to salutary data concerning visually evident congenital anomalies, the rate of chromosomal abnormalities seems increased over age-matched expectations. Bonduelle et al. [22] report is only a modest increase in structural de novo autosomal chromosomal aberrations, 0.36% in ICSI [23] vs. a background [27] of 0.07%. There is a greater increase in sex chromosomal abnormalities, in nine of 1,082 ICSI cases (0.83%) [22] compared to 0.19% background. The Brussels rate is not so high as reported by another Belgium group [28,29], who also found the parental origin in each of six sex chromosomal abnormalities cases to be paternal. This included both 47,XXY as well as 45,X cases.

In conclusion, a trend toward increased de novo sex-chromosomal aberration in ICSI pregnancies is observed, particularly in men with extreme oligoasthenoteratospermia [22]. Otherwise, anomaly rates following ICSI are not increased.

**Biases in surveillance**

*Producing spurious increased rates*

Examination following ART is often more rigorous than that following conventional pregnancies (controls). Unfortunately, this well-meaning medical attention could be scientifically mischievous. If aggressive ART surveillance is not appreciated, the reported anomaly rate might be reported and accepted uncritically as increased (spuriously) compared to the less vigilantly assessed general population. Estimates of anomalies in the latter are usually derived from birth defects registries, which record all major anomalies among neonates born in selected hospitals. Participating neonatologists typically examine every infant carefully but, of necessity, not exhaustively.

We have already presented evidence that more vigorous surveillance exists in ART pregnancies. For example, the UK MRC surveillance recorded many anomalies not necessarily detected in neonatal surveys [13]. Examples cited were mild hypospadias and undescended testes. The international survey of Cohen et al. [3] recorded many minor anomalies that would have either escaped detection or not be considered major in birth defect registries: small umbilical hernia, nonpigmented skin, "hip clicks" that may or may not be indicative of congenital hip dislocation, polydactyly.

Another bias is including internal anomalies that would not be evident solely on external physical exam. If both internal as well as external anomalies in ART offspring are included, more than the 2—3% anomalies expected in the general population would be found because pregnancies in the general population are less likely to undergo comprehensive ultrasound surveys during pregnancy. Included in ART surveillance but almost certainly not in birth defects registries would be these internal anomalies recorded in, as an example, the survey of Cohen [3]: "adrenal hyperplasia", "cardiopathy". Anomalies in the 1990 AFS/SART cohort [17] included periventricular cyst, hydronephrosis, unilateral kidney agenesis, pyloric stenosis, retinopathy of prematurity, and pulmonary hypoplasia.

A more subtle surveillance bias occurs when anomaly assessment following ART is conducted over a prolonged time interval after birth. In the birth defects registries whose data are used to derive the 2—3% anomaly rate in the general population, ascertainment for anomalies is usually restricted to the time of hospitalization after delivery, an interval typically only 1 or 2 days. Completeness of detection of anomalies increases as the length of surveillance after delivery increases; thus, continuing to ascertain anomalies weeks after birth is not comparable to the hospital anomalies ascertained exclusively in the ascertainment characteristic of birth defects registries.

*Biases in surveillance producing spuriously decreased rates*

Biases may also lead to lower than expected ART anomaly rates. In particular, an increased anomaly rate would fail to be appreciated if ART centers do not systematically assess offspring for congenital anomalies. As an example, review of hospital chart review would be a poor way of ascertaining anomalies. Casual surveillance could explain the low anomaly rate recorded in certain surveys, for example, 0.7% in Greek cases recorded by Cohen et al. [3] or 0.9% in the 1990 US AFS/SART cohort [17]. Failure to search systematically for anomalies is a valid concern in almost all ART cohorts, with the notable exceptions of the small IVF case control study of Morin et al. [30] and the ICSI cohort in Brussels [21—24].

Another pitfall arises whenever a significant proportion of a given sample is lost to follow-up. One cannot assume that cases lost to follow-up are comparable to cases remaining for analysis. Moreover, direction of bias is uncertain. Women lost to follow-up might not wish to be troubled because their offspring was healthy and because no personal benefit seemed to accrue from participating in a research protocol. The net effect would be a spuriously increased anomaly rate following ART because normal outcomes had been disproportionately excluded. Conversely, women lost to follow-up who have experienced a bad outcome (pregnancy loss, anomalous infant), may harbor resentment toward the medical and scientific community, leading them to fail to respond to requests for follow-up. If so, the ART anomaly rate would spuriously be decreased.

If only a small proportion of cases from a large cohort are lost to follow-up, the remaining subjects could be assumed to be representative. However, this assumption is not necessarily valid when the outcome sought is infrequent and when a relatively high proportion of cases is lost to follow-up. In ART surveillance the number of cases lost to follow-up may be several fold greater than the background 2—3% anomaly rate. In the 1993 US AFS/SART report [18] 58 anomalies were reported in 3,873 babies, or "1.5 defects per 100 neonates". Yet 447 of 3,873 IVF babies were lost to follow-up (11.4%). If even 10% of the 447 lost cases were anomalous, the overall anomaly rate would have risen to 2.7% (103/3873).

Overlooked on occasion is the problem of insufficient sample size. Sometimes power is lacking to derive any meaningful conclusions concerning whether an increase in anomalies exists over the background rate of 2–3%. As illustrative, detection of a 3-fold increase in anomalies requires 244 cases if the baseline rate were 3% ($\alpha$ = 0.05; 1-$\beta$ = 0.80). If the sample size is only 133 cases, power would be adequate only to exclude a 4-fold increase in anomalies. If one wished to study a specific disorder (e.g., Down syndrome) (1:800 live-borns), a sample size numbering in the thousands would be necessary for reasonable power.

### Effect of including anomalies in liveborns and anomalies in abortuses

A common methodological shortcoming in ART surveillance is pooling anomalies in neonates with anomalies in abortuses (spontaneous or induced). Birth defects registries do not record anomalies in abortuses, induced or spontaneous. Failure to tabulate anomalies in induced abortuses is not based just on fears of incomplete ascertainment, but knowledge that fetuses with anomalies may or may not have survived until birth. The natural history of anomalies is uncertain. For example, considerably fewer than half the trisomy 18 cases detected at amniocentesis persist until birth, and only two-thirds of trisomy 21 cases [31]. Pooling anomalies ascertained during prenatal cytogenetic surveillance (chorionic villus sampling, amniocentesis) with those detected at birth would thus yield data not comparable to the liveborn general population.

### How should anomalies be assessed and recorded?

To assess pregnancy losses and anomalies after ART, Simpson and Liaebers [1] recommend a cohort approach that systematically record data in standard fashion. Data should preferably be recorded on standard forms, designed for ease of computer entry. Prospective evaluation should begin as soon as possible after pregnancy is diagnosed. An intake form might record salient findings: family history, obstetric history, number of prior spontaneous abortions, medical illnesses, exposure to drugs, exposures to toxins like cigarette smoking and alcohol.

The second crucial survey instrument is one for infant evaluation. Forms having over 100 potential anomalies are available and, in fact, have been utilized successfully by the author [32]. However, these lengthy forms usually record presence or absence of not just major, but also minor anomalies whose assessment we have already noted is hazardous. Defining major anomalies is easier. A pragmatic approach is to define a major anomaly as one resulting in death, causing serious handicap, or necessitating surgery. All these outcomes are readily measurable. A vascular malformation requiring surgery is thus defined as a major anomaly, whereas one not requiring surgery is minor. Geneticists and dysmorphologists should be available to confirm abnormal findings and to verify presence or absence of Mendelian disorders or syndromes; however, geneticists should probably not perform examinations routinely because their diagnostic acumen might be greater than that of pediatricians who lack genetic training. Examinations of infants by geneticists or dysmorphologists might show a spuriously increased anomaly rates compared to a group (control) not comparably scrutinized.

As noted previously, one should either restrict surveillance to external anomalies or record separately internal anomalies detectable only by ultrasound. Anomaly assessment should also be restricted to a specified time interval.

## Conclusion

Various pitfalls preclude facile analysis of ART pregnancies, but available data fortunately provide no indication that congenital anomalies are increased in ART pregnancies. Offspring resulting from IVF or ICSI show the same 2–3% anomaly rate as the general population. The sole adverse finding has been the nearly 1% prevalence of sex chromosomal aberrations following ICSI. Guidelines for minimizing surveillance biases in generating data are offered.

## References

1. Simpson JL, Liaebers L. Assessing congenital anomalies after preimplantation genetic diagnosis. J Assist Reprod 1996;13:170–176.
2. Seppala M. The world collaborative report on in vitro fertiliatin and embryo replacement: current state of the art in January 1984. Ann NY Acad Sci 1984;442:558–563.
3. Cohen J, Mayaux MJ, Guihard-Moscato L. Pregnancy outcomes after in vitro fertilization. A collaborative study on 2342 pregnancies. Ann NY Acad Sci 1988;541:1–6.
4. National Perinatal Statistics Unit and The Fertility Society of Australia: IVF and GIFT pregnancies, Australia and New Zealand, 1987, 1995.
5. Steer C, Campbell S, Davies M, Mason B, Collins W. Spontaneous abortion rates after natural and assisted conception. Br Med J 1989;299:1317–1318.
6. Assisted reproductive technology in the United States and Canada: 1995 results generated from the American Society for Reproductive Medicine/Society for Assisted Reproductive Technology Registry: Fertil Steril 1998;69:389–398.
7. Simpson JL. Registration of congenital anomalies in ART populations pitfalls. Hum Reprod 1996;11(Suppl 4);81–88.
8. FIVNAT. French national IVF registry: analysis of 1986 to 1990 data. Fertil Steril 1993;59;587–595.
9. FIVNAT. Pregnancies and births resulting from in vitro fertilization; French National registry, analysis of data 1986 to 1992. Contracept Fertil Sex 1995;23:S141–142.
10. Saunders DM, Lancaster PAL. The wider perinatal significance of the Australian in vitro fertilization data collection program. Am J Perinat 1989;6:252–255.
11. Lancaster PAL. Congenital malformations after in vitro fertilization. Lancet 1987;2:1392–1393.

208

12. Mills JL, Simpson JL, Rhoads GG, Graubard BI, Hoffman H, Conley MR, Lassman M, Cunningham G. Risk of neural tube defects in relation to maternal fertility and fertility drug use. Lancet 1990;336:103—104.
13. Lancaster PAL, Shafir E. High incidence of neural tube effects after assisted conception. Hum Reprod 1996;11:39 (Abstract).
14. Lancaster PAL. Registers of in vitro fertilization and assisted conception. Hum Reprod 1996; 11(Suppl 4);89—104.
15. Beral V, Doyle P. Births in Great Britain resulting from assisted conception, 1978—87, MRC Working Party on Children Conceived by In Vitro Fertilization. Br J Med 1990;300:1229—1233.
16. Rizk B, Doyle P, Tan SL, Rainsburg P, Betts J, Brinsden P, Edwards R. Perinatal outcome and congenital malformations in in vitro fertilization babies from the Bourne-Hallam group. Hum Reprod 1991;6:1259—1264.
17. Medical Research International, Society for Assisted Reproductive Technology (SART), The American Fertility Society: In vitro fertilization-embryo transfer (IVF-ET) in the United States: 1990 results from IVF-ET Registry. Fertil Steril 1992;57:15—24.
18. Society for Assisted Reproductive Technology, American Society for Reproductive Medicine. Assisted reproductive technology in the United States and Canada: 1993 results generated from the American Society for Reproductive Medicine/Society for Assisted Reproductive Technology. Fertil Steril 1995;64:13—21.
19. Palermo GD, Colombero LT, Schattman GL, Davis OK, Rosenwaks Z. Evolution of pregnancies and initial follow-up of newborns delivered after intracytoplasmic sperm injection. JAMA 1996;276:1893—1897.
20. New York State Department of Health. Congenital malformations registry annual report. Statistical summary of children born in 1986 and diagnosed through 1988, 1990.
21. Bonduelle M, Willikens J, Buysse A et al. Prospective study of 877 children born after intracytoplasmic sperm injection, with ejaculated epididymal and testicular spermatozoa and after replacement of cryopreserved embryos obtained after ICSI. Hum Reprod 1996;11(Suppl 4); 131—159.
22. Bonduelle M, Aytoz A, VanAssche E, Devroey P, Liebaers I, Van Steiteghem A. Incidence of chromosomal aberrations in children born after assisted reproduction through intracytoplasmic sperm injection. Hum Reprod 1998;13:781—782.
23. Bonduelle M, Desmyttere S, Buysse A, Van Assche R, Schietecatte J, Devroey P, Van Steirteghem AC, Liebaers I. Prospective follow-up study of 55 children born after subzonal insemination and intracytoplasmic sperm injection. Hum Reprod 1994;9:1765—1769.
24. Bonduelle M, Legein J, Derde MP, Buysse A, Schietecatte J, Wisanto A, Devroey P, Van Steirteghem A, Liebaers I. Comparative follow-up study of 130 children born after ICSI and 130 children born after IVF: Abstracts of the 10th Annual Meeting of the ESHRE, Brussels, 1994;38.
25. Palermo G, Colombero L, Schattman G et al. Evaluation of pregnancies and initial follow-up of newborns delivered after intracytoplasmic sperm injection. J Am Med Assoc 1996;276: 1893—1897.
26. Tarlatzis BC. Report of the ESHRE Task Force on intracytoplasmic sperm injection. Hum Reprod 1996;11(Suppl 4);160—185.
27. Jacobs P, Browne C, Gregson N et al. Estimates of the frequency of chromosome abnormalities detectable in unselected newborns using moderate levels of banding. J Med Genet 1992;29: 103—106.
28. In't Veld P, Brandenburg H, Verhoeff A et al. Sex chromosomal abnormalities and intracytoplasmic sperm injection. Lancet 1995;346:773.
29. Van Opstal D, Los F, Ramlakham S et al. Determination of the parent or origin in nine cases of prenatally detected chromosome aberrations found after intracytoplasmic sperm injection. Hum Reprod 1997;12:682—686.
30. Morin NC, Wirth FH, Johnson DH et al. Congenital malformations and psychosocial development in children conceived by in vitro fertilization. J Pediatr 1989;115:222—227.

31. Hook EB, Hutton DE, Ide R et al. The natural history of Down syndrome conceptuses diagnosed prenatally that are not electively terminated. Am J Hum Genet 1995;57;875−881.
32. Mills JL, Knopp RH, Simpson JL et al. Lack of relation of increased malformation rates in infants of diabetic mothers to glycemic control during organogenesis. N Engl J Med 1988;318: 671−676.

# Clinical applications of preimplantation diagnosis

# Polar body biopsy

Y. Verlinsky, J. Cieslak, S. Rechitsky, V. Ivakhnenko, A. Lifchez, A. Kuliev and the Preimplantation Genetics Group
*Reproductive Genetics Institute, Chicago, Ilinois, USA*

**Abstract.** To avoid fertilization and transfer of genetically abnormal oocytes we have developed an approach for genetic evaluation of human oocytes using the first and second polar body biopsy. We have shown that the polar body biopsy does not affect fertilization and viability of the resulting embryos, as well as pre- and postimplantation development. Our present experience of polar body diagnosis includes about 700 clinical cycles, performed for preimplantation diagnosis for cystic fibrosis, $\alpha$-1-antitrypsin deficiency, retinitis pigmentosa, hemophilia A and B, thalassemia, Alport, Gaucher's, Tay Sach's and sickle cell disease, long-chain acyl-CoA dehydrogenase deficiency, and chromosomal abnormalities. Overall, more than 4,000 oocytes were tested for age-related aneuploidies or the above-listed single gene defects based on the first and second polar body analysis. Over three-quarters of the cycles performed have resulted in embryo transfer, 23% in a clinical pregnancy, from which more than 90 unaffected children have already been born, following confirmation of the polar body diagnosis by prenatal diagnosis. The results demonstrate the reliability of the polar body genetic analysis for preimplantation diagnosis of single gene and chromosomal disorders.

**Keywords:** chromosomal abnormalities, first polar body, FISH, PCR, polar body biopsy, preimplantation genetic diagnosis, second polar body, single gene disorders.

## Introduction

Polar body biopsy provides an option for couples at risk for conceiving a genetically abnormal fetus to avoid birth of an affected child without the need for a selective abortion of an affected fetus following prenatal diagnosis [1–4]. Removing the first and second polar bodies and performing genetic analysis of their DNA make it possible to predict the genotype of the embryos resulting from the corresponding oocytes. This will accordingly involve induction of superovulation to retrieve several follicles, micromanipulation to remove polar bodies (PBR), and subsequent fertilization and transfer of preselected unaffected embryos back to the patient.

Follicular stimulation and oocyte retrieval are performed using a standard IVF protocol. The procedure of PBR has been described elsewhere [5]. Following biopsy, oocytes are washed in IVF medium, inseminated with motile sperm and examined for the presence of pronuclei and for the extrusion of the second polar body, sampled to follow-up the results of the first polar body analysis. To avoid an additional biopsy, sampling of both the first and second polar bodies can be

*Address for correspondence:* Yury Verlinsky PhD, Reproduction Genetics Inst. 836 W. Wellington #4504 Chicago, IL 60657 USA. Tel.: +1-773-296-7095. Fax: +1-773-296-7087.

done simultaneously, following insemination. After an additional 24 h in culture, the oocytes are checked for cleavage, and those which result from the embryos whose first polar body was found to be homozygous for the abnormal gene, are transferred back to the patient to achieve a pregnancy. The second polar body in these cases contains a normal gene. In the cases of heterozygous first polar body, only the embryos resulting from the oocytes whose second polar body contains the abnormal gene are transferred. The affected oocytes subjected to PBR are followed up by a blastomere biopsy or by another possible sampling to confirm the diagnosis. The design of the approach, and a complete description of primers and reaction conditions for preimplantation DNA analysis used in our studies have been described elsewhere [6,7]. Preimplantation polar body analysis for common aneuploidies is performed by the use of the fluorescent in situ hybridization (FISH) technique and application of specific probes for chromosomes 13, 18 and 21 (Vysis, Naperville, IL). The method of applying these probes, scoring criteria of the fluorescence signals and the strategy of the polar body diagnosis of chromosomal disorders have been described previously [8—10].

Our present experience includes a polar body based preimplantation diagnosis in 725 clinical cycles, which were performed for cystic fibrosis (CF), thalassemia, sickle cell anemia, α-1-antitrypsin deficiency, Tay Sach's, Alport and Gauchers disease, retinitis pigmentosa, hemophilia A and B, long-chain acyl-CoA dehydrogenase deficiency and chromosomal abnormalities (Table 1). Indications for chromosomal disorders included age-related aneuploidies in IVF patients and maternal translocations. In the future this can be done for any single gene disorder for which sufficient sequence information is available to design PCR primers, as well as for any chromosomal abnormality, for which chromosome-specific probes exist.

Although the first and second polar bodies have no known biological significance for pre- and postimplantation development, it has been still necessary to

*Table 1.* Preimplantation polar body diagnosis of single gene disorders.

| Condition | Patients | Cycles |
|---|---|---|
| Cystic fibrosis | 11 | 21 |
| Thalassemia | 9 | 17 |
| Tay-Sach's diseases | 1 | 3 |
| Hemophilia A | 2 | 8 |
| Hemophilia B | 1 | 1 |
| Retinitis Pigmentosa | 1 | 1 |
| Sickle cell disease | 3 | 6 |
| Alport disease | 1 | 1 |
| α-1-antitrypsin | 1 | 5 |
| Gaucher | 1 | 1 |
| LCHAD | 1 | 2 |
| Total | 32 | 66 |

follow up and monitor possible developmental changes in the embryos resulting from the oocytes from which the first and second polar bodies were removed. These studies showed no detrimental effect of the procedures on the developmental potential of the resulting embryos, based on the following observations [11,12]:

1) There was no significant decrease in fertilization rate.
2) The proportion of cleaving embryos derived from the oocytes subjected to PBR appeared not to differ from that in control oocytes.
3) No increase was observed in the percentage of polyspermic embryos in the PBR oocytes.
4) About 60% embryos resulted from the PBR oocytes developed to blastocyst stage, similar to nonmanipulated human embryos.
5) There was also no effect of PBR on the implantation rate and the outcome of pregnancy following PBR [8—10].

**Polar body preimplantation diagnosis of Mendelian diseases**

One of the important issues in polar body analysis is its accuracy and reliability for predicting the genotype of the resulting embryos. Initially the method involved the biopsy and genetic analysis of the first polar body only. Although acceptable for a preselection of homozygous normal oocytes following the first meiotic division, this appeared to be limited for those cases where crossover has taken place, resulting in the heterozygous first polar body. This limitation is also true for the polar body diagnosis of chromosomal disorders, as abnormal gametes may result also following errors in the second meiotic division. To overcome the above limitations, sequential analysis of both the first and second polar bodies for single gene disorders, and simultaneous sampling and analysis of both polar bodies for chromosomal disorders have been introduced. As will be demonstrated below, prediction of the genotype of embryos by testing both the first and second polar body is accurate and may be recommended for preimplantation diagnosis of genetic and chromosomal disorders. For example, Table 2 shows that the introduction of a sequential analysis of both the first and second polar bodies allowed us to preselect the normal gametes also from the oocytes heterozygous following the first meiotic division, therefore, almost doubling the number of normal embryos available for transfer [13]. The follow-up PCR analysis of the embryos resulting from the oocytes predicted to be abnormal based on the first and/or second polar testing has been of particular value in this regard, because it made possible to document any potential misdiagnoses, which may have been due to DNA contamination, preferential amplification or allele specific amplification failure, referred as an allele dropout (ADO). As seen from Table 3, ADO is observed in different type of cells, including the first polar bodies, requiring the development of methods for a reliable detection of ADO to avoid misdiagnosis [13,14]. One of such methods appeared to be a simultaneous amplification of the mutant and normal genes together with strongly linked poly-

*Table 2.* Results of two-step polar body analysis in predicting the genotype of oocytes following the first and second meiotic divisions.[a]

| Loci | Total oocytes analyzed by IPB + IIPB | Homozygote after IPB PCR | | Hemizygote after IIPB PCR | | Total oocytes with predicted genotype | |
|---|---|---|---|---|---|---|---|
| | | Normal or A1[b] | Mutant or A2[b] | Normal or A1[b] | Mutant or A2[b] | Normal or A1[b] | Mutant or A2[b] |
| Mutations (3) | 80 | 14 | 14 | 24 | 22 | 38 | 36 |
| STRs (5) | 130[c] | 23 | 28 | 36 | 33 | 59 | 61 |
| Total (8) | 210[c] | 37 | 42 | 60 | 55 | 97 | 97 |

[a]Data includes analysis of three mutations (CFTR Δ F-508, sickle cell disease, and hemophilia B) and 5 STRs (see text); [b]for STR's A1 — maternal allele 1; A2 — maternal allele 2; [c]this does not correspond to the number of oocytes studied as STRs were studied in the same oocytes.

morphic markers, to be designed for each single gene disease for which preimplantation diagnosis is performed. In the first round, PCR is performed with a mixture of outside primers for the gene and polimorphic markers [14]. After 25 cycles, a small quantity of the resulting PCR product is removed and a second round of PCR is performed with inside primers for each individual locus separately. The PCR product resulting from the second round is analyzed by heteroduplex detection, as for CF, or restriction digestion, as for thalassemias and sickle cell disease [14]. The value of linked polymorphic markers in detecting ADO in heterozygous first polar bodies is demonstrated in Table 4, summarizing the results of multiplex PCR for nine loci, including CFTR, β-globin gene, hemophilia B and six polymorphic markers. An overall ADO for all loci was 5.5%, most of which have been detected by multiplex PCR [13]. Table 4 also shows that 97% of the predicted genotypes were confirmed in the follow-up studies of the resulting embryos, demonstrating the accuracy of the multiplex nested PCR analysis for the reliable detection of ADO in polar body preimplantation

*Table 3.* Allele dropout rate in different types of heterozygous single cells.[a]

| Cell type | Heterozygote cystic fibrosis cells (CFTR Δ-F508/n) | | | Heterozygote cells with Sickle cell mutation (s/n) | | |
|---|---|---|---|---|---|---|
| | Total amplified | Both alleles | One allele (ADO) | Total amplified | Both alleles | One allele (ADO) |
| Single blastomeres | 93 | 62 | 31 (33.3%) | 57 | 44 | 13 (22.8%) |
| Single fibroblasts | 1126 | 1046 | 80 (7.1%) | 489 | 451 | 38 (7.7%) |
| First polar bodies | 118 | 111 | 7 (5.9%) | 52 | 47 | 5 (9.6%) |

[a]reference [14].

*Table 4.* Results of two-step polar body analysis in predicting the genotype of oocytes and follow up of the diagnosis in the resulting embryos.[a]

| Locus | Total oocytes obtained | Oocytes with IPB data | | Oocytes with IIPB data | Oocytes with IPB and IIPB data | | Resulting embryos | |
|---|---|---|---|---|---|---|---|---|
| | | Heterozy-gote | Homozy-gote | | Total | ADO | Studied | Con-firmed |
| Mutations[b] (3) | 308 | 166 (59.9%) | 101 (36.5%) | 201 (72.7%) | 153 (55.2%) | 7 (4%) | 130 | 128 (98.5%) |
| STRs[c] (6) | 472[d] | 259 (60.1%) | 165 (38.9%) | 314 (74.0%) | 291 (68.6%) | 18 (6.5%) | 219 | 211 (96.3%) |
| Total | 780[d] | 425 (60.6%) | 266 (37.9%) | 515 (73.5%) | 444 (63.3%) | 25 (5.5%) | 349 | 339 (97.1%) |

[a]reference [14]; [b]CFTR Δ F-508, Sickle cell anemia, Hemophilia B mutations; [c]HumvWf, Hum21S11, HumTHOI, HumFES/FPS, HumF13A1, 5′β Globin STRs; [d]these numbers do not correspond to the number of oocytes, because STRs and mutations were studied simultaneously in the same oocytes.

diagnosis. Our data also show the value of the sequential analysis of both the first and second polar body, which allowed us to detect the presence of ADO. For example, in cases when both the first and second polar bodies show the presence of the same signal for the gene, the results may be interpreted as ADO in the first polar body and confirmed by applying simultaneous amplification of linked polymorphic markers. However, in cases where the first and second polar bodies have different single signals, in the absence of linked polymorphic markers, the ADO in the first polar body will not be detected, and this could lead to the transfer of an affected embryo [13,14]. Therefore, in considering the choices of embryos for transfer, the preference is usually given to those that result from the oocytes with heterozygous first polar body and homozygous mutant second polar body, because this may exclude the possibility of ADO at the locus in question. Of course, it is important to exclude the possibility that the heterozygous status is not due to a contamination by maternal DNA from corona cells or sperm DNA. The risk for the sperm DNA contamination is presently avoided by performing ICSI, while maternal contamination might be detected by the analysis of maternal polymorphic markers [7,13].

We have applied both of these approaches for preimplantation polar body diagnosis for the above-mentioned Mendelian diseases in 32 patients, which resulted in 12 ongoing pregnancies and births of children free of genetic disorder, following confirmation of the polar body diagnosis by prenatal diagnosis (unpublished data). Our follow-up studies now comprise hundreds of embryos resulting from oocytes predicted to be affected, demonstrating the accuracy and reliability of the sequential first and second polar body analysis of oocytes for preimplantation diagnosis of single gene disorders.

## Polar body preimplantation diagnosis of chromosomal disorders

The majority of cases of polar body preimplantation diagnosis, have been performed for chromosomal disorders. A great value of cytogenetic analysis for IVF program is obvious from the data on the rate of chromosomal abnormalities in preimplantation development, which is as high as over 30%, being one of the most important causes of the low success rate of IVF. Analysis of cytogenetic data in oocytes, sperm and early preimplantation embryos also suggests a high relevance of preimplantation chromosomal studies not only for couples at high risk of conceiving a child with chromosomal disorders, such as for couples carrying balanced translocations, but also for couples with any other indication for preimplantation genetic analysis. The human first polar body contains metaphase chromosomes and may be analyzed within 24 h after aspiration [3], but will start degenerating if cultured in vitro for another day. The chromosomes of the first polar body at this stage resemble second metaphase chromosomes, which, however, are more poorly defined. Spectral karyotyping is presently being developed and may allow improving cytogenetic analysis of the first polar body to become acceptable for a standard chromosome analysis. When available, such analysis will be more widely applied in IVF practice to avoid the risk for the production of aneuploid gametes due to maternal age, chromosome translocation, or a previous history of trisomy and recurrent abortions, as the majority of aneuploidies originates from meiosis I errors [15].

Because the second polar body is not at the metaphase stage, the current approaches for its chromosomes visualization involve a nucleous breakdown. Following the activation of oocyte by the sperm penetration (fertilization) or by parthenogenetic activation, the second polar body chromosomes progress from the anaphase and telophase of the second meiotic division to an interphase, forming a visible nucleus, and surviving much longer than the first polar body. Different approaches have been used for the visualization of the second polar body chromosomes [16,17], but the method is still not available for clinical diagnosis. In one of these approaches, to achieve a nucleus breakdown the second polar body nucleus was transferred into a zygote, but the quality of chromosomal preparations was not suitable for karyotyping [16]. In our experiments, the electrofusion instead of nuclear transplantation was applied, resulting in visualization of the second polar body nucleus into mitotic metaphase suitable for cytogenetic analysis [17]. Also we introduced an approach, involving the transformation of the second polar body nucleus into metaphase chromosomes by okadaic acid, which gave more reproducible results, than transplantation or electrofusion [18]. The method is presently being further developed and may soon become available for clinical practice (unpublished data). Preliminary results of the application of this method for testing translocations in the second polar body showed the usefulness of the method in combination with interphase FISH analysis of the first polar body (unpublished data).

In the absence of a reliable method for chromosomal analysis, the current technique for cytogenetic testing of the first and second polar bodies is based on the interphase analysis by FISH. In the past the application of the FISH analysis of blastomeres to preimplantation diagnosis of X-linked disorders, or the age-related aneuploidies were shown to be useful and resulted in a few dozen pregnancies and births of healthy children [19,20]. We have introduced the FISH technique for preimplantation detection of common aneuploidies through the study of the first and second polar bodies [8−10,21]. To investigate the reliability of the technique, the study has initially been undertaken in a series of unfertilized oocytes, to be able to analyze signals simultaneously in both the first polar body and the corresponding oocytes. Using directly labeled fluorescent α-satellite DNA probes which hybridize specifically with centromere region of X-chromosome and chromosome 18, it was possible to identify nondisjunction events which were complementary according to the signals in the first polar body and the oocytes [22]. The data showed that the first meiotic errors can be detected by the first polar body analysis, making possible a preselection of aneuploidy free oocytes for fertilization and transfer in the IVF programs.

The method has presently been applied in 426 IVF patients of advanced maternal age [8−10,21], and those with translocations [23]. The majority of these data were reported elsewhere [8−10,21]. Both the first and second polar bodies were removed and subjected to FISH, using chromosome-specific probes for chromosomes 13, 18 and 21 (Table 5). FISH results of the first and/or second polar bodies were available in 81.6% of biopsied oocytes subjected to FISH analysis. Of 3,217 oocytes with FISH results, both the first and second polar bodies were studied in 2,268 (70.5%) oocytes, the first polar body only in 524 (16.3%) oocytes, and the second polar body only in 424 (13.2%) oocytes. Deviations from the expected normal distribution of FISH signals, were observed in 1,388 (43.1%) oocytes based on the analysis of the first and/or second polar bodies: in 685 (49.4%) oocytes aneuploidy was found only in the first polar body, in 392 (28.2%) − only in the second polar body, and in 311 (22.4%) − both in the first and second polar body. The frequency of chromosomal abnormalities was as high as 35.7% in the first, and 26.1% in the second polar bodies. Most of abnormal first polar bodies were with lack of one or two signals (60.9%), while, in contrast, comparable number of abnormal second polar bodies were with extra (45.9%) or missing signals for the chromosomes studied. The number of polar bodies with complex abnormalities, including the combination of different types of abnormalities for different chromosomes, was also 2 times higher in the first than in second polar bodies.

*Table 5.* Results of preconception FISH analysis for age related aneuploidies.

| Couples | Cycles | Total oocytes studied | Oocytes with FISH results | Normal oocytes | Abnormal oocytes |
|---------|--------|-----------------------|---------------------------|----------------|------------------|
| 425 | 659 | 3943 | 3217 | 1829 (59.9%) | 1388 (43.1%) |

Of 1,829 aneuploidy-free oocytes detected by FISH analysis of the first and/or second polar bodies, 1,558 normal embryos were transferred in 614 treatment cycles, resulting in 131 clinical pregnancies, i.e., yielding a 21.3% pregnancy rate per transfer in the polar body manipulated cycles, well within the pregnancy rate for the routine IVF cycles and even higher than that expected for couples of advanced maternal age. Of 131 clinical pregnancies obtained, 88 resulted in the birth of healthy children, 37 in spontaneous abortions, and 18 are still ongoing confirmed to be unaffected by prenatal diagnosis (unpublished data). The data show that preimplantation diagnosis of common chromosomal aneuploidies by polar body analysis can be useful in avoiding the transfer of cytogenetically abnormal embryos.

## Conclusion

Preimplantation polar body diagnosis makes it possible to detect and avoid genetic and chromosomal disorders before pregnancy. We have shown that the polar body biopsy does not affect fertilization and viability of the resulting embryos. Our present experience of polar body diagnosis includes 725 clinical cycles, performed for preimplantation diagnosis of single gene and chromosomal disorders. Over three-quarters of these cycles have resulted in embryo transfer, about one-quarter in clinical pregnancy and approximately 100 in the birth of unaffected children. The present review describes our current experience on the polar body diagnosis of genetic and chromosomal disorders, demonstrating the reliability of the polar body genetic analysis for preimplantation diagnosis.

## References

1. Verlinsky Y, Kuliev AM (eds). Preimplantation Genetics. New York: Plenum Press, 1991.
2. Edwards RG (ed). Preconception and Preimplantation Diagnosis of Genetic Diseases Cambridge: Cambridge University Press, 1993.
3. Verlinsky Y, Kuliev AM (eds). Preimplantation Diagnosis of Genetic Diseases: A New Technique in Assisted Reproduction. New York: Wiley-Liss, 1993.
4. Verlinsky Y, Kuliev AM. Preimplantation genetic diagnosis. In: Milunsky A (ed) 1998 Genetic Disorders and the Fetus. Baltimore, MD: John Hopkins University Press.
5. Verlinsky Y, Cieslak J. Embryological technical aspects of preimplantation genetic diagnosis. In: Verlinsky Y, Kuliev AM (eds) Preimplantation Diagnosis of Genetic Disorders: A New Technique for Assisted Reproduction. New York: Wiley Liss, 1993;49—67.
6. Strom C, Rechitsky S. DNA analysis of polar bodies and preembryos. In: Verlinsky Y, Kuliev AM (eds) Preimplantation Diagnosis of Genetic Diseases: A New Technique in Assisted Reproduction. New York: Wiley-Liss, 1993;69—91.
7. Rechitsky S, Freidine M, Verlinsky Y, Strom C. Allele drop-out in sequential analysis of single cells by PCR and FISH. J. Assist Reprod Genet 1996;13:115—124.
8. Verlinsky Y, Cieslak J, Freidine M, Ivakhnenko V, Wolf G, Kovalinskaya L, White M, Lifchez A, Kaplan B, Moise J, Ginsberg N, Strom C, Kuliev A. Pregnancies following preconception diagnosis of commom aneuploidies by fluorescent in situ hybridization. Hum Reprod 1995;10: 1923—1927.
9. Verlinsky Y, Cieslak J, Freidine M, Ivakhnenko V, Wolf G, Kovalinskaya L, White M, Lifchez A,

Kaplan B, Moise J, Ginsberg N, Strom C, Kuliev A. Polar body diagnosis of common aneuploidies. J Assist Reprod Genet 1996;13:157—162.

10. Verlinsky Y, Cieslak J, Ivakhnenko V, Lifchez A, Strom C, Kuliev A. Birth of healthy children after preimplantation diagnosis of common aneuploidies by polar body FISH analysis. Fertil Steril 1996;66:126—129.

11. Verlinsky Y, Milayeva S, Evsikov S. Preconception and preimplantation diagnosis for cystic fibrosis. Prenatal Diagn 1992;12:103—110.

12 Verlinsky Y, Rechitsky S, Cieslak J. Reliability of preconception and preimplantation genetic diagnosis. Proceedings of the Eighth International Congress of Human Genetics. Am J Hum Gen 1991;49(Suppl 4):22.

13. Verlinsky Y, Rechitsky S, Cieslak J, Ivakhnenko V, Wolf G, Lifchez A, Kaplan B, Moise J, White M, Ginsberg N, Strom C, Kuliev A. Preimplantation diagnosis of single gene disorders by two-step oocyte genetic analysis using first and second polar body. Biochem Molec Med 1997;62:182—187.

14. Rechitsky S, Strom C, Verlinsky O, Aamet T, Ivakhnenko V, Kukharenko V, Kuliev A, Verlinsky Y. Allele dropout in polar bodies and blastomeres. J Assist Reprod Genet 1998;15:253—257.

15. Antonarakis SE, Petersen MB, McInnis MG et al. The meiotic stage of nondisjunction in trisomy 21: Determination by using DNA polymorphisms. Am J Hum Gen 1992;50:54—550.

16. Modlinski J, McLaren A. A method for visualizing the chromosomes of the second polar body of the mouse egg. J Embryol Exp Morphol 1980;60:93—97.

17. Verlinsky Y, Dozortzev D, Evsikov S. Visualization and cytogenetic analysis of second polar body chromosomes following its fusion with one-cell mouse embryo. J Assist Reprod 1994;11:123—131.

18. Dyban A, De Sutter P, Verlinsky Y. Okadaic acid induces premature chromosome condensation reflecting the cell cycle progression in one cell stage mouse embryos. Molec Reprod Dev 1993;34(4):403—415.

19. Verlinsky Y, Handyside A, Grifo J, Munne S, Cohen J et al. Preimplantation diagnosis of genetic and chromosomal disorders. J Assist Reprod Gen 1994;11(5):236—243.

20. Harper J. Preimplantation diagnosis of inherited disease by embryo biopsy: update of the world figures. J Assist Reprod Genet 1996;13:90—95.

21. Verlinsky Y, Cieslak J, Freidine M, Ivakhnenko V, Evsikov S, Wolf G, White M, Lifchez A, Kaplan B, Moise J, Vally J, Ginsberg N, Strom C, Kuliev A. Preimplantation diagnosis of common aneuploidies by the first- and second-polar body FISH analysis. J Assist Reprod Genet 1998;15:285—289.

22. Dyban A, Fredine M, Severova E, Ivakhnenko V, Verlinsky Y. Detection of aneuploidy in human oocytes and corresponding first polar bodies by FISH. J Assist Reprod Genet 1996;13:72—77.

23. Munné S, Morrison I, Fung J, Márquez C, Weier U, Bahce M, Sable D, Grundfeld L, Schollcraft B, Scott R, Cohen J. Spontaneous abortions are reduced after preconception diagnosis of translocations. J Assist Reprod Genet 1998;15:290—296.

# Cleavage stage embryo biopsy for preimplantation genetic diagnosis

Alan H. Handyside and Alan Thornhill
*Department of Obstetrics and Gynaecology and Institute of Dermatology, UMDS, St Thomas Hospital, London, UK*

**Abstract.** Following in vitro fertilization (IVF), embryos may be biopsied at cleavage stages and single cells prepared for genetic analysis. Over 7 years ago the first pregnancies were established following preimplantation genetic diagnosis (PGD) to diagnose sex in couples at risk of having children with X-linked disease. Currently, fluorescent in situ hybridization (FISH) with sex and autosomal chromosome probe combinations is used to diagnose embryo sex in preference to polymerase chain reaction (PCR) which is generally used to diagnose specific gene defects. PCR and FISH methods are constantly developing for the detection of an increasing range of chromosomal and single gene defects.

Worldwide the PGD cases performed following cleavage stage biopsy have been successful with a pregnancy rate of 26% per embryo transfer. However, polar body biopsy for aneuploidy screening in women of advanced maternal age or after repeated IVF failure may become a major application of PGD. Furthermore, the use of lasers to obtain multiple cells from blastocysts for analysis is under investigation.

However, these alternative approaches await clinical assessment and cleavage stage biopsy remains the main approach to the removal of genomic DNA for genetic analysis at preimplantation stages.

**Keywords:** cleavage stage biopsy, genetic disease, human embryo, preimplantation genetic diagnosis.

## Introduction

It is now over 7 years since the first pregnancies were established following preimplantation genetic diagnosis (PGD) in a series of couples at risk of X-linked disease [1]. Following in vitro fertilization (IVF), embryos were biopsied at cleavage stages on the 3rd day postinsemination and single cells prepared for genetic analysis. In these cases, the polymerase chain reaction (PCR) was used to detect the presence of a Y-chromosome-specific repeated sequence in males. Females identified by the absence of amplified product, which could be carrying the X-linked defect but would not be affected by the disease, were then selectively transferred. The shortcomings of this approach were highlighted by a misdiagnosis in one pregnancy of a male fetus as female, detected by follow-up chorion villus sampling (CVS), which was probably caused by amplification failure from the single biopsied cell. More recently, therefore, fluorescent in situ hybridization

*Address for correspondence:* Dr Alan Handyside, 6th Floor North Wing, Department of Obstetrics and Gynaecology, St. Thomas Hospital, Lambeth Palace Road, London, Se1 7EH, UK. Tel.: +44-171-928-9292 ext. 2728. Fax: +44-171-620-1227.

(FISH) with sex and autosomal chromosome probe combinations have been used almost exclusively to avoid this problem and because they also allow the detection of polyploidy and aneuploidy [2].

PCR and FISH methods are under constant development and have been used extensively for the detection of an increasing range of chromosomal and single gene defects for PGD [3,4].

## Materials and Methods

For successful embryo biopsy it is absolutely essential to have regularly maintained equipment which is both precise and reliable.

### Microscope and micromanipulators

At St Thomas' Hospital we are currently using a combination of Olympus IX70 inverted microscope and micromanipulators specifically designed for embryo biopsy by Research Instruments. Biopsy is performed using $20 \times / 40 \times$ objective and $10 \times$ eyepieces in conjunction with Hoffman Modulation Contrast optics (which are most suitable for use with disposable tissue culture dishes). It is essential that the micromanipulation apparatus should be set up on a vibration-free bench or table (Vibraplane — Kinetic Systems Inc.).

### Preparation of microtools

Successful embryo biopsy is reliant upon high quality microtools. Microtools are commercially available, e.g., Cook (UK) Ltd. Embryo biopsy holding pipette Hammersmith Design: Cook IVF (cat. no. K-HPIP-2135); Embryo Biopsy Pipette: Cook IVF (cat. no. K-EBP-3035); and Assisted Hatching & Zona Drilling Pipette: Cook IVF (cat. no. K-AHP-1035).

However, it is useful to have the option of producing microtools "in-house" owing to possible problems with availability and quality or simply to tailor-make tools for specific requirements. Microtool preparation is time consuming and requires practice. A simple pipette puller based on mechanical tension (Research Instruments, UK) pulls capillary glass to different thicknesses. A microforge (MF-97, Narishige Corp.) is needed to flame polish the pipette tip and bend it to the desired angle (usually 35°). All pipettes are oven sterilized for 2 h at 140°C before use.

Three types of pipettes are used for embryo biopsy: the holding pipette which secures the embryo, acid tyrodes pipette to drill a hole in the zona pellucida and a sampling pipette to aspirate a blastomere from the embryo.

Each pipette can be prepared from the same 1-mm thin-walled borosilicate glass capillary (Clark Electromedical Instruments).

*Holding pipette*

The holding pipette is pulled, cut and heat polished to an external diameter of between 80 and 120 µm and an inner of between 10 and 20 µm using the pipette puller and the microforge.

To break the capillary tube neatly at the desired point, it is positioned horizontally on the microforge so that this point is just in contact with the glass bead on the filament. After heating the filament, the pipette is allowed to fuse with the glass bead before immediately switching off the heat. The sudden contraction of the filament will break the glass neatly. The end of the glass is heat polished until slightly rounded and at the correct internal diameter.

*Acid tyrode pipette*

This has the narrowest lumen of the three pipettes used for biopsy and is produced by pulling a glass capillary to achieve a needle with a short tapering end. The tip of the glass is broken at a diameter of $\leqslant 10$ µm before polishing the tip. The lumen size and taper of this pipette determine the control of acid flow and the ease with which acid is released.

*Sampling pipette*

The size of this pipette is crucial: too large and the entire embryo may be aspirated, too small and blastomeres may lyse during aspiration. The pipette tip is broken at a diameter of 35—40 µm and the tip heat polished to prevent blastomere damage. Since human blastomere size is variable depending on the developmental stage, it is useful to have several different sizes of sampling pipettes for the biopsy procedure.

**Preparation of dishes and medium for biopsy**

*Day 1 ( 1 day after egg collection)*

A culture dish is set up for each normally fertilized embryo by labelling a four-well dish (Nunclon) with the patient's name and embryo number on the base of the dish and on the front panel. Into well 1 0.5 ml of a 50:50 mixture of IVF Universal and M3 medium (Medi-Cult, UK) is dispensed (Fig. 1). Into wells 2—4, 0.5 ml of M3 is dispensed and each well covered with a monolayer (0.6 ml) of washed mineral oil (Squibb, USA) before placing the dishes in the incubator to equilibrate overnight.

*Day 2 ( 2 days after egg collection)*

After scoring the embryos (counting the cells and noting the degree of fragmen-

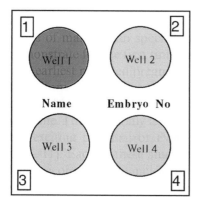

*Fig. 1.*

tation present) each is transferred into well 1 of the appropriately labelled 4-well dish and placed in the incubator for 4 h before transferring each embryo to well 2 and culturing overnight.

Hepes-buffered M3 medium and Nunclon dishes (Marathon Lab Supplies) for the biopsy are placed in the warming oven (37°C) while a sufficient quantity of washed oil for the biopsy procedure (allow 4 ml per embryo) is placed in the incubator. Oil is washed by vigorous mixing with an equal quantity of Earle's Balanced Salt Solution (EBSS — Gibco BRL, UK) and leaving to settle for at least 6 h.

*Day 3 (day of embryo biopsy)*

Cleavage stage embryo biopsy is carried out early in the morning of day 3 postin-semination as previously described [5].

Half an hour before the biopsy, a biopsy dish (Nunclon 60 mm — Marathon) is set up for each embryo and labelled with the patient's name and embryo number. With a Gilson pipette set at 10 µl (P20 or P10 — Anachem, UK) a sterile yellow tip is flushed (× 10) using 25-mM Hepes (Sigma)-buffered M3 medium to remove potential toxic plasticizer residues. Three 15-µl drops of Hepes-buffered M3 medium and one 15-µl drop of Acid Tyrodes (Medicult (UK) Ltd.) are dispensed in the biopsy dish as shown in Fig. 2.

The dish should be oriented as shown below with respect to the position of biopsy micropipettes.

The biopsy dish should be immediately covered with 4 ml of washed and pre-equilibriated mineral oil to avoid evaporation and the prepared dishes put in the warming oven until required.

The appropriately labelled biopsy dish is taken from the warming oven and the corresponding 4-well dish from the holding incubator. The embryo is transferred into the middle droplet of the biopsy dish which is moved to the downflow area and handed over to the person performing embryo biopsy.

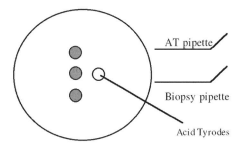

AT pipette

Biopsy pipette

Acid Tyrodes

*Fig. 2.*

*Embryo biopsy*

A biopsy dish is placed on the microscope stage and each of the pipettes filled with the appropriate solution (biopsy medium for holding and sampling pipettes; acid tyrodes for the acid tyrodes pipette). Using a low-power objective the bottom of the medium drop is brought into focus before lowering the pipettes into the drop until they all lie horizontal with respect to the bottom of the dish.

The embryo for biopsy is placed into the medium drop and immobilized using the holding pipette. The embryo should be secured such that the blastomere for biopsy is opposite the holding pipette and accessible for the sampling pipette. One of the smaller blastomeres is selected to minimize the reduction in mass and checked for the presence of a nucleus, as fragments or blebs can be mistaken for blastomeres.

A hole is drilled into the zona by placing the acid tyrodes pipette close to the site of interest and releasing a stream of acid until the zona thins. The sampling pipette is pushed through the hole and the blastomere gently aspirated whilst simultaneously withdrawing from the hole. Once the blastomere is securely out of the zona and inside the pipette it is expelled back into the drop away from the embryo and the sampling pipette removed immediately to prevent back suction. Should compaction have begun in day 3 embryos, a blastomere may be removed by moving the sampling pipette up and down whilst maintaining gentle suction. A second blastomere may be removed from embryos with seven or more cells which may require a modification to the hole or an extra hole. Each biopsied blastomere should be checked for the presence of an interphase nucleus. Biopsy can usually be performed in 5–10 min minimizing the time out of the incubator.

Following biopsy the embryo should be released and washed at least twice to remove acid tyrodes remnants before returning to culture. The blastomere should be washed extensively in handling medium or PBS prior to genetic analysis.

At the end of the biopsy, the embryo is transferred into well 3 of the 4-well culture dish. (This washing stage removes the Hepes-buffered M3 medium). Finally, the embryo is transferred with minimal medium to well 4 and returned to culture.

The biopsy dish containing the isolated blastomeres is returned to the downflow area for sample preparation. The above steps are repeated until all of the embryos have been biopsied.

When the PGD is complete the morphology of each of the embryos is assessed and an accurate cell number count is performed to get an indication of division postbiopsy.

In consultation with the other members of the PGD team and finally with the couple themselves, a maximum of two unaffected embryos with the best morphology is selected for transfer.

## Conclusion

Around 35 centers worldwide are currently offering PGD clinically. To the end of 1996, almost 600 cycles of PGD following cleavage stage biopsy have resulted in over 100 pregnancies and approaching 100 babies born with a pregnancy rate of 26% per embryo transfer (Joyce Harper, personal communication). However, an equal number of cycles involving polar body biopsy for aneuploidy screening in women of advanced maternal age or after repeated IVF failure have already been carried out in a much shorter interval indicating that this may become a major application of PGD [6].

Biopsy of both the first and second polar bodies has been used successfully to screen for maternal mutations in several single gene defects [7]. Also, the use of lasers for zona drilling and excision of herniating trophectoderm cells has allowed FISH analysis of multiple cells [8]. However, the limitations of these two approaches still await clinical assessment and cleavage stage biopsy remains the main approach to the removal of genomic DNA for genetic analysis at preimplantation stages.

## References

1. Handyside AH, Kontogianni EH, Hardy K, Winston RM. Pregnancies from biopsied human preimplantation embryos sexed by Y-specific DNA amplification. Nature 1990;344:768−770.
2. Delhanty JD, Griffin DK, Handyside AH, Harper J, Atkinson GH, Pieters MH, Winston RM. Detection of aneuploidy and chromosomal mosaicism in human embryos during preimplantation sex determination by fluorescent in situ hybridisation (FISH). Hum Mol Genet 1993;2: 1183−1185.
3. Handyside AH, Delhanty JDA. Preimplantation genetic diagnosis: strategies and surprises. Trends Genet 1997;13:270−275.
4. Lissens W, Sermon K. Preimplantation genetic diagnosis: current status and new developments. Hum Reprod 1997;12:1756−1761.
5. Ao A, Handyside AH. Cleavage stage human embryo biopsy. Hum Reprod 1995;Update 1,3.
6. Verlinsky Y, Cieslak J, Ivakhnenko V, Lifchez A, Strom C, Kuliev A. Birth of healthy children after preimplantation diagnosis of common aneuploidies by polar body fluorescent in situ hybridization analysis. Preimplantation Genetics Group. Fertil Steril 1996;66:126−129.
7. Verlinsky Y, Rechitsky S, Cieslak J, Ivakhnenko V, Wolf G, Lifchez A, Kaplan, B, Moise J, Walle J, White M, Ginsberg N, Strom C, Kuliev A. Preimplantation diagnosis of single gene disorders

by two-step oocyte genetic analysis using first and second polar body. Biochem Mol Med 1997;62:182–187.

8.  Veiga A, Sandalinas M, Benkhalifa M, Boada M, Carrera M, Santalo J, Barri PN, Menezo Y. Laser blastocyst biopsy for preimplantation genetic diagnosis in the human. Zygote 1997;5: 351–354.

Fertility and Reproductive Medicine.
R.D. Kempers, J. Cohen, A.F. Haney and J.B. Younger, editors.

231

# Blastocyst biopsy

Sandra Ann Carson

*Associate Professor of Obstetrics and Gynecology, Chief, Baylor Assisted Reproductive Technology, Baylor College of Medicine, Houston, Texas, USA*

**Abstract.** Biopsy at the blastocyst stage is becoming increasingly practical because of advances in vitro culture. Advantages include a higher degree of viability because of natural selection, trophectoderm only biopsy with minimal injury to the inner cell mass, and a much larger number of embryonic cells available for genetic analysis. Disadvantages are the difficulties of removing cells that are adherent to one another and the need to maintain embryos in culture for 2—3 additional days. With the diagnostic advantage that comes from access to a large number of cells for analysis, it is likely that this technique will be used increasingly in preimplantation diagnosis.

**Keywords:** biopsy, blastocyst, embryo, preimplantation diagnosis.

Preimplantation genetic diagnosis remains an exciting technique with little utilization. Until it becomes more efficient and less expensive, or until elective sex selection becomes accepted by society, preimplantation diagnosis is unlikely to become a common procedure. The most recent efforts to increase the efficiency and success of the technique have focused on in vitro culture to, and biopsy of, the blastocyst stage embryo. The blastocyst presents the most opportune stage of embryonic development for biopsy for several reasons:

First, having undergone several cell divisions, the blastocyst survived the initial critical steps of natural selection. Because only the healthiest of the preimplantation embryos become blastocysts, it is not unrealistic to expect higher pregnancy rates per embryo transferred at this stage than from four- to eight-cell embryos. Indeed, this reasoning is reflected by blastocysts recovered from uterine lavage and transferred into synchronized recipients: 60% pregnancy from blastocysts, a rate much higher than that resulting from transferring four-cell embryos [1].

Second, the blastocyst has begun differentiation. Because the cells have divided into a trophectoderm and inner cell mass, the embryo can be biopsied to avoid those cells that will ultimately become the embryo. Although it is unclear as to whether this will increase safety, it does eschew arguments from those questioning the propriety of removing a totipotential cell which theoretically can develop into a fetus and ultimately, baby.

Third, because the blastocyst has started to differentiate and is comprised of over 200 cells, more than just one cell to be safe. More cells and more DNA for

*Address for correspondence:* Sandra A. Carson MD, Baylor College of Medicine, Department of Obstetrics/Gynecology, 6550 Fannin, Suite 801, Houston, TX 77030, USA. Tel.: +1-713-798-8484. Fax.: +1-713-798-8431. E-mail: scarson@bmc.tmc.edu

analysis allow techniques used to amplify and diagnose the DNA to be run in duplicate to confirm the diagnosis.

Finally, blastocysts may be cultured from embryos after in vitro fertilization, but also may be lavaged from the uterus. The former procedure is far less costly, risky, and time consuming than in vitro fertilization. However, this benefit will only become practical if the yield of uterine lavage can be increased [2].

Biopsy at the blastocyst stage does pose certain disadvantages:

1. Differentiation not only provides the advantages listed above, but also poses the disadvantage of cell-to-cell communication. The cells of the trophecto-derm communicate through the formation of gap junctions which are formed of microtubules that allow passage of chemical signals from one cell to its neighbor. This results in cells which are "sticky" and often difficult to separate. In addition, they stick to glass biopsy tools. In our own experience, we found that blastocyst biopsy after a few hours of culture in a Ca/MD-free media allowed easier separation of the cells from the trophectoderm mass [3]. This did not decrease embryo survival. In addition, rinsing biopsy microtools in a silicon solution (Photoflow) aided the prevention of cells sticking to the tools themselves.

2. Blastocysts after in vitro fertilization require 4—5 days of embryo culture. This uses incubator space, which in a busy clinical in vitro fertilization program is limited. Moreover, blastocyst culture requires a different media than early embryo culture. It is not surprising that the larger embryo, physiologically found in the uterus rather than the fallopian tube, has different nutritional demands to the four cell embryo. Indeed, early attempts at blastocyst culture resulted in a much lower pregnancy rate after transfer than the four cell embryo. Other entrepreneurs changed the growth media and had higher success after transfer at the blastocyst stage. However, this media is patented and may be too expensive for preimplantation research budgets [4].

In our early investigation of the blastocyst biopsy, we utilized the murine model [5]. Mouse blastocysts were randomly divided into four groups in an attempt to identify the biopsy technique most useful in removing cells, and maximizing in subsequent embryo survival. The first group was biopsied by inserting a 10-µ aspiration pipette with suction applied. All blastocysts were successfully biopsied, but the survival was 32%. The second technique utilized a microrazor. The tool was made by cutting a corner of a stainless steel razor bade under microscopic vision and gluing it onto a finely pulled glass pipette. The blade was used to excise a protein of the embryo including the zone pellucid. Although cells were successfully removed embryo survival was lowest at 22%. Embryo survival was highest in the groups using the final two techniques. After spontaneous hatching, a finely pulled glass pipette was used to excise the first herniated cells from the blastocyst. The final technique was an adaptation of the previous technique: the zone pellucida of the embryo was first slit with a glass pipette and 4 h later cells were excised as in the previous group. Cells were successfully removed in all embryos using the last two techniques and embryo survival was the highest: 58

and 68%. The final technique offers a bit more laboratory control over the time of hatching and requires less constant checking to determine if hatching has begun. Besides obvious advantages from the personnel standpoint, it prevents repeated exposure to temperature changes from transfer of the embryos from the incubator to the microscope for intermittent checking.

A similar procedure was used in the earliest attempts at human blastocyst biopsy [6]. Dokras biopsied nontransferred human embryos after in vitro fertilization and culture to blastocyst. Indeed this study revealed a 39% embryonic survival after human blastocyst biopsy, not significantly different from the 18% survival in the nonbiopsied controls.

Blastocyst biopsy is feasible for preimplantation diagnosis. Our own group successfully performed the first blastocyst biopsy in a woman undergoing uterine lavage. The diagnosis was made; the embryo affected; and no subsequent transfer was performed. It remains to be seen whether pregnancy can be achieved after preimplantation diagnosis after biopsy of the blastocyst stage embryo.

## References

1. Buster JE, Bustillo M, Rodi I, Cohen SW, Hamilton F, Simon JA, Thorneycroft IA, Marshall JR. Biologic and morphologic development of donated human ova recovered by nonsurgical uterine lavage. Am J Obstet Gynecol 1985;153:211−217.
2. Carson SA, Smith AL, Scoggan JL, Buster JE. Superovulation fails to increase human blastocyst yield after uterine lavage. Prenatal Diagn 1991;11:513−522.
3. Gentry WL, Carson SA, Martin C, Buster JE. Enhanced Survival of Murine Embryos Micromanipulated in Ca++/Mg++ Free Culture Media. 38th Annual Meeting, Society for Gynecologic Investigation, San Antonio, Texas, March 1991.
4. Gardner DK, Vella P, Lane M, Wagley L, Schlenker T, Schoolcraft WB. Culture and Transfer of Human Blastocysts Increases Implantation Rates and Reduces the Need for Multiple Embryo Transfer. 53rd Annual Meeting, American Society for Reproductive Medicine, Cincinnati, October 1997.
5. Carson SA, Gentry WL, Smith AL, Buster JE. Trophectoderm microbiopsy in murine blastocysts: comparison of four methods. Assist Genet 1993;10:427−433.
6. Dokras A. Trophectoderm biopsy in human blastocysts. J In Vitro Fertil Embryo Transfer 1990;7:188.

# Legal and ethical consideration of assisted reproduction

# Regulation of ART: implications for patients. Who decides?

Jean Cohen[1] and Howard W. Jones Jr[2]

[1] Centre de Stérilité de l'hôpital de Sèvres, Paris, France; and [2] The Howard and Georgeanna Jones Institute for Reproductive Medicine, Norfolk, Virginia, USA

**Abstract.** In many countries ART (assisted reproductive technology) has produced the desire for control and regulation of this form of infertility treatment.

The authors compare international laws and regulations or guidelines and examine the implications for patients:
— Who decides on the right to perform ART?
— Who decides which couples may be treated?
— Who decides embryo cryopreservation?
— Who decides the number of embryos to be transferred?
— Who decides on selective reduction?
— Who decides on PID?
— Who decides oocyte donation?
— Who decides if donor sperm can be used?
— Who decides embryo donation?
— Who decides the measures to prevent transmission of diseases in ART?

**Keywords:** ART, international comparisons, regulations.

The development of methods of assisted reproductive technology (ART) has been a major breakthrough in the treatment of infertile couples. This area of assisted reproductive technology interfaces with fundamental issues of life for many people.

One of the basic human rights is that of a woman to be able to decide when and how to conceive. One would imagine that for infertility surgery or medical treatment, ART decisions would be the result of a particular colloquy between women or couples and doctors. But in many countries, ART has produced the desire for control and regulation of this form of infertility treatment. These regulations induce important implications for patients. Such regulations remain open to questioning or discussion since there are not even two countries where regulations are similar.

## Preliminaries to reaching the decision

Even besides regulations which we shall examine further, there are at least two

*Address for correspondence:* Dr Jean Cohen, Directuer du Centre de Stérilité de l'hôpital de Sèvres, 8 rue Marignan, 75008 Paris, France.

other factors which will influence the women or the couples to reach a decision: the level of information and the funding for reproductive therapy.

## The level of information

Conditions for a free choice suppose an adequate knowledge of the elements of choice. Many women are badly informed by the media or lay conversations and they rely on the doctor to make up their minds. We know that, in spite of the obligation in certain countries to hand over a booklet, many centers keep giving false hopes or neglect to speak of possible complications. The value of informed consent depends obviously on the quality of the information which has been received. From this point of view the role of associations of patients becomes all the more significant.

## Funding for reproductive therapy

The reimbursement, total or partial, of the costs of ART by medical insurance must certainly determine the choice of many couples. A woman living in a country that does not support funding for ART, such as the USA or Canada, has not the same choice as the women living in Australia, France or Israel where a certain number of cycles of treatment are sponsored. In the UK sponsoring is totally different from one District Health Authority to another.

## Self-regulation or government regulation?

Do scientists or doctors have to be corralled by legislation or regulations? One could presume that ART is a treatment of infertility as is tubal surgery or ovarian stimulation.

During the first 10 years after Louise Brown was born, there was no legislation in any country. This made possible much progress, such as embryo freezing, coculture, hatching, etc. Nowadays, there are a number of countries which operate under voluntary guideline systems without problems.

The fear to see Man act as God in a field concerning the creation of life has led a certain number of societies to wish to control and regulate this form of treatment of infertility. In addition the newspapers' headlines concerning clonage, selection of sex, posthumous use of human sperm, surrogacy, and errors in laboratories, prompted the authorities to take action.

In many countries, as we shall see, the legislator has defined what is allowed and what is forbidden and has, also, adjusted the structures of control in order to guarantee a quality of care and a protection for couples and children to be. Many doctors and biologists have called for these regulations in order to protect themselves from contingent suing. Many couples — having associations of patients acting for them — have also collaborated to the elaboration of those laws which protect them as well.

However, everybody knows that no law or regulation can stop unscrupulous people from doing unscrupulous things, whether it is in the field of medicine, journalism, business, or education. Nevertheless, everyone feels reassured by regulations.

The result of this evolution on the international level is the existence of multiple attitudes. Certain countries have no regulation. Others have voluntary guidelines that doctors follow. Others have laws voted by their legislative authority.

Legislative regulations are nevertheless often unrealistic and are different from one country to another. We can say that there are no two countries which have adopted the same regulations.

In fact, as far as ART is concerned, the decisions and the choices depend on the country in which one lives and practices; and we know of paradoxical situations which have generated "procreative tourism".

**Divergent laws and practices**

Many authors [1—5] have tried to restate the elements of assisted reproduction practice in different countries, whether it concerns laws (statutes or judge mode), guidelines decided by ethical committees, scientific societies, or even voluntary guidelines accepted by all the ART centers. All of these are extremely diverging and we shall try to describe them looking for who decides.

It is impossible in such a short chapter to study the situation of each country. We shall quote a few of them. The International Federation of Fertilities Societies (IFFS) has elaborated an international statement which is the most recent and the most comprehensive on the subject to this day.

In a compilation of this kind, errors are inevitable. We hope readers will be understanding and call them to our attention.

**Who decides on the right to perform ART?**

A majority of countries operate under laws and voluntary guidelines. A minority such as Belgium, Finland, Greece, Hong Kong, India, and Portugal has no laws nor regulations.

The difference between law and guidelines is that, in the first case, there are regulations governing the centers and the members of the team, and there are sanctions in case of nonapplication of these regulations. In the second case, centers may eventually not respect rules and not be sanctioned. But they could be sued whenever patients wish to do so for complications or incidents in violation of the voluntary guidelines.

It is obvious that laws restrain in general the process of ART. Most of the progress made in ART has been achieved before legislation time and it is no pure chance that many advances made today have originated from Belgium or the USA.

On the contrary the protection of patients is globally more efficient in a country where law controls the efficacy and the activity of centers of ART.

The way agreements to centers are granted varies enormously from one country to another. For example:

- Decision from the Ministry of Health: Australia;
- Decision from the Ministry of Health upon proposition by a national committee consisting of doctors, representatives of scientific organizations, experts, jurists, and family associations: France;
- Decision from Human Fertilization and Embryology Authority (HEFA): 21 members appointed by the Minister of Health: UK;
- Decision from advisory physician body: Israel;
- Decision from committee of the medical associations: Germany;
- Decision from guidelines from religious islamic centers: Egypt; and
- Decision from Gynaecology Society: Japan;

In certain countries, doctors and biologists differ on aspects of the guidelines and/or regulations.

The evaluation of results also varies a lot. Nowadays, national registers exist in many countries. However, besides the fact they are provided by law, only a limited number of countries (e.g., France, UK, Spain, Israel) guarantee their reliability. It is only when an evaluation organization exists which studies each center that we can expect a perfect keeping of the registers.

Moreover, patients find it misleading to obtain results from the registers which allow them to compare centers.

### Who decides which couples may be treated?

Under the European Convention (1978), a single woman or even a lesbian couple is entitled to have children, even though these children might not have a legal father. But, this convention is not applied in most European countries or in the rest of the world.

Most of the countries which have regulations reserve ART to couples with a stable relationship. A certain number of countries, such as Germany, Hungary, Jordan, Poland and Turkey, reserve ART to married couples. Others, the majority of them, accept ART for cohabitant couples, often stating that cohabitation of 2 years fulfills this requirement: Austria, Denmark, and certain states of Australia. In France, nonmarried couples must present a legal certificate of cohabitation. In the UK, single women or lesbian couples are not excluded, provided the "welfare of the child" is guaranteed. In Canada, custom allows professional choice by each center to treat married, common law, single and homosexual couples. In many countries, such as Brazil or Italy, no mention of a specific relationship is required. In Israel, Italy, The Netherlands, Russia, Spain, the UK, and the USA, ART is performed on single women.

Chances for a woman or a couple to have access to IVF are therefore variable, sometimes opposite in two countries, sharing the same boundary. Decision is rarely on the side of patients.

## Who decides embryo cryopreservation and duration of storage?

Cryopreservation of embryos may have a function in enhancing implantation, pregnancy, and birth rates. It is now permitted in most countries for couples to give their consent for storage and use of embryos.

The maximum period of time for storage is very variable. However, a maximum of a 10-year period of time is set in Finland, Israel, Spain, Taiwan, and some states of Australia. A period of 5 years is set in other countries such as France, the UK, Switzerland, and Argentina. On the contrary, in Austria, Sweden, and Denmark, the period of storage has a duration of 1 year. In Japan and the USA, the limit is equal to the reproductive life of the donor.

These different attitudes have obvious consequences concerning the couples. The shorter the duration of storage, the quicker the couples must contemplate a pregnancy.

Differences are even more stressed as far as the future of frozen embryos is concerned. In Austria, Ireland, Israel, and Norway, embryos cannot be donated to another couple nor given to research. In France, they can be donated to another couple but not for research, nor can they be replaced in a woman whose husband died during cryopreservation procedures.

## Who decides the number of embryos to be transferred?

The overall multiple pregnancy rate for ART is 22—28%. This rate increases to 35% when five or more embryos are transferred. Most studies recently published indicate that in order to avoid multiple pregnancies the transfer of no more than three embryos must be contemplated and for young women the transfer of two embryos reduces the risk. However, the study of national registers indicates that the transfer of five or more embryos is still frequent [6].

A certain number of countries has laws or guidelines controlling the number of embryos to be transferred. For example:
- two for Denmark, Sweden, and the UK;
- three for Germany, Japan, and some states of Australia; and
- four for Brazil, Czech Republic.

In many countries, there is still no limit.

Implications for patients is obviously considerable. A high percentage of triple pregnancies and nearly all pregnancies of higher rank are associated with complications, handicaps, and sometimes death of fetuses.

It is also obvious that the patient cannot appreciate the risks of multiple pregnancies. The ART team must bear some responsibility for the choice of the number of embryos.

Too often an excessive number of embryos is transferred to enhance the chances of pregnancy. An international consensus on this matter should help reduce the risks of higher rank pregnancies.

### Who decides on selective reduction in case of multiple pregnancy?

It is now common for women carrying a pregnancy of higher order to have the number of fetuses reduced to one or two (sometimes three) by selective abortion of the fetuses in excess.

Many countries do not mention selective reduction in their laws or guidelines. In that case, it is often practiced except in such countries as Ireland and India. Selective reduction is not allowed in countries such as Mexico or not practiced at all, such as The Netherlands or Portugal.

The situation depends most of the time on the legal status of abortion. In countries where abortion is legal, whatever the reason, there should be no legal barrier to selective reduction. In countries where abortion is illegal or where the medical community is not in favor of abortion, women are led to carry on their multiple pregnancy and to take upon themselves contingent complications.

### Who decides on preimplantation diagnosis?

Preimplantation diagnosis (PID) aims at testing chromosomic or genetic abnormalities in order to prevent transfer of diseased embryos. Parents who know they have an hereditary taint they could pass to their descendants are obviously concerned by the possibility to obtain a PID. If not available, they often turn to an abortion which includes at the same time both normal and abnormal embryos.

In the UK, Spain, and Sweden, PID is allowed and performed. In France, it is theoretically authorized by law but since the publication of the 1994 law, no center has been authorized to perform it. In such countries as Denmark, it is forbidden. In other countries it does not exist for no center ever performs it.

These differences created a "procreative tourism" [7]. French couples, for instance, are directed to the UK or Belgium.

### Who decides oocyte donation?

In some countries such as Austria, Germany, Japan, Norway, and Sweden, oocyte donation is forbidden by law.

Wherever ovum donation is allowed, diverging situations may appear:
- Most of the oocytes available for donation have been obtained from women themselves undergoing IVF (i.e., in the UK and Israel). Some are retrieved from women undergoing tubal sterilization (the USA and UK). Some women volunteer for donation, such as family members or friends (Belgium, The Netherlands). In France, anonymity is mandatory and it is strictly forbidden to ask a patient to bring along a donor. Thus, French patients are obliged to travel to the UK or Belgium.
- No money or any other benefit can be offered for donation in Denmark, France, Israel, Spain, and the UK. In other countries, most of the centers

offer benefits to women donating oocytes.

- Oocyte donation to menopausal women is practiced in several centers (USA and Italy). France has a bioethical law prohibiting ovum donation for those after the age of menopause.

## Who decides if donor sperm can be used?

In comparison with international laws, there is no equivalence between gametes. In nearly all the countries of the world, sperm banks can be found and frozen sperm can be used for ART. This excepts Islamic countries as well as Turkey, where gamete donations are forbidden. In the specific case of postmortem insemination, France forbids it and the UK has allowed it outside its own territory.

## Who decides embryo donation?

Embryo donation is forbidden in countries such as Austria, Jordan, Denmark, Ireland, Germany, Israel, Norway, and Turkey.

The regulations differ in countries where embryo donation is practiced. In some countries, such as the UK, the child will be able to obtain data regarding his conception upon reaching the age of 18. In France, the embryo must be legally adopted via an official deed.

## Who decides the measures to prevent transmission of diseases in ART?

The prevention of the transmission of infections and genetic abnormalities is enforced nearly everywhere in the world as far as sperm donation is concerned. However, it is very different for an oocyte donation.

A certain number of countries, such as Austria, Egypt, Germany, Hungary, Ireland, Poland, Portugal, South Africa, and Turkey have no legislation concerning this prevention. It does not mean though that the centers do not take the appropriate preventive measures individually. These measures may vary following the doctors' decisions.

Other countries have statutes or laws designed to prevent the transmission of diseases. Among them are Denmark, Italy, Israel, Russia, Canada, and The Netherlands. Those regulations, besides genetic abnormalities, generally include HIV, hepatitis, syphilis, and CMV.

However, even in these countries, the list of pathologies varies from one to another. Sometimes, such as in Brazil, no list is provided. The most extreme case is that of artificial insemination and/or IVF for HIV positive couples. AI has been performed in Italy and the USA. But in many countries, hundreds of HIV positive couples are still waiting for a decision.

## Conclusion

The study of the different international legislations shows that the choice of the decision for an ART procedure and its modalities varies considerably. This has an impact on the physician and patient relationship [8].

- Countries where laws exist: theoretically drifts are evaded but at the price of formalities and rules which limit the possibilities of treatment and research.
- Countries where there is no law: patients benefit from medical confidentiality to obtain a treatment but there are less theoretical guarantees on the conditions.
- Countries where ART is funded: social justice is respected for everyone can have access to ART.
- Countries where ART is not funded: only money and private insurance allow someone to be treated, or sometimes the loss of one's own chances when donating oocytes.

However, the other side of a social policy is that there is a cost which leads those who decide to limit ART to certain categories of technics or to certain couples.

The reasons which have led to such contrasting situations are themselves multiple.

- Religious tradition: in countries where Roman catholics are a majority, the Church being opposed to ART, laws are generally restrictive except in Spain where the law has been voted by a Socialist majority. The opposition of the Church does not succeed in forbidding ART but it does limit, for example, cryopreservation or research on the embryo. The Islamic religion opposes strongly the donation of gametes.
- The cultural tradition: plays also an important part. It influences decisions for the benefit of the doctors in Japan or on the contrary privileges the privacy rights in the USA. In Germany the memory of NAZI atrocities limits research on the embryo.
- The politicians: They are the ones who make the laws. In general, they know nothing about ART and its problems and they wish only to please their electorate. They are more concerned about the cost of supplies of government services and try essentially to reduce them. National ethical committees are designated by the governments then in power and they reflect in the end the wishes of the political power they represent.
- The evolution of the role of the practitioners: of course, in the beginning the first teams took upon themselves initiatives which led to the first IVF pregnancies, GIFT, cryopreservation of embryos, and donation of gametes. But very quickly a great fear overcame a majority of doctors or biologists, afraid of the possible drift. Professional scientific groups could have then set limits for ART, proposed self-regulation but they faded and let representatives of the Society take over.

The actual situation has no coherence.

- An infertile woman with a hydrosalpinx can refer to a public or private center and obtain a salpingoplasty without any formality and in general be funded.

The same woman suffering from a hydrosalpinx of severe prognosis will be asked to be married, young, and have no disease in order to benefit from ART which she will nevertheless have to pay for.

- Moreover, different legislations from one country to another raise problems.
- Two progenitors living in two different jurisdictions in the same nation may be controlled by different rules (e.g., in Australia).
- Transportation and use of frozen embryos has no consistency.
- Doctors are often obliged to send patients to other countries (e.g.; France).
- Patients are required to undertake "procreative tourism" such as those from the Northern European countries which set a perfect example.

The Nordic Committee on Assisted Reproduction has published in the ESHRE newsletter (1996) a survey of the differences in legislation and practice of ART in the Nordic countries (Denmark, Finland, Norway and Sweden) and has paid special attention to the consequences of these differences on the treatment of infertile couples. Despite a long tradition of cooperation between the Nordic countries on political and other levels, there are still prominent differences in legislation on ART. The reproductive problems facing the infertile couples in these countries are very similar and there exists a great deal of medical consensus. The question therefore arises whether the Nordic people really are so different in their moral and ethical standpoints as the legislation suggests. To what degree have the legislators discussed these important issues across the international borders?

Iceland and Finland have no ART legislation today. In Iceland, a limited ART practice is regulated by a hospital ethics committee, but clinicians eagerly wait for politicians to lay down concrete guidelines. Finland has had several papers on proposed ART legislation but they have never been presented to the parliament. Laws on ART have been passed in Denmark, Norway and Sweden and the legislative differences between these countries are remarkable.

Sperm donors may be anonymous in Denmark and Norway. In Sweden, offspring resulting from donor insemination have an established legal right to information on the identity of the sperm donor. Oocyte freezing is allowed in Denmark and Sweden, but not in Norway. Oocyte donation is forbidden in Norway and Sweden, but allowed in Denmark, but only if IVF oocyte aspiration is the source of the oocyte. Donor insemination in connection with IVF is allowed in Denmark but this is forbidden in both Norway and Sweden.

These differences created by the politicians and regulators have resulted in a sizeable traffic of infertile couples seeking treatment across legislative borders, the import and export of ART. Swedish couples seek sperm donor insemination (IAD) in Denmark and Finland to escape the lack of anonymity demanded for sperm donor practice in Sweden. Norwegian couples seek microinsemination in Denmark and Sweden because of a temporary ban on the method in Norway. The ban was recently lifted but clinics now face a formidable backlog of treatment demands. Norwegian couples also seek treatment with egg donation in Denmark and Finland. Icelandic couples seek advanced forms or ART abroad while clinicians wait for the political go ahead.

In Finland, clinicians have stopped waiting for legislative guidelines and now practice the widest range of ART services in the Nordic countries. Preimplantation diagnosis is allowed in Sweden, where the authorities have recently decided not to legislate on this issue, but a restrictive use of this method under governmental control is demanded. Legislation on Denmark and Norway on this issue requires state controlled licensing subject to application. In Denmark, permission must be granted in parliament. Neither country has a preimplantation service today. In Finland, this service is not yet available but is allowed in the papers on proposed legislation existing to this date.

Legislation on embryo research varies from total prohibition in Norway to permission under strict conditions in Denmark and Sweden.

Since there are so many difficulties and as we are dealing with a field in continuous development, control of ART by parliamentary legislation is less desirable. The nature of law is that it is susceptible to be revised only relatively slowly compared with developments of medical science and the public perception of the latter.

We strongly believe that medical and biological communities acting in ART should express minimum thresholds of regulations. These common international guidelines, whether technical or ethical, should express for each given situation the minimal aims, means, and risks, as well as individual and social costs. Each individual and each government would then be able to make up its own mind and decide accordingly to its own imperatives.

Such a consensus has been prepared by a group of international experts of IFFS and is published on the occasion of the San Francisco meeting 1998.

## References

1.  Baird PA. The role of society in assisted reproduction in IVF and ART. In: Gomel V, Leung P (eds) Proceedings of the 10th World Congress on In Vitro Fertilization and Assisted Reproduction, Vancouver. Bologna, Italy: Monduzzi Editore, 1997;1119—1126.
2.  Cohen J. Regulations of assisted reproductive technologies international comparisons in IVF and ART. In: Gomel V, Leung P (eds) Proceedings of the 10th World Congress on In Vitro Fertilization and Assisted Reproduction, Vancouver. Bologna, Italy: Monduzzi Editore, 1997; 1131—1136.
3.  Jones HW Jr. The time has come. Fertil Steril (Editor's Corner) 1996;65:1090.
4.  Jones HW Jr. The many faces of morality. In: Mori T, Aono T, Tominaga T, Hiroi M (eds) Frontiers in Endocrinology: Perspectives on Assisted Reproduction, Proceedings of VIIIth World Congress of In Vitro Fertilization, Kyoto. Rome, Italy: Ares-Serono Symposia Publication, 1994;13—18.
5.  Schenker J. Assisted reproductive practice in Europe: legal and ethical aspects. Hum Reprod (Update) 1997;3(2):173—184.
6.  Cohen J. How to avoid multiple pregnancies in ART. Hum Reprod 1998;(In press).
7.  Evans D, Evans M. Fertility, infertility and the human embryo: ethics, law and practice of human artificial procreation. Hum Reprod (Update) 1996;2(3):208—224.
8.  Nisker JA. Rachel's ledders or how societal situation determines reproductive therapy. Hum Reprod 1996;11(6):1162—1167.

# How far should we go with genetic screening in assisted reproduction?

Inge Liebaers[1], Maryse Bonduelle[1], Elvire Van Assche[1], Willy Lissens[1], Paul Devroey[2] and André Van Steirteghem[2]
*Centers for [1]Medical Genetics, and [2]Reproductive Medicine, Dutch-speaking Brussels Free University, Brussels, Belgium*

**Abstract.** Genetic screening refers to tests which are offered to a population because the incidence of a particular genetic aberration is elevated. The persons who are tested do not have any prior medical problems. Infertile men and women do have a problem and often specific genetic tests have to be performed as part of the diagnostic work-up before assisted reproduction techniques will eventually be offered. This has nothing to do with screening. During assisted reproduction, situations occur in which genetic tests are performed on the embryo to establish a diagnosis of a particular disease because the parents were previously shown to be carriers of a genetic defect. Also the womens' age may be a reason to look for a chromosomal aberration in the embryos before transfer. If, however, all IVF-embryos would in the future be analyzed for chromosomal aneuploidies one can refer to it as genetic screening. After assisted reproduction and in particular after intracytoplasmic sperm injection embryos or foetuses can be screened for sex chromosomal anomalies. Performing adequate genetic tests in assisted reproduction is on the one hand part of good medical practice and on the other hand part of ongoing research into the causes of infertility.

**Keywords:** assisted reproductive technology, genetic counselling.

## Introduction

Assisted reproductive technology (ART) has been developed over the last 20 years and is still being developed, mainly to alleviate infertility. Causes of infertility are nongenetic, genetic or unknown. Within the group of unknown causes of infertility, certainly more genetic defects will be found with time. So far, different genetic aberrations have already been observed in men and in women presenting with infertility.
1. Numerical chromosomal anomalies as in Turner syndrome (45,X) or Klinefelter syndrome (47,XXY); the link between a 47,XXX or a 47,XYY-karyotype and infertility is not yet clearly established [1—4].
2. Structural chromosomal aberrations as para- or pericentric inversions and balanced single segment or double segment translocations; they are observed with a higher frequency in infertile men and women and in couples with recurrent miscarriages than in the general population [1—6].
3. Microdeletions such as these on the long arm of the Y-chromosome at the q11

---

*Address for correspondence:* Prof Inge Liebaers, Center for Medical Genetics, AZ-VUB, Laarbeeklaan 101, B-1090 Brussels, Belgium. Tel.: +32-2-477-60-71. Fax: +32-2-477-60-72.

locus and microtranslocations such as the one leading to the presence of the SRY-gene on the short arm of an X-chromosome in an XX-male; a routine karyotype will not identify these aberrations but molecular techniques will [1,2,4,7–10].

4. Gene mutations have been identified and will be identified in several monogenic conditions in which infertility can be a feature [11,12].

To identify these anomalies, adequate genetic tests have to be performed. The aim of these tests is to find the cause of the infertility and thus establish a more precise diagnosis. Genetic screening is something different. Genetic screening can be offered to a population because the incidence of a particular autosomal recessive gene mutation is elevated. For instance, in the Caucasian population or in the Ashkenazi Jewish population, carriers of a cystic fibrosis or Tay-Sachs mutation may be identified through a screening program; these individuals have no disease, but if two carriers want to have children, they know now that they have a 1/4 risk of having a child with cystic fibrosis or with Tay-Sachs disease [13,14]. In other words, to establish a causal diagnosis of infertility, one performs tests among which genetic tests and thus one does not screen. One could enumerate here, a list of genetic tests which may help in finding out why somebody is infertile. However, to be more practical and more precise, the genetic tests to be done will be discussed in relation to the clinical situation.

**Genetic testing of in- or subfertile couples before artificial reproduction**

A careful history should be taken. This history should not only include a personal history but also a detailed family history looking for miscarriages or the birth of a child with multiple malformations pointing to a possible familial chromosomal balanced translocation or looking for sibs also presenting with infertility pointing to a possible monogenic cause of infertility such as immotile cilia syndrome, Kallman syndrome or cystic fibrosis [11,12]. It is furthermore important to do a thorough clinical examination, not only to diagnose Turner and Klinefelter patients but also to eventually recognize symptoms which may point to other transmissible diseases such as myotonic dystrophy, an autosomal dominant disease that may also include subfertility, or another dominant disease such as neurofibromatosis, not causing infertility but characterized by multiple visible café au lait spots among other symptoms and a recurrence risk to offspring of 1/2 [15,16]. Complementary investigations will have to be done next. The genetic tests to be performed should take into account results of other investigations which will allow differential diagnosis.

In infertile women, karyotyping should be performed if a chromosomal aberration is suspected such as in premature menopause, recurrent first trimester abortions and also in cases of unexplained infertility. Other specific genetic tests may be indicated according to the history, physical examination and other available information, i.e., analysis of the fragile X-gene in case of family history of mental retardation [17].

In infertile men, genetic testing will also vary according to the available information. The knowledge whether the man has obstructive or nonobstructive azoospermia or extreme oligoasthenoteratozoospermia (OAT) will guide the geneticist. In most of the cases of male infertility it is indicated to do a karyotype of peripheral lymphocytes; it is certainly indicated in case of nonobstructive azoospermia and severe OAT [3,4,6]. It is also indicated to look for AZF a,b,c deletions on the long arm of chromosome Y in men with severe OAT [4,8–10]. In men with obstructive azoospermia due to congenital bilateral absence of the vas deferens (CBAVD) a DNA analysis of the CFTR-gene should be performed [18,19]. More specific testing is indicated if conditions such as Kallman syndrome, Kennedy disease or Steinert's myotonic dystrophy are suspected [11,12]. In other conditions such as the immotile cilia syndrome genetic testing should be done as soon as it is available. As in women, other genetic tests can and should be performed if indicated according to the available information. More advanced or more complex genetic tests can be indicated and performed in specialized centers investigating male or female infertility for research purposes such as meiotic studies in testicular biopsies or chromosome studies in sperm [4,20–23].

Finally genetic screening tests such as for cystic fibrosis or Tay-Sachs disease can also be offered at this point and should certainly be performed before treatment starts or even before treatment is planned [13,14].

## Genetic testing during assisted reproduction

Preconceptional or preimplantation genetic diagnosis (PGD) has to be performed during treatment because the procedure is based on the genetic analysis of one or two polar bodies of the oocyte or of one or two blastomeres of the cleaving embryo and eventually on trophectoderm cells from the blastocyst [24–26]. The indication for PGD can be a high-risk situation for a monogenic disease [27]. The most prominent example within the group of patients facing infertility is the risk for cystic fibrosis in a couple where the man has congenital bilateral absence of the vas deferens due to one or two mutations in the CFTR gene and his wife happens to be the carrier — before genetic testing her a priori risk to be a carrier is 1/25. The risk for the couples to have a child with CF is between 1/4 and 1/2 [18,19,27]. Depending on the mutations detected in the couple PGD can readily be offered by specialized centers or a custom-designed single cell polymerase chain reaction (PCR)-assay will have to be developed. In case PGD is not available, conventional prenatal diagnosis should be offered to these couples in case of pregnancy. PGD has been performed for other high-risk monogenic conditions but most of the time for fertile couples. Recently techniques are being developed to also offer PGD to couples carrying structural chromosomal aberrations, often the cause of in- or subfertility. In this case the single cell analysis is based on the fluorescent in situ hybridization (FISH) technique [28].

A question for debate is whether PGD should, from now on, also be offered to all women over 35 years having IVF without or with ICSI with the aim to avoid the birth of children with trisomy 13, 18, 21 or a sex chromosomal aberration [29—31]. Another aim may be to screen the embryos for aneuploidy to increase the success rate of ART in older women by eliminating, for example, trisomy 16 and trisomy 22, as well as triploid embryos. Techniques are indeed being developed to identify by FISH at the single cell level up to 10 chromosomes in two rounds of FISH or even all chromosomes in one round of FISH [32]. Even the idea of screening all IVF embryos for the most common aneuploidies does exist. And finally, the fear exists, that one day the technology will be available to screen embryos for all possible chromosome abnormalities as well as for all possible gene defects and that at the end ART will replace natural reproduction [33,34].

**Genetic testing after assisted reproduction**

From existing studies, it is known that, after IVF with ICSI, an increase in de novo chromosomal aberrations has been observed when compared to the general population. In one prospective study a total of 28 chromosomal aberrations were detected in 1,082 foetal karyotypes from CVS or amniotic cells. Ten of these were inherited, mainly from the fathers and only one of these was unbalanced and led to termination of pregnancy. From the other 18 anomalies, nine were autosomal aberrations and either trisomies, often in mothers over 35 years, or apparently balanced translocations. All of the trisomic pregnancies were terminated while none of the translocation pregnancies were. Finally the remaining nine chromosomal aberrations were sex chromosome aneuploidies of different kinds and half of these led to pregnancy termination [35]. At least one other study has observed an increase in sex chromosomal aberrations after ICSI [36]. The most probable but not proven explanation for this observation is an increase in sex chromosome aneuploidies in the sperm of subfertile males [21,37]. It is intended, based on the above knowledge, to inform the couples who will be treated and to offer them the possibility of prenatal diagnosis or, for the time being, in a limited number of situations PGD.

Within the same study as mentioned above a further pregnancy follow-up and more importantly a baby follow-up have taught us that after IVF with ICSI the incidence of 2.3% of major congenital malformations in 1966 live born infants is not increased when compared to general population based surveys. To be sure that the use of epididymal or testicular sperm as well as the transfer of cryopreserved embryos after ICSI are as safe as ICSI with ejaculated sperm, further evaluations are necessary [38].

**Discussion and Conclusions**

Performing genetic tests before, during and eventually after assisted reproduction has in the first place to do with good clinical practice. These tests not only allow the establishment of a correct diagnosis, they also allow adequate genetic counselling to the couple and eventually also to their respective families as discussed in the following examples [39].

1. A women with a 45,X karyotype may now become pregnant with donated oocytes, fertilized by her partner, however, before treating her a complete checkup for possible Turner syndrome complications should be done [40].

2. Some men with a 47,XXY karyotype may now father a child with testicular sperm but since it is not clear whether the few spermatozoa present in their testes bear a normal sex chromosome complement, preimplantation genetic diagnosis should be performed on the embryos obtained [41,42]. The couple should know that the success rate of the treatment remains low and is dependent on the number of spermatozoa recovered.

3. If a man or a woman are carriers of a structural chromosomal aberration it is most probable that their infertility or subfertility or recurrent miscarriages are related to that problem. Unless PGD is performed to exclude "unbalanced" embryos the success rate of their treatment will be decreased due to nonimplantation or miscarriages [28]. After PGD as well as when no PGD was performed prenatal diagnosis should be performed to either confirm the results of the PGD or to exclude the presence of an unbalanced foetus in an ongoing pregnancy possibly leading to the birth of a child with multiple congenital anomalies. In these cases it has also been indicated to suggest to the patients to inform sibs in the first place that they may carry a translocation as well.

4. In case the man carries a Yq11 deletion he should be informed that his sons will most probably carry the same mutation and will therefore have a high risk of being in- or subfertile. If the couple want to avoid that risk only XX-embryos, identified through PGD, can be transferred. If not, certainly in the male children, a follow-up is indicated by first analyzing the Yq11 region in cord blood and later on by trying to collect information on his fertility. On the other hand useful information could be obtained by looking at the Yq11 deletion in the father and the brothers of the patients.

5. If a man with CBAVD has a partner who is a carrier of a CFTR mutation, several possible risks may come forward according to the man's CFTR-gene sequences. Certainly a number of these couples will have a risk of 1/4, even 1/2. In these cases PGD should be performed, and if not, certainly prenatal diagnosis. Also family counselling is indicated [18,19,27].

Of course other situations may come up depending on the cause of the infertility. Myotonic dystrophy may lead to oligoastenozoospermia and other problems. The risk of transmitting the disease is 1/2 and the severity of the symptoms may increase in the next generation [15]. Here also PGD is indicated [27]. Finally ART and PGD may be a solution to couples at risk for chromosomal or monogenetic diseases without fertility problems. Moreover, in a number of situations with increased genetic risk oocyte or embryo donation may bring the solution but these situations are not within the scope of this paper [27,40].

Another reason to carry out genetic investigation in the case of infertility treatable by ART is to understand more about the causes of premature menopause, polycystic ovary disease, abnormal spermatogenesis, etc. However these investigations do not fall within the scope of routine clinical care but have to be part of research programs.

Performing genetic testing during treatment, in other words evaluating the embryo before transfer is of course indicated in the high-risk situations mentioned above. From the ongoing age-related aneuploidy screening programs we will learn whether indeed the miscarriage rate decreases while the pregnancy rate increases [29–31]. On the other hand we also want to be sure that while the risk of a trisomy 13, 18, 21 pregnancy is reduced, the IVF success rate does not decrease because of the manipulation of the embryo. If the preliminary data are confirmed, caution should still be made about extending the aneuploidy screening to all IVF-embryos [43–46].

Genetic testing after ART either prenatally or postnatally has to be discussed with the couples involved. Efforts should be made to continue or start follow-up studies to further evaluate the safety of ART.

In conclusion it should be said that genetic testing has to be part of the work-up of patients who might be treated by ART if we want to meet good clinical standards. Genetic screening may be offered to them as it may be offered to other couples who want to reproduce. Doing research within the field of infertility is important to learn more about its causes and this is even more true in the light of ART [47–49].

## References

1. Robinson A, de la Chapelle A. Sex chromosome abnormalities. In: Rimoin DL, Connor JM, Pyeritz RE (eds) Emery and Rimoins's Principles and Practice of Medical Genetics. Vol 1. New York: Churchill Livingstone, 1996;973–997.
2. Simpson JL, Golbus MS (eds). Genetics in Obstetrics and Gynecology, 2nd edn. Philadelphia: W.B. Saunders Company, 1992.
3. Van Assche E, Bonduelle M, Tournaye H, Joris H, Verheyen G, Devroey P et al. Cytogenetics of infertile men. In: Van Steirteghem A, Devroey P, Liebaers I (eds) Genetics and Assisted Human Conception. Vol 11, (Suppl 4) Hum Reprod. Oxford, UK: Oxford University Press, 1996;1–26.
4. Chandley AC. Chromosome anomalies and Y chromosome microdeletions as causal factors in male infertility. In: Devroey P, Tarlatzis B, Van Steirteghem A (eds) Current Theory and Practice of ICSI. Vol 13 (Suppl 1), Hum Reprod. Oxford, UK: Oxford University Press, 1998;45–50.
5. Spinner NB, Emanuel BS. Deletions and other structural abnormalities of the autosomes. In: Rimoin DL, Connor JM, Pyeritz RE (eds) Emery and Rimoins's Principles and Practice of Medical Genetics. Vol 1. New York: Churchill Livingstone, 1996;999–1025.
6. Yoshida A, Miura K, Shirai M. Cytogenetic survey of 1,007 infertile males. Urol Int 1997;58: 166–176.
7. Bogan J, Page D. Ovary? testis? – A mammalian dilemma. Cell 1994;76:603–607.
8. Reijo R, Lee TY, Salo P, Alagappan R, Brown LG, Rosenberg M et al. Diverse spermatogenic defects in humans caused by Y-chromosome deletions encompassing a novel RNA-binding protein gene. Nature Genet 1995;10:383–393.
9. Vogt PH, Edelmann A, Kirsch S, Henegariu O, Hirschmann P, Kiesewetter F et al. Human Y

chromosome azoospermia factors (AZF) mapped to different subregions in Yq11. Hum Mol Genet 1996;5:933–943.

10. Vogt PH. Genetics of idiopathic male infertility: Y chromosomal azoospermia factors (AZFa, AZFb, AZFc). In: Van Steirteghem A, Devroey P, Tournaye H (eds) Male Infertility. London: Baillière Tindall, Clin Obstet Gynaecol 1997;4:773–796.

11. Mak V, Jarvi KA The genetics of male infertility. J Urol 1996;156:1245–1257.

12. Meschede D, Horst J. The molecular genetics of male infertility. Molec Hum Reprod 1997; 3:419–430.

13. Brock D. Heterozygote screening for cystic fibrosis. Eur J Hum Genet 1995;3:2–13.

14. Paw Bh, Tieu Pt, Kaback MM, Lim J, Neufeld EF. Frequency of three Hex A mutant alleles among Jewish and nonJewish carriers identified in a Tay-Sachs screening program. Am J Hum Genet 1990;47:689–705.

15. Ptacek LJ, Johnson KJ, Griggs RC. Genetics and physiology of the myotonic muscle disorders. N Engl J Med 1993;328:482–489.

16. Riccardi V. Neurofibromatosis, Phenotype, Natural History and Pathogenesis, 2nd edn. Baltimore: The Johns Hopkins University Press, 1992.

17. Oostra BA, Jacky PB, Brown WT, Rousseau F. Guidelines for the diagnosis of fragile X syndrome. J Med Genet 1993;30:410–413.

18. Lissens W, Mercier B, Tournaye H, Bonduelle M, Férec C, Seneca S et al. Cystic fibrosis and infertility caused by congenital bilateral absence of the vas deferens and related clinical entities. In: Van Steirteghem A, Devroey P, Liebaers I (eds) Genetics and Assisted Human Conception, Vol 11, (Suppl 4) to Hum Reprod. Oxford, UK: Oxford University Press, 1996;55–80.

19. Lissens W, Liebaers I. The genetics of male infertility in relation to cystic fibrosis. In: Van Steirteghem A, Devroey P, Tournaye H (eds) Male Infertility. London: Baillière Tindall, Clin Obstet Gynaecol 1997;4:797–818.

20. Downie SE, Flaherty SP, Matthews CD. Detection of chromosomes and estimation of aneuploidy in human spermatozoa using fluorescence in-sity hybridization. Molec Hum Reprod 1997;3:585–598.

21. Martin R. Genetics of human sperm. J Assist Reprod Genet 1998;15:240–245.

22. Barlow AL, Hultén MA. Combined immunocytogenetic and molecular cytogenetic analysis of meiosis I human spermatocytes. Chromosome Res 1996;4:562–573.

23. Hunt P. The control of mammalian female meiosis: factors that influence chromosome segregation. J Assist Reprod Genet 1998;15:246–252.

24. Tarin JJ, Handyside AH. Embryo biopsy strategies for preimplantation diagnosis. Fertil Steril 1993;59:943–952.

25. Lissens W, Sermon K. Preimplantation genetic diagnosis: current status and new developments. Hum Reprod 1997;12:1756–1762.

26. Verlinsky Y, Kuliev A. Preimplantation genetics. J Assist Reprod Genet 1998;15:215–218.

27. Liebaers I, Sermon K, Staessen C, Joris H, Lissens W, Van Assche E et al. Clinical experience with preimplantation genetic diagnosis and intracytoplasmic sperm injection. In: Devroey P, Tarlatzis B, Van Steirteghem A (eds) Current Theory and Practice of ICSI. Vol 13 (Suppl 1). Hum Reprod. Oxford, UK: Oxford University Press, 1998;186–195.

28. Munné S, Morrison L, Fung J, Marquez C, Weier U, Bahçe M et al. Spontaneous abortions are reduced after preconception diagnosis of translocations. J Assist Reprod Genet 1998;15: 290–296.

29. Verlinsky Y, Cieslak J, Ivakhnenko V, Evsikov S, Wolf G, White M et al. Preimplantation diagnosis of common aneuploidies by first- and second-polar body FISH analysis. J Assist Reprod Genet 1998;15:285–296.

30. Gianaroli L, Magli MC, Ferraretti AP, Fiorentino A, Garrisi J, Munné S. Preimplantation genetic diagnosis increases the implantation rate in human in vitro fertilization by avoiding the transfer of chromosomally abnormal embryos. Fertil Steril 1997;68:1128–1131.

31. Magli MC, Gianaroli L, Munné S, Ferrarreti AP. Incidence of chromosomal abnormalities from

a morphologically normal cohort of embryos in poor-prognosis patients. J Assist Reprod Genet 1998;15:297–301.

32. Fung J, Hyun W, Dandekar P, Pedersen PA, Weier U. Spectral imaging in preconception/preimplantation genetic diagnosis of aneuploidy: multicolor, multichromosome screening of single cells. J Assist Reprod Genet 1998;15:323–330.

33. Testart J, Sèle B. Opinion. Towards an efficient medical eugenics: is the desirable always the feasible? Hum Reprod 1995;10:3086–3090.

34. Handyside AH. Opinion. Common sense as applied to eugenics: response to Testart and Sèle. Hum Reprod 1996;11:707.

35. Bonduelle M, Aytoz A, Van Assche E, Devroey P, Liebaers I, Van Steirteghem A. Incidence of chromosomal aberrations in children born after assisted reproduction through intracytoplasmic sperm injection. Editorial, Hum Reprod 1998;13:781–782.

36. In't Veld P, Brandenburg H, Verhoeff A, Dhont M, Los F. Sex chromosomal abnormalities and intracytoplasmic sperm injection. Lancet 1995;346:773.

37. Van Opstal D, Los F, Ramlakhan S, Van Hemel JO, Van Den Ouweland AMW, Brandenburg H et al. Determination of the parent of origin in nine cases of prenatally detected chromosome aberrations found after intracytoplasmic sperm injection. Hum Reprod 1997;12:682–686.

38. Bonduelle M, Aytoz A, Wilikens A, Buysse A, Van Assche E, Devroey P, Van Steirteghem A, Liebaers I. Prospective follow-up study of 1987 children born after intracytoplasmic sperm injection (ICSI). In: Filicori M (ed) Treatment of Infertility: The New Frontiers. Communications Media for Education, Inc. (In press) 1998.

39. Harper P. Practical Genetic Counselling. 4th edn. Cambridge UK: Butterworth-Heinemann Ltd, 1993.

40. Pados G, Camus M, Van Steirteghem A, Bonduelle M, Devroey P. The evolution and outcome of pregnancies from oocyte donation. Hum Reprod 1994;9:538–542.

41. Staessen C, Coonen E, Van Assche E, Tournaye H, Joris H, Devroey P et al. Preimplantation diagnosis for X and Y normality in embryos from three Klinefelter patients. Hum Reprod 1996;11:1650–1653.

42. Tournaye H, Staessen C, Liebaers I, Van Assche E, Devroey P, Bonduelle M, Van Steirteghem A. Testicular sperm recovery in nine 47,XXY Klinefelter patients. Hum Reprod 1996;11: 1644–1649.

43. Reubinoff BE, Shushan A. Debate. Preimplantation diagnosis in older patients. To biopsy or not to biopsy? Hum Reprod 1996;11:2071–2075.

44. Verlinsky Y, Kuliev A. Debate. Preimplantation diagnosis inolder patients. Preimplantation diagnosis of common aneuploidies in infertile couples of advanced maternal age. Hum Reprod 1996;11:2076–2077.

45. Egozcue J. Debate. Preimplantation diagnosis in older patients. Of course, not. Hum Reprod 1996;11:2077–2078.

46. Munné S, Cohen J. Debate concluded. Preimplantation diagnosis in older patients but of course! Hum Reprod 1997;12:413–414.

47. St. John J, Cooke ID, Barratt Ch. Mitochondrial mutations and male infertility. Letters to the Editor. Nature Med 1997;3:124–215.

48. Tesarik J, Adel F, Brami C, Sedbon E, Thorel J, Tibi C, Thébault A. Spermatid injection into human oocytes II. Clinical application in the treatment of infertility due to non-obstructive azoospermia. Hum Reprod 1996;11:780–783.

49. Tesarik J, Mendoza C. Genomic imprinting abnormalities: a new potential risk of assisted reproduction. Molec Hum Reprod 1996;2:295–298.

# Posthumous reproduction

John A. Robertson

*Law School, University of Texas at Austin, Austin, Texas, USA*

**Abstract.** The question of posthumous reproduction arises with increasing frequency in assisted reproduction. Such situations can involve stored gametes or embryos with or without prior consent of the deceased for posthumous reproductive use, as well as postmortem retrieval of gametes without prior consent. Three sets of interests are involved in these cases: that of the deceased, the next of kin requesting positive use, and resulting children. Analysis of these interests shows that physicians and clinics may ethically and legally (in the USA) accede to requests of persons with proper dispositional authority to effectuate posthumous reproduction with the reproductive material at issue.

**Keywords:** assisted reproduction, harm to offspring, posthumous reproduction, postmortem gamete retrieval, stored gametes.

Technical advances in assisted reproduction have enabled both the living and the dead to reproduce. The prospect of posthumous reproduction arises in several different settings [1]. Most common is the situation in which gametes or embryos have been stored with the prospect of posthumous conception or implantation and reproduction clearly contemplated and intended. In some cases, gametes or embryos have been stored without specific instructions that they may be used after death, but the person with legal control over the stored material wishes to use them, thus bringing about the deceased's posthumous reproduction. Finally, it is possible to retrieve sperm (and possibly in the future eggs) posthumously from a deceased person and use them to effectuate reproduction by the deceased [2].

As with many advances in assisted reproduction, there is not yet a clear and precise set of rules for how each of these situations of posthumous reproduction should be handled. Yet there is a clear emerging consensus about more basic principles of law and ethics for reproductive decisions which can be drawn upon to deduce what the likely response or rule for situations of posthumous reproduction should be, as the following discussion will show [1,3].

In assessing the three situations identified, three different sets of interests must be balanced [1]. One is the interest of the deceased person, if any, in whether reproduction occurs posthumously. An essential aspect of this interest is whether the deceased person when alive gave directions about reproduction or disposition

*Address for correspondence:* John A. Robertson JD, Law School, University of Texas at Austin, 727 East 26th Street, Austin, TX 78705, USA.

of stored gametes or embryos or their body after their death. Second is the interest of the person with legal authority over the deceased person's gametes, embryos, or body in using that material for reproduction, thereby causing the posthumous reproduction of the deceased. In most instances the person with legal authority will be the spouse of the deceased or a parent or sibling who wishes the deceased's gametes to be used by another for the deceased's posthumous reproduction. Third is the interest of the child who is born as a result of posthumous reproduction. Although that child will have been conceived (or embryos implanted in the uterus if conception has already occurred) after the death of a genetic parent, the situation of the child is similar to that of a child conceived by an unmarried woman who is brought into the world without a known rearing father. In both cases but for the unmarried or posthumous conception or birth, the child in question would not have been born. Because living without the company of one biological parent does not render that person's life full of irremediable suffering, the resulting child is not harmed by posthumous reproduction, for that child has no alternative to being born posthumously.

**Storage of gametes or embryos with prior directive for posthumous reproduction**

The strongest case for posthumous reproduction arises when a person stores his or her gametes prior to treatment for cancer so that their gametes will escape the toxicities of treatment and be viable for reproductive uses. Although the person's intent in this situation ordinarily is to preserve viable gametes so that they may be used after treatment has successfully cured or arrested the disease, the person storing the gametes understands that use of the gametes may not occur during their lifetime, and gives explicit written directions that his or her spouse or family may use the stored reproductive material to effectuate his or her posthumous reproduction. May a physician or clinic faced with this situation comply with the survivors' request to use the stored material for reproduction, including the posthumous reproduction of the deceased?

There is growing ethical and legal recognition that posthumous reproduction may occur in this situation [1,3,5]. The deceased has consented when competent to posthumous reproduction. The person wishing to use the stored reproductive material to reproduce is likely to be the surviving spouse. It could also be the parents or siblings of the deceased, who wish to donate the material to a companion of the deceased or, in the case of stored embryos, would like to hire a surrogate so that posthumous reproduction of the deceased may occur. Nor is the child injured by being conceived or born posthumously. If posthumous conception or birth does not occur, the child will never come into existence. Once alive, the child clearly has interests in continuing to live, despite the absence of a biological parent whose death preceded the childs conception or implantation. The absence of this biological parent is to be regretted, but there is no alternative way for this child to have come into existence, and his or her present existence appears to be no worse than that of children born to single women.

The legality of posthumous reproduction when a prior directive for posthumous use of stored gametes or embryos exists will depend on the jurisdiction. In the USA no law would prohibit or penalize a physician or clinic that acceded to a surviving spouse or family members request to use the stored material to enable reproduction, including the posthumous reproduction of the deceased to occur [1]. Neither concerns about the single parent situation of the child (which may only be temporary) or the wishes of already existing children who object to the birth of another sibling would operate as a legal barrier to use of the stored reproductive material, if the person wishing its posthumous use otherwise has the legal authority to control its disposition [4].

**Storage of gametes or embryos without prior directive for posthumous use**

What then about the posthumous use of gametes or embryos that have been stored without an explicit prior directive from the deceased that they may be used posthumously for reproduction? Such a situation is likely to be quite common. Men who store sperm prior to cancer treatment may assume that they will live to use the stored material and not give instructions concerning disposal after death. Couples undergoing IVF may store surplus embryos without specifying that they may be used after death. May a physician or clinic accede to the request of the surviving spouse or family member to release or use stored gametes or embryos to be used for conception or implantation, thereby causing the posthumous reproduction of the deceased, even when the deceased has not given prior consent for that use?

A crucial issue in this situation is that the person who wishes to use the gametes or embryos for conception or implantation has the legal right to control their postmortem disposition. If the person has that authority, then the issue posed is whether the deceased's failure to make an explicit directive in favor of posthumous use should operate as a limit or check on that dispositional authority.

Some persons, asserting that no reproduction should occur without consent, have argued that posthumous reproduction should never occur without the explicit prior consent of the deceased [3,5]. In their view, deceased persons still have interests, and those interests include not having posthumous offspring without consent. Others have argued that the principle of no reproduction without consent, while important for reproduction occurring during a persons lifetime, should not apply when a person is deceased. In their view deceased persons, being dead, no longer have interests, and thus posthumous reproduction can neither harm nor benefit them. Even if they concede that certain interests, such as attorney–client confidentiality, should survive death because of the effect that survival of that privilege has on ones interests in planning ones life when alive, they might still plausibly distinguish posthumous reproduction as not falling into that category because the prospect of unconsented to posthumous reproduction will affect few decisions when alive.

Philosophers and ethicists are likely to continue to debate whether deceased persons have interests at all, and if so, whether those interests extend to post-humous reproduction. However, given the plausibility of concluding that persons no longer have reproductive interests once they are dead, and the strong interest of persons with legal dispositional authority over the reproductive material to use the stored material for their own or anothers reproduction, it should be ethically and legally acceptable to use the stored material without the deceased's prior consent. Although still debated and denied by some commentators, such a position is likely to be legally accepted in the USA, though other countries might take a different view of the matter [1,3,5].

## Postmortem retrieval of gametes without prior directive

The most controversial case involving posthumous reproduction — the question of postmortem gamete retrieval with prior consent — arises with increasing frequency. A person who has not previously stored gametes or embryos suffers unexpected trauma and dies. That person's spouse or family requests that gametes be retrieved from the deceased's body so that they or another might use them to reproduce, thus also causing the posthumous reproduction of the deceased. Surveys show that such requests are increasingly common, and that physicians and programs often satisfy them [4]. Should urologists faced with requests for postmortem sperm retrieval or gynecologists who in the future are asked to remove and preserve ovarian tissue be free on ethical and legal grounds to accede to such requests?

Although clear lines for this practice have not yet emerged and some bioethicists oppose the practice, the ethical and legal issues are similar to those that arise in the second situation discussed above — whether stored gametes and embryos may be used for posthumous reproduction without the deceased's prior consent. The only difference between the two situations is the timing of gamete retrieval — premortem in one case and postmortem in the other. But the timing of gamete retrieval is irrelevant to the ethical and legal analysis of whether posthumous reproduction may occur. As long as the person requesting postmortem gamete retrieval has the legal authority to make such a request, the fact that gametes must first be retrieved, as opposed to removed from storage and thawed, should not matter [1].

The acceptability of postmortem gamete retrieval without prior consent of the deceased will thus depend on ones position on posthumous reproduction with stored gametes or embryos when the deceased has not given prior consent for posthumous use. If one finds that such use is acceptable because the deceased lacks interests in whether or not posthumous reproduction occurs (as one might reasonably conclude), then retrieving gametes postmortem to enable posthumous reproduction to occur implicates no additional interests of the deceased. Indeed, postmortem retrieval without prior consent would enable the person requesting it (or their designee) to reproduce, and would not harm the resulting child anymore than posthumous reproduction with stored gametes or embryos but no prior directive for postmortem use would harm the child. On the other hand, if one objects to posthumous use of stored gametes when there is no prior directive for postmortem use, then one should object to postmortem gamete retrieval without consent as well [3,5].

Legally, the crucial issue in this scenario is whether the person requesting postmortem gamete retrieval has the legal authority to authorize removal of gametes or ovarian tissue from the deceased's body. In the USA the Uniform Anatomical Gift Act (UAGA) in effect in every state gives the next of kin, in designated order of closeness, the right to make anatomical gifts of the body without limiting the uses that can be made of the gift. Although the precise question of whether that authority would extend to retrieving gametes to be used by the kin or their designee for their own reproduction or that of others has not yet been faced by the courts, it is both plausible and reasonable to read the UAGA as granting that authority. Whether or not an anatomical gift can be made to the person with decisional authority over the body, it certainly could be made to a physician or other person who then donates that material to the person with original decisional authority. If this interpretation is correct, then physicians and hospitals may retrieve gametes from deceased persons at the request of that legally authorized person and use them for postmortem conception as that person directs, even though the deceased issued no prior instructions for postmortem gamete retrieval.

## Conclusion

The analysis of three main situations involving posthumous reproduction shows that although posthumous reproduction is still controversial, physicians and clinics have reasonable grounds for thinking that they may ethically and legally (at least in the USA) participate in posthumous reproduction in the three situations discussed. Of course, no physician or clinic is obligated to participate. But if they think that the person requesting posthumous use would be a responsible parent and has legal authority to direct the use of stored gametes or embryos or dispose of the deceased's body, they may ethically accede to their wishes and effectuate the requested reproduction, thus causing the posthumous reproduction of the deceased to occur.

## References

1. Robertson JA. Posthumous reproduction. Indian Law J 1994;69:1027–1065.
2. Kerr SM, Caplan A, Polin G, Smugar S, O'Neill K, Urowitz S. Postmortem sperm procurement. J Urol 1997;157:2154–2158.
3. Schiff AR. Arising from the dead: challenges of posthumous reproduction. N Carolina Law Rev 1997;75:901–955.
4. Hecht V. Kane, 50 Cal. App. 4th 1289, 59 Cal. Rptr. 2d 222 (1996).
5. The New York State Task Force on Life and the Law, Assisted Reproductive Technologies: Analysis and Recommendations for Public Policy 1998; 294–298.

# Polycystic ovarian disease

# Polycystic ovarian disease: obesity and insulin resistance

Zeev Shoham and Ariel Weissman

*Department of Obstetrics and Gynecology, Hebrew University and Hadassah Medical School, Jerusalem, Israel*

**Abstract.** Polycystic ovarian disease is a heterogeneous disorder, consisting mainly of menstrual dysfunction, hirsutism, infertility, obesity, elevated basal LH levels, hyperandrogenemia and polycystic appearance of the ovaries, which may all present in various combinations. It is considered the most common cause of anovulatory infertility. Obese women with PCOD often express insulin resistance, but it can also be demonstrated in lean PCOD patients. The resulting hyperinsulinemia may stimulate androgen production by theca cells, through a direct effect of insulin on theca cells, or through the action of the intraovarian growth factors (IGFs) or their binding proteins. Hence, for a specific subgroup of patients, insulin resistance may play a major role in the pathophysiology of PCOD. Weight loss should be considered as a first option for women who are obese and present with either infertility or any of the other metabolic disturbances characteristic of PCOD. In anovulatory patients with insulin resistance who present with infertility, ovulation induction with either clomiphene citrate or gonadotropins merits specific considerations, since while success rates may be compromised, the risk for ovarian hyperstimulation syndrome is increased. Modern trends in PCOD management include medical therapy with insulin sensitizing agents, and surgical ovarian diathermy. Long-term consequences of PCOD, obesity and insulin resistance may include an increased risk for diabetes and cardiovascular disease. Weight loss should be encouraged as it may also limit the remote risks associated with this condition.

**Keywords**: hyperinsulinemia, infertility, insulin, insulin resistance, obesity, polycystic ovarian disease, weight loss.

## Introduction

Polycystic ovarian disease (PCOD) has been one of the most discussed, controversial and explored areas in reproductive medicine. The etiology of the disease is uncertain, as there is a spectrum of disorders encompassed by the diagnosis of PCOD.

Sclerocystic changes in the human ovary were clearly described by Chereau in 1845, and Gusserow, Martin, Wiedow, Zweifel, and others were practicing wedge resection of such ovaries in Europe before 1897. In the USA, Findley described wedge resection for "cystic degeneration" of the ovary as early as 1904. Occasional reports continued to appear over the years. In 1935, in their original paper, Stein and Leventhal described seven hirsute and infertile women with amenorrhea or oligomenorrhea in whom bilateral cystic ovarian enlargement was found

---

*Address for correspondence:* Zeev Shoham, Department of Obstetrics and Gynecology, Kaplan Medical Center, Rehovot 76100, Israel.

at laparotomy [1].

PCOD may appear with minimal signs of hyperandrogenism in lean women with regular menses or in obese, very hirsute, oligo- or amenorrheic women, as originally described by Stein and Leventhal, representing, respectively, the mild and the severe ends of the diagnostic spectrum.

Despite the fact that a vast amount of clinical, laboratory and experimental data has been accumulated, the etiology of PCOS has remained the subject of interest and ongoing controversy for almost 60 years. Various mechanisms, involving numerous organ systems, have been postulated over the years in the pathogenesis of the common form of PCOD. These include abnormalities in the ovaries, hypothalamic-pituitary unit, thyroid gland, adrenals and/or adipose tissue [2]. No underlying cause, however, has been clearly identified.

Polycystic ovaries (PCOs) are thought to be the most common cause of anovulatory infertility and menstrual irregularity. The ability to detect PCO on pelvic ultrasonography has led to the re-evaluation of the prevalence and the etiology of this disorder. However, neither the site nor the nature of the primary lesion in women with PCO is known, and there is no complete agreement as to how infertile or hirsute women with PCO should be treated. Similarly, because of the clinical heterogeneity of patients presenting with PCO and the variation in ovarian size and morphology, uniform diagnostic criteria have not been established.

Clinical PCOD is characterized in its purest form by menstrual dysfunction, hirsutism, infertility, obesity, and polycystic ovaries. Although not all women with PCOD have all components of this syndrome, the frequency of obesity is high (around 50%), and insulin resistance and hyperinsulinemia appear to be almost universal findings.

Obesity has been associated with PCOD since the syndrome was first described [1]. In 1952, Roger and Mitchell [3] found a high incidence (45%) of obesity in amenorrheic patients. In subjects with PCOD, the body mass index (BMI) is correlated with an increased rate of hirsutism, cycle irregularities and infertility [4,5]. Body fat distribution (increased waist:hip ratio), rather than body weight alone, appears to have an important affect on fecundity [6]. Weight loss in obese women with PCOD, has been shown to bring about the reduction in estrone concentrations, and resumption of normal gonadotropin secretion and regular menstrual cycles [7]. In one of the largest studies ever published, focusing on the clinical spectrum of the disorder, Balen and his colleagues [5] were able to show that of 1,741 women with PCOS, who all had PCO on pelvic ultrasound, 38.4% were overweight ($BMI > 25$ kg/m$^2$) (Fig. 1).

In their study, Balen and his colleagues [5] also found that the patients' BMI was significantly correlated with ovarian volume. A higher BMI was associated with a rise in serum testosterone concentration and with the prevalence of hirsutism. Obesity was also significantly associated with an increased rate of infertility and menstrual disturbances. The rates of primary (15%) and secondary (8%) infertility were fairly constant with BMIs of $20-10$ kg/m$^2$ but rose to 26 and 14%, respectively, when the BMI was $> 30$ kg/m$^2$.

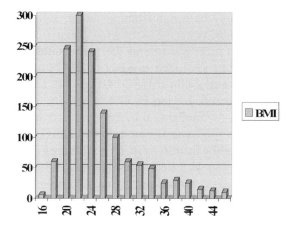

*Fig. 1.* Frequency distribution of BMI (kg/m$^2$) of 1,741 women with PCOS. (Reproduced, with permission from [5].)

Burghen et al. in 1980 [8] were the first to suggest that insulin resistance and PCOD were closely linked, and that there was a correlation between serum concentrations of insulin and androgens in obese women. Nestler el al. [9] subsequently proposed that obesity plays a central role in the development of PCOD by leading to hyperinsulinaemia in susceptible individuals. In recent years, substantial evidence has accumulated suggesting that insulin and growth hormone (GH) may have gonadotropin-augmenting effects with regard to ovarian function. The localization of GH, insulin, and insulin-like growth factors receptors and their gene expression to specific ovarian compartments has led to the establishment of the concept of an endocrine role for these extraovarian factors in the pathophysiology of PCOD. The association between hyperandrogenemia and PCOD with disorders of insulin resistance has been well-documented [10]. Mild insulin resistance has been noted to exist in both obese and nonobese women with PCOD [8,11].

**Obesity and insulin resistance**

Although the pathophysiology of PCOD has long remained elusive, there is an increasing amount of evidence that the primary abnormality in PCOD is excessive ovarian androgen production. While only 35–50% of patients with PCOD are obese, obesity has consistently been shown to increase the prevalence of hirsutism and anovulation when compared to lean women with PCOD. The association of hyperandrogenemia and PCOD with disorders of extreme insulin resistance has been documented extensively [10] following the first report by Burghen et al. [8]. It was therefore hypothesized that obesity and the consequent hyperinsulinemia might lead to the genesis of PCOD in susceptible individuals [9]. However, mild insulin resistance has also been noted in nonobese women with PCOD [11], and therefore, obesity may be a contributing factor, but certainly not a prerequisite for insulin resistance.

In obese women, hyperinsulinemia plays a central role in the pathogenesis of the PCOD [12] by both stimulating ovarian androgen production [13] and by decreasing the serum sex hormone-binding globulin (SHBG) levels [14]. Obese women with PCOD also demonstrate increased ovarian P450c17a activity, a key enzyme in the biosynthesis of androgens, as demonstrated by an increased secretion of serum 17 a-hydroxprogesterone in response to stimulation by GnRH agonists [15]. P450c17a appears to be stimulated by insulin in PCOD. Reducing insulin release with metformin [16] or weight loss [17] decreases ovarian P450c17a activity and serum-free testosterone concentrations in obese women with the disorder. In vitro, insulin can enhance pituitary LH and FSH release [18]. This phenomenon suggests a role for excess stimulation of the gonadotrope by insulin, thus inducing an abnormal gonadotropin secretion pattern in PCOD.

Since obesity is associated with insulin resistance [19], the development of PCOD in obese patients may be caused not only by abnormal gonadotropin secretion induced by hyperinsulinemia but also by the amplification of the action of LH on the ovary in the presence of elevated insulin levels [13]. It might therefore be speculated that any cause of insulin resistance that results in hyperinsulinemia might lead to the development of PCOD in a susceptible individual through several endocrine pathways (Fig. 2).

The ovary expresses receptors for both insulin and insulin-like growth factor I (IGF-I) and there appears to be cross-reactivity between these hormones and

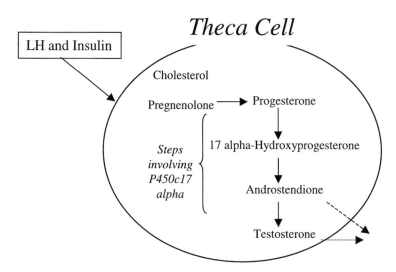

*Fig. 2.* Possible mechanisms of insulin and LH stimulation of ovarian cytochrome P450c17α activity and androgen production. In the theca cells, insulin may stimulate ovarian cytochrome P450c17α, resulting in increase 17α-hydroxylase and, to a lesser extent, 17,20-lyase activity. This would lead to an increase in androgen production. Alternatively, insulin enhances LH pulses, which stimulate ovarian P450c17α activity. (Reproduced, with permission from [34].)

their receptors. Thus, hyperinsulinemia may lead to direct stimulation of insulin receptors in the ovary. IGF-I has been shown to potentate the stimulating effect of FSH on ovarian aromatase activity, on estradiol and progesterone secretion, and on the expression of LH receptors [20].

Fasting insulin levels correlate positively with serum IGF-I levels and inversely with insulin-like growth factor binding protein I (IGFBP-I) concentrations in lean women with PCOD. IGFBP-I plays a central role in regulating the bioavailability of IGF-II and to a lesser extent IGF-I, and is known to be regulated by insulin. Insulin decreases the circulating concentration of IGFBP-I and thus increases the potential for IGF-I to stimulate the ovary. IGF-I augments the action of LH in stimulating the theca and interstitial compartments of the ovary [21]. This synergistic effect may lead to increased activity of cytochrome P450c-17-$\alpha$ hydroxylase, which is an important intermediary in the production of androgens. LH regulation of cytochrome P450 steroidogenic enzymes catalyses the final rate-limiting step in testosterone and androstendione biosynthesis, which are than used as substrates by ovarian granulosa cells for the conversion of androgenic precursors to estrogens.

It has been shown [22] that a major effect of insulin on androgen secretion is mediated through changes in SHBG levels. In addition, a study by Hamilton-Fairley et al. [23] has shown that the level of insulin was not significantly raised in the PCOD group as a whole, but was found to be elevated in anovulatory compared with ovulatory women despite having similar androgen levels. This may indicate that insulin resistance in the ovary contributes to the mechanism of anovulation, and that insulin may not be directly involved in increased androgen production in these women.

Insler and colleagues [24] found that serum IGF-I concentration was inversely correlated with insulin concentration and was significantly lower in obese PCOD subjects than in nonobese. They have also demonstrated significantly lower SHBG serum levels in obese women, compared to nonobese. It may thus be postulated that in obese women, hyperinsulinemia is a secondary disorder, resulting in a decrease in SHBG and IGFBP-I levels. This, in turn further leads to an increase in free androgens, which are subsequently converted to estrone due to the presence of excessive amounts of adipose tissue. Insulin inhibits IGFBP-I gene expression, and this observation may reflect insulin sensitivity at the hepatic level, despite insulin resistance in other tissues in the majority of PCOD patients. Concurrent with the decrease IGFBP-I, there is an increase in the levels of the free IGF-I, which may synergistically act with LH to stimulate thecal androgen production in PCOS women (Fig. 3).

**Treatment implications**

Obesity plays a central role in the development of PCOD, leading to hyperinsulinemia in susceptible individuals. This hyperinsulinemia may alter androgen metabolism through a variety of mechanisms, all leading to hyperandrogenism.

268

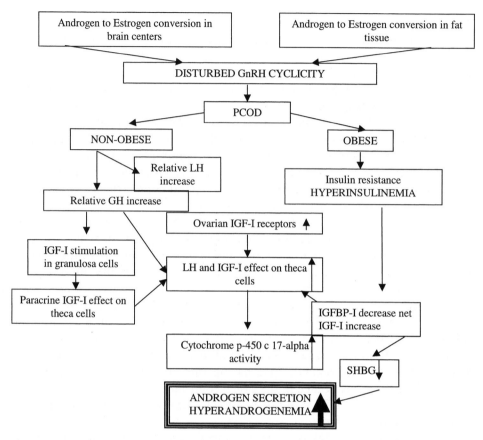

*Fig. 3.* Possible mechanisms leading to PCOS in obese and nonobese women. (Reproduced, with permission from [24]).

Since obesity has an adverse effect on rates of ovulation and miscarriage, weight loss alone may improve the symptoms of PCOD and the patient's endocrine profile and result in spontaneous ovulation and successful pregnancies [25]. Out of 13 obese and anovulatory patients who underwent a weekly program of behavioral change in relation to exercise and diet over a 6 months period, ovulation resumed in 12 and 11 conceived, five of them spontaneously [25]. Fasting insulin and testosterone levels dropped significantly, while SHBG concentrations rose. Thus, the importance of weight reduction is straight forward, and it should be used as the first therapeutic strategy, irrespective of whether the patient has originally presented with infertility, menstrual disturbances or even hirsutism. It should be emphasized, however, that the metabolic status in obese PCOD patients may be genetically predetermined, and therefore, achieving weight reduction may be extremely difficult.

Weight reduction should also be encouraged prior to ovulation induction therapy, as it appears to be lees effective when the BMI is greater than $28-30$ kg/m$^2$

[26]. While clomiphene citrate remains the first line of therapy for induction of ovulation in patients with PCOD, resistance to clomiphene ovulation induction is common with obesity and hyperinsulinemia, resulting from peripheral insulin resistance [27,28]. It has been shown that the dose of clomiphene citrate must be increased with increasing body weight [29]. Polson et al. [30], however, have demonstrated that obese patients who fail to respond to 100 mg of daily clomiphene will not ovulate on a higher dose. Since response to ovulation induction with hMG or pulsatile GnRH affected by body weight to a lesser extent, a direct central effect of insulin at the hypothalamus or pituitary level cannot be ruled out. At present, it is unknown whether treatments focusing on improving insulin sensitivity without weight loss will also improve the response to clomiphene in clomiphene resistant women.

Response to induction of ovulation with gonadotropins may also be affected by obesity, as demonstrated by Hamilton-Fairley et al. [26], who showed a blunted response to gonadotropin therapy in PCOD patients with moderate obesity ($BMI < 28$ kg/m$^2$) as compared to nonobese women. Obese patients were less likely to ovulate, and required larger daily doses and total amount of exogenous gonadotropins. Obese patients were also characterized by increased risk for miscarriage. Fulghesu et al. [31] compared the response to FSH therapy in normo- and hyperinsulinemic PCOD patients. Insulin levels seemed to influence the ovarian response to FSH, as evidenced by enhancement of recruitment of antral follicles and higher rate of ovarian growth and the ovarian hyperstimulation syndrome (OHSS) in the hyperinsulinemic patients. In contrast to the findings of Hamilton-Fairley et al. [26], insulin levels or BMI had no influence on the total dose of gonadotropins required for ovulation induction. Hyperinsulinemia and obesity may also interfere with the response to pulsatile GnRH therapy, and a positive correlation has been demonstrated between insulin response to a glucose challenge and ovarian volume in PCOD patients who failed to ovulate with pulsatile GnRH [32].

Recently, due to the close relationship between PCOD and insulin resistance, insulin sensitizing agents have become an increasingly popular treatment modality. Metformin enhances the sensitivity of peripheral tissues to insulin and decreases hepatic glucose production, thus decreasing insulin secretion [33]. In subjects with PCOD, metformin ameliorates hyperandrogenism and abnormal gonadotropin secretion and can restore menstrual cyclicity and fertility [34—37]. Troglitazone, another insulin sensitizer which also appears to improve significantly the endocrine and metabolic abnormalities, has been associated with spontaneous return of ovulation and enhancement of fertility in PCOD subjects without changes in weight [38,39]. This agent, however, has been withdrawn recently because of reports of death from hepatotoxicity. New preparations of insulin sensitizers are currently being investigated.

Laparoscopic ovarian surgery has the advantages of a single treatment that restores ovulation, with the correction of many of the associated endocrine abnormalities and an apparent low rate of miscarriage [40—42]. The success of this treatment modality is difficult to predict based on patients' pretreatment characteristics. In one study [43], no correlation could be demonstrated between patients' BMI, ovarian volume, and testosterone levels with treatment outcome. There are, however, increased risks associated with laparoscopy and anesthesia, and long-term concerns of adhesion formation and loss of functional ovarian tissue, and these should be weighed against the benefits.

Routine measurement of circulating insulin levels in patients with PCOD is rarely necessary, as it adds little, if any, to the management. However, since the prevalence of type II diabetes in obese patients with PCOD may be as high as 11% [44], a glucose tolerance test may be indicated.

In the long term, due to the observation that women with PCOD and insulin resistance may be at increased risk for type II diabetes, cardiovascular disease, or both, obese women (BMI > 30 kg/m$^2$) with PCOD should be encouraged to lose weight in an effort to limit the remote risks associated with this condition.

## References

1. Stein IF, Leventhal ML. Amenorrhea associated with bilateral polycystic ovaries. Am J Obstet Gynecol 1935;29:181–191.
2. Rosenfield RL, Barnes RB, Cara JF, Lucky AW. Dysregulation of cytochrome p450c17a as the cause of polycystic ovarian syndrome. Fertil Steril 1990;53:785–791.
3. Roger J, Mitchell GW. The relation of obesity to menstrual disturbances. N Engl J Med 1952; 247:53–56.
4. Kiddy DS, Hamilton-Failey D, Bush A, Anyaoku V, Reed MJ, Franks S. Improvement in endocrine and ovarian function during dietary treatment of obese women with polycystic ovary syndrome. Clin Endocrinol 1992;36:105–111.
5. Balen AH, Conway GS, Kaltsas G, Techatraisak K, Manning PJ, West C, Jacohs HS. Polycystic ovary syndrome: the spectrum of the disorder in 1741 patients. Hum Reprod 1995;10: 2107–2111.
6. Zaadstra BM, Seidell JC, Van Noord PA te Velde ER, Habbema JD, Vrieswijk B, Karbaat J. Fat and female fecundity: prospective study of effect of body fat distribution on conception rates. Br Med J 1993;306:484–487.
7. Harlass FE, Plymlate SR, Fariss BL, Belts RP. Weight loss is associated with correction of gonadotropin and sex steroid abnormalities in the obese anovulatory female. Fertil Steril 1984; 42:649–652.
8. Burghen GA, Givens JR, Kitabchi AE. Correlation of hyperandrogen with hyperinsulinism in polycystic ovarian disease. J Clin Endocrinol Metab 1980;50:113–116.
9. Nestler JE, Clore JN, Blackard WG. The central role of obesity (hyperinsulinemia) in the pathogenesis of the polycystic ovary syndrome. Am J Obstet Gynecol 1989;161:1095–1097.
10. Poretsky L, Kalin MF. The gonadotropic function of insulin. Endocr Rev 1987;8:132–141.
11. Chang RJ, Nakamura RM, Jndd HL, Kaplan SA. Insulin resistance in nonobese patients with polycystic ovarian disease J Clin Endocrinol Metab 1983;57:356–359.
12. Nestler JE. Role of obesity and insulin in the development of anovulation. In: Filicori M, Flamigni C (eds) Ovulation Induction: Basic Science and Clinical Advances. Amsterdam: Elsevier, 1994;103–114.
13. Barbieri RL, Makris A, Randall RW, Daniels G, Kristner RW, Ryan KJ. Insulin stimulates androgen accumulation in incubations of ovarian stroma obtained from women with hyperandrogenism. J Clin Endocrinol Metab 1986;62:904–910.
14. Nestler JE, Powers LP, Matt DW et al. A direct effect of hyperinsulinemia on serum sex-hor-

mone binding globulin levels in obese women with the polycystic ovary syndrome. J Clin Endocrinol Metab 1991;72:83–89.

15. White D, Leigh A, Wilson C, Donaldson A, Franks S. Gonadotropin and gonadal steroid response to a single dose of a long-acting agonist of gonadotropin-releasing hormone in ovulatory and anovulatory women with polycystic ovary syndrome. Clin Endocrinol (Oxf) 1995; 42:475–481.

16. Nestler JE, Jakubowicz DJ. Lean women with polycystic ovary syndrome respond to insulin reduction with decreases in ovarian P450c17 α activity and serum androgens. J Clin Endocrinol Metab 1997;82:4075–4079.

17. Jakubowicz DJ, Nestler JE, Nestler JE. 17 alpha hydroxyprogesterone response to leuprolide and serum androgens in obese women with and without polycystic ovary syndrome after dietary weight loss. J Clin Endocrinol Metab 1997;82:556–560.

18. Adashi EY, Hsueh AJ, Yen SS. Insulin enhancement of luteinizing hormone and follicle-stimulating hormone release by cultured pituitary cells. Endocrinology 1981;108:1441–1449.

19. Glass AR, Burman KD, Dahma WT, Boehm TM. Endocrine function and human obesity. Metabolism 1981;30:89–104.

20. Adashi EY, Resnick CE, Bernandez ER et al. Insulin-like growth factor I as an amplifier of follicle stimulating hormone action: studies on mechanisms and sites of action in cultured rat granulosa cells. Endocrinology 1988;122:1583–1591.

21. Care JF, Fan J, Azzraello J, Rosenfield RL. Insulin like growth factor I enhances luteinizing hormone binding to rat ovarian theca-interstitial cells. J Clin Invest 1990;86:560–565.

22. Sharp PS, Kiddy DS, Reed MJ, Anyaoku V, Johanstone DG, Franks S. Correlation of plasma insulin and insulin like growth factor-I with indices of androgen transport and metabolism in women with polycystic ovary syndrome. Clin Endocrinol 1991;35:253–257.

23. Hamilton-Fairley D, Kiddy D, Anyaoku V, Koistinen R, Seppala M, Franks S. Response of sex hormone binding globulin and insulin-like growth factor binding protein-1 to an oral glucose tolerance test in obese women with polycystic ovary syndrome before and after caloric restriction. Clin Endocrinol 1993;39:363–367.

24. Insler V, Shoham Z, Barash A, Koistiner R, Seppala M, Hen M, Lunenfeld B, Zadik Z. Polycystic ovaries in non-obese and obese patients: possible pathophysiological mechanism based on new interpretation of facts and findings. Hum Reprod 1993;8:379–384.

25. Clark AM, Ledger W, Galletly C, Tomlinson L, Blaney F, Wang X, Norman RJ. Weight loss results in significant improvement in pregnancy and ovulation rates in anovulatory obese women. Hum Reprod 1995;10:2705–2712.

26. Hamilton-Fairley D, Kiddy D, Watson H, Paterson C, Franks S. Association of moderate obesity with poor pregnancy outcome in women with polycystic ovary syndrome treated with low dose gonadotrophins. Br J Obstet Gynaecol 1992;99:128–131.

27. Espinosa de los Monteros A, Ayala J, Sanabria LC et al. Serum insulin in clomiphene responders and nonresponders with polycystic ovarian disease. Rev Invest Clin 1995;47:347–353.

28. Armstrong AB, Hoeldtke N, Weiss TE et al. Metabolic parameters that predict response to clomiphene citrate in obese oligo-ovulatory women. Military Med 1996;161:732–734.

29. Shepard MK, Balmaceda JP, Lelia CG. Relationship of weight to successful induction of ovulation with clomiphene citrate. Fertil Steril 1979;32:641–645.

30. Poslon DW, Kiddey DS, Mason HD et al. Induction of ovulation with clomiphene citrate in women with polycystic ovary syndrome: the difference between responders and non-responders. Fertil Steril 199;51:30–34.

31. Fulghesu AM, Villa P, Pavone V et al. The impact of insulin secretion on the ovarian response to exogenous gonadotrophin in polycystic ovary syndrome. J Clin Endocrinol Metab 1997;2: 644–648.

32. Filicori M, Flamigni C, Cognini G et al. Increased insulin secretion in patients with multifollicular and polycystic ovaries and its impact on ovulation induction. Fertil Steril 1994;62: 279–85.

33. DeFronzo RA, Barzilai N, Simonson DC. Mechanism of action of metformin in obese and lean noninsulin-dependent diabetic subjects. J Clin Endocrinol Metab 1991;73:1294–1301.

34. Nestler JE, Jakubowicz DJ. Decreases in ovarian cytochrome P450c17alpha activity and serum free testosterone after reduction of insulin secretion in polycystic ovary syndrome. N Engl J Med 1996;335:617–623.

35. Velazquez EM, Mendoza S, Hamer T, Sosa F, Glueck CJ. Metformin therapy in polycystic ovary syndrome reduces hyperinsulinaemia, insulin resistance, hyperandrogenaemia and systolic blood pressure, while facilitating normal menses and pregnancy. Metabolism 1994;43:647–654.

36. Velazquez EM, Mendoza SG, Wang P, Glueck CJ. Metformin therapy is associated with a decresae in plasminogen activator inhibitor-1, lipoprotein(a) and immunoreactive insulin levels in patients with PCOS. J Clin Endocrinol Metab 1997;82:524–530.

37. Velazquez EM, Acosta A, Mendoza SG. Menstrual cyclicity after metformin therapy in PCOS. Obstet Gynecol 1997;90:392–395.

38. Dunaif A, Scott D, Finegood D, Quintana B, Whitcomb R. The insulin-sentizing agent troglitazone improves metabolic and reproductive abnormalities in polycystic ovary syndrome. J Clin Endocrinol Metab 1996;81:3299–3306.

39. Ehrmann DA, Cavaghan MK, Imperial J, Sturis J, Rosenfield RL, Polonsky KS. Effects of metformin on insulin secretion, insulin action and ovarian steroidogenesis in women with polycystic ovary syndrome. J Clin Endocrinol Metab 1997;82:1241–1247.

41. Gjoannaess H. The course and outcome of pregnancy after ovarian electrocautery with PCOS: the influence of body weight. Br J Obstet Gynaecol 1989;96:714–719.

42. Armar NA, McGarrigle HHG, Honour JW, Holownia P, Jacobs HS, Lachelin GCL. Laparoscopic ovarian diathermy in the management of anovulatory infertility in women with polycystic ovaries: endocrine changes and clinical outcome. Fertil Steril 1990;53:45–49.

43. Abdel Gadir A, Alnaser HMI, Mowafi RS, Shaw RW. The response of patients with polycystic ovarian disease to human menopausal gonadotrophin therapy after ovarian electrocautery or a luteinizing hormone-releasing hormone agonist. Fertil Steril 1992;57:309–313.

44. Conway GS. Insulin resistance and the polycystic ovary syndrome. Contemp Rev Obstet Gynecol 1990;2:34–39.

273

# Polycystic ovarian disease: genetic aspects

P.G. Crosignani

*I Department of Obstetrics and Gynecology, University of Milano, Italy*

**Abstract.** In view of the high prevalence of affected individuals, a genetic cause of the syndrome has been suggested. The studies on the familial clustering of polycystic ovary syndrome (PCOS) cases show a substantial increased risk in the first degree relatives of PCOS patients and are consistent with an autosomal dominant model of genetic transmission. The high prevalence of PCOS in twins has been explained by the presence of prenatal causative factors. Recently genetic studies have been shown that the steroid synthesis gene CYP 11α is an important locus for the susceptibility of the hyperandrogenemia frequently present in PCOS patients. A single molecular defect leading to the activation of a serine kinase may explain both the increased steroidogenetic activity and the insulin resistance observed in PCOS patients. Finally a defective VNTR 5′ region to the insulin gene is a major locus for PCOS-associated hyperinsulinemia.

Prenatal and postnatal environmental risk factors are of critical importance for the initiation and the maintenance of the syndrome.

**Keywords:** hirsutism, hyperandrogenism, insulin resistance, obesity, oligomenorrhea.

## Prevalence

The polycystic appearance of the ovary is the essential sign of polycystic ovary syndrome (PCOS) characterized by a wide heterogeneity of additional clinical and biochemical features. The presence of polycystic ovaries (PCO) has often been observed in healthy women but it is more frequently reported in women with abnormal cycles and hyperandrogenism (Table 1).

Since these symptoms are found in up to 10% of young women, PCOS is certainly the most frequent endocrine disorder diagnosed in these subjects. Despite the high prevalence of the isolated polycystic ovarian morphology (22%), the syndrome may be accompanied by minimal clinical manifestation and in particular no uniformly deleterious effect on fertility has been reported [1]. Similarly, a controlled comparative study of patients undergoing an IVF program found no significant difference in pregnancy and live birth rates between PCOS and non-PCOS women [4].

Nevertheless in a large group of PCOS patients, Balen et al. [5] found a high prevalence of hirsutism (66%) and primary and secondary infertility rates of 46 and 26%, respectively. Conception and miscarriage rates in PCOS patients were directly related to hypersecretion of LH (Table 2).

*Address for correspondence:* P.G. Crosignani MD, Clinica Ostetricia E Ginecologica I, Faculty of Medicine, University of Milan, Via Commenda 12, 20122 Milan, Italy. Tel.: +39-2-55193176. Fax: +39-2-55187146. E-mail: pgcros@imiucca.csi.unimi.it

Table 1. Prevalence of the polycystic appearance of the ovary in different groups of premenopausal women.

| Study | Women | Prevalence (%) |
|---|---|---|
| R.N. Clayton et al., 1992 [1] | Healthy women | 22 |
| J. Adams et al., 1986 [2] | Amenorrheic | 26 |
| J.B. O'Driscoll et al., 1994 [3] | Hirsute with normal cycles | 52 |
| J.B. O'Driscoll et al., 1994 [3] | Hirsute with abnormal cycles | 81 |
| J. Adams et al., 1986 [2] | Oligomenorrheic | 87 |

A consistent proportion of PCOS women have impaired glucose tolerance, hyperinsulinemia and/or decreased insulin sensitivity. These conditions are frequently associated with obesity (Table 3). Since insulin resistance in PCOS patients is predominantly extrasplanchic [8], the fasting blood sugar is normal.

According to Franks [9] ovarian morphology is the essential marker of the syndrome while the wide range of related phenotypes can be explained by the interaction of a small number of key genes with environmental factors.

## Studies of PCOS phenotypes in various populations

In view of the high prevalence of affected individuals, a genetic cause of the syndrome has been suggested over the past 30 years [10]. In order to study the existence of this mechanism, several studies on the presence of PCOS phenotypes in different populations have been carried out.

### Families

Ovarian morphology, menstrual irregularities and signs of hyperandrogenism were the main symptoms taken into account by the studies on the familial clustering of PCOS cases, while premature balding was the male phenotype frequently found in the male relatives. All the studies show a substantial increased risk of PCOS in first degree female relatives of PCOS patients (Table 4).

Most of the reports are consistent with an autosomal dominant model of genetic transmission.

Recently Franks published the largest study in this field including 23 informa-

Table 2. Conceptions and miscarriages in PCOs patients according to their plasma LH concentration [6].

| LH (mIU/ml) | No. patients | Conceptions | | Miscarriages | |
|---|---|---|---|---|---|
| | | No. | % | No. | % |
| < 10 | 147 | 147 | 88 | 20 | 65 |
| > 10 | 46 | 31 | 67 | 15 | 12 |

*Table 3.* Impaired glucose tolerance and decreased insulin sensitivity in PCOS patients [7].

| Subjects studied (No.) | Glucose intolerance | | Insulin sensitivity |
|---|---|---|---|
| | No. | % | |
| Nonobese controls (15) | 0 | 0 | Reference group |
| Obese controls (14) | 0 | 0 | Decreased vs. nonobese |
| Nonobese PCOS (13) | 1 | 7 | Decreased vs. controls |
| Obese PCOS (15) | 6 | 38 | Decreased vs. controls |

tive PCOS pedigrees. One is illustrated in Fig. 1 (reproduced with permission). The condition appears to be passed down through either sex. The symptomatic heterogeneity observed between the proband and her sisters is clear. The data of this study are not incompatible with an autosomal dominant model not excluding otherwise different modes of inheritance [9].

*Races*

Carmina et al. [15] studied 75 PCOS women, 25 each from the USA, Italy and Japan, and their conclusion was that although obesity and hirsutism vary according to genetic and environmental factors, the prevalence of adrenal androgen excess and insulin resistance appear to be fairly uniform among the various ethnic groups. More recent studies found, however, that ethnicity and PCOS are associated with independent and additive decrease of insulin action in Caribbean-Hispanic women [8]. There were differences in insulin and glucose

*Table 4.* Familial clustering of PCOS cases.

| Publication | Population studied (No.) | Collection of the data | Ovarian imaging | Findings |
|---|---|---|---|---|
| Ferriman and Purdie, 1979 [11] | • Hirsute women (284) (188 with enlarged ovary) • Oligomenorrheic with enlarged ovary (45) | Questionnaire | Gynecography | Compared to controls (179) higher prevalence of: • hirsutism • oligomenorrhea and infertility in the first degree female relative |
| Lunde et al., 1989 [12] | PCO women after wedge resection (132) | Questionnaire | Observation during surgery | PCO phenotype in 31.4% of first degree relatives (3.2% in the controls) |
| Hague et al., 1988 [13] | PCOs women and their relatives (50) | Direct interview | US | • 51% risk of PCOs in the first degree female relatives • Association with congenital adrenal hyperplasia |
| Carey et al., 1993 [14] | PCOS family pedigrees (10) | Direct interview | US | 67% of mothers and 87% of sisters affected |

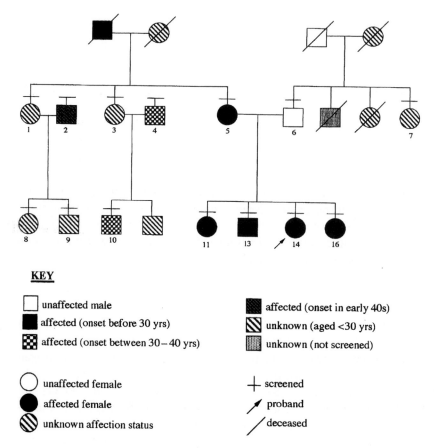

**KEY**

| | |
|---|---|
| ☐ unaffected male | ▨ affected (onset in early 40s) |
| ■ affected (onset before 30 yrs) | ◩ unknown (aged <30 yrs) |
| ▦ affected (onset between 30–40 yrs) | ▥ unknown (not screened) |

| | |
|---|---|
| ◯ unaffected female | ┼ screened |
| ● affected female | ↗ proband |
| ◉ unknown affection status | ╱ deceased |

*Fig. 1.* A large pedigree with familial polycystic ovary syndrome. Numbers below and horizontal bars above symbols indicate individuals who were fully screened by interview, examination, ovarian ultrasound (females) and biochemical testing. Affected status in other family members was assigned by history and/or photographic evidence.

responses to the glucose provocative tests between white and Indian women with the syndrome [16].

*Twins*

PCOS has been occasionally reported in identical twins [17,18]. A recent Australian study found a 50% incidence of PCOS in 34 female–female twins studies. The high degree of discordance in sonographic ovarian imaging between twins suggests a complex inheritance pathway and/or an important role of environmental factors in the genetic transmission mechanism [19].

The authors suggest that the high prevalence of PCOS in the twins may be explained by prenatal causes.

## Genetic mechanism of inheritable vulnerability

*Ovarian hyperandrogenism*

While the secretion of androgens by adrenals may be increased, the main source of androgen excess in PCOS is the ovary [20].

In these patients the theca cells of the ovarian stroma produce higher than normal amounts of progesterone and androgen. This hypersecretion is related to an intrinsic abnormality of the theca cells rather than to abnormal gonadotropin stimulation [21—23].

This finding prompted the study of the .cholesterol side chain cleavage gene (CYP 11α) as a possible cause of the deranged steroidogenesis. Gharani et al. [24], in a large case-controlled study, followed the segregation of CYP 11α in 20 PCOS families. The most common polymorphism of the gene (indicated as 216−) was reported to be significantly associated with PCOS families. A non-parametric linkage analysis carried out by the use of polymorphic markers in that region similarly suggested that steroid synthesis gene CYP 11α is a very important locus for the genetic susceptibility of PCOS hyperandrogenism (NPL score = 3.03, p = 0.003) [24].

*Hyperandrogenism and insulin resistance*

The increased ovarian and adrenal steroidogenetic activity observed in PCOS can also be caused by augmented lyase activity, exclusively performed by the cytochrome P450C17α. Serine phosphorylation of this enzyme system selectively increases its lyase activity, leading to secretion of ovarian and adrenal androgen without a rise in ACTH or other steroidogenetic activity [25].

Insulin resistance is another common feature of women with PCOS. The causes of the conditions are still unknown.

One explanation could be the increased concentration of free fatty acid induced by the central obesity frequently present in these patients; nevertheless there are also data supporting the existence of a genetic target cell defect as a cause of the metabolic condition [26].

The same hyperphosphorylation process described for cytochrome P450C17 lyase activity has been implicated as the cause of a specific postreceptor defect of transduction of the insulin signal in fibroblast [27].

In these patients the autophosphorylation of the serine residue (rather than tyrosine autophosphorylated) impairs insulin signal transduction and contributes to the observed 50% insulin resistance.

Thus a single molecular defect leading to the activation of a serine kinase could explain the two main biochemical disturbances in these patients: hirsutism and insulin resistance.

*Abnormality in insulin secretion*

Hyperinsulinemia has been reported in patients with PCOS and the syndrome is one of the major risk factors for noninsulin dependent diabetes mellitus (NIDDM) [28].

The β cell dysfunction is not obesity-dependent and in the majority of PCOS women is not associated with glucose intolerance [7].

The direct role of the insulin gene in the etiology of hyperinsulinemia has been recently investigated in three groups of PCOS patients (one of which included 17 families with several affected individuals). All three different populations showed an association between class III alleles at the VNTR 5′ to the insulin gene and PCOS [29].

The association was stronger in anovulatory patients in whom hyperinsulinemia is more frequently seen. A nonparametric linkage analysis performed in the PCOS families showed excess allele sharing at the same locus (NPL score 3.250, p = 0.002) [30].

The authors concluded that the VNTR 5′ region to the insulin gene is a major locus for PCOS- associated hyperinsulinemia.

Table 5 summarizes the pathophysiology for the inherited genetic susceptibilities.

## Environmental risk factors for PCOS

*Prenatal life*

Cresswell et al. [31] recently carried out a retrospective study on fetal growth of patients who were found to have polycystic ovaries in adult life. The analysis suggests the existence of specific prenatal risk factors for the later expression of the PCOS phenotype. According to the authors, PCOS obese women have higher than normal ovarian secretion of androgens causally associated with maternal obesity and high birth weight. Thin women with polycystic ovaries are postulated

*Table 5.* PCOS: pathophysiology for the inherited susceptibility.

| Gene | Molecular lesion | Target | Phenotype |
|------|-----------------|--------|-----------|
| Insulin gene 11 p 15.5 locus | Class III alleles at VNTR | Pancreatic β cells | Hyperinsulinemia |
| Gene encoding cholesterol side chain cleavage CYP 11α locus | 216 genotype | Ovarian theca cells | Hyperandrogenism |
| Autosomal dominant gene | Point mutation encoding serine hyperphosphorilation | • Adrenal and ovarian P450 C17αLYASE | Hyperandrogenism |
| | | • Activated insulin receptor | Insulin resistance |

to have altered hypothalamic control of LH release resulting from their prolonged gestations.

*Postnatal risk factors*

*Obesity.* Obesity is an independent risk for chronic anovulation [32]. Body fat distribution (waist-to-hip ratio) seems more important than weight per se [33].

In obese women, the two main mechanisms leading to anovulation are similar to those observed in patients with PCOS: 1) excess of LH and androgen secretion; and 2) hyperinsulinemia and insulin resistance. In fact, short-term fasting reduces LH secretion in normal weight women [34]. In overweight women caloric restriction lowers insulin levels and increases SHBG (sex hormone binding globulin) concentrations [35] while in severely obese patients, postgastroplasty recovery of ideal weight restores normal glucose and insulin metabolism [36].

In contrast, in women with PCO, obesity worsens the syndrome: in these patients insulin resistance appears to be directly related to BMI [37] while weight reduction in obese PCO results in decreased LH hypersecretion and reversal of insulin insensitivity [38,39]. Recent experimental data also suggest the existence of genetic control of appetite, body weight and reproductive function [40].

*Chronic anovulation*
The role of chronic anovulation as an environmental risk factor for PCOS is suggested by several pathophysiological mechanisms where androgen, LH and SHBG play the key roles.

A subgroup of patients with polycystic ovaries and showing hypogonadotropic anovulation has been described. Interestingly, in eight out of 20 of the investigated patients, BMI was above the normal range [41].

## Disease risk for familial PCOs patients

Through the inherited alteration of insulin secretion there is an obvious link between PCOS and type 2 diabetes [30].

In a study carried out on 33 wedge resected women 22—31 years following surgery, Dahlgren et al. [42] showed that PCOS women had a marked increase in prevalence of central obesity, higher basal serum insulin concentrations, higher prevalence of diabetes mellitus (15% in PCOS and 2.3% in the controls) and hypertension (39% in PCOS and 11% in the controls). In addition, a considerably increased risk (RR 7.4) of developing myocardial infarction has been predicted in the same group of PCOS patients [43].

More recently Pierpoint et al. [44] in a large study found that despite the presence of cardiovascular risk factors the chance of dying before the age of 75 for PCOS patients is not higher than average.

## Conclusion

PCOS can be considered a complex metabolic syndrome potentially affecting fertility and influencing the health of many individuals. The syndrome is initiated or maintained by the combined effect of inheritable genetic susceptibilities and additional environmental risk factors. To date, the complicated panel of genetic and postconceptional mechanisms leading to PCOS are still not fully understood.

## Acknowledgements

I gratefully acknowledge Howard Jacobs and Steve Franks for their constructive and critical revision of the manuscript and Ms Simonetta Vassallo for her secretarial assistance.

## References

1. Clayton RN, Ogden V, Hodgkinson J, Worswick L, Rodin DA, Dyer S, Meade TW. How common are fertility in the general population? Clin Endocrinol 1992;37:127—134.
2. Adams J, Polson DW, Franks S. Prevalence of polycystic ovaries in women with anovulation and idiopathic hirsutism. Br Med J 1986;293:355—359.
3. O'Driscoll JB, Mamtora H, Higginson J, Pollock A, Kane J, Anderson DC. A prospective study of the incidence of clear-cut endocrine disorders and polycystic ovaries in 350 patients with hirsutism or androgenic alopecia. Clin Endocrinol 1994;41:231—236.
4. MacDougall MJ, Tan S-L, Balen A, Jacobs HS. A controlled study comparing patients with and without polycystic ovaries undergoing in-vitro fertilization. Hum Reprod 1993;8:233—237.
5. Balen AH, Conway GS, Kaltsas G, Techatraisak K, Manning PJ, West C, Jacobs HS. Polycystic ovary syndrome: the spectrum of the disorder in 1,741 patients. Hum Reprod 1995;10: 2107—2111.
6. Regan L, Owen EJ, Jacobs HS. Hypersecretion of luteinising hormone, infertility, and miscarriage. Lancet 1990;336:1141—1144.
7. Dunaif A, Finegood DT. β cell dysfunction independent of obesity in the polycystic ovary syndrome. J Clin Endocrinol Metab 1996;81:942—947.
8. Dunaif A, Segal KR, Shelley DR, Green G, Dobrjanski A, Licholai T. Evidence for distinctive and intrinsic defects in insulin action in the polycystic ovary syndrome. Diabetes 1992; 41:1257—1266.
9. Franks S, Gharani N, Waterworth D, Batty S, White D, Williamson R, McCarthy M. The genetic basis of polycystic ovary syndrome. Hum Reprod 1997;12:2641—2648.
10. Cooper H, Spellacy W, Prem K, Cohen W. Hereditary factors in the Stein-Leventhal syndrome. Am J Obstet Gynecol 1968;100:371—387.
11. Ferriman D, Purdie AW. The inheritance of polycystic ovarian disease and a possible relationship to premature balding. Clin Endocrinol 1979;11:291—300.
12. Lunde O, Magnus P, Sandvik L, Hoglo S. Familial clustering in the polycystic ovarian syndrome. Gynecol Obstet Invest 1989;28:23—30.
13. Hague WM, Adams J, Reeders ST, Peto TE, Jacobs HS. Familial polycystic ovaries: a genetic disease? Clin Endocrinol (Oxf) 1988;29:593—605.
14. Carey AH, Chan KL, Short F, White D, Williamson R, Franks S. Evidence for a single gene effect in polycystic ovaries and male pattern baldness. Clin Endocrinol 1993;38:653—658.
15. Carmina E, Koyama T, Chang L, Stanczyk FZ, Lobo RA. Does ethnicity influence the preva-

lence of adrenal hyperandrogenism and insulin resistance in polycystic ovary syndrome. Am J Obstet Gynecol 1992;167:1807—1812.

16. Norman RJ, Mahabeer S, Masters S. Ethnic differences in insulin and glucose response to glucose between white and Indian women with polycystic ovary syndrome. Fertil Steril 1995; 63:58—62.

17. McDonough PG, Mahesh VB, Ellegood JO. Steroid, follicle stimulating hormone, and luteinizing hormone profiles in identical twins with polycystic ovaries. Am J Obstet Gynecol 1972; 113:1072—1078.

18. Hutton C, Clark F. Polycystic ovarian syndrome in identical twins. Postgrad Med J 1984;59: 64—65.

19. Jahnfar S, Eden JZ, Warren P, Seppala M, Hgyun TV. A twin study of polycystic ovary syndrome. Fertil Steril 1995;61:478—486.

20. Franks S. Polycystic ovary syndrome: a changing perspective. Clin Endocrinol 1989;31:87—120.

21. Gilling-Smith C, Willis DS, Beard RW, Franks S. Hypersecretion of androstenedione by isolated theca cells from polycystic ovaries. J Clin Endocrinol Metab 1994;79:1158—1165.

22. Gilling-Smith C, Story EH, Rogers V, Franks S. Evidence for a primary abnormality of thecal cell steroidogenesis in the polycystic ovary syndrome. Clin Endocrinol 1997;47:93—99.

23. Ibañez L, Hall JE, Potau N, Carrascosa A, Prat N, Taylor AE. Ovarian 17-hydroxyprogesterone hyperresponsiveness to gonadotropin-releasing hormone (GnRH) agonist challenge in women with polycystic ovary syndrome is not mediated by luteinizing hormone hypersecretion: evidence from GnRH agonist and human chorionic gonadotropin stimulation testing. J Clin Endocrinol Metab 1996;81:4103—4107.

24. Gharani N, Waterworth DM, Batty S, White D, Gilling-Smith C, Conway GS, McCarthy M, Franks S, Williamson R. Association of the steroid synthesis gene CYP11α with polycystic ovary syndrome and hyperandrogenism. Hum Mol Genet 1997;6:397—402.

25. Zhang LH, Rodriguez H, Ohno S, Miller WL. Serine phosphorylation of human P450c17 increases 17,20-lyase activity: implications for adrenarche and the polycystic ovary syndrome. Proc Natl Acad Sci USA 1995;92:10619—10623.

26. Holte J. Disturbances in insulin secretion and sensitivity in women with the polycystic ovary syndrome. Clin Endocrinol Metab 1996;10:221—247.

27. Dunaif A, Xia J, Book CB, Schenker E, Tang Z. Excessive insulin receptor serine phosphorylation in cultured fibroblasts and in skeletal muscle. A potential mechanism for insulin resistance in the polycystic ovary syndrome. J Clin Invest 1995;96:801—810.

28. Holte J, Bergh T, Berne C, Wide L, Lithell H. Restored insulin secretion after weight loss in obese women with polycystic ovary syndrome. J Clin Endocrinol Metab 1995;80:2586—2593.

29. Bennett ST, Lucassen AM, Gough SCL, Powell EE, Undlien DE, Protchard LE, Merriman ME, Kawaguchi Y, Dronsfield MJ, Pociot F et al. Susceptibility to human type 1 diabetes at IDDM2 is determined by tandem repeat variation at the insulin gene minisatellite locus. Nature Genet 1995;9:284—292.

30. Waterworth DM, Bennett ST, Gharani N, McCarthy MI, Hague S, Batty S, Conway GS, White D, Todd JA, Franks S, Williamson R. Linkage and association of insulin gene VNTR regulatory polymorphism with polycystic ovary syndrome. Lancet 1997;349:986—990.

31. Cresswell JL, Barker DJP, Osmond C, Egger P, Phillips DIW, Fraser RB. Fetal growth, length of gestation, and polycystic ovaries in adult life. Lancet 1997;350:1131—1135.

32. Grodstein F, Goldman MB, Cramer DW. Body mass index and ovulatory infertility. Epidemiology 1994;5:247—250.

33. Zaadstra BM, Seidell JC, Van Noord PA, te Velde ER, Habbema JD, Vrieswijk B, Karbaat J. Fat and female fecundity: prospective study of effect of body fat distribution on conception rates. Br Med J 1993;306:484—487.

34. Olson BR, Cartledge T, Sebring N, Defensor R, Nieman L. Short-term fasting affects luteinizing hormone secretory dynamics but not reproductive function in normal-weight sedentary women. J Clin Endocrinol Metab 1995;80:1187—1193.

282

35. Kiddy DS, Hamilton-Farley D, Bush A, Short F, Anyaoku V, Reed MJ, Franks AD. Improvement in endocrine and ovarian function during dietary treatment of obese women with polycystic ovary syndrome. Clin Endocrinol Oxf 1992;36:105—111.

36. Letiexhe MR, Scheen AJ, Gerard PL, Desaive C, Lefebvre PJ. Postgastroplasty recovery of ideal body weight normalizes glucose and insulin metabolism in obese women. J Clin Endocrinol Metab 1995;80:364—369.

37. Pasquali R, Fabbri R, Venturoli S, Paradisi R, Antenucci D, Melchionda N. Effect of weight loss and antiandrogenic therapy on sex hormone blood levels and insulin resistance in obese with polycystic ovaries. Am J Obstet Gynecol 1986;154:139—144.

38. Bützow TL, Lehtovirta MT, Väinämö U, Siegberg R, Hovatta O, Apter D. The effect of weight reduction on gonadotrophin, insulin and androgen metabolism in hyperandrogenic overweight infertile women. Abstract book of the 12th Annual Meeting of the European Society of Human Reproduction and Embryology, Maastricht, The Netherlands, 30 June to 3 July 1996, Hum Reprod 1996;11:Abstract Book 1, 47—48.

39. Kiddy DS, Sharp PS, White DM, Scanlon MF, Mason HD, Bray CS, Polson DW, Reed MJ, Franks S. Differences in clinical and endocrine features between obese and nonobese subjects with polycystic ovary syndrome: and analysis of 263 consecutive cases. Clin Endocrinol Oxf 1990;32:213—220.

40. Friedman JM. The alphabet of weight control. Nature 1997;385:119—120.

41. Shoham Z, Conway GS, Patel A, Jacobs HS. Polycystic ovaries in patients with hypogonadotropic hypogonadism: similarity of ovarian response to gonadotropin stimulation in patients with polycystic ovarian syndrome. Fertil Steril 1992;58:37—45.

42. Dahlgren E, Johansson S, Lindstedt G, Knutsson F, Odén A, Janson PO, Mattson L-Å, Crona N, Lundberg P-A. Women with polycystic ovary syndrome wedge resected in 1956 to 1965: a long-term follow-up focusing on natural history and circulating hormones. Fertil Steril 1992; 57:505—513.

43. Dahlgren E, Janson PO, Johansson S, Lapidus L, Oden A. Polycystic ovary syndrome and risk for myocardial infarction. Evaluated from a risk factor model based on a prospective population study of women. Acta Obstet Gynecol Scand 1992;71:599—604.

44. Pierpoint T, McKeigue PM, Isaacs AJ, Wild SH, Jacobs HS. Mortality of women with polycystic ovary syndrome at long-term follow-up. J Clin Epidemiol 1998;(In press).

Fertility and Reproductive Medicine.
R.D. Kempers, J. Cohen, A.F. Haney and J.B. Younger, editors.

# PCO — What is it? How is it diagnosed?

Violanda Grigorescu

*ACCES — Romanian Association of Embryology and Human Reproduction, 1st Clinic of Obstetrics and Gynecology, Targu Mures, Romania*

**Abstract.** Polycystic ovary syndrome (PCOS) is probably the most prevalent endocrinopathy in women and by far the most common cause of anovulatory infertility, yet its pathogenesis still remains an enigma.

This syndrome has produced an abundance of theories and a plethora of treatment regimes. It is no longer a mere rare gynecological curiosity but an endocrinopathy with multisystem sequelae.

Obtaining a consensus on such a controversial issue as the diagnostic criteria, nomenclature and pathogenesis of PCOS, is a virtual impossibility.

However, a near consensus of opinion is about all that already exists. The future direction of research is to clarify this puzzle which is PCOS.

Recent progress in the diagnosis, pathophysiology, long-term ramifications and treatment of PCOS has been rapid but the pathogenesis remains a challenging enigma and the treatment symptomatic.

**Keywords:** free testosterone index, histological features of PCO (polycystic ovary), hyperandrogenia, LH:FSH ratio, PCOS (polycystic ovary syndrome), ultrasound.

## Introduction

This syndrome has produced an abundance of theories and a plethora of treatment regimes. It is no longer a mere rare gynecological curiosity but an endocrinopathy with multisystem sequelae. To obtain a consensus on the diagnostic criteria nomenclature and pathogenesis of polycystic ovary syndrome (PCOS) is a virtual impossibility. However, a near-consensus of opinion is about all that already exists. The future direction of research is to clarify this puzzle which PCOS is. Recent progress in the diagnosis, pathophysiology, long-term ramifications and treatment of PCOS has been rapid but the pathogenesis remains a challenging enigma and the treatment symptomatic. PCOS is probably the most prevalent endocrinopathy in women and by far the most common cause of anovulatory infertility, yet its pathogenesis still remains an enigma.

## History

Chereau described in 1844 sclerocystic changes in the human ovary (Chereau,

*Address for correspondence:* Dr Violanda Grigorescu, 200 Carman Ave Ap. 7B, East Meadow, NY 11224, USA. Tel.: +1-516-357-8757. Fax: +1-516-357-8757. E-mail: postavaru@aol.com

1844) some 90 years before the classic paper of Stein–Leventhal (1935).

Elevated luteinizing hormone (LH) concentrations were first reported in 1958 and created a criterion for diagnosis. The introduction of radioimmunoassays in 1971 stimulated reliance on biochemical diagnosis. Although it was clear as early as 1962 that there was a wide variety of clinical presentation, it was only in 1976 that the concept of PCOS with normal LH concentrations was conceived (Rebar et al. 1976). A further milestone was the discovery of the association of PCOS and insulin resistance by Kahn et al. (1976) and Burghen et al. (1980). Swanson et al. (1981) first described the ultrasound findings of women with PCOS in 1981. However, only after Adams et al. (1985) [1] refined and critically defined diagnostic criteria in their seminal paper did the ultrasound diagnosis of PCOS become accepted throughout the world.

## Definition

The typical ultrasound features of the PCO in the presence of oligomenorrhea and/or clinical symptoms of hyperandrogenism such as hirsutism define PCOS.

## Prevalence

Adams et al. (1986) [2] using ultrasound criteria, found PCO in 87% of women with oligomenorrhea and in a similar proportion of women with hirsutism and regular ovulatory menstruation.

Adams et al. (1986) [2] discovered PCO in 30–40% of women with amenorrhoea. Adams et al. (1986) [2] and Hull (1987), found PCOs associated with 75% of cases with anovulatory infertility. Polson et al. (1988) [3] assessed the prevalence of PCO in the general healthy female population of fertile age using 257 volunteers. PCOs were found in 22%. In a similar study on 100 normal Arab women, Abdel Gadir et al. (1992) found a prevalence of 16%.

## Diagnosis

For many years following the original description by Stein Leventhal (1935), the diagnosis was purely clinical and relied on the presence of obesity, hirsutism, amenorrhoea and enlarged ovaries. It is clear today that this description represents extreme or advanced cases and if judgement was made purely on these clinical symptoms alone, many less blatant but nevertheless clinically significant cases would be missed. The diagnosis of PCOS was mainly based upon the three chief criteria: clinical presentation, biochemical characterization, and characterization of ovarian abnormalities.

*Clinical presentation*

- Patient history (initiation symptoms before/during puberty),
- family history, and
- signs and symptoms (menstrual cycle disturbances, hirsutism, obesity, acne, insulin resistance, anovulation-infertility).

*Biochemical characterization*

Hormone estimates in peripheral blood:
- high androgen levels (testosterone, T/SHBG (sex hormone binding globulin) ratio, androstenedione);
- augmented LH/FSH ratio;
- elevated free oestradiol, oestrone;
- hyperprolactinemia;
- insulin resistance;
- reduced concentration of SHBG;
- hormone estimates in follicular fluid; and
- Granulosa cell function in vitro by culturing cell or ovarian tissue.

*Characterization of ovarian abnormalities*

- Classical morphology,
- laparoscopic inspection, and
- ultrasonography.

Because in routine clinical practice diagnostic criteria should be simple and easy to implement, specific signs and symptoms together with hormone estimates in peripheral blood are considered to be of major importance.

**Clinical presentation of PCOS**

*Clinical history*

Most patients exhibiting chronic hyperandrogenic anovulation have a distinct clinical history with a normal menarcheal age, excessive hair growth and overweight before, and irregular menstrual cycles directly after menarche.

Within families of patients with PCOS there seems to be dominant transmission. PCOS is transmitted by a single gene in an autosomal dominant pattern, and a male phenotype in families of probands has been identified by premature balding associated with an elevation of serum androgens (Carey et al. 1993). The same group (Carey et al. 1994) have identified a new single base change in the 5′promoter region of CYP17, the gene encoding for P450c17α on chromosome 10q24,3 in individuals with PCOS/male pattern baldness. While this variation in the A2 allele of CYP17 may cause modification of expression, it has been excluded as the primary genetic defect for which the search continues.

A further genetic influence is that of a postreceptor defect, unique to PCOS, causing a resistance to insulin action.

PCOS has a variable type and degree of expression of symptoms, and hirsutism and oligomenorrhea as the main complaints. In addition, hypertension, diabetes, insulin resistance and obesity occur more often in families of PCOS patients, with endocrine abnormalities and disturbed testis function in male family members.

## Symptoms

Women with PCO may display a wide range of clinical symptoms. At the extreme end of this range are the women who are practically normal, have no signs of hyperandrogenism and who are amenorrhoeic but have PCO on ultrasound examination, and the women who have the full-blown expression of the classical Stein-Leventhal syndrome.

Several concepts are important in order to understand this heterogeneity of clinical presentation. PCOs are there for life and only the clinical expression may change, while the typical ultrasonic findings will remain identifiable. If accepting that PCOS is basically a disorder of ovarian function, symptomatology is dictated by extraovarian factors.

Hirsutism and menstrual cycle disturbances have been found to be significantly more common in obese than nonobese women with PCOS. Alopecia may occur in severe PCOS untreated women and acanthosis nigricans is a rare but a pathognomonic finding associated with obesity and insulin resistance.

### Infertility

Population-based calculations of the prevalence of PCOS presenting with infertility and oligomenorrhea have been published by Hull (Epidemiology of infertility and polycystic ovarian disease endocrinological and demographic studies, Gynecol Endocrinol, 1987). The annual incidence of infertility presenting with the classical PCOS including hirsutism and oligo-amenorrhoea is 41 per million.

### Obesity

Obesity is considered to be an important clinical diagnostic criterion since it represents the capacity to convert androgen to estrogens in peripheral fat tissue.

Weight is often expressed as BMI (body mass index; weight divided by height), and overweight is defined as BMI > 25. However, there is discussion as to what extent BMI adequately represents body fat content. Skinfold thickness or underwater body weight may be more suitable for the accurate assessment of body composition.

It was noted that more than 80% of patients found to have PCOS were obese prior to puberty. Moreover, several studies have noted that obesity is associated with elevated androgen production and an increased incidence of amenorrhea.

These observations have led to speculation that obesity plays a role in the pathogenesis of PCOS. However, obesity occurs in only 35—60% of women with PCOS, and, clearly, all obese women do not have hormonal disturbances.

Nonetheless, there are several mechanisms by which obesity has been postulated to play a role in the development of chronic hyperandrogenic anovulation characteristics of PCOS.

First, gonadal steroid feedback changes could result from obesity because of increased extraglandular aromatization of androgen to estrogen, and decreased sex hormone binding globulin (SHBG) levels. These changes may play a role in the development of PCOS by causing chronic inappropriate estrogen feedback on the hypothalamic-pituitary axis, leading to distorted gonadotropin release and anovulation, and by increasing androgen production which may directly inhibit follicular maturation.

Zhang and colleagues found (and published in 1984 in J Clin Endocrinol Metab) similarly low levels of SHBG in both ovulatory and nonovulatory obese women. However, only the anovulatory women had increased serum androgen levels, suggesting that obesity is not the only factor contributing to chronic anovulation.

Second, neuroendocrine abnormalities, such as a central lesion involving the putative feeding center of the ventromedial hypothalamus and the anatomically closely related neurones in the arcuate nucleus involved in pulsatile gonadotropin releasing hormone (GnRH) secretion, might explain the association of PCOS and obesity.

Shelley and Dunaif showed in 1989 that obese and nonobese women with PCOS have similar patterns of pulsatile gonadotropin release. This strongly suggests that obese women with PCOS do not have a distinct neuroendocrine disorder.

Lesions of the ventromedial hypothalamus in animals can lead to obesity and hyperinsulinemia. Hence, the association of hyperinsulinemia and obesity of PCOS might be secondary to an abnormality in the ventromedial hypothalamus. Nonobese women with PCOS are hyperinsulinemic, but to a lesser degree than their obese counterparts. Obesity and insulin resistance do occur without PCOS, and nonobese women with PCOS usually have no history of obesity.

It is possible that other hormonal abnormalities that occur in obese PCOS women, such as hyperinsulinemia, could produce neuroendocrine and ovarian steroidogenesis changes. A correlation between hyperinsulinemia and hyperandrogenism has been shown in PCOS, and obese women with PCOS are significantly more hyperinsulinemic than nonobese women with PCOS.

Third, obesity might be secondary to metabolic changes such as androgenic-mediated increases in body weight, or a decrease in energy expenditure. A defect in energy expenditure in obese subjects may be secondary to insulin resistance.

It was demonstrated that both normal and obese women with PCOS had blunted postprandial thermogenesis.

There is little evidence that hyperandrogenism, or a defect in energy expenditure, is the primary cause of obesity in PCOS.

In conclusion, obesity is not associated with discernible changes in gonadotropin release or gonad steroid levels in chronic hyperandrogenic anovulation. Despite significant insulin resistance, in obese women with PCOS, there is no additional defect in energy expenditure. Weight reduction can improve menstrual function in some obese hyperandrogenic amenorrheic women. Thus, obesity may contribute to the hormonal abnormalities of PCOS by an unknown mechanism. A common neuroendocrine change, closely linked genetic abnormalities, could explain the association of obesity and PCOS.

## Hirsutism

Hirsutism as a clinical sign of hyperandrogenia is also a main diagnostic criterion and can be quantified according to criteria set by Ferriman and Gallway. This score usually takes the equivalent of their "hormonal" hair score of more than 12 to indicate hirsutism. However, hair growth on some parts of the body may be dependent mainly on genetic factors and therefore racial differences do occur.

### Biochemical characterization

*Hormone estimates in peripheral blood*

— high androgen levels (testosterone, "free androgen index" = $T \times 100/SHBG$, androstenedione),
— augmented LH and LH:FSH ratio elevated or normal free estradiol and estrone,
— hyperprolactinemia,
— insulin resistance, and
— reduced concentration of SHBG.

Hyperandrogenemia is known to be involved in anovulation and the occurrence of PCOs in various clinical states such as congenital adrenal hyperplasia, androgen-producing tumors, Cushing's disease and long-term androgen treatment in female-to-male transsexuals. Controversy still exists, however, as to what extent androgen screening should be performed clinically for proper diagnosis of hyperandrogenism. It could be performed by the assays of testosterone and other steroids as: androstenedione, dihydroepiandrostendione, dihydrotestosterone, or 17-hydroxyprogesterone. The determination of dihydroepiandrosterone sulfate (DHEAS) as an exclusive marker of adrenal androgen production is a useful addition, and it can distinguish between ovarian and adrenal androgen production with important therapeutic consequences.

The "free androgen index" ($T \times 100/SHBG$) represents adequate androgen activity. For its calculation it is necessary to also determine SHBG.

Augmented luteinizing/follicle stimulating hormone (LH/FSH) ratios have also been considered a key biochemical criterion for the diagnosis of PCOS. Yen and colleagues have done an extensive work on this and it is now known that altered gonadotropin output mainly represents increased pituitary sensitivity due to altered steroid feedback. Absolute values for LH/FSH ratios, however, may depend on applied radioimmunoassays as well.

The critical levels taken for diagnostic are: LH 10 IU/l, LH:FSH ratio > 2.0 and testosterone 2.5 nmol/l.

Hyperprolactinemia and insulin resistance can also be observed in a proportion of patients suffering from PCOS.

The endocrine profile of women with PCOS tends to vary with the symptomatology. Diagnostic accuracy of hormonal methods, published by Hull in 1989:
— 89% progesterone challenge test to assess estrogen status,
— 65% assessment of hirsutism,
— 93% Combination of both tests,
— 67% LH of 10 IU/l (above or below that critical level),
— 51% LH/FSH ratio of 3.0,
— 58% LH/FSH ratio of 2.5,
— 70% LH/FSH ratio of 2.0, and
— 83% testosterone of 2.5 nmol/l.

**Hormone estimates in follicular fluid**

These estimates may involve androstenedione/estradiol ratios as an index of granulosa cell function, estimates of radioimmunoactive and bioactive FSH levels as an indication of granulosa cell stimulation, and determination of various growth factors (such as insulin-like growth factor) as potential intraovarian regulators.

Estrogen levels in PCOS follicular fluid are low, similar to those in fluid from follicles of a similar size in normal ovaries.

This is consistent with the lack of estrogen-secretory preovulatory follicle development in PCOs. Androgen levels in PCOS follicular fluid are either slightly elevated or within the ranges observed for normal and atretic follicles of equivalent sizes in "normal ovaries".

Granulosa cell function could be characterized in vitro by culturing cells or ovarian tissue

**Characterization of ovarian abnormalities**

*Morphology: histological features*

The histological features of PCOs compared with the normal ovary are:
1) increased volume (2 × cross-sectional area);
2) same number of primordial follicles;

3) double the number of ripening and atretic follicles;
4) increased and more collagenized tunica;
5) slight increase in cortical stromal thickness;
6) greatly increased (5×) subcortical stroma with increased vascularity and innervation; and
7) frequent occurrence of hilar cell nests.

It remains unclear whether the increased androgen production from the PCO is simply a feature of the increased number of (LH-responsive) theca-interstitial cells or whether the cells themselves are qualitatively different, in their steroidogenic capacity, from those in the normal ovary.

Classical morphological ovarian criteria of Stein–Leventhal are:
— stroma hyperplasia,
— hypertecosis,
— capsule thickening, and
— cystic degeneration of follicles.

*Laparoscopic inspection*

A description of the distinct ovarian appearance of PCOs during laparoscopy is also rarely applied as a diagnostic procedure.

The typical appearance of PCOs at laparoscopy, with or without confirmation by ovarian biopsy, is still regarded as a *sine qua non* for diagnosis by a number of clinicians.

*Ultrasonography*

Ultrasound assessment of ovarian morphology should be the gold standard for the diagnosis of PCO.

The ultrasound appearance of the PCO first defined by Swanson at al. in 1981 were refined by Adams et al. in 1985 [1]. Based on the criteria of Adams et al. (1985) [1], PCO should be diagnosed when more than 10 discrete follicles of < 10 mm diameter are seen in the ovary, usually peripherally arrayed around an enlarged, hyperechogenic, central stroma. Less commonly, multiple small follicles are distributed throughout the expanded stromal compartment in a random arrangement. As few as (but not fewer than) 10 follicles may be present in each ovary.

Objective estimates of the size of the stroma are difficult but stroma occupying more than 25% of the ovarian volume has been suggested as the criterion. In those cases with only a moderate increase in follicularity, the identification of the increased stromal content by its prominent echoes helps to distinguish polycystic from normal and multifollicular ovaries (MFO).

Ultrasonography is a noninvasive technique for the characterization of ovarian morphology which has a high concordance rate with laparoscopic examination (Eden, 1988) and histological examination [4].

The advent of high-resolution, transvaginal ultrasound examination of the ovaries has provided the biggest single contribution to the diagnosis of PCOs and that this examination, performed by an experienced operator, should be the basis of the diagnosis.

Recently, Dewailly et al. (1994) have described an objective quantitative method of ovarian stromal assessment by using a computerized ultrasonic technique in measuring stromal and cyst areas. By using this computerized ultrasonic technique, a much more objective, standardized diagnosis of PCO can be obtained.

Multicystic ovaries represent weekly active ovaries that are typical of early puberty and of the recovery phase of amenorrhoea, due to a hypothalamic disorders caused by weight loss and/or psychological disturbance. It is associated with a slowing of LH pulses.

In functional terms, multicystic ovaries should be categorized with the inactive ovarian group in which there is no evident follicular development (being associated with lack of oestrogen production).

The specific ultrasound appearance of multicystic ovaries are of only a small number of follicles, 6—10 per ovary, ranging up to 10 mm in diameter and distributed anywhere within the ovary, often far below the surface. Where follicles abut there is little stroma to be seen between them, and the stromal echoes generally are weak. It would seem that the follicles are in various stages of weak activity or atresia. It is now preferable to call such ovaries "multifollicular". Indeed, it would be more preferable to call PCOs "polymicrofollicular", or something similar, because the present term is simply inaccurate and misleading.

The three types of ovary (normal, MFO and PCO) also differ significantly in their average volume but the ranges overlap such that the volume is not a useful individual criterion of PCOS.

The criteria for the diagnosis of PCOs described above may need to be revised for the assessment of PCOs by vaginal ultrasonography. Histological studies have now confirmed the morphological diagnosis of PCOS suggested by ultrasonography [4].

**Late sequelae**

- Hypertension
- Cardiovascular disease
- Diabetes melitis
- Endometrial carcinoma

As a final conclusion of all studies performed and all new discoveries about clinical and laboratory features of PCO, it can be concluded with what Hull said in 1989: "For the moment, what needs to be appreciated of PCOD appears rather like an iceberg, having largely remained out of sight below the clinical surface until now, but that part is still generally easily managed as before. It fills a big gap that has existed in our understanding and classification of ovulatory disorder".

# References

1. Adams J, Polson DW, Mason HD, Abdulwahid NA, Tucker M, Morris DV, Price J, Jacobs HS. Multifollicular ovaries: clinical and endocrine features and response to pulsatile gonadotrophin releasing hormone. Lancet 1985;2:1375—1378.
2. Adams J, Polson DW, Franks S. Prevalence of polycystic ovaries in women with anovulation and idiopathic hirsutism. Br Med J 1986;193:355—359.
3. Polson DW, Adams J, Wadsworth J, Franks S. Polycystic ovaries — a common finding in normal women. Lancet 1988;1:870—872.
4. Saxton DW, Farquhar CM, Rae T, Beard RW, Anderson MC, Wadsworth J. Accuracy of ultrasound measurements of female pelvic organs. Br J Obstet Gynecol 1990;97(8):695—699.
5. Willemson WN, Franssen AM, Rolland R, Vemer HM. The effects of Buserelin on the hormonal states in PCOD. [Review] [36 refs] Prog Clin Biol Res 1986;225:377—389.
6. Cooke ID, Lunenfeld B. Current Understanding of Polycystic Ovarian Disease. Proceedings of a meeting held at the Royal Society of Medicine London, 1989.
7. Erickson GF, Magoffin DA, Dyer CA, Hofeditz C. The ovarian androgen producing cells: a review of structure/function relationship. Endocrine Rev 1985;6:371—399.
8. Homburg R. Polycystic ovary syndrome — from gynaecological curiosity to multisystem endocrinopathy. Hum Reprod 1996;11:1,29—39.
9. Mason HD, Sagle M, Polson DW, Kiddy D, Debriansky D, Adams J, Franks S. Reduced frequency of luteinizing hormone pulses in women with weight loss-related amenorrhoea and multifollicular ovaries. Clin Endocrinol 1988;28:611—618.
10. Rosenfeld RL, Barnes RB, Cara JF, Lucky AW. Dysregulation cytochrome P450c 17 alpha as the cause of polycystic ovary syndrome. Fertil Steril 1990;53:785—791.
11. Rowe PJ, Comhaire FH, Hargreave TB, Mellows HJ. WHO manual for the standardized investigation and diagnosis of the infertile couples, 1992.

# Contraception

# Long-acting hormonal contraception

Biran Affandi

*Klinik Raden Saleh, Department of Obstetrics and Gynecology, Faculty of Medicine, University of Indonesia, Jakarta, Indonesia*

**Abstract.** Steroids can be administered in at least five different ways: injectables, hormone-releasing IUDs, implants, vaginal rings and pills. Progestins — synthetic steroids — are used as the main bioactive substance. Different progestins are effective for different periods of time; progestins in daily oral pills are effective for 24 h. The effectiveness of progestins can be prolonged by incorporating them in a sustained release system that gradually releases the hormone, thus they can be effective for up to 5 years or more. Two progestin-only injectables are widely available in the family planning programs, DMPA and NET-EN, beside two combined injectables: Cyclofem (DMPA+EC), and Mesigyna (NETEN+EV). Injectable microspheres and microcapsules, suspended in solution, are administered with a hypodermic needle. The tiny particles of different sizes, consisting of hormones in a polymer carrier, dissolve and release hormones at various rates, providing a nearly constant dose that prevents pregnancy for 1 to 6 months. The vaginal ring is placed by the woman in her vagina, where it gradually releases hormones. Implantable contraceptives are placed just under the skin on the inside of a woman's arm. Implant capsules release the progestin at a slow, steady rate. There are three implantables available on the market: Implanon, Norplant and Jadelle. For 1—5 years they prevent nearly all pregnancies. After this time they must be replaced. Biodegradable implants are also placed under the skin, but they eventually dissolve and disappear. Natural and synthetic progestins were first added to IUDs in the early 1970s. Its main advantages over nonhormonal IUDs are less menstrual bleeding per cycle and less painful menstruation.

**Keywords:** contraceptives, hormonal, long-acting.

## Introduction

Sustained release systems have proved useful in various medical applications, among them treatment of ophthalmologic disorders and heart disease. However, probably in no area have research efforts been greater than in contraception.

Folkman and Long in 1964 [1] published their findings that silastic tubes could serve as a reservoir for the prolonged administration of a drug. Two years later, Dziuk and Cook found that the in vitro release of steroids from silastic capsules was practically constant and independent of the drug concentration inside the tube. Based on the above studies Segal and Croxatto, during the XXIII Annual Meeting of the American Fertility Society, proposed the concept of a reversible, long-acting contraceptive method using a silastic capsule which is implanted under the skin and which has a slow and constant release of contraceptive ster-

*Address for correspondence:* Biran Affandi, Klinik Radeh Saleh, Department of Obstetrics and Gynecology, Faculty of Medicine, University of Indonesia, JL. Raden Saleh Raya 49, Jakarta 10330, Indonesia.

oids. This is now well known as Norplant [2].

Apart from implant administration, contraceptive steroids can also be administered by several other routes; orally, intramuscularly, intravaginally, intrauterinely, intracervically, rectal, intranasally and transdermally. Some of these routes of administration have been developed into contraceptive methods that are widely used and others are still under clinical trial. On the market today at least three different sustained release systems for steroid contraception are available: injectables, hormone-releasing IUDs and implants.

Several other systems for sustained release of steroids are being developed and some will probably come into widespread use within the next few years or so [3].

The objectives of this paper are: 1) to review the mechanisms of sustained release systems; 2) to discuss the status contraceptive methods; and 3) to outline the problem and research needs.

## Mechanism of sustained release systems

Although physical characteristics of a system are often used to classify drug formulations, here we shall use the mechanism-controlling release as a basis for characterizing polymeric drug delivery systems. The mechanisms at present include [4]:
1. Diffusion controlled systems:
    a) reservoir systems,
    b) matrix systems;
2. Chemically controlled systems:
    a) bioerodible systems,
    b) pendant chain systems;
3. Solvent-activated systems:
    a) swelling-controlled systems,
    b) osmotic systems; and
4. Magnetically controlled systems:

The analyses presented in each section are for simplified cases. More complex phenomena or combinations of two mechanisms (e.g., diffusion plus swelling) are also possible.

### Diffusion-controlled systems

### Reservoir systems
In these type of system, a core of drugs is surrounded by a polymer and diffusion of the drug through the polymer is threat-limiting step. These systems would include membranes, microcapsules, liposomes, and hollow fibers. Either porous or nonporous polymer systems may be used.

### Matrix systems
In matrix systems the drug is uniformly distributed throughout a solid polymer.

As in reservoir systems, drug diffusion throughout the polymer is the rate-limiting step.

## Chemically controlled systems

### Bioerodible systems

In chemically controlled systems, the drug is distributed throughout a polymer in the same way as in reservoir or matrix systems. The difference is, however, that while the polymer phase in those systems remains unchanged with time and drug is released by diffusion, the polymer phase in bioerodible systems (in this paper, the words "bioerodible" and "biodegradable" are used interchangeably) decreases with time. Biodegradation begins after drug release has been almost completed. In the bioerodible matrix, as the polymer surrounding the drug is eroded, the drug escapes. This property offers a significant advantage over non-erodible systems in many applications because biodegradable polymers are eventually absorbed by the body, obviating the need for surgical removal. However, this advantage must be weighed against the potential disadvantage that the absorption products may be toxic, immunogenic, or carcinogenic.

### Pendant chain systems

In pendant chain systems, a drug is chemically bound to a polymer backbone chain and is released by hydrolytic or enzymatic cleavage. In its simplest form, the pendant chain system consists of drug attached to a polymer backbone. The polymer system can be either soluble or insoluble. Soluble backbone-chains are generally used for transport functions such as cell targeting; insoluble forms are more desirable for long-term controlled-release implants. The backbone may also be biodegradable or nonbiodegradable. For in vivo use, it is important that the polymers do not cause immunology reactions and that the drugs, when coupled to the polymers, do not induce allergic reactions.

## Solvent-activated systems

### Swelling-controlled systems

Swelling-controlled release of potent drugs may be achieved by using the glassy/rubbery transition of polymers in the presence of a penetrate and by the macro-molecule relaxation associated with this transition. In these systems the drug is originally dissolved or dispersed in a polymer solution; the solvent is then evaporated, leaving the drug dispersed in a glassy (solvent-free) polymer matrix. There is no drug diffusion in the solid phase. As the dissolution medium penetrates the matrix, the polymer swells and its glass transition temperature is lowered below the temperature of the experiment. Therefore, the swollen polymer is in a rubbery state, and it allows the drug contained in it to diffuse outward.

*Cosmetically controlled systems*

An osmotic system comprises of a core which contains a bioactive agent. The core is surrounded by a semipermeable film that, when placed in contact with water, causes water to be transported through the membrane to ward the core, resulting in the solute being pumped out of the matrix.

*Magnetically controlled systems*

In magnetically controlled systems, drug and small magnetic beads are uniformly dispersed within a polymer matrix. On exposure to aqueous media, drug is released in a fashion typical of diffusion-controlled matrix systems. However, on exposure to an oscillating external magnetic field, drug is released at a much higher rate.

The mechanism responsible for this magnetic modulation is unclear. It may be that the beads cause alternating compression and expansion of the pores within the matrix, thus facilitating drug release. This magnetic delivery system allows external control of drug release rates and permits a modulated release pattern to occur.

**Present status of long-acting contraceptive methods**

Progestin prevents pregnancy is several ways: it suppresses ovulation, makes cervical mucus hostile, suppresses cyclic development of endometrium and delays ovum transport.

Progestins can be administered as long-acting contraceptive agents by incorporating them in a sustained release systems. There are at least five different routes to administer them [5]: 1) injectables, 2) implantables, 3) steroids-releasing IUDs, 4) vaginal rings, and 5) once-a-month pills.

**Injectable contraceptives**

Approximately 22 million women around the world are currently using long-acting injectable and implantable steroid contraceptives, mostly in developing countries, and the number of users is increasing. It is generally believed that the popularity of such methods would considerably increase if they were further improved. Table 1 describes the current status of injectable contraceptives which are either available on the market or being developed.

Injectable hormonal contraceptives, when properly used, are amongst the most effective methods of contraception available today. They combine almost complete effectiveness with reliable reversibility. Most clinical trials report less than one pregnancy per 100 women in the 1st year.

Thus they should be included among the family planning methods available at any clinic or other health facility offering an integrated family planning service. It is estimated that over 35 million women worldwide have used this method

*Table 1.* Status of injectable contraceptive, 1998.

| Type | Duration | Existing systems | Status |
|---|---|---|---|
| Injectable | Monthly | 1. 25 mg DMPA + 5 mg EC | Market |
| | | 50 mg NET-EN + 5 mg EV | Market |
| | | 250 mg HPC + 5 mg EV | Phase IV |
| | | 4. 150 mg DHPA + 10 mg EE | Phase IV |
| Injectable | 2—3 months | 1. 200 mg NET-EN | Market |
| | | 2. 150 mg DMPA | Market |
| | | 3. 100 mg NET microcapsules | Phase I-II |
| Injectable | 6 monthly | 1. 450 mg DMPA | Market |
| | | 2. 200 mg net microcapsules | Phase I |

and approximately 17 million are using it currently. It is licensed for contraceptive use in more than 106 countries [5,6].

Only about 10% of DMPA users have normal cycles in the 1st year of use. DMPA users can expect to have irregular bleeding in the first 6 months and then infrequent bleeding or amenorrhoea in the next 6 months and beyond. By comparison, in a WHO tiral of six OCs, 59—87% of women had normal bleeding patterns after 1 year.

NET EN has somewhat less effect on bleeding patterns than DMPA. In a comparative trial bleeding episodes in the first 6 months were significantly shorter among NET EN users than among DMPA users. Bleeding patterns after 6 months were similar, however, amenorrhoea lasting more than 90 days was significantly less common among NET EN users [6].

In 1988, the World Health Organization reported a phase III multicentre comparative study of Cyclofem and Mesigyna. A total of 2,320 women were recruited into a 17-centre random allocation clinical trial. Over 1 year of follow up 10,969 woman-months of use were collected for Cyclofem and 10,608 woman-months for Mesigyna. Two pregnancies occurred, both with Mesigyna, one in the second and one in the third injection interval, giving a life table rate of 0.18 per 100 woman-years. Heavy, prolonged, irregular bleeding or a combination of these accounted for a discontinuation rate of 6.3% with Cyclofem and 7.5% with Mesigyna, while discontinuation rates for amenorrhoea were low at 2.1% (Cyclofem) and 1.6% (Mesigyna). The overall total discontinuation rates were 35.5% for Cyclofem and 36.8% for Mesigyna at 1 year. Discontinuations for other medical reasons were low for both preparations [7].

**Implantable contraceptives**

There are three implantable contraceptives available for large-scale introduction into family planning programs: Norplant, Implanon and Jadelle. The other implantable contraceptives are still in the phase I—III clinical trial (Table 2).

300

*Table 2.* Status of implantable contraceptives, 1998.

| Implants | Duration | Existing systems | Status |
|----------|----------|------------------|--------|
| 6 Rods | 5 years | Norplant-6 | Market |
| 2 Rods | 3 years | Jadelle | Market |
| 1 Rod | 3 years | Implanon | Market |
| 1 Rod | 1 year | Uniplant | Phase III—IV |

## Norplant

Norplant consists of six 2.4 mm × 3.4 cm subdermal capsules releasing LNG during some 6—7 years. The initial release rate is rather high, approximately 80 µg/24 h during the first 6—18 months of use, after which the system will deliver 30 µg/24 h during a minimum of 5 years. Norplant provides a high contraceptive efficacy during 5 years; a study involving 437 woman indicates a gross cumulative pregnancy rate of 1.8 per 100 women at 5 years and another study, a continuation rate of 49 per 100 women at 4 years. The safety of Norplant, like that of DMPA and NET-EN, has been carefully assessed; after reviewing all animal and clinical data, the participants of a WHO consultation concluded that "Norplant provides an effective and reversible long-term method of fertility regulation". It certainly provides an important option for women desiring long-term contraception. Like with any other progestogen-only system, bleeding irregularities occur also in Norplant users [8] (Table 3).

Compared to IUD and DMPA, Norplant has a higher continuation rate (Table 4).

## Implanon®

NV Organon (Oss, The Netherlands) has developed a single-rod implant (Implanon7) with a length of 40 mm and a diameter of 2 mm, which is applied subdermally by a disposable sterile inserter. The rod is made of an ethylene vinyl acetate copolymer (EVA) with a core containing approximately 68 mg 3-ketodesogestrel or etonogestrel (ENG).

The initial release rate of the implant is approximately 67 µg/day which slowly

*Table 3.* Cumulative rate per 100 Norplant acceptors by year.

| Rates/year | 1 | 2 | 3 | 4 | 5 |
|------------|-----|-----|-----|-----|-----|
| Pregnancy | 0.0 | 0.2 | 0.5 | 0.5 | 1.8 |
| Expulsion | 0.0 | 0.0 | 0.0 | 0.0 | 0.0 |
| Bleeding | 2.3 | 5.3 | 6.9 | 8.0 | 9.2 |
| Medical | 1.1 | 1.4 | 1.8 | 3.4 | 3.9 |
| Personal | 1.1 | 1.6 | 2.5 | 6.4 | 6.9 |
| Continuation | 95.5 | 91.5 | 88.3 | 81.7 | 78.2 |

*Table 4.* One-year cumulative rate per 100 acceptors.

| Rate | Implant | IUD | Injectable |
|------|---------|-----|------------|
| Pregnancy | 0.0 | 0.4 | 0.3 |
| Expulsion | 0.0 | 4.4 | 0.0 |
| Bleeding | 2.3 | 1.0 | 5.7 |
| Medical | 1.1 | 7.6 | 6.7 |
| Personal | 1.1 | 18.6 | 27.3 |
| Continuation | 95.5 | 68.2 | 60.0 |

decreases over time. The constant release profile results in sufficiently high plasma ENG concentration ($> 90$ pg/ml) to inhibit ovulation for at least 3 years.

ENG is a progestin, structurally derived from 19-nortestosterone, it is the biologically active metabolite of desogestrel (DSG). DSG is the progestin component of a number of widely used oral contraceptives with a well-established efficacy and safety profile. The characteristics of the implant's EVA membrane, combined with the high specific progestin activity of ENG, allow the use of a single-rod system with a low and almost zero-order release. As a consequence of these properties, dose-related side effects are minimized.

No pregnancy occurred during the 4-year use (Table 5), making the life table cumulative discontinuation rate at year 4 for pregnancy among users of Implanon7 is 0.0 per 100 women-years.

The continuation rates are shown in Table 5, being year 1: 98.5%, year 2: 96.5%, year 3: 84.7% and year 4: 65.3%.

A multicentred study was conducted in Indonesia to compare the efficacy, acceptability and safety of Implanon and Norplant.

At 3 years follow-up, none of the subjects became pregnant in both groups. One-year continuation rates were 97.3 per 100 women for Implanon® and 97.6 per 100 women for Norplant®. After 3 years the continuation rates were 90.6 and 92.0, respectively. In the Implanon® group 42 subjects discontinued the method use. The reasons were: bleeding irregularities (four subjects), amenorrhoea (one subject), other medical reasons (four subjects), nonmedical reasons

*Table 5.* Net cumulative termination and continuation rates per 100 women.

| Type of termination | Year-1 | Year-2 | Year-3 | Year-4 |
|---------------------|--------|--------|--------|--------|
| Pregnancy | 0.0 | 0.0 | 0.0 | 0.0 |
| Amenorrhea | 0.5 | 0.5 | 0.5 | 0.5 |
| Bleeding irregularities | 0.0 | 0.0 | 0.0 | 0.0 |
| Other medical | 0.0 | 0.5 | 1.0 | 1.5 |
| Planning pregnancy | 0.5 | 1.5 | 10.5 | 27.2 |
| Other personal | 0.5 | 1.0 | 3.5 | 5.5 |
| Total termination | 1.5 | 3.5 | 15.7 | 34.7 |
| Continuation | 98.5 | 96.5 | 84.3 | 65.3 |
| No. of woman-years | 197 | 386.0 | 505.8 | 658.4 |

(24 subjects) and lost to follow-up (nine subjects). In the Norplant® group 36 subjects discontinued the method use. The reasons were bleeding irregularities (four subjects), other medical reasons (five subjects), nonmedical reasons (11 subjects), and lost to follow-up (16 subjects). There were no statistically significant differences between the groups. None of the subjects in both groups suffered from serious side effects (Table 6).

## Jadelle

A second generation system consisting of two 2.4 mm × 4.4 cm rods each containing 70 mg LNG has been available on the market for some time. Jadelle delivers amounts of LNG equivalent to those released by Norplant; at the end of 6 years of use there is still no evidence for a decline in release rates. As with other progestin-only contraceptives the major reasons for discontinuations were menstrual irregularities (28.5%).

During the first 3 years of Norplant-2 use, side effects profile, continuation rates, and contraceptive effectiveness are comparable to Norplant. After 3 years of use, the contraceptive effectiveness of Norplant-2 markedly declines to such extremes that the system should be removed. As with Norplant, Norplant-2 does not appear to have a clinically significant effect on lipoprotein profile, hepatic transaminases, or glucose tolerance [11,12].

## Uniplant (nomegestrol acetate implant)

Uniplant (Theramex, Monaco) is a second-generation single silastic implant containing 55 mg nomegestrol acetate with contraceptive effectiveness of 1-year duration. In a multicenter study involving 1,598 women enrolled in 10 countries and covering 15,201 woman-months of observation, the main complaint was menstrual-related; only 56% of the women had normal cyclical menstruation.

*Table 6.* Cumulative life-table discontinuation and continuation rates at 3 years.

| Reasons for terminating study | Cumulative rates | | | | | |
|---|---|---|---|---|---|---|
| | Implanon7 (n = 448) | | | Norplant7 (n = 450) | | |
| | Year-1 | Year-2 | Year-3 | Year-1 | Year-2 | Year-3 |
| Pregnancy | 0.0 | 0.0 | 0.0 | 0.0 | 0.0 | 0.0 |
| Amenorrhea | 0.0 | 0.0 | 0.2 | 0.0 | 0.0 | 0.0 |
| Bleeding irregularities | 0.2 | 0.7 | 0.9 | 0.0 | 0.7 | 0.9 |
| Other medical | 0.2 | 0.4 | 0.9 | 0.4 | 0.9 | 1.1 |
| Nonmedical | 1.1 | 2.6 | 5.1 | 0.7 | 1.1 | 2.4 |
| Lost to follow-up | 1.1 | 1.6 | 2.0 | 1.3 | 1.8 | 3.6 |
| Discontinuation | 2.6 | 5.3 | 9.1 | 2.4 | 4.5 | 8.0 |
| Continuation | 97.4 | 94.7 | 90.9 | 97.6 | 95.5 | 92.0 |

The 12 months gross cumulative discontinuation rate was 20.47 + 1.33%. Nine pregnancies occurred in subjects with normal weight: height ratio resulting in a Pearl index of 0.7. The average weight gain was 1.0 kg; both systolic and diastolic blood pressure decreased significantly at 12 months, whereas both hematological and clinical biochemistry profiles during 12 months of observation were within the normal range. The antifertility effect of Uniplant is due to impairment of follicular development, endometrial growth and cervical mucus characteristics. Uniplant use did not have any adverse effect on breast-feeding or infant health or gain in weight, while homozygous sickle cell patients showed significant improvement in their clinical wellbeing due to an increase in F-cell levels and fetal hemoglobin. This symptomatic improvement has also been documented with the use of depot medroxy-progesterone and Norplant [11,13].

**Capronor**

This consists of a single biodegradable capsule that delivers LNG for approximately 12—18 months. It is at an early stage of development: preliminary clinical trials have been completed. Since the biodegradation takes several years until no more steroid is released, this implant system seems to combine the advantages of retrievable and biodegradable implants [6,8].

The Research Triangle Institute currently is developing two new versions of its biodegradable implant Capronor. Capronor 2 and Capronor 3. Capronor 2 is a 4-cm capsule of the polymer caprolactone filled with 18 mg of levonorgestrel. Recent studies have shown that two capsules may be required with this formulation. Capronor 3 is a single 4-cm copolymer capsule (a caprolactone and trimethylenecarbonate blend) filled with 32 mg of levonorgestrel. Thus far, no human trials have been conducted with these new formulations, but nonhuman primate studies are encouraging and indicate very steady release rates in both versions. The copolymer blend releases the drug more readily, allowing a thicker capsule that produces a steadier release of the hormone. The copolymer also biodegrades more quickly than the single polymer.

In earlier formulations of Capronor-which consisted of levonorgestrel suspended in an oily solution of ethyl oleate within caprolactone tubing-clinical studies on women showed promising results for a biodegradable implant. It was effective for only 8 to 10 months, however, in part because of an unsteady release rate caused by the ethyl oleate vehicle, now eliminated. The Capronor tubing appears to be easier to insert and remove than Norplant's Silastic tubes in part because the caprolactone polymer has a slippier surface and offers less resistance in body tissues. The capsule remains intact through the 12-month period of levonorgestrel release. Thus it may be removed during this interval if desired. Later, however, over several years the capsule biodegrades gradually to E-hydroxycaproic acid, then to carbon dioxide and water, which are absorbed by the body [6].

**Fused pellets**

These are subcutaneous, bioabsorbable pellets fused with cholesterol, releasing NET. The insertion of three or four pellets (containing approximately 35 mg NET each) seems to result in predominantly anovulatory cycles. Single implants releasing NET or LNG are also under evaluation; the present systems do not appear to have as yet a reliable contraceptive potential [14,15].

Capsules releasing ST-1435: ST-1435 (16-methylene-17-acetoxy-19-norprogesterone) has a high progestational potency when given parenterally but is practically inactive when given orally. At least theoretically, it is an ideal steroid for postpartum contraception. Preliminary clinical results are encouraging, although the system may require certain modifications because of the too rapid steroid release [14,15].

*Progesterone implants*

In this method six $3.2 \times 11.8$ mm pellets containing 100 mg progesterone each are implanted subdermally in nursing women 6 weeks after delivery; the duration of effective life is 5 months, during which the peripheral progesterone levels remain around $10-15$ nmol/l. One pregnancy occurred in 1,614 woman-months of observation, compared to 19 pregnancies in 677 woman-months in an untreated lactating group [14,15].

**IUD-releasing hormones, vaginal rings, and once-a-month pills** (Table 7)

*Vaginal rings*

The major advantages of these systems are that they can be inserted and removed by the subject; they achieve a good contraceptive effect through the constant release of small amounts of steroids by the systemic route, avoiding thereby any first-pass effect on the liver [14,15].

**Rings for continuous use**

*Rings releasing LNG*

This system developed by WHO releases 20 µg LNG/24 h and provides an

*Table 7.* Status of IUD-releasing hormones, vaginal rings and once-a-month pill.

| Type | Duration | Systems | Status |
|------|----------|---------|--------|
| IUD | 8 years | LNG-IUD | Market |
| IUD | 1 year | Progestasert | Market |
| Vaginal ring | 2−3 months | 1. LNG | Phase III-IV |
| | | 2. Prog | Phase II-III |
| Pill | 1 month | Sev. Form | China |

acceptable contraceptive efficacy with a minimal steroid load of 600 µg per month. The drug is released continuously with a near zero order rate and provides constant blood levels for at least 3 months. The device is used continuously and is removed during menstruation. In a phase III clinical trial conducted in 13 countries, there were 21 pregnancies (one ectopic) in more than 700 woman-months and the discontinuation for bleeding irregularities was 15.7 per 100 women at 390 days of use. A similar ring releasing 25 µg LNG by a different polymeric system has been developed by a European pharmaceutical house and tested clinically. Compared to the WHO ring, this system provides higher LNG levels and inhibits ovulation more frequently [14,15].

*Rings releasing progesterone*

Preliminary trials of rings releasing 2.4—4.8 mg/24 h progesterone in normally menstruating women were unsuccessful because of unacceptable bleeding profiles. However, the pharmacokinetic and pharmacodynamic properties of these rings and the success of rings releasing 5—10 progesterone/24 h may represent an ideal, long-acting contraceptive for postpartum women. Such studies are now in progress.

*Rings releasing NET*

Rings releasing 200 µg/24 h NET exhibited excellent pharmacokinetic and pharmacodynamic properties but produced unacceptable bleeding profiles.

**Rings for discontinuous use**

A delivery system releasing 280 µg/24 h LNG together with 180 µg estradiol has been tested in an international clinical trial. The rings are inserted for 3 continuous weeks and then removed for 1 week (as in contraception with OCs). The use of these large steroid doses results in almost complete inhibition of ovulation; at the same time headache and nausea are less common than with OC use.

**IUD-releasing hormone**

The levonorgestrel-releasing intrauterine device LNg IUD is a new contraceptive method that combines the advantages of both hormonal and intrauterine contraception. It gives users noncontraceptive health benefits and can also be used as an effective therapy for menorrhagia.

The local release of LNg within the endometrial cavity results in strong suppression of endometrial growth as the endometrium becomes insensitive to ovarian estradiol. The endometrial suppression is the reason for a significant reduction in menstrual blood loss or amenorrhoea, and for the disappearance of dysmenorrhoea.

The bleeding pattern during the use of the LNg IUD is characterized by a reduction in the blood loss and in the 3 months of use, however, irregular spotting is common. The removal of the device results in a quick return of menstrual bleeding and fertility.

The failure rate of copper-releasing IUDs, as with other methods of fertility regulation, is higher in young women and decreases with age. The LNg IUD, on the other hand, has the same low pregnancy rate in every age group of the users. The LNg IUD also gives protection against ectopic pregnancy and pelvic inflammatory disease and, by reducing menstrual blood loss, increases the body iron stores.

The LNg IUD can be used to effectively treat menorrhagia. This has been demonstrated in studies with quantitative determination of menstrual blood loss. During the 1st year of use, the LNg IUD reduced menstrual blood loss by 90% from pretreatment levels.

Comparative clinical trials with the LNg IUD cover more than 10,000 women-years of follow-up during use over 5 to 7 years. The Pearl pregnancy rate in studies has been 0.0–0.2 per 100 women-years. The overall ectopic Pearl pregnancy rate is 0.02 per 100 woman-years [16].

*Progesterone-releasing devices*
A device releasing 65 μg/24 h progesterone (Progestasert) has been marketed in several countries.

The use of Norplant and other long-acting progestin contraceptive methods is increasing, especially in the developing countries. Since bleeding problems are the main problems of these methods, research on endometrial bleeding should be considered a priority.

The causes of bleeding problems are not understood, and simple and reliable treatment regimens have not yet been adequately investigated. An improved knowledge of the underlying endometrial events and biochemical mechanisms could be expected to lead to improved long-acting methods with reduced bleeding disturbances, and to improve means of treatment of the disturbances [17].

## References

1. Dziuk PJ, Cook B. Passage of steroids through silicone rubber. Endocrinology 1966; 78:208–211.
2. Segal SJ. Contraceptive subdermal implants. In: Mishell DR Jr (ed) Advances in Fertility Research, vol. I. New York: Raven Press, 1982;117–127.
3. Odlind V. New delivery systems for hormonal contraception. Acta Obstet Gynecol Scand 1986;134(Suppl.):15–20.
4. Langer RS. Polymers and drug delivery systems. In: Zatuchni GI, Goldsmith A, Shelton JD, Sciarra JJ (eds) Long-Acting Contraceptive Delivery Systems. Philadelphia: Harper & Row Publishers, 1984;23–32.
5. Population Reports. Long-acting progestins – promise and prospects, Series K, Number 2, 1983.

6. Population Reports, New Era for Injectables, Series K, Number 5, 1995.
7. WHO. A multicentered phase III comparative study of two hormonal contraceptive preparations given once-a-month by intramuscular injection: I. Contraceptive efficacy and side effects. Contraception 1988;37:1—20.
8. Affandi B. Clinical, pharmacological and epidemiological studies on a levonorgestrel implant contraceptive. Dissertation, University of Indonesia, 1987.
9. Affandi B, Korver T, Paul Geurts TB, Coeling Bennink HJT. A phase II study with single implant contraceptive containing 3-ketodesogestrel. Contraception (In press).
10. Affandi B, Hoesni HM, Barus RP et al. A multicentred phase III study between Implanon and Norplant. Contraception (In press).
11. Ladipo O, Cautinho EM. Contraceptive implants. Curr Opin Obstet Gynecol 1994;6:564—569.
12. Cullins VE. Injectable and implantable contraceptives. Curr Opin Obstet Gynecol 1992;4:536—543.
13. Cautinho EM, de Souza JC, Athaide C et al. Multicenter clinical trial on the efficacy and acceptability of Uniplant. Contraception 1996;53:121—125.
14. Population Reports. Hormonal contraception: new long acting methods, Series K, Number 3, 1988.
15. Diczfalusy E. New developments in oral, injectable and implantable contraceptives, vaginal rings and intrauterine device: A review. Contraception 1986;33:7—22.
16. Luukkainen T, Toivonen J. Levonorgestrel-releasing IUD as a method of contraception with therapeutic properties. Contraception 1995;52:269—276.
17. Fraser IS. Towards a better understanding of the effects of progestogens on the mechanisms of endometrial bleeding. Recommendations for Research. Presented at the Symposium on Contraception and Mechanisms of Endometrial Bleeding, 28 November—2 December, Geneva, 1988.

Fertility and Reproductive Medicine.
R.D. Kempers, J. Cohen, A.F. Haney and J.B. Younger, editors.

# Third-generation oral contraceptives and venous thromboembolism: is the association a real effect?

Walter O. Spitzer

*Stanford University, Palo Alto, California, USA; and McGill University, Montreal, Canada*

**Abstract.** The Bradford-Hill criteria, to diagnose causality from an observed estimate of association from clinical and epidemiological associations, were used to consider whether or not third-generation oral contraceptives (OCs) are associated with an increased risk of venous thromboembolism (VTE) compared with second-generation OCs. This review also examines whether, or not, bias may have spuriously increased the odds ratio for third-generation OCs compared to second-generation OCs as references reported in studies published in December 1995 and January 1996.

The nine Bradford-Hill criteria have not been met. No causality can therefore be elucidated from the apparent association of third-generation OCs with occurrence of VTE. There is considerable evidence of systematic error or bias in the 1995—1996 studies which led to the "pill scare" focused on third-generation OCs.

**Keywords:** bias, Bradford-Hill: causality, cardiovascular, myocardial infarction, oral contraceptives, stroke, venous thromboembolism.

## Introduction

In October 1995, The British Committee on Safety of Medicines (CSM 1995) warned that oral contraceptives (OCs) containing the third-generation progestogens, desogestrel or gestodene, were associated with an increased risk of venous thromboembolism (VTE) in younger women compared with OCs that contained the second-generation progestogen, levonorgestrel. The warning was based on data from four studies, which at the time were unpublished. A major pill scare resulted, the effects of which still persist.

The four studies: the WHO Collaborative Study of Cardiovascular Disease and Steroid Hormone Contraception [1]; the Transnational Study of Oral Contraceptives and the Health of Young Women [2]; the Boston Collaborative Drug Surveillance Program (BCDSP) [3]; and the Leiden Thrombophilia Study [4] were finally published in December 1995 and January 1996. The general interpretation of the data, at that time, heightened the pill scare based on statistically significant odds ratios (OR) or relative risks (RR) of 2.4, 2.2, and 1.5 reported for the WHO, BCDSP and Transnational studies, respectively. The results of the Leiden study were not statistically significant.

A question of high relevance to any clinician confronted with such findings is:

---

*Address for correspondence:* Professor W.O. Spitzer, Department of Medicine, Stanford University, 10707 La Honda Rd, Star Rte 172A, Woodside, CA 94062-3751, USA.

from the observed association between the defined exposure factor and a clinical outcome can one determine causality? ORs and RRs are estimates of association. They are not sufficient proof of causality, even when statistically significant. A relative risk of 2.0 means that a baseline incidence for venous thromboembolism (VTE) of approximately one in 10,000 women using OCs containing second-generation progestogens would increase to two per 10,000 in women taking OCs containing third-generation progestogens.

Since the original publications, a further four studies have been published: the Danish case-control study [5], a MediPlus-based study in the UK [6], a MediPlus-based study in Germany [7], and an advanced analysis of the earlier Transnational Study [8].

Later studies suggest that the 1995–1996 data may have failed to address adequately the questions of "bias", i.e., preferential prescribing, selective referral, healthy user effect, and "confounders", particularly duration of use.

A revised interpretation is now proposed based on the advanced analyses of the 1995–1996 data and an updated synthesis of all findings since 1995 [9]:
1) there is no difference in the risk of VTE between first-time users of second- or third-generation OCs;
2) the difference in the risk of VTE associated with third- and second-generation OCs is more likely to be explained by bias than by a causal relationship;
3) absolute rates of VTE for third-generation OC users reported in 1995–1996 are lower than those for users of second-generation OCs in 1988–1991;
4) the risk of MI is lower in users of third-generation OCs;
5) the risk of stroke remains low for both second- and third-generation OC users, and there is no difference between generations in incidence rate; and
6) ORs or relative risks of about 2.0 for VTE are not clinically important and are of no significance to public health or drug safety.

The question that remains, however, and which this review addresses is: can "causality" be elucidated from any observed third-generation OC association with an excess of VTE, based on an apparent relative risk of around 2.0? The question will be addressed within the framework of the Bradford-Hill [10] criteria for causality in a systematic synthesis of the published data. Sources of bias based on empirical findings in the data of the Transnational Study will also be examined.

**Bradford-Hill criteria of causality**

In the USA, these criteria are often referred to as the "Surgeon General's criteria", since they were used when interpreting the evidence of association between cigarette smoking and lung cancer. The Bradford-Hill criteria are guidelines and not a checklist. Ultimately, clinical and epidemiological judgement needs to be invoked. There is no automatic formula or algorithm that will lead to a "verdict" of causality.

The nine Bradford-Hill criteria are: 1) experiment, 2) strength, 3) consistency,

4) gradient, 5) biological and clinical plausibility, 6) specificity, 7) coherence, 8) temporality, and 9) analogy.

## Experiment

Experimental evidence, i.e., a properly designed, randomized, controlled clinical study, is the "gold standard" method for demonstrating causation. However, no such experiments have been done with OCs, because it would be neither feasible (a minimum of 400,000 women per arm would be needed in a randomized controlled trial) nor ethical (women could not be randomized once concerns about the newer products had been raised). Accrual to such a study would also take several years, and would make such an "experiment" untimely. Regulators need to make decisions rapidly. There is no experimental evidence of an association between VTE and third-generation OCs.

## Strength

The strength of an association is measured by the size of the odds ratio or relative risk. ORs or RRs of 1.0 mean that there is "no association". Values of $> 1.0$ mean that the exposure factor (e.g., third-generation OCs) are associated with a higher risk than the reference (e.g., second-generation OCs), while RRs $< 1.0$ mean the exposure factor is "protective" or conveys "benefit".

The odds ratios for third- vs. second-generation OCs in the 1995–1996 studies and the later 1997 studies range from 0.7–2.2. The estimates indicate that the strength of association between third-generation OCs and VTE is weak. For example, the RR reported for cigarette smoking and lung cancer have been found to be as high as 23.0, and that for short acting $\beta$-agonists and premature death due to asthma is as high as 90.0 [11]. An OR of 2.0 for third-generation OCs is very weak.

## Consistency

Although the odds ratios for the 1995–1996 studies are consistent in direction and magnitude (i.e., 1.5–2.2, all above 1.0), they are consistently weak. Again, while the ORs in the later 1997 cohort and case-control studies are also consistent, they are all lower with some values $< 1.0$.

## Gradient

Evidence that increased exposure to a risk factor increases the rate of occurrence of a disorder or its severity suggests causality. An example of this is the increased risk of VTE with the higher doses ($> 50$ µg) of estrogen used in early first-generation OCs. However, in four of the studies, when the dose of estrogen was reduced from 30 to 20 µg ethinylestradiol (EE) or from 50 to 35 µg of EE com-

*Table 1.* Inverse dose–effect for oral contraceptives (OCs) containing desogestrel or cyproterone acetate and different doses of ethinylestradiol (EE).

| Study | Type of OC | Comparison group | OR (95% CI) |
|---|---|---|---|
| WHO (WHO, 1995) | 150 μg desogestrel +30 μg EE | Nonusers | 7.6 (3.9 – 14.7) |
| | 150 μg desogestrel +20 μg EE | Nonusers | 38.2 (4.5 – 325) |
| BCDSP (Jick et al. 1995) | 150 μg desogestrel +30 μg EE | Levonorgestrel OCs | 2.7 (not reported) |
| | 150 μg desogestrel +20 μg EE | Levonorgestrel OCs | 1.9 (not reported) |
| Transnational (Lewis et al. 1996) | 150 μg desogestrel +30 μg EE | Levonorgestrel OCs | 1.5 (0.9 – 2.5)[a] |
| | 150 μg desogestrel +20 μg EE | Levonorgestrel OCs | 2.8 (1.3 – 6.5)[a] |
| MediPlus UK (Farmer et al. 1997) | 150 μg desogestrel +30 μg EE | Levonorgestrel OCs | 0.6 (0.3 – 1.5) |
| | 150 μg desogestrel +20 μg EE | Levonorgestrel OCs | 2.9 (0.9 – 10.0) |
| WHO (WHO 1995) | 2 mg cyproterone acetate + 50 μg EE | Nonusers | 3.8 (1.4 – 10.7) |
| | 2 mg cyproterone acetate + 35 μg EE | Nonusers | 14.9 (3.7 – 59.4) |

WHO = World Health Organization; BCDSP = Boston Collaborative Drug Surveillance Program; OR = Odds ratio; CI = Confidence interval. [a]Subgroup of women aged 25–44 years.

bined with cyproterone acetate there was an inverse dose gradient of relative risks in relation to VTE (Table 1). These inverse paradoxical gradients, therefore, not only fail to support causality but militate against a causal interpretation of an association between third-generation OCs and VTE.

*Biological and clinical plausibility*

A critical assessment of prospective, controlled, randomized hematological studies has not shown any differences between third- and second-generation OCs that would indicate a higher thrombotic potential [12], and there is no known biologically plausible mechanism which can account for the observed difference in these VTE rates.

Although Rosing et al. [13] suggested that OCs (particularly those containing third-generation progestogens) might induce a thrombophilic state similar to the one associated with the Leiden mutation, it has not been possible to reproduce their results. Methodological flaws resulting from the lack of randomization in the study and the inconsistency of the findings using a new assay {based on activated protein C (APC) sensitivity ratio compared with results from the traditional measurements of activated partial thromboplastin time (APTT)} make the clinical relevance of these data difficult to interpret.

*Table 2.* Summary of lack of evidence for diagnosing the causality of third-generation oral contraceptives for VTE.

| Bradford-Hill criteria | Status |
| --- | --- |
| Experiment | Not done |
| Strength | Very weak |
| Consistency | Consistently weak |
| Gradient | Inverse |
| Biological plausibility | Absent |
| Specificity | Lacking |
| Coherence | Missing |
| Temporality | Noncontributory |
| Analogy | Not found |

## Specificity

Specificity of an association occurs when the exposure factor concerned is known to be exclusive to the target outcome, and when the target outcome is known to have no other risk factors associated with it. For example, the only adverse event known to be associated with thalidomide is focomelia. Conversely, focomelia is not associated with any other risk factor. In contrast, risk factors other than OC use are associated with an increased risk of VTE, including obesity and pregnancy. Similarly, stroke and myocardial infarction (MI) are both associated with smoking and hypertension, while MI is also associated with increased levels of low-density-lipoprotein-cholesterol. Thus, OCs in general, and third-generation OCs in particular, cannot be shown to be specifically and exclusively associated with the occurrence of adverse cardiovascular or cerebrovascular events, and particularly not with VTE.

## Coherence

Evidence from different disciplines and different sources which "hangs well together" is considered to be coherent. In the alleged association of third-generation OCs with an excess of VTE, there is a paradoxical gradient in the incidence of VTE in relation to estrogen dose. Further, there is no laboratory evidence to be marshalled if one wished to claim coherence.

## Temporality

All the studies relating to the association of VTE with OC use were designed to ensure that exposure to OCs preceded the target event. Therefore, temporality is noncontributory in this assessment of causal implications of the associations.

314

*Analogy*

Analogy only supports causation if similar associations or causal relationships can be found in other relevant areas of epidemiology. No apposite examples of analogy have been found to date.

*Summary*

None of the nine Bradford-Hill criteria have been met (Table 2), and causality and overall profile with respect to the alleged association of third-generation OCs with an excess of VTE is not consistent with a causal interpretation of the known evidence.

## Bias

Observational, epidemiological research is inherently and unavoidably affected by systematic error or bias since the design is not experimental. Many important biases may have distorted the estimates of effect of VTE associated with the use of third-generation OCs in the 1995–1996 studies. For three of those, healthy user bias, prescribing bias and referral bias, there is empirical evidence that it occurred [8]. One category of systematic error, healthy user bias alone could explain the difference between the estimates of ORs found and 1.0 which would have indicated "no association". In this paper, only that bias is presented in detail.

## Healthy user bias

In theoretical pharmacoepidemiological terms, "the healthy user effect", also known as "the prudent doctor bias", "play the winner bias" and "attrition of susceptibles", occurs when patients who have been treated with a drug that has been available for some time, but who are considered clinically to be "at higher risk" in some way, are switched to a newer drug, ostensibly safer, because their prudent physician feels that this will be better for them. Any comparison of the effects of the two drugs is therefore biased since comparisons done for OCs used by higher risk patients (i.e., women who are thought to be more susceptible to VTE and who were given the newer third-generation OCs) and OCs used by lower risk patients (i.e., women who are not thought to be susceptible to VTE and thus were maintained on the older second-generation OCs). As a result, the newer drug appears to be associated with a higher rate of occurrence of VTE than the older drug. In reality the differences observed are due to differences in the risk profiles of the women in each group compared and not to differences in the OCs.

This effect was demonstrated in the Transnational Study [14], in which a brand-specific analysis revealed that the risk of VTE was significantly correlated with the timing of that brand's introduction into a market. In that analysis there were remarkably paradoxical findings in all the studies contrasting third- and second-generation combined OCs. For instance, norgestimate is largely metabolized to levonorgestrel. Therefore in terms of clinical and biological plausibility, the two should exhibit similar risks for VTE, which is not the case. Norgestimate is almost twice as high as levonorgestrel. Attrition of susceptible bias also explains the inverse paradoxical gradient wherein the OR with desogestrel 20 µg is twice that with desogestrel 30 µg. Higher ORs with lower doses of ethynylestradiol are biologically implausible.

It deserves emphasis that the bias of a "healthy user effect" alone easily explains a small increase from 1.0 to 1.5 in the Transnational Study and even the difference from 1.0 to 2.2 in the WHO Study. The existence of this bias has been demonstrated empirically.

*Prescribing and referral bias*

There is also empirical evidence that these two forms of systematic error occurred in European countries when the Transnational studies were being conducted [8]. Prescribing bias distorts epidemiological studies when doctors prescribe OCs perceived to be safer (i.e., third-generation pills) to women at higher risk of a cardiovascular adverse event (e.g., women more obese or smokers). Referral bias occurs when women suspected clinically of VTE and known to have taken more controversial third-generation OCs are referred to hospital more readily for investigation than women with a similar clinical presentation but who take the more established less controversial second-generation OCs. Referral bias is particularly important because both the Transnational and the WHO case-control studies were hospital-based.

In-depth discussions of prescribing and referral systematic error have been published [8].

## Conclusions

None of the nine Bradford-Hill criteria for causality have been met. Causality cannot be elucidated for the observed association between third-generation OCs and VTE. Three biases have been shown empirically to affect estimates of case-control studies examining the association of third-generation OCs and VTE: healthy user bias, prescribing bias and referral bias. The healthy user effect (or attrition of susceptible bias) by itself could explain the ORs reported in recent research. It is concluded that the apparent difference in risk ratios between third- and second-generation OCs is more likely to be due to bias than to represent a true causal effect.

316

## References

Committee on Safety of Medicines. Combined oral contraceptives and thromboembolism. London: Committee on Safety of Medicines, 1995.

1. WHO Collaborative Study of Cardiovascular Disease and Steroid Hormone Contraception. Effect of different progestogens in low oestrogen oral contraceptives on venous thromboembolic disease. Lancet 1995;346:1582—1588.

2. Spitzer WO, Lewis MA, Heinemann LA, Thorogood M, MacRae KD. Third generation oral contraceptives and risk of venous thromboembolic disorders: an international case-control study. Transnational Research Group on Oral Contraceptives and the Health of Young Women. Br Med J 1996;312:83—88.

3. Jick H, Jick SS, Gurewich V, Myers MW, Vasilakis C. Risk of idiopathic cardiovascular death and non-fatal venous thromboembolism in women using oral contraceptives with differing progestogen components. Lancet 1995;346:1589—1593.

4. Bloemenkamp KWM, Rosendaal FR, Hemerhorst FM, Buller HR, Vandenbroucke JP. Enhancement by factor V Leiden mutation of risk of deep-vein thrombosis associated with oral contraceptives containing a third-generation progestagen. Lancet 1995;346:1593—1596.

5. Lidegaard O. The influence of thrombotic risk factors when oral contraceptives are prescribed. A control only study. Acta Obstet Gynecol Scand 1997;76:252—260.

6. Farmer RDT, Lawrenson RA, Thompson CR, Kennedy JG, Hambleton IR. Population-based study of risk of venous thromboembolism associated with various oral contraceptives. Lancet 1997;349:83—88.

7. Farmer RDT, Lawrenson RA, Lewis MA et al. A German population-based study of risks of venous thromboembolism. BMJ (In press).

8. Suissa S, Blais L, Spitzer WO, Cusson M, Lewis S, Heinemann L. First-time use of newer oral contraceptives and the risk of venous thromboembolism. Contraception 1997;56:141—146.

9. Spitzer WO. The 1995 pill scare revisited: anatomy of a non-epidemic. Hum Reprod 1997;12: 2347—2357.

10. Bradford-Hill A. The environment and disease: association or causation. Proc Roy Soc Med 1965;58:295—300.

11. Spitzer WO, Suissa S, Ernst P, Horwitz RI, Habbick B, Cockcroft D, Boivin JF, McNutt M, Buist AS, Rebuck AS. The use of β-agonists and the risk of death and near death from asthma. N Engl J Med 1992;326:560—561.

12. Winkler UH, Schindler AE, Endrikat J, Dusterberg B. A comparative study of the effects of the hemostatic system of two monophasic gestodene oral contraceptives containing 20μg and 30μg ethinylestradiol. Contraception 1996;53:75—84.

13. Rosing J, Tans G, Nicolaes GAF et al. Oral contraceptives and venous thrombosis: different sensitivities to activated protein C in women using second- and third-generation oral contraceptives. Br J Haematol 1997;97:233—238.

14. Lewis MA, Heinemann LAJ, MacRae KD, Bruppacher R, Spitzer WO with the Transnational Research Group on Oral Contraceptives and the Health of Young Women. The increased risk of venous thromboembolism and the use of third-generation progestagens: role of bias in observational research. Contraception 1996;54:5—13.

# Emergency contraception: no longer the nation's best kept secret

Paul F.A. Van Look

*UNDP/UNFPA/WHO/World Bank Special Programme of Research, Development and Research Training in Human Reproduction, World Health Organization, Geneva, Switzerland*

**Abstract.** Emergency contraception, defined as "methods that women can use after intercourse to prevent pregnancy", has the potential to prevent tens of millions of unintended pregnancies throughout the world but, until a few years ago, this potential remained largely unknown and hence unrealized. A series of events during the last 3 to 4 years, however, is gradually lifting the veil off the "nation's best kept secret" in many countries around the world.

**Keywords:** intrauterine devices, levonorgestrel, mifepristone, oral contraceptives, postcoital contraception, Yuzpe regimen.

Multinational randomized clinical trials supported by our program have led to the development of two alternative hormonal regimens for emergency contraception. These two new approaches involve the use of either a single, low (10 mg) dose of the antiprogestogen mifepristone or two doses of 750 µg levonorgestrel taken 12 h apart. Both regimens are associated with significantly less nausea and vomiting as well as a reduced frequency of some other side effects compared to the current standard approach of giving an elevated dose of combined oral contraceptive pills (the Yuzpe regimen). Contraceptive efficacy of these new hormonal regimens may also be superior to the Yuzpe regimen.

Increasing efforts are being made by health and family planning organizations to bring emergency contraception into the mainstream of reproductive health care. These efforts include, among others, the issuance, by several organizations, of revised clinical guidelines that have removed all past contraindications to the use of emergency contraceptive pills, with the exception of pregnancy; the initiation of media campaigns in several countries to increase public awareness; the establishment of a multiagency Consortium for Emergency Contraception dedicated to identify, through model introductions and operations research, the specific "best practices" needed to broaden access to hormonal emergency contracep-

*Address for correspondence:* Paul F.A. Van Look, UNDP/UNFPA/WHO/World Bank Special Programme of Research, Development and Research Training in Human Reproduction, World Health Organization, 1211 Geneva 27, Switzerland.

***

[1]The views expressed in this paper are those of the author and do not necessarily represent those of the cosponsoring agencies and of the other governmental and nongovernmental agencies, organizations and foundations that support the UNDP/UNFPA/WHO/World Bank Special Programme of Research, Development and Research Training in Human Reproduction.

tives and the testing of innovative service delivery models such as prescribing by pharmacists on behalf of physicians.

## Introduction

In 1995, Hatcher et al. [1] published their popular book "Emergency Contraception: The Nation's Best Kept Secret". In it the authors describe the deplorable lack of knowledge and resulting infrequent use of emergency contraception, a method of contraception that, until that time, had remained very much in the shadows of reproductive health care, with its use restricted, in the USA like in many other countries, to rape victims and university health centers. Yet, calculations suggested that, in the USA alone, emergency contraception could potentially prevent up to 1.7 million unintended pregnancies, or nearly half of the estimated 3.5 million unplanned pregnancies that occur annually in that country [2]. In nearly all other countries in the world, a similar situation prevailed with the possible exception of The Netherlands and the UK.

In The Netherlands, emergency contraception was widely known and used, no doubt because of the influence of Ary Haspels who, together with Morris and van Wagenen [3,4], was the first to introduce in the 1960s the postcoital use of a high dose of estrogen for prevention of unwanted pregnancy in the human [5]. In the UK following publication of the Government's "Health of the Nation" paper in 1992 [6], countrywide efforts were initiated to increase awareness of emergency contraception among health care personnel and the general public, in particular young people, as one of the key strategies to lower the high teenage pregnancy rate. Promotion of emergency contraception was facilitated by the fact that the UK was one of the few industrialized countries where a dedicated product (PC4) was specifically registered since 1984 for use in emergency contraception. However, in the UK as well as in the other countries where this product was on the market (e.g., Germany, Finland, Norway, Sweden, New Zealand), the manufacturing company made little or no effort to inform prescribers and potential users about its availability. As a result of the government-sponsored campaign, however, both knowledge [7,8] and use became more widespread with the number of packets of PC4 sold in the UK rising to about 1 million in 1997. To this number must be added an unknown, but likely to be substantial, number of "home made" emergency contraceptive pill doses prepared by family planning providers and clinics through cutting up monthly strips of oral contraceptive pills with the appropriate ethinylestradiol/levonorgestrel (or dl-norgestrel) composition.

In developing countries, particularly in the People's Republic of China, a variety of progestogen-only containing pills, the so-called "visiting pills" or "vacation pills", are being used as a method of contraception by couples who are living apart for most of the year and can have intercourse only intermittently, during brief visiting spells and vacation periods [9]. In general, these pills are used on several successive days and this approach is not truly, therefore, a form of emergency contraception. Tablets of 750 µg levonorgestrel are marketed for "occasional" postcoital use in some 20 countries around the world under the trade name of Postinor® [10]. The recommended regimen of this preparation is to take one tablet as soon as possible after intercourse. In case of more than two successive acts of intercourse a second tablet must be taken 8 h later. For any given cycle the manufacturing company recommends that the total dose should not exceed four tablets. Although this regimen is not typically an emergency contraceptive regimen, and Postinor® was not registered in any country for this indication until very recently, the results of recent clinical trials described below indicate that this preparation can be used very effectively and with few side effects for this purpose.

In this paper I will review some of the important developments that have taken place during the last 2 to 3 years and which are gradually lifting the veil of the "nation's best kept secret". These developments have been grouped under two headings: 1) clinical advances, and 2) rising international interest. Greater detail on some of the issues discussed in this paper can be found in other reviews on emergency contraception recently written by the author [11–13].

## Clinical advances

At a Consensus Conference in April 1995 a group of experts defined emergency contraception as "methods that women can use after intercourse to prevent pregnancy" [14]. It is sometimes referred to as "morning-after" or "postcoital" contraception but these descriptions are somewhat misleading and their use should be avoided for two reasons. First, these terms do not accurately convey the correct timing of use. The currently used methods of hormonal emergency contraception need not be given the "morning-after" but are effective as long as treatment is commenced within 72 h of the act of unprotected intercourse, and a copper-releasing intrauterine device (IUD) can be inserted for up to 5 days after the calculated earliest day of ovulation [13]. Second, neither of the two terms, "morning-after" and "postcoital", convey the important message that emergency contraception should not be used regularly but that it is for emergency use only, as its name implies.

The origin of today's hormonal methods of emergency contraception can be traced back to the mid-1920s when it was demonstrated for the first time that ovarian extracts with estrogenic activity had an antifertility effect in several species of lower mammals. Human trials of postcoitally administered estrogen were initiated in the 1960s. The first users were rape victims who received 50 mg of the nonsteroidal estrogen, diethylstilbestrol (DES), for 4–6 days [3]. In a subsequent study the same workers gave a daily dose of 25–50 mg of DES or 0.5–2.0 mg of ethinylestradiol for 5 days to women volunteers following unprotected intercourse [4]. No pregnancies occurred in over 100 midcycle exposures. (Without information about the day of unprotected intercourse relative to the estimated day of ovulation, it is not possible to predict how many pregnancies would have occurred if no treatment had been given; a conservative estimate would be about 10 per 100 women.) Since the original two trials, many studies have confirmed the effectiveness of a high dose of estrogen given postcoitally in preventing unplanned pregnancy [15]. DES and ethinylestradiol have been used most frequently for this purpose, but other estrogens (oral and intravenous conjugated estrogen, intramuscular estradiol benzoate and estradiol phenylpropionate) have also been employed on occasion.

As one might expect, use of estrogen in the high doses recommended for emergency contraception is associated with a high incidence of unpleasant side effects, nausea and vomiting in particular. This, and the finding that DES administration during pregnancy can lead to vaginal adenosis and malignancy in the female offspring, as well as to other genital abnormalities in both male and female offspring, has led to an abandonment of high-dose estrogen in favor of the Yuzpe regimen.

The Yuzpe regimen, named after its inventor the Canadian gynecologist Albert Yuzpe, involved in its original form the administration of two oral contraceptive tablets each containing 50 µg ethinylestradiol and 500 µg dl-norgestrel followed, 12 h later, by a second dose of two such tablets [16,17]. Thus, the total doses of steroid given amounted to 200 µg ethinlyestradiol and 2 mg dl-norgestrel, the latter being equivalent to 1 mg of the biologically active enantiomer, levonorgestrel. Since several of the pill brands currently on the market have only about half the steroid hormone content of the pills used in the original Yuzpe regimen, they need to be given in double doses (twice four pills instead of twice two pills).

As is the case also for high-dose estrogen, it is generally recommended that, for maximum effectiveness, treatment with the Yuzpe regimen must start within 72 h of the act of unprotected intercourse (or within 72 h of the first act if there have been several). Under those conditions a review of published data indicated a pregnancy rate of 1.8% among 3,802 women [18]. An analysis of 10 published trials of the Yuzpe regimen, which included data on the cycle day of unprotected intercourse and thus permitted comparison of the observed and expected pregnancy rates, yielded an average effectiveness rate of 74%, i.e., the Yuzpe regimen prevents about three-quarters of the pregnancies that would occur without treatment [19]. Although this and a subsequent analysis of nine of the trials [20] did not indicate a declining effectiveness with increasing delay, within the 72-h window, between the time of unprotected intercourse and the start of treatment, and Grou and Rodrigues [21] have even suggested that the Yuzpe regimen may remain effective beyond 72 h, the data from our recent WHO trial described below do not support this proposition.

Although the Yuzpe regimen is associated with a somewhat reduced incidence of side effects compared to high-dose estrogen, nausea (about 50% of women) and vomiting (15−20% of women) remain common and this may affect compliance and, thus, efficacy of the regimen. For this reason, our program has been engaged for several years in the search for alternative treatments with equal or better efficacy but fewer side effects than the Yuzpe regimen. This research has resulted in two novel options, one of which is now being registered in several countries around the world. These new approaches involve the use of either a single dose of the antiprogestogen mifepristone or two doses of 750 μg levonorgestrel.

## Mifepristone

Our program started to investigate the potential of mifepristone for emergency contraception in 1989 following the reports that this antiprogestogen blocks ovulation when given in the days preceding ovulation and retards endometrial development when administered shortly after ovulation. Two randomized controlled trials were supported in the UK [22,23]; in both trials, a single dose of 600 mg of mifepristone was compared with the Yuzpe regimen when given within 72 h after unprotected coitus. Mifepristone proved to be more effective: in the two trials combined, three pregnancies were reported among 597 women who received mifepristone, in contrast to nine pregnancies among 589 women who received the Yuzpe regimen. In addition, women who used mifepristone had significantly less nausea and vomiting. However, they were more likely to have a delay in the onset of next menses, presumably because administration of mifepristone in the preovulatory phase blocked or delayed ovulation [24]. Such delay can worry women already fearful of an unintended pregnancy. Also, delayed ovulation means conception risk later in this prolonged cycle if no contraception is used; in fact, in one of the above-mentioned two trials the three pregnant women were reported to have conceived 10−15 days after mifepristone treatment [23].

The results from these two studies clearly suggested that mifepristone has potential for use in emergency contraception. However, the dose of 600 mg employed would not be practical for at least two reasons. First, this dose can be used to induce abortion and hence would not be acceptable in countries with restrictive abortion legislation. Second, this high dose would be too expensive for routine use. Results from studies on the mechanisms of action of mifepristone suggest that, in fact, much lower doses of mifepristone than 600 mg may confer protection against pregnancy when used for emergency contraception [25]. To test this assumption our program recently completed a multicenter, randomized controlled trial to compare the efficacy and side effects, including the timing of the subsequent menstrual period, of single doses of 600, 50 and 10 mg of mifepristone when the treatment was given within 120 h (5 days) of unprotected coitus [26].

The trial was conducted in 11 family planning clinics in Australia, China, Finland, Georgia, the UK and the USA. It included 1,717 healthy women with regular menstrual cycles who were randomly assigned to the three different treatment groups (600, 50 and 10 mg). Thirty-two women (1.9%) were lost to follow up and excluded from the analysis.

Baseline characteristics of the women assigned to the three treatment groups

322

were similar (Table 1). Between 26 and 31% of women had previously used emergency contraception and 56—58% gave condom failure as the reason for requesting emergency contraception on this occasion. The number of pregnancies was similar among women receiving 10, 50 and 600 mg of mifepristone with pregnancy rates of 1.2, 1.3 and 1.3%, respectively (Table 2). Expressed in terms of the proportion of expected pregnancies prevented, the three doses had effectiveness rates of 82, 80 and 81%, respectively. Two of the observed pregnancies (both in the 50-mg group) were tubal pregnancies. No major side effects occurred during the study, except a delay in the onset of next menses which was significantly related to dosage: the higher the mifepristone dose, the longer the mean delay to resumption of menses. Also, women receiving the higher dose were more likely to experience vaginal bleeding within the first 5 days of drug administration. In view of these favorable findings a new multicenter trial has been initiated by our program to compare the 10-mg dose of mifepristone with the levonorgestrel regimen described below.

*Levonorgestrel*

As mentioned earlier, levonorgestrel is marketed in a number of countries for "occasional postcoital contraception" in packs containing 750 µg tablets. A previous study supported by our program in Hong Kong tested the efficacy and side effects of these tablets as an alternative hormonal emergency contraceptive [27]. The tablets were compared with the Yuzpe regimen in a randomized controlled trial involving women requesting emergency contraception within 48 h after unprotected coitus. Women assigned to levonorgestrel took 750 µg and a repeat dose of 750 µg 12 h later. Among the 834 who started treatment, the pregnancy rate with the Yuzpe regimen was 3.5% compared with 2.9% in the levonorgestrel group. After exclusion of women with further acts of intercourse in the cycle, the pregnancy rates were 2.7% (95% CI 1.0—4.1%) and 2.4% (95% CI 0.8—4.1%), respectively. In addition, the incidence of vomiting with levonorgestrel was much lower (2.7 vs. 22.4%), a highly significant and clinically important difference. In view of these promising results in a single center, our program recently conducted a larger multicenter trial to compare the regimens when

*Table 1.* Selected characteristics of participants in three-dose study of mifepristone.

| Characteristic | Treatment group | | |
|---|---|---|---|
| | 10 mg (n = 565) | 50 mg (n = 561) | 600 mg (n = 559) |
| Previous use of emergency contraception | 31.0% | 26.6% | 25.9% |
| Reason for requesting emergency contraception | | | |
| - no method use | 40.9% | 40.6% | 40.8% |
| - condom failure | 56.8% | 58.1% | 55.6% |
| - other contraceptive failure | 2.3% | 1.3% | 3.6% |

*Table 2.* Pregnancy rates by treatment group in three-dose study of mifepristone.

| Group | No. of subjects | Observed pregnancies | | |
|---|---|---|---|---|
| | | No. of cases | Rate (%) | 95% CI |
| 10 mg | 565 | 7 | 1.24 | 0.50−2.54 |
| 50 mg | 561 | 7 | 1.25 | 0.50−2.55 |
| 600 mg | 559 | 7 | 1.25 | 0.50−2.56 |
| Total | 1685 | 21 | 1.25 | 0.77−1.90 |

started within 72 h of unprotected coitus [28].

This double-blind, randomized, controlled trial recruited 1,998 women at 21 centers around the world; outcome was unknown for 43 women (2.2%), most of whom (39) were lost to follow up. The randomization produced similar baseline characteristics of women in both treatment groups (Table 3). About one-fifth had used emergency contraception in the past and somewhat less than half of the women sought treatment because of barrier method failure. Nearly half of the women in each group started treatment within 24 h, and somewhat more than 80% within 48 h, of unprotected coitus.

The pregnancy rate among women who received the Yuzpe regimen (31/979) was 3.2% (95% CI 2.2−4.5%), in contrast to 1.1% (11/976; 95% CI 0.6−2.0%) among those who received levonorgestrel. Expressed in terms of the proportion of expected pregnancies prevented, the effectiveness rates were 57 and 85% for the Yuzpe regimen and levonorgestrel, respectively. Nausea, vomiting, dizziness and fatigue were significantly less frequent among women in the levonorgestrel group (Table 4), and the efficacy of both treatments declined with increasing time since unprotected coitus (p = 0.01).

Thus, both the earlier trial by Ho and Kwan [27] and this new study have found levonorgestrel to be superior in side-effect profile to the Yuzpe regimen, the current standard for emergency contraception. The efficacy of levonorgestrel also

*Table 3.* Selected characteristics of participants in trial of Yuzpe regimen versus levonorgestrel.

| Characteristic | Treatment group | |
|---|---|---|
| | Yuzpe regimen (n = 979) | Levonorgestrel (n = 976) |
| Prior use of emergency contraception | 23.2% | 20.8% |
| Barrier method failure prompting enrollment | 44.0% | 43.5% |
| Delay of treatment (h) | | |
| ⩽24 | 46.9% | 46.1% |
| 25−48 | 37.8% | 34.7% |
| 49−72 | 15.1% | 19.0% |
| >72 | 0.2% | 0.2% |

324

*Table 4.* Side effects by treatment group in trial of Yuzpe regimen vs. levonorgestrel.

| Side effect | Treatment group | |
|---|---|---|
| | Yuzpe regimen (n = 979) | Levonorgestrel (n = 977) |
| Nausea[a] | 50.5% | 23.1% |
| Vomiting[a] | 18.8% | 5.6% |
| Dizziness[a] | 16.7% | 11.2% |
| Fatigue[a] | 28.5% | 16.9% |
| Headache | 20.2% | 16.8% |
| Breast tenderness | 12.1% | 10.8% |
| Low abdominal pain | 20.9% | 17.6% |
| All other complaints[b] | 16.7% | 13.5% |

[a]$p \leqslant 0.01$; [b]mostly diarrhoea and some irregular bleeding or spotting.

appears greater. A comparative trial of levonorgestrel and the 10-mg dose of mifepristone is currently under way.

**Rising international interest**

Within the last 3 to 4 years many health and family planning organizations have undertaken efforts to bring emergency contraception into the mainstream of reproductive health care [11].

For instance, in October 1994, the International Medical Advisory Panel of the International Planned Parenthood Federation issued substantially liberalized guidelines [29] designed to make emergency contraceptive pills more easily accessible through "the most practical delivery systems" and to remove virtually all contraindications for their use. The nearly complete lifting of contraindications was prompted by WHO's review of medical eligibility criteria for contraceptive use which concluded that there are no absolute medical contraindications to the use of the Yuzpe regimen with the exception of pregnancy [30]. In this last situation, emergency contraceptive pills should not be used, not because they are thought to be harmful to either the mother or the early pregnancy, but because they are no longer effective.

Second, in April 1995, experts from around the world meeting in Bellagio (Italy) produced a "Consensus Statement on Emergency Contraception", which calls on family planning providers to educate themselves about the regimens and to ensure that women everywhere "have access to these safe and effective ways to prevent unwanted pregnancy" [14]. The experts recommended, among other things, that emergency contraceptives be added to essential drug lists, a recommendation acted upon in December 1995 by the WHO Expert Committee on the Use of Essential Drugs [31].

Third, to test new strategies for expanding knowledge and appropriate use of emergency contraceptive pills and to work with industry to make dedicated products widely available at reasonable cost, seven major organizations established, in late 1995, the Consortium for Emergency Contraception. The member organizations of the Consortium are the Concept Foundation, the International Planned Parenthood Federation, the Pacific Institute for Women's Health, Pathfinder International, the Population Council, the Program for Appropriate Technology in Health, and our program at WHO. The Consortium's goal is to identify, through model introductions and operations research, the specific "best practices" needed to broaden access to hormonal emergency contraceptives while ensuring their safe and appropriate use. Model introduction programs sponsored by the Consortium are currently under way in four countries (Indonesia, Kenya, Mexico and Sri Lanka) and, depending upon the availability of funds, similar programs will be initiated in a further 10–12 countries. Introduction of emergency contraception into national programs is also being undertaken by our program, independent of the Consortium, in South Africa and Zambia.

Fourth, as a result of the research supported by our program on the use of levonorgestrel in emergency contraception, the manufacturers of Postinor® are now producing Postinor-2®, a two-pill pack of 750 µg levonorgestrel tablets. This new preparation is being used by the Consortium for Emergency Contraception in its introductory programs and, at the time of writing, has been formally registered in Hungary, Kenya and Sri Lanka. An application for marketing of this product in the USA is being considered by the US Food and Drug Administration (USFDA).

Fifth, national campaigns have been launched in several countries (e.g., the UK, Sweden, USA) to educate women and providers about emergency contraception. In the USA, an Emergency Contraception Hotline was launched on Valentine's Day 1996. The toll-free Hotline provides callers with information about methods of emergency contraception and offers a list of health care providers in each caller's area who can prescribe emergency contraception. Information about emergency contraception and the more than 2,000 practitioners across the USA who are providing it can also be found on the World Wide Webb (http://opr.princeton.edu/ec/). More recently, a pilot project was started in the state of Washington in which specially trained pharmacists can directly supply emergency contraceptive pills through a collaborative drug therapy agreement. The agreement, which includes a "prescribing protocol", is signed between the pharmacist and a health care provider with independent prescribing authority such as a physician, and serves to delegate prescribing authority to the pharmacist. The success of this pilot project in the USA has given new impetus to the debate in the UK about the introduction of a similar scheme of distribution by pharmacists.

Sixth, in June 1996, an Advisory Committee of the USFDA, on an unusual initiative, declared the Yuzpe method safe and effective and urged its wider availability. This action should facilitate approval of a Yuzpe-type preparation in the USA. In early 1997, a newly established company announced its intention to apply to the USFDA for registration of such a product. However, it would appear that this has not yet happened and, as described earlier, approval for marketing of a Yuzpe-type product may be overtaken by registration of levonorgestrel. Registration of a drug or device in the USA is required before government agencies such as the US Agency for International Development can supply them to developing countries.

Finally, the American College of Obstetricians and Gynecologists (ACOG) issued, in October 1996, Practice Patterns on Emergency Contraception. A revised version was published in December 1996 [32]. Because ACOG issues Practice Patterns so infrequently, these guidelines are highly influential and serve to mainstream new and innovative medical practices. Also, in its clinical standards and guidelines, the Planned Parenthood Federation of America now includes advance provision of emergency contraceptive pills for later use (adopted in 1996) or, for established clients, prescription given over the telephone (adopted in 1997). Family planning clinics in the federally funded Title X programme received explicit authorization to provide emergency contraceptive treatment in April 1997 [33]. All these new developments provide further encouragement for health care professionals in the USA to prescribe emergency contraception.

**Conclusion**

Unplanned pregnancies occur — and will continue to occur — irrespective of the quality and accessibility of family planning services, the prevalence of contraceptive use, and the degree of motivation of contraceptive users to avoid such pregnancies. In some instances these pregnancies are entirely unexpected, such as when a woman conceives with an intrauterine device in situ or following sterilization. Many unintended pregnancies in contraceptive users, however, are due to a failure of the contraceptive method in use that was recognized at the time when it occurred. Typical examples of such situations include the breakage or slippage of a condom, or displacement of a diaphragm, during intercourse; or failed coitus interruptus with ejaculation in the vagina or on the external genitalia. In these instances, as well as in all situations in which sexual intercourse took place without using any method of family planning, emergency contraception offers a last chance, secondary method of contraception to avoid unplanned pregnancy.

Given that current hormonal methods of emergency contraception rely on technology that has been available for some 30 years, family planning programs and practitioners not yet offering this effective means of preventing unplanned pregnancy should seriously consider doing so.

**References**

1. Hatcher RA, Trussell J, Stewart F, Howell S, Russell CR, Kowal D. Emergency contraception: the nation's best kept secret. Decatur GA: Bridging the Gap Communications, 1995.

2. Trussell J, Stewart F, Guest F, Hatcher RA. Emergency contraceptive pills: a simple proposal to reduce unintended pregnancies. Fam Plan Perspect 1992;24:269—273.

3. Morris JMCL, van Wagenen G. Compounds interfering with ovum implantation and development. III. Role of estrogens. Am J Obstet Gynecol 1966;96:804—815.

4. Morris JMcL, van Wagenen G. Postcoital oral contraception. In: Hankinson RKB, Kleinman RL, Eckstein P, Romero H (eds) Proceedings of the Eight International Conference of the International Planned Parenthood Federation 1967;256—259.

5. Haspels AA. Interception: postcoital estrogens in 3016 women. Contraception 1976;14: 375—381.

6. Anonymous. Health of the Nation. London: HM Stationery Office, 1992.

7. Graham A, Green L, Glasier AF. Teenagers' knowledge of emergency contraception: questionnaire survey in southeast Scotland. Br Med J 1996;312:1567—1569.

8. Smith BH, Gurney EM, Aboulela L, Templeton A. Emergency contraception: a survey of women's knowledge and attitudes. Br J Obstet Gynecol 1996;103:1109—1116.

9. Prasad MRN. Postcoital agents and menses-inducers. In: Diczfalusy E, Diczfalusy A (eds) Research on the Regulation of Human Fertility. Needs of Developing Countries and Priorities for the Future. Copenhagen: Scriptor, 1983;678—711.

10. Task Force on Postovulatory Methods for Fertility Regulation. Postcoital contraception with levonorgestrel during the periovulatory phase of the menstrual cycle. Contraception 1987; 36:275—286.

11. Van Look PFA. Emergency contraception: a brighter future? In: Ottesen B, Tabor A (eds) New Insights in Gynecology and Obstetrics. Research and Practice. Carnforth: The Parthenon Publishing Group Ltd., 1998;174—183.

12. Van Look PFA, Stewart FH. Emergency contraception. In: Hatcher RA, Trussell J, Stewart F, Stewart GK, Kowal D, Guest F, Cates W Jr (eds) Contraceptive Technology, 17th revised edn. New York, NY: Irvington Publishers, 1998;(In press).

13. Van Look PFA. Emergency contraception: the Cinderella of family planning. In: Rodriguez O, Hedon B, Daya S (eds) Clinical Infertility and Contraception. Carnforth: The Parthenon Publishing Group Ltd., 1998;(In press).

14. Anonymous. Consensus statement on emergency contraception. Contraception 1995;52: 211—213.

15. Van Look PFA. Postcoital contraception: a cover-up story. In: Diczfalusy E, Bygdeman M (eds) Fertility Regulation Today and Tomorrow. New York, NY: Serono Symposia Publications from Raven Press, 1987;29—42.

16. Yuzpe AA, Lancee WJ. Ethinyl-estradiol and dl-norgestrel as a postcoital contraceptive. Fertil Steril 1977;28:932—936.

17. Yuzpe AA, Smith RP, Rademaker AW. A multicenter clinical investigation employing ethinylestradiol combined with dl-norgestrel as a postcoital contraceptive agent. Fertil Steril 1982; 37:508—513.

18. Fasoli M, Parazzini F, Cecchetti G, La Vecchia C. Postcoital contraception: an overview of published studies. Contraception 1989;39:459—468,699—700.

19. Trussell J, Ellertson C, Stewart F. The effectiveness of the Yuzpe regimen of emergency contraception. Fam Plan Perspect 1996;28:58—64,87.

20. Trussell J, Ellertson C, Rodriguez G. The Yuzpe regimen of emergency contraception: how long after the morning after? Obstet Gynecol 1996;88:150—154.

21. Grou F, Rodrigues I. The morning-after pill — how long after? Am J Obstet Gynecol 1994;171: 1529—1534.

22. Glasier A, Thong KJ, Dewar M, Mackie M, Baird DT. Mifepristone compared with high-dose estrogen and progestogen for emergency postcoital contraception. N Engl J Med 1992;327: 1041—1044.

23. Webb AMC, Russell J, Elstein M. Comparison of Yuzpe regimen, danazol, and mifepristone (RU 486) in oral postcoital contraception. Br Med J 1992;305:927—931.

328

24. Liu JH, Garzo G, Morris S, Stuenkel C, Ulmann A, Yen SSC. Disruption of follicular maturation and delay of ovulation after administration of the antiprogesterone RU 486. J Clin Endocrinol Metab 1987;65:1135—1140.
25. von Hertzen H, Van Look PFA. Research on new methods of emergency contraception. Int Fam Plan Perspect 1996;22:62—68.
26. Task Force on Postovulatory Methods of Fertility Regulation. A randomized controlled trial comparing three single doses of mifepristone in emergency contraception. Lancet 1998 (Submitted).
27. Ho PC, Kwan MSW. A prospective randomized comparison of levonorgestrel with the Yuzpe regimen in postcoital contraception. Hum Reprod 1993;8:389—392.
28. Task Force on Postovulatory Methods of Fertility Regulation. Levonorgestrel versus the Yuzpe regimen of combined oral contraceptives for emergency contraception: a randomized controlled trial. Lancet 1998;(In press).
29. International Planned Parenthood Federation. Statement on Emergency Contraception. London: International Planned Parenthood Federation, 1994.
30. World Health Organization. Improving access to quality care in family planning. Medical eligibility criteria for contraceptive use, Document. WHO/FRH/FPP/96.9. Geneva: World Health Organization, 1996.
31. World Health Organization. The use of essential drugs. Seventh report of the WHO expert committee (including the revised model list of essential drugs), WHO technical report series 867. Geneva: Word Health Organization, 1997.
32. American College of Obstetricians and Gynecologists. Emergency Oral Contraception. ACOG Practice Patterns. Washington DC: The American College of Obstetricians and Gynecologists, 1996.
33. Kring T. OPA Program Instruction Series, OPA 97—2: Emergency Contraception, 23 April 1997 (memorandum).

# Reproductive surgery in the female

# Laparoscopic surgery to enhance fertility

Guillermo Marconi

*Instituto de Ginecología y Fertilidad (IFER) Buenos Aires, Argentina*

**Abstract.** Laparoscopic surgery can improve fertility as a primary treatment of tuboperitonial factor. To achieve best results, the same criteria that govern microsurgery must be followed: adequate training, correct technique and patient selection. The tube can be damaged by different organisms, compromising cell vitality. Alteration of cell membrane allows passage of certain anilines, which can color the nucleus. A total of 310 tubes from 163 patients who underwent a surgical or diagnostic laparoscopy during fertility studies were analysed by salpingoscopy. A previous injection of 20 ml of a 10% solution of methylene blue in saline was used to dye cellular nuclei. The evaluation of nuclear staining with methylene blue, adhesions, vascular alterations and flattening of folds in relation to pregnancy achievement was performed. Quantification of salpingoscopic findings was carried out according to a score. Flattening of folds and vascular alterations yielded no difference in the pregnant and nonpregnant group. On the other hand, adhesions and nuclear staining were significantly greater in the nonpregnant group. Methylene blue staining is a new tool to evaluate in vivo the cytohistological tubal damage, and is a helpful method to determine the prognoses for tubal function.

**Keywords:** stained nuclei, fertility, salpingoscopy.

The idea of increasing fertility by means of laparoscopic surgery can be considered from different points of view: 1) the sequelae that the technique can leave behind, which can affect fertility, or 2) as a primary treatment of tuboperitoneal adhesions of endometriotic, iatrogenic or infectious origin.

We will focus our interest on laparoscopic surgery as a therapeutic technique in tuboperitoneal factor of postsurgical or infectious origin. We will not include endometriosis, which will be discussed in other lectures in the congress.

In most cases, treatment of tuboperitoneal factor is undoubtedly surgical. Tulandi et al. in 1990 [1] confirmed the efficiency of surgical treatment in the pathology of this factor. He analyzed 147 patients with tuboperitoneal factor. Sixty-nine of them underwent surgery, and the rest were not treated. He observed a global pregnancy rate of 59.4% in treated patients vs. 15.4% in the nontreated group. The cumulative pregnancy rate at 12 and 24 months follow-up was 32 and 45% in the treated group and 11 and 16% in the nontreated group, respectively. The degree of adhesions in women who conceived was milder than in those who did not conceive, whether treated or not.

*Address for correspondence:* Guillermo Marconi MD, Instituto de Ginecología y Fertilkidad, Marcelo T. De Alvear 2259, 7mo. Pisa (1122) Buenos Aires, Argentina. Fax: +54-1-821-1130.
E-mail: gmarconi@intramed.net.ar

*Table 1.* Distribution of women with pregnancies after tubal surgery. (Adapted from [2].)

| Hydrosalpinx | Grade I | Grade II | Grade III | Grade IV |
|---|---|---|---|---|
| No. | 100 | 109 | 64 | 18 |
| % Full-term pregnancies | 33 | 22 | 7.8 | 5.6 |

The importance of surgical treatment is well reflected in the article of Winston and Margara [2]. They describe an overall pregnancy rate of 33% in hydrosalpinx, when tubal lesions were mild (Table 1). They show that surgical correction of tubal pathology is definite, and therefore in properly selected patients using an adequate microsurgical technique, treatment by salpingostomy yields better results than multiple cycles of in vitro fertilization.

Nevertheless surgery is not useful with tubal blockages in which the possibility of reconstruction is very low, and relapses of pelvic infection high. Neither can it be applied in hydrosalpinx with pachysalpingitis, or in proximal tubal obstructions in which the endosalpinx is severely damaged.

In the 1960s, microsurgery became the treatment selected for tuboperitoneal disease, providing fundamental data regarding the pathology of surgical gynecology. It emphasized the importance of adequate treatment and care of the female pelvis during the surgery, whether patients were sterile or not. It became clear that an inadequate technique could cause adhesions, and sterility might ensue. On the other hand it emphasized a conservative approach to surgery. Total extirpations were techniques of the past, and the new motto of meticulous surgeries was the conservation of organs. As Gomel suggests [3], more than a surgical technique it became a "surgical philosophy".

Microsurgery can be performed by laparotomy or by laparoscopy. Laparoscopic surgery began to be frequently used in gynecological treatment in the late 80s, even though in the late 70s and early 80s some publications can be found [4,5]. As with every new technique, it had followers and opponents. The benefits of one technique over another was for a long time a matter of extensive debate, it seems nowadays that global results are similar using laparotomy or laparoscopy (Tables 2 and 3). Selection of technique will depend on the expertise of each surgeon, keeping in mind that the beneficiary is the patient. Rock and Moutos [7] suggest that nowadays there is considerable pressure on physicians, by both patients and peers, to perform gynecological procedures endoscopically.

Is there any unique type of laparoscopic surgery that enhances fertility? Decidedly not. In order to be considered an efficacious technique surgical laparoscopy must meet certain criteria, which have been held in microsurgery for more than 30 years in relation to: 1) surgical training, 2) surgical technique, and 3) selection of pathology.

*Table 2.* Overall pregnancy rate comparing both techniques. (Adapted from [6].)

|  | Laparotomy (59) | Laparosopy (22) |
|---|---|---|
| Full-term pregnancy | 21 (36%) | 7 (32%) |
| Ectopic pregnancy | 3 (5%) | 2 (9%) |

## Surgical training

The fact that all gynecological surgeons perform diagnostic endoscopy does not necessarily qualify them to perform operative endoscopy. Experience can be obtained through formal training during residency, postgraduate educational programs, and preceptorships with experienced endoscopists, or fellowships in either reproductive endocrinology or reproductive surgery [7]. In a recent workshop held in Buenos Aires, Liu [8] claimed that only 25% of the surgeons who start their training in endoscopic surgery attain a degree of excellence.

Once a physician has been credentialed in endoscopic surgery, there should be a system to monitor his or her performance periodically [7]. This should be done by the professional societies that grant credentials. It must be borne in mind that the percentage of complications decreases with increasing expertise, and that the most severe complications occur at the beginning of training.

## Surgical technique

We will emphasize the importance of instrumentation. It is not necessary to purchase every endoscopic equipment in the commercial stands, only adequate instrumentation. Good scissors, correct forceps, appropriate coagulation systems, are all indispensable. This means not more than a dozen instruments.

If we analyze results of most authors (Tables 4 and 5), there does not seem to be any differences in overall pregnancy rate whether the surgeon uses scissors, monopolar current, or lasers. In Table 6 we have summarized the relevant published data.

## Selection of pathology

Success in medical practice implies that a precise diagnosis must be achieved in order to apply the correct treatment. In surgical treatment of tuboperitoneal

*Table 3.* Cumulative pregnancy rate. (Adapted from [6].)

|  | Laparotomy | Laparoscopy |
|---|---|---|
| 12 months | 36% | 57% |
| 24 months | 40% | 57% |

*Table 4.* Results of pregnancy rate in laparoscopy according to different techniques.

| Author | Technique | No. | % Pregnancies |
|---|---|---|---|
| Mettler (1997) | S/TC | 44 | 29 |
| Madalenat (1979) | S | 144 | 24 |
| Mintz (1979) | S | 65 | 37 |
| Gomel (1983) | S | 92 | ·62 |
| Fayez (1983) | S | 50 | 56 |
| Bruhat (1983) | S/EC | 93 | 52 |
| Reich (1987) | S/EC | 27 | 81 |
| Serour (1989) | S/EC | 25 | 12 |
| Donnez (1989) | $CO_2L$ | 186 | 58 |
| Marconi (1996) | S/TC/EC | 191 | 52 |

S: scissors, TC: endocoagulation, EC: electrocoagulation, L: laser.

pathology, experience and expertise is important not only in relation to the surgeon and the technique to be applied, but also in the analysis and evaluation of the pathological findings. A mistake in data interpretation of complementary studies is also a failure.

Diagnostic hysterosalpingography and laparoscopy are still in use. But in spite of their intrinsic value both evaluate only patency and integrity of tubal mucosa, however, functionality is beyond these studies.

With the introduction of salpingoscopy in Fallopian tube evaluation a new aspect is introduced: the morphology of intratubal components. Many authors suggest that salpingoscopy should be routinely performed when studying the tubal factor [9—14].

The endosalpingeal alterations most frequently described are related to the trophism of folds of the mucosa, to the presence of adhesions which occlude the lumen of the tube or folds, and to alterations in salpingeal vascularization. The presence in the endosalpinx of nuclei stained with methylene blue has also been mentioned as of potential prognostic value in evaluating the physiology or the organ [9].

Taking into consideration the degree and type of alteration of the components of the endosalpinx, different classifications have been suggested to quantify and interpret lesions from the anatomical point of view. Unfortunately none of them

*Table 5.* Results of salpingostomies using surgical laparoscopies.

| Author (year) | Technique | No. | % Pregnancies |
|---|---|---|---|
| Mettler (1979) | S/TC | 36 | 26 |
| Gomel (1983) | S | 9 | 44.4 |
| Fayez (1983) | S | 19 | 10 |
| Donnez (1989) | $CO_2/L$ | 25 | 20 |
| Daniel (1989) | $CO_2/L$ | 21 | 24 |
| Marconie (1996) | S/TC/EC | 101 | 28 |

S: scissors, TC: endocoagulation, EC: electrocoagulation, L: laser.

evaluate tubal physiology [15—17].

In such classifications, nuclear staining is not considered, and as this parameter is important in evaluating the vitality of tubal cells, a new system of classification has been devised in order to quantify salpingoscopic findings (Table 6). A score of one to four was applied to quantify the intensity of each type of pathology: flattening of folds, adhesions, nuclear staining and vascular alterations. One corresponded to absence of a lesion and four to maximal intensity. Therefore a normal tube would have a score of four, and a severely damaged one would add to a score of 16.

*Results of different scores (considering both oviducts) were grouped into three categories*

- Type A epithelium: score between eight and 10. Normal tubes, or tubes with only one parameter mildly affected.
- Type B epithelium: score between 11 and 17. Tubes are not normal, and pathology is generally combined.
- Type C epithelium: score between 18 and 32. Severe damage or destruction of the endosalpinx.

Using salpingoscopy we evaluated 310 tubes from 163 patients who had to undergo a surgical or diagnostic laparoscopy during fertility evaluations. The rigid optic of the colpomicrohisterocope (R. Wolff, GMBH, Knittligen, Germany) was used. It was inserted in the abdominal cavity through a second laparoscopic via. Methodology as well as morphological results have been previously described [9].

Before salpingoscopy, 20 ml of a 10% solution of methylene blue in saline solution (NaCl 10%) was injected through the cervical cannula. Through the same via 50 ml of saline solution was subsequently injected in order to wash away exceeding dye and achieve a better vision.

When introducing the optic into the tube through the fimbrial ostium, in some

*Table 6.* Classification in salpingoscopy.

| Score | Folds | Adhesions | Nuclear staining | Vascular alterations |
|---|---|---|---|---|
| 1 | Free, flexus, trophic | Absent | Absent | Absent |
| 2 | Mild flattening | Few; no compromise of tubal lumen. | Some isolated nuclei, 25% of the mucosa is stained. | Altered morphology (approximately 25%). |
| 3 | Marked flattening, rigidity. Folds can be absent in some areas. | Moderate compromise of lumen, greater consistency and size of adhesions. | Greater concentration of stained nuclei (25—50% of the mucosa). | Altered vessels (50% or more). Areas with vessels of neoformation. |
| 4 | Absent | Great compromise of tubal lumen. | Very high concentration. Greater than 50% of the mucosa stained. | Scarce and thin capillaries in the tubal wall. Vessels of neoformation in the whole tube. |

patients intense blue dotting could be observed. Increasing the magnifying power it could be assessed that dotting corresponded to staining of cell nuclei. Stained nuclei were evenly aligned along the edge of the endosalpingeal major folds probably indicating coloring of tubal cells. Dispersed inflammatory cells (such as lymphocytes) with great affinity for vital dyes could also be observed.

Of the 163 patients, 107 had a type A epithelium, 43 had type B and 13 type C. Forty patients presented a normal laparoscopy. Of these, 92.5% of them had a type A epithelium and 7.5% type B. Similarly of the 33 patients with endometriosis, 93.9% were type A and 6.1% type B.

Sixty patients (36.8%) had an altered peritoneal factor. Of these, 50% belonged to type A epithelium, 38.3% to type B, and 1.7% to type C. And in 30 patients with damaged tubes, 30% were type A, 50% type B and 20% type C. Differences between tubal mucosa pertaining to normal laparoscopies and the endometriotic group with those who had infectious alterations in their tubes or peritoneum were highly significant ($p < 0.01$) (Table 7)

Sixty-seven patients became pregnant (41.1%). Of these pregnancies 74.6% (50) belonged to group A, 23.9% (16) to group B and 1.4% to group C. Analysis of tubal damage was performed taking into consideration the total score. The average score of tubes of patients who got pregnant was 9.7 ± 3.9 and of those who did not 12.1 ± 6.3 ($p < 0.0001$) (Table 8).

If we analyzed tubal damage per tube in pregnant patients, scores were 5.1 ± 1.7 and 5.1 ± 2.5 for the left and right tubes, respectively. In the not pregnant group scores were 6.1 ± 3.1 and 6.0 ± 3.3, respectively, for left and right tubes. There were no significant differences between tubes within groups, but the differences between pregnant and nonpregnant patients were highly significant ($p = 0.02$).

In order to better evaluate tubal damage, data were regrouped into healthy tubes or less damaged tubes in one column and, in the other column, the contralateral more severely damaged tube. Results are presented in Table 9 and show that pregnant patients had a score of 4.6 ± 1.0 and 5.9 ± 2.6 (healthier vs. more damaged tube $p < 0.001$), while in the nonpregnant group the difference was not significant (5.8 ± 3.1 and 6.4 ± 3.3). There was no significant difference in the more damaged tube between the pregnant and nonpregnant group.

*Table 7.* Laparscopic diagnosis and epithelium types.

| Epithelium | Laparoscopies | | | |
| --- | --- | --- | --- | --- |
| | Normal[a] n: 40 (24.5%) | Endometriosis[b] n: 33 (20.2%) | Peritoneal factor[c] n: 60 ( 36.8%) | Tubal factor[d] n: 30 (18. 4%) |
| Type A | 92.5% | 93.9% | 50% | 30% |
| Type B | 7.5% | 6.1% | 38.3% | 50% |
| Type C | – | – | 11.7% | 20% |

[a,b] vs. [c,d] $p < 0.001$.

*Table 8.* Global results.

| | Pregnant | Not pregnant |
|---|---|---|
| Patients | 67 | 96 |
| Tubes | 129 | 181 |
| Score | 9.7 ± 3.9 | 12.1 ± 6.3[a] |

[a]$p < 0.0001$.

It can be observed that in less damaged tubes in the pregnant group, the pathology was mild (score 5.9 ± 2.6). This score was significantly different from contralateral tubes and both tubes in the nonpregnant group. Therefore, these results suggest that a patient with at least one healthy or mildly damaged tube can achieve pregnancy successfully.

Analysis of frequency of altered patterns of salpingoscopic pathology revealed that flattening of folds and vascular alterations were not different between groups (31.3 and 20% in the pregnant group and 37.5 and 21.7% in the nonpregnant group). On the other hand, the presence of adhesions and nuclear staining were significantly greater in the nonpregnant group (adhesions 13.6 vs. 26.8% $p < 0.004$, and nuclear staining: 25.0 vs. 41.7% $p < 0.009$, pregnant vs. nonpregnant) (Table 10).

Different degrees of nuclear density could be observed, from isolated to highly concentrated nuclei, which occupied most of the mucosa. Lower concentrations of nuclear coloring and percentage of stained epithelium in pregnant and nonpregnant patients was reflected in the scores for these parameters which were 1.6 ± 0.8 and 2.2 ± 1.14, respectively ($p = 0.02$).

Differences in the presence of adhesions and nuclear staining were also found when tubes were grouped according to laparoscopic diagnosis. In normal or endometriotic laparoscopies, the score was 2.0 ± 0.7 and 1.9 ± 0.2 for adhesions, and 2.1 ± 0.6 and 2.2 ± 0.7 for nuclear staining, respectively. In peritoneal factors and tubal obstructions, the score was 3.1 ± 1.9 and 3.1 ± 2 for adhesions and 3.9 ± 2.3 and 4.2 ± 2 for staining, respectively. Normal and endometriotic groups were not different, whereas scores in normal laparoscopies vs. peritoneal and tubal factors were significantly different ($p < 0.002$ and $p < 0.0001$ for adhe-

*Table 9.* Results grouped according to the degree of tubal pathology.

| | Pregnant | | Not pregnant | |
|---|---|---|---|---|
| | Less damaged tube[a] n: 65 | More damaged tube[b] n: 64 | Less damaged tube[c] n: 97 | More damaged tube[d] n: 84 |
| Score | 4.6 ± 1 | 5.9 ± 2.6 | 5.8 ± 3.1 | 6.4 ± 3.3 |

[a,b]$p < 0.001$; [a,c]$p < 0.003$.

*Table 10.* Frequency of different pathologies.

|  | Flattening of folds | Adhesions | Vascular alterations | Nuclear staining |
|---|---|---|---|---|
| Pregnant | 31.3% | 13.6% | 20.8% | 25.0% |
| Not pregnant | 37.5% | 26.8% | 21.7% | 41.7% |
|  | n.s. | $p < 0.004$ | n.s. | $p < 0.009$ |

sions and staining, respectively) (Table 11).

The tube can be damaged by different organisms, and infections represent the most severe injuries, leaving behind sequelae with a poor prognostic. Infections attack the functionality of cells [18—20] acting on four ultrastructural systems which are fundamental for cell vitality: 1) the cell membrane, which regulates ionic homeostasis and osmotic equilibrium; 2) aerobic respiration, fundamental for oxidative phosphorylation and production of ATP; 3) protein synthesis; and 4) the integrity of genetic information and translation.

If alterations are irreversible, they produce cell death (necrosis or apoptosis) and the prognoses will depend of the percentage of dead cells [18]. Subtle lesions cannot be appreciated other than by histology, and there are practically no in vivo studies to demonstrate such damage [18,19].

Irreversible changes, such as necrosis or apoptosis, increase cytoplasmic eosinophilia, which is reflected in electron microscope studies as a discontinuity in the cellular membrane and in the organelles, with intense alteration of mitochondriae. In the nucleus, picnosis is apparent, with nuclear constriction and an increase in basophilia [3].

Methylene blue is a basic vital dye that can color the neuronal axes and nerve terminals. This dye can enter the cell when there are structural alterations in the cell membrane induced by irreversible lesions. Nuclear basophilia found is the result of picnosis in the nucleus.

Hershlag et al. [2] compared salpingoscopic and histological findings in tubes and found a significant correlation between the techniques. In electron microscopy studies, tubes with normal or mildly altered mucosa presented a homogenous cytoplasm, abundant mitochondriae, normal nuclei and a conserved ciliary apparatus. By contrast, in more severely injured tubes there was a rupture of the plasma membrane, digested mitochondriae, and vacuolization of the cytoplasm.

*Table 11.* Score of adhesions and nuclear staining in relation to laporoscopic diagnosis.

| Laparoscopic finding | Normal[a] | Endometriosis[b] | Peritoneal factor[c] | Tubal factor[d] |
|---|---|---|---|---|
| Adhesions | $2 \pm 0.7$ | $1.9 \pm 0.2$ | $3.0 \pm 1.9$ | $3.1 \pm 2.03$ |
| Nuclear staining | $2.1 \pm 0.6$ | $2.2 \pm 0.7$ | $3.9 \pm 2.3$ | $4.2 \pm 2.05$ |

[a,c]$p < 0.002$; [a,d]$p < 0.0001$.

These are signs of irreversible cellular injury, which allow the entry of methylene blue. Therefore we can suggest that nuclear staining with methylene blue is the expression of damage of the tubal cells which would not be detected using a simple salpingoscopic observation. Severity and prognosis of the organ will depend on the percentage of epithelium that is altered, and of the intensity of the phenomenon.

Vazquez [18] describes that there is a poor prognosis when inflammatory cells are present in the wall of the hydrosalpinges. The presence of inflammatory cells in the submucosa or the muscularis has even a worse prognosis. These cells, which are generally lymphocytes, have nuclei with great affinity for methylene blue due to their high chromatin content.

We have previously described that in salpingoscopy after chromotubation, not only lymphocytes but also cells of the tubal mucosa were colored by methylene blue. This phenomenon was evidenced especially in patients who had suffered inflammatory processes [5]. When comparing the presence of adhesions and stained nuclei according to pathology described by laparoscopy, we found that normal or endometriotic laparoscopies presented a practically normal score, whereas in laparoscopies with peritoneal factors or tubal obstructions scores was significantly higher. Such data shows the impact that infections have on tubal epithelium. An irreversible cellular damage was detected which would probably influence the future of the organ.

Vazquez [21] affirms that in order to have a good prognosis in hydrosalpinx surgery, the epithelial injury must be minimal. She reports only a 7% pregnancy rate with more than 50% of damaged tubal mucosa, as determined by the microscope during microsurgery; and between 50 and 69% of pregnancies in patients with healthy mucosa (more than 50 and 70% of undamaged mucosa, respectively). In concordance, we show that pregnant patients presented the lowest degree of nuclear staining, which is a reflection of a lower degree of cellular damage of the mucosa.

In summary, normal tubal epithelium does not regularly take up methylene blue, but a previous process to injury of cellular ultrasctructures allows the passage of the supravital dye into the cytoplasm, and consequently into the nucleus. Therefore nuclear staining with methylene blue is a useful method to evaluate in vivo the cytohistological injury which an inflammatory process leaves behind, and it allows a prognosis of the tube by means of an endoscopic procedure.

Laparoscopic surgery can enhance fertility if it is performed by highly trained surgeons with appropriate techniques and instrumentation and with a correct analysis of the pathology involved.

Salpingoscopic evaluation of tubal mucosa is a useful method in the prognosis for tubal function. It questions the reconstruction of the tube in patients with severe alterations of the tube, as the possibility of restoration of function and pregnancies are remote. Staining with methylene blue is an additional tool for evaluating in vivo the cytohistological damage produced by an infection that has altered the integrity of the cell. It is a helpful method to characterize the prognosis for tubal function. It is easy to perform, easily identifies the pathology and can be simply quantified.

Salpingoscopy together with nuclear staining of the endosalpingial cells provides the morphological aspect of evaluating the tube, and adds the functional aspect, improving the diagnosis which cannot be determined by indirect studies such as radiology, laparoscopy or simple salpingoscopy.

Finally, it must be emphasized that intraluminal adhesions and nuclear staining are the highlights of the study. Intratubal adhesions are the luminal sequelae of an inflammatory process, while nuclear staining is the cellular sequelae of the injury, the expression of the functional alteration of the tubal cell.

## References

1. Tulandi T, Collins JA, Burrows E et al. Treatment-dependent and treatment independent pregnancy among women with periadnexal adhesions. Am J Obst Gynecol 1990;162:354.
2. Winston RML, Margara R. Microsurgical salpingostomy is not an obsolete procedure. Br J Obstet Gynaecol 1991;98:637.
3. Gomel V. Te Linde's Operative Gynecology, 8th edn. Philadelphia: Lippincott-Raven Publishers, 1997.
4. Gomel V. Laparoscopic tubal surgery in infertility. Obstet Gynecol 1975;46:47.
5. Mettler L, Giesel H, Semm K. Treatment of female infertility due to tubal obstruction by operative laparoscopy. Fertil Steril 1979;32:384.
6. Saravelos H, Li T-C, Cook I. An analysis of outcome of microsurgical and laparoscopic adhesiolysis for infertility. Hum Reprod 1995;10:2887.
7. Rock J, Moutos DM. Endoscopic Management of Gynecologic Diseases. Philadelphia: Lippincott-Raven Publishers, 1996.
8. Liu CY. International Workshop of Gynecologic Laparoscopic Surgery. 1998; Buenos Aires-Argentina.
9. Marconi G, Augé L, Sojo E, Young E, Quintana R. Salpingoscopy: systematic use in diagnostic laparoscopy. Fertil Steril 1992;57:742−746.
10. De Bruyne F, Jürgens H, Reinhart W. The prognostic value of the salpingoscopy. Hum Reprod 1997;12,266−271.
11. De Bruyne F, Puttemans P, Boeckx W, Brosens I. The clinical value of salpingoscopy in tubal infertility. Fertil Steril 1989;51:339−340.
12. Marana R, Rizzi M, Muzzi L. Correlation between the American Fertility Society classification of adnexal adhesion and distal tubal occlusion, salpingoscopy, and reproductive outcome in tubal surgery. Fertil Steril 1995;64:924−929.
13. Heylen SM, Brosens IA, Puttemans PJ. Clinical value and cumulative pregnancy rates following rigid salpingoscopy during laparoscopy for infertility. Hum Reprod 1995;10:2913−2916.
14. Shapiro B, Diamond M, De Charney A. Salpingoscopy: an adjunctive technique for evaluation of the fallopian tube. Fertil Steril 1988;49:1076−1079.
15. Kerin J, Williams D, San Romano G, Pearlstone A, Grundfest W, Surrey E. Falloscopy classification and treatment of fallopian tube diseases. Fertil Steril 1992;57:731−741.
16. Brosens I, Boeckx W, Delattin Ph, Puttemans P, Vázquez G. Salpingoscopy: a new pre-operative diagnostic tool in tubal infertility. Br J Obstet Gynaecol 1987;94:768−773.
17. Scudamore IW, Dumphy BC, Bowman W, Jenkins J, Cooke ID. Comparison of ampullary assessment by falloscopy and salpingoscopy. Hum Reprod 1994;9:1516−1518.
18. Vázquez G, Winston RML, Boeckx W. The epithelium of human hydrosalpinges: a light optical and scanning microscopy study. Br J Obstet Gynecol 1983;90:764−770.

19. Hershlag A, Seifer DB, Carcangiu ML. Salpingoscopy: light microscopic and electron micro-scopic correlation. Obstet Gynecol 1991;77:399—405.
20. Cotran RS, Kumar V, Robbins SL. Pathologic Basis of Disease. WB Saunders Company 1994;1—55.
21. Vázquez G, Boeckx W, Brosens, Prospective study of mucosal lesion and fertility in hidrosal-pinges. Hum Reprod 1995a;10:1075—1078.

Fertility and Reproductive Medicine.
R.D. Kempers, J. Cohen, A.F. Haney and J.B. Younger, editors.

343

# Hysteroscopy for reproductive surgery in the female

Jacques E. Hamou

*Hopital Antoine Beclere, Universite de Paris, Paris, France*

**Abstract.** Operative hysteroscopy offers in most organic and Müllerian defects a very effective treatment and a less invasive approach as an alternative to laparotomy.

A total of 24 patients with a septum have been treated by operative hysteroscopy and 16 pregnancies have occurred within 18 months with 10 term deliveries. Miscarriages have dropped from 81% before treatment to 13% following treatment.

For 69 patients treated for adhesions, 60 pregnancies were reported: 75% had a term delivery, however, there was a 25% miscarriage rate.

Concerning submucous fibroids, we have treated 48 patients yielding 27 pregnancies, with five miscarriages. This study includes interstitial fibroids resected after enucleation in the cavity by a new technical approach (hydromassage and controlled irrigation by the endomat).

Also, 21 DES (diethylstilbestrol)-exposed patients who had undergone plastic hysteroscopic enlargement surgery are reported, with six pregnancies obtained within 12 months, and four term deliveries.

**Keywords:** in vitro fertilization, laparoscopic tubal microsurgery, microsurgery, operative laparoscopy, tubal infertility, tuboplasty.

The main indication for operative hysteroscopy remains metrorrhagia. Infertility is second at 28% in our center. Hysteroscopy, used first as a diagnostic tool in infertility, becomes a significant conservative therapeutic instrument.

Whether it concerns Müllerian defects, synechiae, polyps, fibroids or other pathology such as DES (diethylstilbestrol)-exposed patients, bony metaplasia or endometrial dystrophies, operative hysteroscopy affords a less invasive approach and in many instances an alternative to laparotomy.

The importance of infertility as an hysteroscopic indication is variable and related to the orientation of the gynaecologist.

The rate of infertility for hysteroscopic indications varies from 10 [1] to 38% [2].

Evaluation of infertility by hysteroscopy identifies 33—65% of patients with abnormalities (Table 1).

### Materials and Methods

A prior diagnostic hysteroscopy was always performed whether it was related to septums (24 patients), adhesions (69 patients), myomas (48 patients) or plastic

---

*Address for correspondence:* Dr Jacques E. Hamou, Attaché des Hopitaux de Paris, Maternités Tenon, Port Royal et A. Béclere, 31, Rue Robert de Flers, 75015 Paris, France.

*Table 1.*

|  | Valle [3] | Snowden et al. [4] | Taylor [5] | Hamou et al. [6] |
|---|---|---|---|---|
| Number | 142 | 77 | 400 | 128 |
| Normal | 38% | 84% | 55% | 42% |
| Malformations | 6% | 1% | 11% | 2% |
| Adhesions | 20% | 8% | 21% | 25% |
| Polypes-myomas | 32% | 3% | 4% | 10% |
| Other | 4% | 1% | 9% | 21% |

uterine enlargement in DES-exposed patients (21 patients).

No special premedication was given except for seven patients with large fibroids > 3 cm who had had gonadotropin releasing hormone analogues (GnRH-a) for 2 months. Patients were discharged the same day of the hysterosurgery except for two patients who remained overnight (one perforation, one hemorrhage). A control diagnostic hysteroscopy at 2 months was performed. The Hamou micro-hysteroscope No. 2 of 4 mm with a double flow resectoscope of 9.3 mm (Storz Tuttlingen, Germany) was used. Irrigation with glycine 1.5% through a pump with an electronic control of flow and pressure was used (Hamou endomat, Storz Tuttlingen, Germany).

**Septums**

A uterine septum is the most frequent malformation (60%) related to Müllerian defects. It is found in 1.9—3% of the female population [7]. When this defect is present, Fedele et al. [8] report 30—75% of miscarriages of first trimester, with also a high rate of late miscarriages, in utero deaths, fetal hypotrophy and toxemia, dystocia presentation in 30%, and 15—58% premature deliveries. Overall, 33% will not have a term delivery. Infertility that is related to a septum is still controversial.

Preoperative evaluation involves a mandatory transvaginal ultrasound to assess the thickness and size of the septum. If the ultrasound cannot rule out a bicornuate uterus, a laparoscopy is performed.

Resection is performed with the 7-mm endoscopic electrical knife. Ostiums are used as reference to realign the fundus and to avoid uterine wall thinning. A residual thickness of the fundus of 8—9 mm should be respected.

Therapeutic efficiency is evaluated for a population with a past history of obstetrical pathology. Table 2 gives our results compared to other studies.

Deliveries of a living child have significantly increased and the rate of miscarriages prior to resection of 81% will drop to 13% after operative hysteroscopy.

*Table 2.*

|  | Decherney [9] | Bautrant [1] | Zioua [10] | Hamou [11] |
|---|---|---|---|---|
| Number | 72 | 15 | 23 | 24 |
| Pregnancies | 68 | 11 | 19 | 16 |
| Miscarriages before | — | — | 36 | 23 |
| Miscarriages after | 5 | 1 | 1 | 6 |
| Term delivery | 58 | — | 9 | 10 |
| Complications | 1 | — | 1 | — |

## Adhesions

The prevalence rate of adhesions is not easy to assess since if adhesions are present, they are very often, asymptomatic. Fayez et al. [12] have evaluated 400 infertile patients and reported 82 with adhesions (20.5%):
1. Synechiaes of less than 3 months, not yet organised can be easily freed by the distal end of the hysteroscope during a diagnostic procedure.
2. Extensive and older adhesions usually become fibrous requiring a hysteroscopic operative resection under anesthesia. Prior reliable ultrasound evaluation is mandatory. It will assess a residual cavity and the importance of the remaining endometrium, which determines the final result.

Endoscopic resection using the electric knife was facilitated by visualisation of a least one ostium. It was used as a reference to reconstitute the cavity. If no ostium is located, the resection is more hazardous and a preoperative ultrasound or laparoscopy can be helpful. Estrogens were given for 2 months after surgery.

Table 3 shows comparative results with the literature. When compared to results in patients presenting synechiae without treatment (17), 46% will become pregnant, 30% will have a term delivery and 13% will present with a placenta accreta. After treatment by laparoscopy and hysteroscopy, 50% will become pregnant of which 55% will have a term delivery and 8% a placenta accreta.

## Submucous fibroids

An impact of fibroids on reproduction is uneasy to define. Such pathology is frequently observed with an incidence of 20% for females who are older than 40

*Table 3.*

|  | March [13] | Valle [14] | Lamcet [15] | Hamou [16] |
|---|---|---|---|---|
| Number | 38 | 187 | 185 | 69 |
| Pregnancies obtained | 39 | 143 | 135 | 60 |
| Miscarriages | 14% | 18% | 26% | 25% |
| Living children | 87% | 79% | 71% | 75% |
| Placenta accreta | — | 1 | — | 1 |

years of age.

They are not frequently implicated as the exclusive cause of primary infertility. Generally, they are identified by hysterosalpingogram, ultrasound or diagnostic hysteroscopy when evaluating infertility.

Conventionally, only submucous fibroids of less than 4 cm are resected by operative hysteroscopy. Actually, newer techniques permit resection of interstitial myomas of less than 3 cm. The fibroid capsule is opened after ultrasound localisation and the myoma is enucleated into the uterine cavity by hydromassage and resected.

To evaluate the impact of hysteroscopic resection of a fibroid on infertility, only patients with a prior history of miscarriages or premature deliveries are shown in Table 4. Therefore, fibroid resection in infertile patients is indicated since it increases statistically the rate of living children.

**DES-exposed patients**

DES-exposed patients will generally present a hypoplastic uterine cavity. In France, between 1950 and 1977, 200,000 women were given DES. Kaufman [21] reported 70% abnormalities in exposed patients. Cabau [22] in a retrospective study of 258 patients reported 9.4% ectopic pregnancies vs. 1.8% for nonexposed sisters, 12.8% premature deliveries vs. 0%, and 14.6% first-trimester miscarriages.

The technique of hysteroscopic plastic surgery to enlarge the cavity also uses the electric endoscopic knife. Prior precise assessment of ultrasound assessed the exact thickness of marginal and fundus of the myometrium is required. If its thicker than 12 mm, operative hysteroscopy is indicated and a tailored resection is performed to leave a residual myometrium thickness of 8—9 mm.

A total of 21 patients were treated between June 1994 and May 1997, 20 of which were infertile (eight primary infertility, and 12 secondary), and four had associated pathology. With a mean follow up of 13 months, six patients became pregnant, two had a miscarriage at 5 and 10 weeks and four had a term delivery. One case of placenta accreta occurred.

This procedure may be indicated only when no other associated pathology is found in the infertile patient or a patient with repeat miscarriages.

*Table 4.*

|                      | Loffer [18] | Corson [19] | Mergui [20] | Hamou [6] |
|----------------------|-------------|-------------|-------------|-----------|
| Number               | 15          | 13          | 15          | 48        |
| Pregnancies obtained | 8           | 13          | 6           | 27        |
| Miscarriages         | —           | 3           | 2           | 5         |
| Living children      | 7           | 10          | 4           | 20        |

# References

1. Bautrant E, Boubsi L, Blanc B. La résection endo-utérine transcervicale: efficacité et innocuité d'une technique opératoire. A propos d'une série de 129 cas. Gynécologie 1991;42(2):115−120.
2. Hamou J, Salat-Baroux J. Hystéroscopie et microhystéroscopie opératoire. Mise à jour en Gynecol Obstet. Paris: Vigot, 1988;171−197.
3. Valle RF. Hysteroscopy in the evaluation of female infertility. Am J Obstet Gynecol 1980; 137:425−431.
4. Snowden EU, Jarrett JC, Dawood MY. Comparison of diagnostic accuracy of laparoscopy, hysteroscopy and hysterosalpingography in evaluation of female infertility. Fertil Steril 1984; 41:709−713.
5. Taylor PJ. Correlations in infertility: symptomatology, hysterosalpingography, laparoscopy and hysteroscopy. J Reprod Med 1977;8:339−342.
6. Hamou J, Salat-Baroux J. L'endocol en microhystéroscopie. In: Netter A, Gorins A (eds) Actualités Gynécologiques. Paris: Masson, 1984;1−11.
7. Simon C, Martinez L, Pardo F, Tortajada M, Pellicer A. Mullerian defects in women with normal reproductive outcome. Fertil Steril 1991;56(6):1192−1193.
8. Fedele L, Marchini M, Baglioni A, Carinelli SG, Candiani GB. Endometrial reconstruction after hysteroscopic incisional metroplasty. Obstét Gynécol 1989;73(3) part 2:492−494.
9. Decherney AH, Russel JB, Graebe RA, Polan ML. Resectoscopic management of müllerian fusion defects. Fertil Steril 1986;45(5):726−728.
10. Zioua F, Mouelhi C, Lhamdoun A, Ferchiou F, Meriah S. Les métroplasties hystéroscopiques des cloisons utérines. Gynecol Obstet Biol Report 1993;22:600−604.
11. Hamou J. Hysteroscopy and Microcolpohysteroscopy: Text and Atlas. East Norwalk, Connecticut, USA: Appleton and Lange, 1991;115−125.
12. Fayez JA, Mutie G, Schneider PJ. The diagnostic value of hysterosalpingography and hysteroscopy in infertility investigation. Am J Obstet Gynecol 1987;156(3):558−560.
13. March CM, Israel R. Gestational outcome following hysteroscopic lysis of adhesions. Fertil Steril 1981;36(4):455−458.
14. Valle RF, Sciarra JJ. Intrauterine adhesions: hysteroscopic diagnosis, classification, treatment and reproductive outcome. Am J Obstet Gynecol 1988;158(6,1):1459−1470.
15. Lamcet M, Kessler I. Analyse du syndrome d'Asherman et résultats de son traitement moderne. Contr Fertil Sex 1989;17(3):247−255.
16. Hamou J, Salat-Baroux J, Siegler AM. Diagnosis and treatment of intrauterine adhesions by microhysteroscopy. Fertil Steril 1983;39(3):321−325.
17. Schenker JG, Margalioth EJ. Intrauterine adhesions: an update appraisal. Fertil Steril 1982; 37(5)593−610.
18. Loffer FD. Removal of large symptomatic intrauterine growths by the hysteroscopic resectoscope. Obstet Gynecol 1990;76:836−840.
19. Corson SL, Brooks PG. Resectoscopic myomectomy. Fertil Steril 1991;55(6):1041−1044.
20. Mergui JL, Renolleau C, Salat-Baroux J. Hystéroscopie opératoire et fibromes. Gynecology 1993;1(6):326−337.
21. Kaufman RH et al. Upper genital tract changes and pregnancy outcome in offspring exposed in utero to DES. Am J Obstet Gynecol 1988;137:299−307.
22. Cabau A, Lion O. Accidents de la reproduction et stérilité ches les femmes exposées au DES in utéro. Contr Fertil Sex 1996;24(4):253−258.

# Tubal surgery in the era of ART

Paul Devroey

*Centre for Reproductive Medicine, Dutch-speaking Brussels University, Brussels, Belgium*

**Abstract.** In the presence of tubal pathology, similar pregnancy rates are obtained after microsurgery and laparoscopic surgery. Salpingolysis, salpingoneostomy and fimbrioplasty are the first line therapies. If the fallopian tubes are irreparably damaged, in vitro fertilization (IVF) is the treatment of choice and is indicated after failed reconstructive surgery. In case of irreparably damaged fallopian tubes including hydrosalpinges, salpingectomy is indicated. Reduced implantation and pregnancy rates are observed in the presence of hydrosalpinges. Reconstructive and excisional surgery, and IVF are complementary.

**Keywords:** in vitro fertilization, laparoscopy, microsurgery, pregnancy rates.

## Introduction

Since in vitro fertilization (IVF) became available, tubal pathology is currently one of the frequent indications. Moreover, IVF is usually performed to circumvent sterility due to tubal pathology. It is obvious that all women with tubal pathology can be helped by IVF.

The origin of the tubal dysfunction can vary from minor disease of the fallopian tubes to major damage. Occasionally both fallopian tubes can also be absent. It is of paramount importance to diagnose correctly the health or the disease of the fallopian tubes. A correct understanding and an accurate evaluation of the extent of the disease is needed. A correct diagnosis is needed to define further treatments. If both fallopian tubes are absent or severely damaged, only IVF can be offered. The value of microsurgery for any given case has to be judged by well-defined criteria. If surgery offers an acceptable option, the preferred choice is surgery. In this chapter the therapeutic outcome of surgery for different pathologies will be discussed.

It is impossible to judge the effectiveness of the different surgical approaches since no evidence-based data are available. No prospective randomized studies have been performed comparing the laparoscopic approach vs. laparotomy. Also no data are available comparing surgery with IVF.

Indeed, the interpretation of tubal findings has to be analyzed in relation to the sperm parameters of the male partner. The sense of assessing the function of the

*Address for correspondence:* Prof Dr P. Devroey, Centre for Reproductive Medicine, AZ VUB, Laarbeeklaan 101, 1090 Brussels, Belgium. Tel.: +32-2-4776501. Fax: 32-2-4776549.
E-mail: fertility@az.vub.ac.be

fallopian tube in severe male factor infertility has to be questioned. Since intracytoplasmic sperm injection became a viable solution, the indication for a diagnostic and therapeutic laparoscopy has to be reconsidered.

Besides therapeutic reconstructive surgery, the debate on extripative surgery is still open. Which are the indications to perform a unilateral or bilateral salpingectomy?

## Methodology

Before evaluating the fallopian tubes it seems logical to perform a semem analysis. If by repetition, the sperm function is considered to be extremely impaired, there is no place to perform invasive diagnostic procedures in the female partner. In view of intracytoplasmic sperm injection the most important evaluation relates to the normality of the uterine cavity.

If the sperm parameters are normal, or close to normal, diagnostic evaluation of the female partner is needed. Different investigations can be carried out. The most frequently used ones are salpingography and laparoscopy. Salpingoscopy and falloposcopy are other options.

Many tubal pathologies can be detected and various treatments are available such as: (ovario)salpingolysis, tubal uterine implantations, tubotubal anastomosis, salpingoneostomy and fimbrioplasty.

## Results

Unfortunately no prospective randomized data are available compairing microsurgery and endoscopic surgery (Tables 1–5).

1. *Microsurgical and laparoscopic ovariosalpingolysis* [1–7]. In the presence of peritubal adhesions comparable pregnancy rates have been reported.

*Table 1.* Outcome after microsurgical and laporascopic ovariosalpingolysis.

| Microsurgical | | | Laparoscopical | | |
|---|---|---|---|---|---|
| Reference | n | Pregnancy rate (%) | Reference | n | Pregnancy rate (%) |
| Fayez (1982) [1] | 8 | 75 | Gomel (1983) [6] | 92 | 67 |
| Frantzen (1982) [2] | 49 | 41 | Fayez (1982) [1] | 50 | 60 |
| Donnez (1986) [3] | 42 | 67 | Donnez (1989) [8] | 186 | 58 |
| Tulandi (1986) [4] | 63 | 57 | | | |
| Singhal (1991) [5] | 78 | 46 | | | |

2. *Salpingoneostomy* [1,3,7—17]. In the presence of various degress of hydrosalpinx formation, tubal dysfunction is almost in all cases present. The degree of mucosal damage indicates the severity. Salpingoneostomy aims to create a new ostium.

*Table 2.* Outcome after microsurgical salpingoneostomy and laparoscopic salpingoneostomy.

Salpingoneostomy

| Microsurgical | | | Laparoscopical | | |
|---|---|---|---|---|---|
| Reference | n | Pregnancy rate (%) | Reference | n | Pregnancy rate (%) |
| Gomel(1978) [9] | 41 | 39 | Fayez (1983) [7] | 19 | 11 |
| Fayez (1982) [1] | 20 | 40 | Daniell (1984) [14] | 21 | 24 |
| Tulandi (1985) [10] | 67 | 27 | Donnez (1989) [8] | 25 | 20 |
| Donnez (1986) [3] | 83 | 38 | Canis (1994) | 87 | 40 |
| Schlaff (1990) [11] | 95 | 27 | Dubuisson (1994) [16] | 81 | 37 |
| Singhal (1991) [5] | 97 | 40 | Dlugi (1994) [17] | 20 | |
| Winston (1991) [12] | 323 | 43 | | | |
| Strandell (1995) [13] | 109 | 36 | | | |

3. *Fimbrioplasty* [1,3,18—20]. Fimbrial agglutination is associated with endosalpingeal damage and fimbrial stenosis. Fimbrioplasty aims to incise the fibrotic fimbrial bands and to dilate the stenosis.

*Table 3.* Outcome of microsurgical and laparoscopical fimbrioplasty.

Fimbrioplasty

| Microsurgical | | | Laparoscopical | | |
|---|---|---|---|---|---|
| Reference | n | Pregnancy rate (%) | Reference | n | Pregnancy rate (%) |
| Fayez 1982 [1] | 7 | 57 | Gomel 1983 [6] | 12 | 50 |
| Donnez 1986 [3] | 132 | 61 | Fayez 1983 [7] | 14 | 35 |
| Lavy 1987 [18] | 134 | 60 | Dubuisson 1990 [20] | 31 | 35 |

**Discussion**

Since no prospective data are available comparing the results of microsurgery with the ones of endoscopic surgery, it is almost impossible to indicate the most suitable approach. If with both approaches similar pregnancy rates are obtained, laparoscopic surgery is the preferred method because of the decreased invasiveness. In these retrospective reviews, a significant increased pregnancy rate was observed after microsurgical fimbrioplasty compared with the laparoscopic approach (p < 0.05). In general, a close relationship can be observed between the health of the fallopian tube and the mucosal appearance, and the pregnancy rates. All aim to judge the functionality of the fallopian tubes [21,22]. In this respect, salpingoscopy can provide additional information [23]. If intratubal adhesions are present the pregnancy rate after microsurgical salpingoneostomy drops to 0%. The mucosal status appears to be the predictive factor. If the mucosal score indicates excessive lesions, no pregnancies are observed [14,17,18,24]. According to the above-described findings, surgical treatment should not be performed in case of excessive tubal damage. In the presence of severely damaged fallopian tubes or after unsuccessful reconstructive surgery, IVF has to be considered. Several studies have analyzed the pregnancy outcomes after IVF in tubal infertility. Different cumulative pregnancy rates have been observed varying from 55 to 70%. It is extremely difficult to evaluate cumulative pregnancy rates especially with respect to the drop-outs and the number of cycles performed [25–27]. It is of paramount importance by evaluating cumulative delivery rates to express the results in the real cumulative and theoretical cumulative pregnancy rates. A substantial number of patients abandon the treatment, especially for psychological reasons. It has been reported that after 10 cycles the real cumulative pregnancy rates after IVF for tubal infertility is 47% and the theoretical one is 80% [28].

An intriguing question remains in relation to the place of extirpative surgery and there are probably two indications to excise the fallopian tubes. It has been reported that in the case of damaged fallopian tubes, the ectopic pregnancy rate is significantly increased to approximately 10% [29,30]. Doubtlessly, if an ectopic pregnancy occurs after IVF, a salpingectomy should be performed. A more difficult question is in the case of irritable tubal damage, is whether to perform a salpingectomy. A salpingectomy prior IVF aims to avoid ectopic pregnancies after IVF-ET. So far, a general consensus has not yet been reached.

Special attention has to be given to the presence of large hydrosalpinges. In this condition, retrograde flow of hydrosalpinx liquid into the uterine cavity could

*Table 4.* Comparison of pregnancy rates after IVF in patients with or without hydrosalpinges.

| Reference | Pregnancy rate/ET (%) | | Delivery rate/ET (%) | |
|---|---|---|---|---|
| | Hydrosalpinx | Control group | Hydrosalpinx | Control group |
| Strandell 1994 [32] | 13 | 26 | 7 | 18 |
| Andersen 1994 [33] | 10 | 30 | 7 | 21 |
| Kassabji 1994 [34] | 18 | 31 | 10 | 25 |
| Vandromme 1995 [35] | 10 | 23 | 10 | 21 |
| Katz 1996 [36] | 17 | 37 | | |
| Blazar 1995 [37] | 39 | 45 | | |
| Sharara 1996 [38] | 25 | 33 | | |
| Chelton 1996 | 3 | 42 | | |
| Muray 1998 [40] | | | 8 | 39 |

adversely affect the embryonic implantation rates [31]. There is some evidence that pregnancy rates are reduced in the presence of a hydrosalpinx. These data are not prospective and not randomized [32–40].

Retrospective data on implantation rates demonstrate reduced implantation rates in the presence of hydrosalpinges.

It seems apparent that if, in the presence of a hydrosalpinx, salpingoneostomy cannot be performed, it is indicated to perform salpingectomy.

*Table 5.* Reduced embryonic implantation rates in the presence of hydrosalpinges.

|  | Implantation rate (%) | |
| --- | --- | --- |
|  | Hydrosalpinx | Control group |
| Andersen 1994 [33] | 3 | 10 |
| Kassabji 1994 [34] | 8 | 12 |
| Vandromme 1995 [35] | 4 | 10 |
| Katz 1996 [36] | 4 | 11 |
| Sharara 1996 [38] | 10 | 13 |
| Murray 1998 [40] | 3 | 16 |

## Conclusion

In the presence of tubal damage, reconstructive surgery is the first choice. If a hydrosalpinx is irreparably damaged, salpingectomy is indicated. In the case of unsuccessful reconstructive surgery, a salpingectomy prior to IVF has to be considered. If tubal damage is irreparable, or after failed reconstructive surgery, IVF is indicated.

## References

1. Fayez JA, Suliman SO. Infertility surgery of the oviduct: comparison between macrosurgery and microsurgery. Fertil Steril 1982;37:73–78.
2. Frantzen C, Schlosser HW. Microsurgery and postinfectious tubal infertility. Fertil Steril 1982; 38:397–402.
3. Donnez J, Casanas-Roux F. Prognostic factors of fimbrial microsurgery. Fertil Steril 1986; 46:200–204.
4. Tulandi T. Salpingo-ovariolysis: a comparison between laser surgery and electrosurgery. Fertil Steril 1986;45:489–491.
5. Singhal V, Li TC, Cooke ID. An analysis of factors influencing the outcome of 232 consecutive tubal microsurgery cases. Br J Obstet Gynecol 1991;98:628–636.
6. Gomel V. Salpingo-ovariolysis by laparoscopy in infertility. Fertil Steril 1983;40:607–611.
7. Fayez JA. An assessment of the role of operative laparoscopy in tuboplasty. Fertil Steril 1983;39:476–479.
8. Donnez J, Nisolle M, Casanas-Roux F. CO2 laser laparoscopy in infertile women with adnexal adhesions and women with tubal occlusion. J Gynecol Surg 1989;5:47–53.

9. Gomel V. Salpingostomy by microsurgery. Fertil Steril 1978;29:380—387.
10. Tulandi T, Vilos GA. A comparison between laser surgery and electrosurgery for bilateral hydrosalpinx: a 2 year follow-up. Fertil Steril 1985;44:846—847.
11. Schlaff WD, Massiakos DK, Damewood MD, Rock JA. Neosalpingostomy for distal tubal obstruction: prognostic factors and impact of surgical technique. Fertil Steril 1990;54:984—990.
12. Winston RML, Margara RA. Microsurgical salpingostomy is not an obsolete procedure. Br J Obstet Gynecol 1991;98:637—642.
13. Strandell A, Bryman I, Janson PO, Thorburn J. Background factors and scoring systems in relation to pregnancy outcome after fertility surgery. Acta Obstet Gynecol Scand 1995;74:281—287.
14. Daniell JF, Herbert CM. Laparoscopic salpingostomy utilizing the CO2 laser. Fertil Steril 1984;41:558—563.
15. Canis M, Mage G, Pouly JL, Manhes H, Wattiez A, Bruhat MA. Laparoscopic distal tuboplasty: report of 87 cases and a four year experience. Fertil Steril 1991;56:616—621.
16. Dubuisson JB, Chapron C, Morice P, Aubriot FX, Foulot H, Bouquet de Jolinière J. Laparoscopic salpingostomy: fertility results according to the tubal mucosal appearance. Hum Reprod 1994;9:334—339.
17. Dlugi AM, Reddy S, Saleh WA, Mersol-Barg MS, Jacobsen G. Pregnancy rates after operative endoscopic treatment of total (neosalpingostomy) or near total (salpingostomy) distal tubal occlusion. Fertil Steril 1994;62:913—920.
18. Lavy G, Diamond MP, De Cherney AH. Ectopic pregnancy: its relationship to tubal reconstructive surgery. Fertil Steril 1987;47:543—556.
19. Gomel V. Salpingo-ovariolysis by laparoscopy in infertility. Fertil Steril 1984;40:607—611.
20. Dubuisson JB, Bouquet de Jolinière J, Aubriot FX, Daraï E, Foulot H, Mandelbrot L. Terminal tuboplasties by laparoscopy: 65 consecutive cases. Fertil Steril 1990;54:401—403.
21. Mage G, Pouly JL, Bouquet de Jolinière J, Chabrand S, Riouallon A, Bruhat MA. A preoperative classification to predict the intrauterine and ectopic pregnancy rates after distal tubal microsurgery. Fertil Steril 1986;46:807—810.
22. Boer-Meisel ME, te Velde ER, Habbema JDF, Kardaun JWPF. Predicting the pregnancy outcome in patients treated for hydrosalpinx: a prospective study. Fertil Steril 1986;45:23—29.
23. De Bruyne F, Puttemans P, Boeckx W, Brosens I. The clinical value of salpingoscopy in tubal infertility. Fertil Steril 1989;51:339—340.
24. Marana R, Rizzi M, Muzii L, Catalano GF, Carvana P, Mancuso S. Correlation between the American Fertility Society classifications of adnexal adhesions and distal tubal occlusion, salpingoscopy and reproductive outcome in tubal surgery. Fertil Steril 1995;64:924—929.
25. Fivnat. French national IVF registry: analysis of 1986 to 1990 data. Fertil Steril 1993;59:587—595.
26. Alsalili M, Yuzpe A, Tummon I, Parker J, Martin J, Daniel S, Rebel M, Nisker J. Cumulative pregnancy rates and pregnancy outcome after in-vitro fertilization: > 5000 cycles at one centre. Hum Reprod 1995;10:470—474.
27. Benadiva CA, Kligman I, Davis O, Rosenwaks Z. In vitro fertilization versus tubal surgery: is pelvic reconstructive surgery obsolete? Fertil Steril 1995;64:1051—1061.
28. Pouly JL, Janny L, Pouly-Vye P, Boyer C, Canis M, Bassil S, Chapron C, Zambrano R, Moussali F, Boucher D, Bruhat MA. Cumulative delivery rate after in vitro fertilization for tubal infertility. Références en Gynecologie Obstetrique — Experts conference — Satellite Symposium IFSS 1995, Vichy, France 1995;224—230.
29. Dubuisson JB, Aubriot FX, Mathieu L, Foulot H, Mandelbrot L, Bouquet de Jolinière J. Risk factors for ectopic pregnancy in 556 pregnancies after in vitro fertilization: implications for preventive management. Fertil Steril 1991;56:686—690.
30. Zouves C, Erenus M, Gomel V. Tubal ectopic pregnancy after in vitro fertilization and embryo transfer: a role for proximal occlusion or salpingectomy after failed distal tubal surgery? Fertil Steril 1991;56:691—695.
31. Meyer WR, Beyler SA. Deleterious effects of hydrosalpinges on in vitro fertilization and endo-

metrial integrin expression. Ass Reprod Rev 1995;5:201—203.

32. Strandell A, Waldenström U, Nilsson L, Hamberger L. Hydrosalpinx reduces in- vitro fertilization/embryo transfer pregnancy rates. Hum Reprod 1994;9:861—863.

33. Andersen AN, Yue Z, Meng FJ, Petersen K. Low implantation rate after in vitro fertilization in patients with hydrosalpinges diagnosed by ultrasonography. Hum Reprod 1994;9:1935—1938.

34. Kassabji M, Sims JA, Butler L, Muasher SJ. Reduced pregnancy outcome in patients with unilateral or bilateral hydrosalpinx after in vitro fertilization. Eur J Obstet Gynecol Reprod Biol 1994;56:129—132.

35. Vandromme J, Chasse E, Lejeune B, Van Rysselberge M, Delvigne A, Leroy F. Hydrosalpinges in-vitro fertilization: an unfavorable prognostic feature. Hum Reprod 1995;10:576—579.

36. Katz E, Akman M, Damewood MD, Garcia JE. Deleterious effect of the presence of hydrosalpinx on implantation and pregnancy rates with in vitro fertilization. Fertil Steril 1996;66:122—125.

37. Blazar AS, Alexander K, Seifer DB, Frishman GF, Wheeler CA, Haning RV Jr. Absence of an Effect of Hydrosalpinx on Pregnancy Rate in In Vitro Fertilization. In: 51st Annual Meeting of the American Fertility Society. Seattle, WA: American Society for Reproductive Medicine, 1995 (Abstract).

38. Sharara FI, Scott RT, Marut EL, Queenan JT Jr. In-vitro fertilization outcome in women with hydrosalpinx. Hum Reprod 1996;11:526—530.

39. Shelton KE, Butler L. Toner JP, Oehninger S. Muasher SJ. Salpingectomy improves the pregnancy rate in-vitro fertilization patients with hydrosalpinx. Hum Reprod 1996;11:523—525.

40. Murray DL, Sagoskin AW, Widra EA, Levy MJ. The adverse effect of hydrosalpinges on in vitro fertilization pregnancy rates and the benefit of surgical correction. Fertil Steril 1998;69:41—45.

# Endometriosis

# Should you treat minimal/mild endometriosis?

Rodolphe Maheux[1], Sylvie Marcoux[2] and Sylvie Bérubé[2]

[1]Department of Obstetrics-Gynecology, and [2]Epidemiology Research Group, Laval University Quebec City, Canada

**Abstract.** *Objectives.* Minimal or mild endometriosis is frequently diagnosed in infertile women. Resection or ablation of endometriosis though often employed has not been rigorously evaluated for efficacy. This randomized controlled trial examined whether surgical laparoscopy enhanced fecundity in infertile women with minimal/mild endometriosis.

*Methods.* Participants were infertile women with minimal or mild endometriosis between the ages of 20 and 39 without any other factors to explain their infertility. Recruitment occurred between October 1992 and April 1996 in 25 clinics across Canada. Women were centrally randomized during the laparoscopy to resection/ablation of visible endometriosis (n = 172) or diagnostic laparoscopy only (n = 169). They were followed for 36 weeks after the laparoscopy or, for those who became pregnant during that interval, up to 20 weeks of pregnancy.

*Results.* The probability of becoming pregnant in the first 36 weeks following laparoscopy, and for that pregnancy to reach 20 weeks, was 31.20% in women who had resection/ablation of endometriosis compared to 18.10% in the control group (log-rank test, p = 0.006). Corresponding fecundability rates were 4.82 and 2.51 per 100 person-months (relative rate, 1.92; 95% confidence interval, 1.22–3.03). Fetal losses occurred in 20.6 and 21.6% of all recognized pregnancies from the surgery group and the control group, respectively (p = 0.91). Four minor operative complications were reported (three in the surgery group and one in the control group).

*Conclusions.* Resection/ablation of minimal and mild endometriosis enhances fecundity in infertile women and can be safely performed by laparoscopic surgeons.

**Keywords:** fecundity, infertility, minimal/mild endometriosis, resection/ablation of endometriosis.

Endometriosis is a pathologically benign disorder characterized by the presence of functional endometriotic implants outside the uterus. These implants are often associated with inflammatory reaction and may lead to the formation of adhesions and to anatomical distortions. Dysmenorrhea, dyspareunia and infertility are commonly reported with endometriosis. The diagnosis of endometriosis requires direct visualization. This is most commonly done by laparoscopy, which is now routinely performed in women with infertility. The prevalence of endometriosis varies between 4 and 33% among infertile women undergoing a diagnostic laparoscopy [1].

The etiology of endometriosis is still debated. The frequent location of endometriotic implants either on the ovaries, near the fimbriated ends of the fallopian tubes or in the posterior cul-de-sac supports the theory that retrograde menstruation plays a key role in the physiopathology of the disease [2]. This phenom-

*Address for correspondence:* Rodolphe Maheux MD, Hôpital St. Francois D'assis, 10 Rue De L'aspinay, Quebec, Canada G1l-3l5. Tel.: +1-418-525-4307. Fax: +1-418-525-4481.

enon could result either in direct peritoneal implantation of endometrial cells [3] or metaplasia of the local coelomic epithelium [4]. Immunologic factors may also be involved [5,6]. Occasionally, endometriotic implants may be spread by lymphatic or vascular diffusion to distant sites. Finally, clinical and experimental observations [7,8] support the role of estrogens in the pathogenic process, although the exact mechanism of the hormonal dependence of endometriotic implants is still unknown.

The most widely used classification of endometriosis is that of the American Fertility Society (AFS). This classification was last revised in 1985 [9]. It has replaced previous scoring systems developed by Acosta [10] and Kistner [11]. According to the R-AFS, endometriosis is classified in four stages. Stages I (minimal) and II (mild) are characterized by the presence of peritoneal or superficial ovarian endometriotic implants, with or without filmy adhesions. Stages III (moderate) and IV (severe) usually imply either deep ovarian implants, dense adhesions or complete cul-de-sac obliteration.

It is easily conceivable that an endometrial cyst or an anatomical distortion caused by dense adhesions, as seen in stages III or IV endometriosis, may interfere with tubo-ovarian function and cause infertility. However, whether and how stages I and II endometriosis are related to infertility is more debated. Several explanations have been put forward. First, increased peritoneal prostaglandins concentrations are found in women with endometriosis [12,13]. These prostaglandins may interfere with ovulation [14], alter tubal peristalsis, affect corpus luteum function, reduce sperm motility, or increase uterine contractility thus interfering with implantation of the blastocyst [12,13]. Second, endometriosis is associated with a higher concentration of peritoneal macrophages, increasing the risk of sperm phagocytosis [15]. Finally, autoimmunity [16] and deficient cellular immunity [5] may also play a role in endometriosis-associated infertility.

Although the literature on treatment modalities for endometriosis is abundant, well-designed studies on the effectiveness of these treatments on fertility are rare. Subjects in such studies are often heterogeneous with regard to the stage of endometriosis and presence of other infertility factors. Sample sizes are small. Although the duration of follow up often varies among subjects, few studies used life-table analysis. Most authors only report a crude pregnancy "risk" (number of women who became pregnant over the total number of treated subjects), which does not take into account the length of the observation period. There are very few randomized controlled trials. From 1982 to 1989, Evers [17] identified 286 articles which discussed the results of endometriosis therapy; only 15 were randomized controlled trials; of these, seven included a no treatment arm. Only four of the latter had pregnancy rates as one of their endpoints [18–21], all reporting no increase in pregnancy rates with medical treatment. The inclusion of an untreated group is an important and acceptable issue in trials on endometriosis, for at least two reasons: first, there is currently no standard effective treatment for minimal or mild endometriosis; second, a relatively high and unpredictable proportion of women become pregnant under expectant management.

Treatment of infertility associated with mild endometriosis has focused on drug-induced reduction or surgical destruction of endometriotic implants. Medical treatments take advantage of the hormonal dependence of endometriotic implants. The most commonly used medication for endometriosis today is danazol, an isoxazole derivative of 17-α-ethinyltestosterone which inhibits ovulation and alters ovarian steroidogenesis. Danazol produces atrophy of endometriotic implants [22] and relieves pelvic pain and dyspareunia [23] but is associated with significant androgenic side effects. Moreover, none of the randomized [18,20,21] or nonrandomized studies [24] which compared danazol to expectant management could demonstrate a beneficial effect of danazol on fertility. Randomized trials comparing a medical treatment to expectant management are available for only two other medications, gestrinone [19] and medroxyprogesterone acetate [21], both of which were found ineffective. Pregnancy rates comparable to those observed with danazol have been reported following the use of buserelin [25] and nafarelin [26], two GnRH agonists, as well as following Enovid [27], an oral contraceptive. Finally, estrogens [28], androgens [29,30] and gossypol [31] have also been used in patients with endometriosis. However, poor efficacy combined with important side effects have limited their acceptability. In brief, no medical treatment of endometriosis-associated infertility has yet been found superior to expectant management.

Conservative surgery for minimal or mild endometriosis consists of laparotomy during which all active endometriotic implants are removed and damaged areas are reperitonalized. This may be associated with a variety of additional surgical techniques such as uterine suspension, presacral neurectomy, uterosacral ligament transection or lysis of adhesions. Only three studies [32—34] have compared conservative surgery to expectant management but none of them was a randomized trial. These authors reported similar [32,34] or lower [33] pregnancy rates in patients treated by conservative surgery than in untreated patients. Combined medical and surgical treatment has been advocated by some investigators. In one study, a combined approach did not appear more effective than expectant management [35]; in four out of five [36—40] nonrandomized studies, combined therapy was found better than either danazol alone [36—38] or surgery alone [40].

Laparoscopic surgical treatment of endometriosis most frequently consists in electrocauterization or laser vaporization of endometriotic implants and lysis of adhesions. Complications of laparoscopic surgery are rare but include uncontrollable bleeding necessitating a laparotomy, intestinal or ureteral injuries [41]. Compared to conservative surgery, laparoscopic surgery offers several advantages: it is less invasive, it does not require hospitalization, operating time and recovery period are shorter, less blood is lost, the likelihood of postoperative adhesions is reduced. Another important advantage of laparoscopy is that treatment can be undertaken at the same time as diagnostic laparoscopy, a routine procedure in infertility work-up. Although in theory laser produces less tissue damage than cautery [42], this has not been substantiated. Moreover, laser is costly and has no proven advantage over cautery in terms of subsequent fertility. Electrocautery and laser are considered as two equivalent and acceptable technical modalities. Either one or the other is used, depending on surgeons' preference and on availability.

Since the early reports by Eward in 1978 [43] and Bruhat in 1979 [44] on the use of cautery and laser laparoscopy for the treatment of endometriosis, several case series were published [45–59]. Keye et al. estimated that the percentage of women who became pregnant following laser lapararoscopy reached 52% [42], a figure similar to the crude pregnancy risk observed after laparoscopic cauterization (53%) [60]. As these reports do not include a comparison group, they provide no valid information on the efficacy of laparoscopic treatment for endometriosis-related infertility.

Several studies have compared laparoscopic treatment of endometriosis with other therapeutic modalities [39,61–63]. Treatment allocation was not randomized and therefore these studies are prone to selection bias. Chong et al. [61] treated 167 patients harboring minimal endometriosis with either laser laparoscopy (n = 83), danazol (n = 47) or both approaches combined (n = 37). Groups differed with respect to age, duration of infertility and the presence of other risk factors for infertility. Only uncorrected pregnancy probabilities are available. In each group 49, 44.6 and 51.4% of the patients became pregnant, respectively. Ronnberg et al. [39] treated 90 patients with conservative surgery, 59 with danazol only, 44 with surgery and danazol postoperatively, and 18 with laparoscopic electrocoagulation. The mean score according to the AFS-R classification was 8.1, 15.2, 6.0 and 1.9 in the four groups, respectively. Despite these differences in the severity of endometriosis, the uncorrected pregnancy probability was lower among women treated with laparoscopic electrocoagulation (17%) than among patients treated with conservative surgery (43%), surgery combined with danazol (32%) or danazol only (56%). Seiler et al. [63] treated 45 patients with laparoscopic electrocauterization and 41 with danazol. All subjects had moderate endometriosis according to Acosta classification. Treatment was alternated every 2 or 3 months, so that calendar months determined the patient's treatment. Age, duration of infertility, presence of other infertility factors were not different in the two groups. After 7 months of observation, the pregnancy probability was similar for subjects treated with laparoscopic cauterization (44%) or danazol (39%). Fayez et al. [62] studied 238 patients with minimal or mild endometriosis who had no other major causes of infertility. Women were treated either with danazol alone (n = 76), operative laparoscopy and danazol (n = 80) or operative laparoscopy alone (n = 82). Age, duration of infertility and parity were similar in the three groups. Uncorrected pregnancy probabilities in this study appeared higher with operative laparoscopy alone (73.2%) or combined with danazol (53.8%) than with danazol alone (26.3%). Cumulative pregnancy probabilities based on life-table analysis also favoured patients treated with operative laparoscopy.

To properly evaluate the effect of laparoscopic surgery in infertilie patients har-

*Table 1.* Base-line characteristics of infertile women with minimal or mild endometriosis and operative complications according to study group[a].

| Characteristics | Laparoscopic surgery group (n = 172) | Diagnostic laparoscopic group (n = 169) |
|---|---|---|
| Age (years) | 31 ± 3 | 30 ± 4 |
| < 30 | 36% | 45% |
| 30–34 | 49% | 44% |
| > 35 | 15% | 11% |
| BMI (kg/m$^2$) | 23 ± 4 | 23 ± 4 |
| Education (years) | 14 ± 3 | 14 ± 3 |
| Caffeine intake (mg/day) | 271 ± 238 | 302 ± 291 |
| Smoking status | | |
| Nonsmoker | 72% | 71% |
| Smoker, < 20 cig./day | 19% | 16% |
| Smoker, > 20 cig./day | 9% | 13% |
| Primary infertility[b] | 66% | 75% |
| Duration of infertility (months) | 31 ± 16 | 31 ± 16 |
| 12–24 | 44% | 42% |
| 25–36 | 34% | 35% |
| > 36 | 22% | 23% |
| Coital frequency (last 3 months) (No./month) | 10 ± 4 | 10 ± 4 |
| Motile sperm count ($\times 10^6$) | 181 ± 154 | 197 ± 196 |
| Less than 14% normal forms in semen (No.) | 3 | 1 |
| Cycle length (last 6 months) (days) | 29 ± 2 | 29 ± 2 |
| Laparoscopic findings | | |
| Median R-AFS score[c] | 4 | 4 |
| Minimal endometriosis | 62% | 67% |
| Superficial lesions only | 52% | 57% |
| Lesions on peritoneum only | 60% | 70% |
| Adhesions | 16% | 18% |
| Fibroid | 11% | 7% |
| Partial tubal occlusion | 8% | 5% |
| Intraoperative complications (no.) | | |
| Intestinal contusion | 1 | 0 |
| Slight tear of tubal serosa | 1 | 0 |
| Difficult pneumoperitoneum | 1 | 0 |
| Vascular trauma | 0 | 1 |
| Duration of anesthesia (min) | 46 ± 19 | 33 ± 13 |
| Postoperative complications (No.) | | |
| Wound infection or hematoma | 7 | 5 |
| Urinary tract infection | 3 | 1 |

[a]± Values correspond to mean ± SD; [b]defined as no previous pregnancy; [c]R-AFS denotes the Revised American Fertility Society classification of endometriosis. Endometriotic implants on the peritoneum or ovaries are given a score according to diameter and depth whereas adhesions are scored taking into account density and degree of enclosure. Total (implants and adhesions) R-AFS scores from 1–5, 6–15, 16–40 or 41–150 correspond to minimal (stage I), mild (stage II), moderate (stage III) and severe (stage IV) endometriosis, respectively.

boring minimal or mild endometriosis, we conducted the Endocan Studies (Table 1).

We studied 341 infertile women aged between 20 and 39 years with minimal or mild endometriosis. During diagnostic laparoscopy the women were randomly assigned to resection or ablation of visible endometriosis or diagnostic laparoscopy only. They were followed up for 36 weeks after the laparoscopy or, for those who became pregnant during that interval, up to 20 weeks of pregnancy.

Among the 172 women who had resection or ablation of endometriosis, 50 became pregnant and had 20-week or longer pregnancies, as compared with 29 of the 169 women in the diagnostic laparoscopy group (cumulative probabilities, 30.7 and 17.7%, respectively; log-rank test, $p = 0.006$). The corresponding rates of fecundability were 4.7 and 2.4 per 100 person-months (rate ratio, 1.9; 95% confidence interval 1.2–3.1). Fetal losses occurred in 20.6 and 21.6% of all recognized pregnancies in the laparoscopic surgery group and the diagnostic laparoscopy group, respectively ($p = 0.91$). Four minor operative complications (intestinal contusion, slight tear of tubal serosa, difficult pneumoperitoneum and vascular trauma) were reported (three in the surgery group and one in the control group).

We found that resection or ablation of minimal and mild endometriosis increases the likelihood of pregnancy in infertile women as compared with diagnostic laparoscopy alone. The shape of the incidence curves suggests that this difference would have remained the same had the follow up been longer. The women were assigned to a treatment group during the laparoscopy after the staging of endometriosis was completed in order to prevent exclusion of women after randomization and biased staging of endometriosis due to knowledge of the treatment group.

Four of the 79 women whose pregnancies reached 20 weeks, all in the diagnostic laparoscopy group, reported a cointervention during the cycle of conception (clomiphene citrate therapy in two women, superovulation/intrauterine insemination in one woman or in the preceding cycle (cyst excision in one woman). Had these cointerventions contributed to the occurrence of the pregnancy, this would result in slight underestimation of the effect of the laparoscopic surgery.

We did not require histologic confirmation of suspected endometriotic lesions because it is not routine practice to obtain histologic diagnosis before proceeding to the destruction of lesions. Furthermore, removal of lesions by biopsy, especially in women who have few lesions, is a form of surgical treatment. In order to reduce the risk that women without endometriosis were enrolled in the trial, we required that typical lesions be seen. If some women without endometriosis had nevertheless been included, the results would underestimate the efficacy of laparoscopic surgery in women who had endometriosis because women without endometriosis would be unlikely to benefit from the intervention.

Fetal losses occurred in approximately 20% of recognized pregnancies irrespective of the study group. These results do not support the view that the treatment of endometriosis reduces the risk of spontaneous abortion in infertile women [64—66].

Several observations support the validity of our results. The ratio of minimal to mild endometriosis (1.8) in the women we studied is close to those reported in other studies of infertile women (2.0 to 2.4) [67—69]. The fecundability rate in the diagnostic laparoscopy group (3.2 per 100 person-months) is similar to the rate (3 per 100 person-months) estimated in four groups of untreated infertile women with mild endometriosis [70].

Our results have important implications. First, they provide infertile couples and their physicians with useful figures on which to base decisions about laparoscopy. The absolute increase in the 36-week probability of pregnancy beyond 20 weeks attributable to laparoscopic surgery was 13%. Stated differently, one out of eight women [71] with minimal or mild endometriosis should benefit from resection or ablation of endometriosis when considering that outcome of pregnancy. Second, operative laparoscopy can be performed at the same time as the diagnostic laparoscopy, prolongs the laparoscopy by only a few minutes, entails few risks, and can be done on an outpatient basis. We recommend therefore that minimal or mild endometriosis diagnosed during laparoscopy for infertility be resected or ablated at that time. Third, the monthly fecundability rate among women who underwent laparoscopic surgery (6.1%) remains much lower than that expected in fertile women (20%) [72]. This indicates that the destruction of visible endometriotic implants and adhesiolysis do not affect all factors by which minimal and mild endometriosis contribute to infertility, such as tissular growth factors, prostaglandin concentrations and macrophage activity in the peritoneal fluid, or that factors other than endometriosis interfere with fertility.

In conclusion, laparoscopic surgery in infertile women with minimal or mild endometriosis is effective in increasing fecundity in these women while incurring minimal risk.

## References

1. Pauerstein CJ. Clinical presentation and diagnosis. In: Schenken RS (ed) Endometriosis. Contemporary Concepts in Clinical Management. Philadelphia: Lippincott, 1989;127.
2. Sampson JA. Perforating hemorrhagic (chocolate) cysts of the ovary. Arch Surg 1921;3:245.
3. Sampson JA. Peritoneal endometriosis due to dissemination of endometrial tissue into the peritoneal cavity. Am J Obstet Gynecol 1927;14:422.
4. Meyer R. Metaplasia theory with inflammation as a primary inducing factor: adenomyosis, adenofibrosis and adenomyoma. In: Von Walter H (ed) Veit-Stockel Handbuch der Gynakologic. Munchen, Bergmann, 1930.
5. Dmowski WP, Steele RW, Baker GF. Deficient cellular immunity in endometriosis. Am J Obstet Gynecol 1981;141:377.
6. Steele RW, Dmowski WP, Marmer DJ. Immunologic aspects of human endometriosis. Am J Reprod Immunol 1984;6:33.
7. Dizerega GS, Barber DL, Hodgen GD. Endometriosis: role of ovarian steroids in initiation, maintenance, and suppression. Fertil Steril 1980;33:649.
8. Vernon M, Rush M, Wilson E. Effect of pregnancy and steroids on endometrial implants in rats with surgically induced endometriosis. Fertil Steril 1984;41:10S.

9. American Fertility Society. Revised American Fertility Society Classification of endometriosis. Fertil Steril 1985;43:351.
10. Acosta AA, Buttram VC, Besch PK et al. A proposed classification of pelvic endometriosis. Obstet Gynecol 1973;42:19.
11. Kistner RW. Gynecology, Principles and Practice, 2nd edn. Chicago: Year Book Medical Publishers, 1979;432.
12. Drake TS, O'Brien WF, Ramwell PW et al. Peritoneal fluid thromboxane $B_2$ and 6-keto prostaglandin $F_1$ alpha in endometriosis. Am J Obstet Gynecol 1981;140:401.
13. Badawy SZA, Cuenca V, Marshall L et al. Cellular components in peritoneal fluid in infertile patients with and without endometriosis. Fertil Steril 1984;42:704.
14. Marik J, Hulka J. Luteinized unruptured follicle syndrome: a subtle cause of infertility. Fertil Steril 1978;29:270.
15. Muscato JJ, Haney AF, Weinberg JB. Sperm phagocytosis by human peritoneal macrophages: a possible cause of infertility in endometriosis. Am J Obstet Gynecol 1982;144:503.
16. Meek SC, Hodge DD, Musich JR. Autoimmunity in infertile patients with endometriosis. Am J Obstet Gynecol 1988;158:1365.
17. Evers JLH. The pregnancy rate of the no-treatment group in randomized clinical trials of endometriosis therapy. Fertil Steril 1989;52:906.
18. Seibel MM, Berger MJ, Weinstein FG et al. The effectiveness of danazol on subsequent fertility in minimal endometriosis. Fertil Steril 1982;38:534.
19. Thomas EJ, Cooke ID, Successful treatment of asymptomatic endometriosis: does it benefit infertile women? Br Med J 1987;294:1117.
20. Bayer SR, Seibel MM, Saffan DS et al. Efficacy of danazol treatment for minimal endometriosis in infertile women, a prospective randomized study. J Reprod Med 1988;33:179.
21. Telimaa S. Danazol and medroxyprogesterone acetate inefficaceous in the treatment of infertility in endometriosis. Fertil Steril 1988;50:872.
22. Floyd WS. Danazol: endocrine and endometrial effects. Int J Fertil 1980;25:75.
23. Buttram VC, Belue JB, Reiter R. Interim report of a study of danazol for the treatment of endometriosis. Fertil Steril 1982;37:478.
24. Hull ME, Moghissi KS, Magyar DF et al. Comparison of different treatment modalities of endometriosis infertile women. Fertil Steril 1987;47:40.
25. Fedele L, Bianchi S, Viezzoli T et al. Gestrinone versus danazol in the treatment of endometriosis. Fertil Steril 1989;51:781.
26. Henzl MR, Corson SL, Moghissi K et al. Administration of nasal nafarelin as compared with oral danazol for endometriosis. A multicenter double-blind comparative clinical trial. N Engl J Med 1988;318:485.
27. Noble AD, Letchworth AT. Medical treatment of endometriosis: a comparative trial. Postgrad Med J 1979;55:37.
28. Bickers W. Stillbestrol in endometriosis. South Med J 1949;42:229.
29. Creadick RM. The nonsurgical treatment of endometriosis: a preliminary report on the use of methyltestosterone. NC Med J 1950;11:576.
30. Preston SN, Campbell HB. Pelvic endometriosis treatment with methyltestosterone. Obstet Gynecol 1953;2:152.
31. Han M. Preliminary results of the gossypol treatment in the menopausal functional uterine bleeding, muyoma, and endometriosis. Acta Med Chin Acad Med Sci 1980;2:167.
32. Garcia C-R, David SS. Pelvic endometriosis: infertility and pelvic pain. Am J Obstet Gynecol 1977;129:740.
33. Olive DL, Lee KL. Analysis of sequential treatment protocols for endometriosis-associated infertility. Am J Obstet Gynecol 1986;154:613.
34. Schenken RS, Malinak RL. Conservative surgery versus expectant management for the infertile patient with mild endometriosis. Fertil Steril 1982;37:183.
35. Wong PC, Heng SH, Kumar J et al. Expectant treatment versus conservative treatment in the

management of mild endometriosis. Asia-Oceania J Obstet Gynaecol 1986;12:43.

36. Badawy SZA, ElBakry MM, Samuel F et al. Cumulative pregnancy rates in infertile women with endometriosis. J Reprod Med 1988;33:757.

37. Buttram VC, Reiter RC, Ward S. Treatment of endometriosis with danazol: report of a 6-year prospective study. Fertil Steril 1985;43:353.

38. Federici D, Conti E, Costantini W et al. Endometriosis and infertility: our experience over the five years. Hum Reprod 1988;3:109.

39. Ronnberg L, Jarvinen PA. Pregnancy rates following various therapy modes for endometriosis in infertile patients. Am J Obstet Gynecol Scand 1984;123(Suppl):69.

40. Wheeler JM, Malinak LR. Postoperative danazol therapy in infertility patients with severe endometriosis. Fertil Steril 1981;36:460.

41. Gomel V, James C. Intraoperative management of ureteral injury during operative laparoscopy. Fertil Steril 1991;55:416.

42. Keye WR. Laparoscopic treatment of endometriosis. Obstet Gynecol Clin North Am 1989;16:157.

43. Eward RD. Cauterization of stages I and II endometrisis and the resulting pregnancy rate. In: Philip JM (ed) Endoscopy in Gynecology. California: Downey, 1978;276.

44. Bruhat M, Mage C, Manhes M. Use of carbon dioxide laser via laparoscopy. In: Kaplan I (ed) Laser Surgery III. Proceedings of the Third Congress for the International Society for Laser Surgery. Tel Aviv: International Society for Laser Surgery, 1979;275−282.

45. Daniell JF, Pittaway DE. Use of the $CO_2$ laser in laparoscopic surgery: initial experience with the second puncture technique. Infertility 1982;5:15.

46. Kelly RW, Roberts DK. $CO_2$ laser laparoscopy: a potential alternative to danazol in the treatment of stage I and II endometriosis. J Reprod Med 1983;28:638.

47. Martin DC. $CO_2$ laser laparoscopy for the treatment of endometriosis associated with infertility. J Reprod Med 1985;30:409.

48. Daniell JF. Operative laparoscopy for endometriosis. Semin Reprod Endocrinol 1985;3:353.

49. Feste JR. Laser laparoscopy: a new modality. J Reprod Med 1985:30:413.

50. Davis GD. Management of endometriosis and its associated adhesions with the $CO_2$ laser laparoscope. Obstet Gynecol 1986;68;422.

51. Nehzat C, Crowgey SR, Garrison CP. Surgical treatment of endometriosis via laser laparoscopy. Fertil Steril 1986;45:778.

52. Donnez J. Carbon dioxide laser laparoscopy in infertile women with adhesions or endometriosis. Fertil Steril 1987;48:390.

53. Olive DL, Martin DC. Treatment of endometriosis-associated infertility with $CO_2$ laser laparoscopy. The use of one- and two-parameter exponential models. Fertil Steril 1987;48:18.

54. Paulson JD, Asmer P. The use of $CO_2$ laser laparoscopy for treating endometriosis. Int J Fertil 1987;32:237.

55. Gast MJ, Tobler R, Strickler RC et al. Laser vaporization of endometriosis in an infertile population. The role of complicating infertility factors. Fertil Steril 1988;49:32.

56. Nehzat C, Crowgey S, Nezhat F. Videolaseroscopy for the treatment of endometriosis associated with infertility. Fertil Steril 1989;51:237.

57. Sutton C, Hill D. Laser laparoscopy in the treatment of endometriosis. A 5-year study. Br J Obstet Gynaecol 1990;97:181.

58. Sulewski JM, Curcio FD, Bronitsky C, Stenger VG. The treatment of endometriosis at laparoscopy for infertility. Am J Obstet Gynecol 1980;138:128.

59. Murphy AA, Schlafl WD, Hassiakos D, Durmosoglu F, Damewood F, Rock JA. Laparoscopic cautery in the treatment of endometriosis-related infertility. Fertil Steril 1991;55:246.

60. Olive DL, Haney AF. Endometriosis-associated infertility: a critical review of therapeutic approaches. Obst Gynecol Surv 1986;41:538.

61. Chong AP, Keene ME, Thornton NL. Comparison of three modes of treatment for infertility patients with minimal pelvic endometriosis. Fertil Steril 1990;53:407.

62. Fayez JA, Collazo LM, Vernon C. Comparison of different modalities of treatment for minimal and mild endometriosis. Am J Obstet Gynecol 1988;159:927.
63. Seiler JC, Gidwani G, Ballard L. Laparoscopic cauterization of endometriosis for fertility: a controlled study. Fertil Steril 1986;46:1098.
64. Groll M. Endometriosis and spontaneous abortion. Fertil Steril 1984;41:933—935.
65. Wheeler JM, Johnston BM, Malinak LR. The relationship of endometriosis to spontaneous abortion. Fertil Steril 1983;39:656—660.
66. Naples JD, Batt RE, Sadigh H. Spontaneous abortion rate in patients with endometriosis. Obstet Gynecol 1981;57:509—512.
67. Gruppo italiano per lo studio dell'endometriosi. Prevalence and anatomical distribution of endometriosis in women with selected gynaecological conditions: results from a muticentric Italian study. Hum Reprod 1994;9:1158—1162.
68. Koninckx PR, Meuleman C, Demeyere S, Lesaffre E, Cornillie FJ. Suggestive evidence that pelvic endometriosis is a progressive disease, whereas deeply infiltrating endometriosis is associated with pelvic pain. Fertil Steril 1991;55:759—765.
69. Matorras R, Rodiguez F, Pijoan JI, Ramon O, de Teran GG, Rodriguez-Escudero F. Epidemiology of endometriosis in infertile women. Fertil Steril 1995;63:34—38.
70. Hull MGR. Infertility treatment: relative effectiveness of conventional and assisted conception methods. Hum Reprod 1992;7:785—796.
71. Laupacis A, Sackett DL, Roberts RS. An assessment of clinically useful measures of the consequences of treatment. N Engl J Med 1988;318:1728—1733.
72. Cramer DW, Walker AM, Schiff I. Statistical methods in evaluating the outcome of infertility therapy. Fertil Steril 1979;32:80—86.
73. Nowroozi K, Chase JS, Check J, Wu CH. The importance of laparosocopic coagulation of mild endometriosis in infertile women. Int J Fertil 1987;32:442.
74. American Fertility Society. Revised American Fertility Society classification of endometriosis: 1985. Fertil Steril 1985;43:351—352.
75. Kaplan E, Meier P. Nonparametric estimation from incomplete observations. J Am Stat Assoc 1958;53:457—481.
76. Mantel N. Evaluation of survival data and two rank order statistics arising in its consideration. Cancer Chemother Rep 1966;50:163—170.
77. Cox DR. Regression models and lifetables. J R Stat Soc 1972;34:184—220.

Fertility and Reproductive Medicine.
R.D. Kempers, J. Cohen, A.F. Haney and J.B. Younger, editors.

# Management of advanced endometriosis

Paolo Vercellini, Anna Pisacreta, Olga De Giorgi, Lara Yaylayan, Barbara Zàina and Pier Giorgio Crosignani

*Clinica Ostetrica e Ginecologica "Luigi Mangiagalli", University of Milan, Milan, Italy*

**Abstract.** It is perhaps logical to consider "advanced endometriosis" simply as a stage IV of the American Society for Reproductive Medicine classification. However, the definition "advanced endometriosis" should also include the infiltrative forms that involve vital structures such as bowel, ureters, and bladder, or forms such as many rectovaginal lesions that might greatly alter the quality of life because of severe pain at menstruation and intercourse but that are given little or no weight in the current staging system. Drugs do not cure endometriosis but only induce temporary quiescence of active lesions and may be useful in selected circumstances. Due to their tolerable side effects and limited cost, progestins with or without estrogens should be seriously considered as first-line medical treatment for temporary pain relief. However, in most cases of severe disease, surgery is the final solution. The pelvis affected by advanced endometriosis can be divided into four distinct sectors with specific anatomical and pathological characteristics each requiring a particular surgical approach. In a sagittal view, the presence of an anteverted uterus delimits two dependent areas in which the regurgitated endometrial cells may collect, implant and grow: the anterouterine and posterouterine pouches, the former being the site of origin of bladder detrusor endometriosis and the latter of rectovaginal endometriosis. Also, the two adnexal regions are anatomically different, the left one being "hidden" by the sigmoid colon and the right one being completely exposed to the pelvic environment as the cecum is anatomically more cranial. The left ovary is more frequently affected by an endometrioma than the right, and likewise, ureteral involvement by endometriosis is more frequent on the left side than the right. No consensus has been reached regarding the efficacy of adjuvant therapy. There are practical advantages inherent in the use of medical treatment before conservative surgery for advanced endometriosis, but whether this translates into better conception rates and reduced pain recurrence rates is unproven. Likewise, the available data do not support the notion that suppressing ovarian activity postoperatively increases the pregnancy rate or reduces the long-term pain and disease recurrence rates. Finally, great importance must be given to complete and balanced counseling, as awareness of the real possibilities of different treatments will enhance the patient's collaboration, facilitating acceptance of what may be considered a reasonable compromise but might otherwise appear as a partial therapeutic failure.

**Keywords:** endometriosis, infertility, medical treatment, pelvic pain, surgery.

## Introduction

What is advanced endometriosis? It is tempting to consider it simply as the fourth stage of the American Society for Reproductive Medicine (ASRM) classification [1]. However, it might also be argued that the definition "advanced endo-

---

*Address for correspondence:* Paolo Vercellini MD, Clinica Ostetrica e Ginecologica "Luigi Mangiagalli", Università di Milano, Via Commenda 12, 20122 Milano, Italy. Tel.: +39-2-55193176. Fax: +39-2-55187146.

metriosis" should also include the infiltrative forms that involve vital structures, e.g., bowel, ureters and bladder, or forms such as many rectovaginal lesions that might greatly alter the quality of life because of severe pain at menstruation and intercourse [2—5]. Unfortunately, all the above disease patterns are not specifically addressed in the ASRM scheme which was devised mainly with the object of stratifying patients with a different reproductive prognosis [6—8]. In the ASRM staging system great weight is given to ovarian endometriomas so that, for example, a woman with bilateral endometriotic cysts of 4 cm in diameter is considered as having severe disease [1]. From a practical standpoint, these clinical conditions can often be managed easily as operative laparoscopy has almost replaced laparotomy in the surgical approach to adnexal lesions and the mere presence of ovarian cysts usually does not pose particularly difficult technical problems [9—14]. Endoscopic enucleation of a large endometrioma is gratifying for both the surgeon and the patient viewing the operation recorded on a videotape, but the real difficulties are usually found to lie elsewhere and are not necessarily proportional to cyst diameter, whereas score attribution is [1,15]. We consider that management of severe endometriosis should be viewed in perspective, giving greater importance to aspects that pose the most difficult surgical problems independently of stage classification. As these situations are not very frequent, no formal comparative trial on the most effective treatment exists. Consequently, most of the considerations and suggestions that follow are unfortunately not "evidence-based" but again the result of opinions based on clinical experience.

**Medical management**

It is well-established that hormonal drugs do not cure endometriosis but only induce temporary quiescence of active lesions [16,17], and that in most cases of advanced disease, surgery is the final solution [14]. However, there are several situations in which medical treatments are still useful. Some women who have already undergone several operations might prefer to avoid further surgery but need pain relief, and others may want only to postpone surgery because of study, work or family problems. Furthermore, ovarian inhibition may be helpful to confirm a preoperative diagnosis when the presenting symptoms are unusual or not clearly attributable to endometriosis. Prompt resolution of disturbances during a short course of medical therapy indicates that endometriosis is in fact the cause and might tip the balance in favor of surgery. Temporary suppression of ovulation may help to distinguish an endometrioma from a luteal cyst, avoiding an untimely intervention in the presence of a functional formation. Drugs may be chosen as an alternative to surgery in the rare very difficult case in which the risks of morbidity and complications outweigh the benefits of a radical operation. However, surgery for ovarian cysts or pelvic lesions of doubtful nature should never be deferred on the assumption that they are endometriotic in origin. The results of transvaginal ultrasonography as a test for the diagnosis of endometriotic cyst are impressive but obtained by expert observers working in tertiary-care, referral centers. Moreover, although elevated CA 125 serum levels are not unusual in the presence of endometriosis, they may be associated with ovarian cancer even in a young woman [18]. In general, prolonged drug treatments for endometriomas are unwarranted also because their resolution has been demonstrated to be highly unlikely [19]. When long-term pain relief is the main objective, great care should be paid to the choice of drug. There is no conclusive evidence that danazol, GnRH agonists or gestrinone produce significantly better antalgic results than progestins or estrogen-progestogen combinations although the considerable differences in safety and tolerability should obviously be taken into account [20]. Recently, several studies have been published on the comparison of the effect of GnRH agonist treatment with or without different types of steroidal add-back therapy [21]. The combination schemes were better tolerated and consistently induced less side effects, as well as limited, or no, bone resorption, but convincing evidence is still lacking that these schedules yield better results than those obtainable with progestins alone. The use of GnRH agonists plus add-back regimens in routine practice would greatly increase the cost of therapy and may limit patients' compliance. Finally, medical therapies should no longer be prescribed with the aim of increasing the chance of pregnancy because it has been repeatedly and definitively demonstrated that hypoestrogenizing drugs do not influence reproductive prognosis [22–26].

**Surgical debulking: a four-quadrant approach**

Although the pathogenesis of endometriosis is still controversial, most available data support the notion that retrograde menstruation is a key factor [27–30]. In fact, the distribution and pattern of lesions seem to be determined mainly by gravity, proximity to the site of abdominal entry and anatomicophysiological variables [31]. In this respect, the pelvis affected by endometriosis could be divided into four distinct sectors with specific anatomical and pathological characteristics each requiring a particular surgical approach. In a sagittal view, the presence of an anteverted uterus delimits two dependent areas in which the regurgitated endometrial cells may collect, implant and grow, the anterouterine and posterouterine pouches, the former being the site of origin of bladder endometriosis [31–33] and latter of rectovaginal endometriosis [3,33]. Also the two adnexal regions are anatomically different, the left one being "hidden" by the sigmoid colon, as is well known to those who perform gynecologic laparoscopic surgery. Not only does this portion of the large bowel lean on the left tube and ovary but it is very often fixed to the pelvic brim by filmy adhesions which are so frequently observed as to be considered a paraphysiological finding. A microenvironment is established around the left adnexa, the boundaries of which are the pelvic side wall, the lateral aspect of the sigmoid and the left broad ligament [34]. Furthermore, involvement of the sigmoid in endometriotic lesions of the left ovary is much more common than involvement of the cecum, which is anatomically more cranial, in endometriomas of the right gonad [34].

A general consideration to be kept in mind is that usually very little ectopic endometrium is found even in the most devastating forms of endometriosis. In fact, the so-called infiltrating endometriotic lesions consist mostly of dense, reactive fibrotic tissue. The pathogenetic pathway leading to anatomic distortion begins with superficial implantation of endometrial cells. This constitutes a strong inflammatory stimulus which triggers a common "protective" response: pelvic structures adhere to the site of ectopic implants with the "aim" of circumscribing the irritating lesion and excluding it from the peritoneal environment [33]. Fibroblasts participate in the "burial" of endometrial foci, but any ensuing scar retraction may cause duplication and invagination of adjacent surfaces. If this occurs, the result differs according to the affected site. When the ovary is involved, an endometriotic cyst may develop [35,36] whereas duplication of the anterouterine pouch peritoneum initiates bladder detrusor endometriosis [32]. When the process involves the sigmoid, the surgeon may have the impression of a distinct, large, hard nodule, but often most of the palpated lesion consists of duplicated and invaginated intestinal wall with only very limited endometriotic tissue [3]. Paradoxically, it seems that the abdominopelvic host response, more than regurgitated endometrial cells per se, is the real cause of the severe anatomic damage (adhesions and fibrosis) observed in advanced endometriosis [33,37,38].

*The anterouterine pouch*

Deep nodules at this site usually involve the bladder dome [32]. However, it must be remembered that there are two distinct forms of bladder detrusor endometriosis, spontaneous and iatrogenic [39] (after a cesarean section), with clearly different pathogenesis and clinical implications. In the former case the vesical nodule represents only one site of a more generalized disease [32,40,41], whereas in the latter the lesion is usually isolated and it may be caused by intraoperative dissemination of endometrial cells or a suboptimal surgical technique for closure of the low transverse uterine incision [32,39]. About 1% of women with spontaneous pelvic endometriosis have urinary tract lesions, involving the bladder in 84% of the cases [40,42]. Vesical endometriosis may present with variable symptoms and insidious onset, often mimicking recurrent cystitis [43]. The classic clinical features are catamenial frequency, urgency, and pain at micturition with vesical tenesmus of varying severity [32,40–43]. Urine cultures are usually negative. Endometriosis rarely infiltrates and ulcerates the mucosal layer of hollow viscera. Consequently, cystoscopy may not reveal the true nature of the lesion because the typical endometriotic bluish nodules are visible in only a minority of patients and biopsies may be nonspecific [32,40–43]. However, cystoscopy should always be performed to rule out epithelial cancer or other nonendometriotic tumors. Ultrasonography with full bladder, although nondiagnostic, reveals the intraluminal nature of the lesion and identifies a cleavage plane between the detrusor nodule and the uterine wall, excluding an anterior leiomyoma [44]. MRI does not normally provide different or more precise information than ultrasound scans, and we do not recommend its routine performance. Intravenous urography is useful to rule out any ureteral strictures and hydroureteronephrosis. Prompt recognition of the condition is important to avoid prolonged morbidity and erroneous treatments, and to limit further involvement of the bladder wall. All antiendometriosis medical treatments are temporarily successful but recurrence of symptoms is the rule at drug withdrawal [45]. However, a preoperative course of medical therapy may be helpful to support the diagnosis in doubtful cases [32]. The definitive solution for bladder endometriosis is transperitoneal abdominal surgery at laparoscopy [46,47] or laparotomy [32], although the latter modality is preferable if a very expert endoscopist is not available. Because of the full-thickness nature of the nodule we never suggest a transurethral resection, which, if complete, has a high risk of bladder perforation and, if partial, would result in short-term recurrence. The procedure begins with careful identification of the limits of the nodule which is generally anterior to the uterine isthmus along the midline. First, any adhesions between the anterior uterine wall and the vesicouterine fold peritoneum must be lysed. As it is not possible to remove the detrusor nodule without opening the bladder lumen, an intentional sagittal incision through the vesical dome is suggested. This exposes the surgical field, making the procedure easier, safer and faster. The lesion is excised with mechanical scissors or electric scalpel and the bladder is finally oversewn with two watertight fine synthetic absorbable sutures. At first-line surgery, the endometriotic vegetation is usually located on the posterior bladder wall well above the trigonal area. Consequently, ureteral cannulation is not indispensable. A very different situation may exist in patients with recurrent lesions which may infiltrate down the bladder approaching the ureteral meatuses. It is our strong conviction that surgical eradication of recurrent bladder detrusor endometriosis should be performed by a urologist. Finally, due to its position far from the adnexa, isolated bladder detrusor endometriosis may not always interfere with fertilization processes. Consequently, it is not unusual to observe conceptions also in nonoperated women. However, in the event that a cesarean section is indicated, one should not be tempted to schedule partial cystectomy on the same occasion as the considerable increase in blood flow renders the procedure hemorrhagic. Furthermore, unexpectedly, pregnancy status does not facilitate development of cleavage planes between the uterus and the bladder due to the firm fibrotic nature of the adhesions. Unfortunately, symptoms usually reappear when ovulation resumes, and surgery is only deferred.

*The posterouterine pouch*

Some authors suggest that deep endometriotic nodules involving the posterior vaginal and anterior rectal walls should be considered a different disease from peritoneal endometriosis and called rectovaginal septum adenomyosis [48,49].

According to this theory, the histopathogenesis is not related to implantation of regurgitated endometrial cells but to metaplasia of Müllerian remnants [49]. Alternatively, these forms could be the most severe manifestation of peritoneal disease, and the label of rectovaginal "septum" lesions should be reconsidered based on anatomical considerations. In fact, the vast majority of these nodular fibrotic placques are found in the retrocervical area, sometimes extending laterally along the parametrium. The rectovaginal septum is located caudally with respect to the posterior vaginal fornix and is usually not the real site of deep nodular endometriosis [50]. Partial obliteration of the pouch of Douglas by the anterior rectal wall may give a false impression of a subperitoneal lesion when it is not. Furthermore, various extensions of intraperitoneal disease were present in all cases of vaginal endometriosis observed by us, suggesting that the pathogenesis may not be completely different [3,5]. There are not sufficient data to discard the hypothesis that the inflammation triggered by bleeding intraperitoneal endometriotic papules in the most dependent portion of the pouch of Douglas results in adhesion between adjacent peritoneal surfaces, that is, the anterior rectal wall and posterior vaginal fornix [33]. The ectopic implants become nodular when embedded by firm, scar-like connective tissue resulting from reactive proliferation of fibroblasts, which also infiltrate the muscular layers of the rectum and vagina giving origin to a sort of desmoid tumor [51]. In other words, what it is called rectovaginal septum endometriosis is instead massive disease of the deepest portion of the pouch of Douglas which has been buried and excluded from the remaining pelvis by adhesions [33]. The semilunar hard crest protruding through the posterior fornix, which is frequently palpated and observed in these situations, is a fibrotic "cast" of what was the bottom of the posterouterine pouch. Consequently, excision of these lesions implies removal of the fibrotic cast of the cul-de-sac which may or may not involve the entire vaginal wall thickness and the rectal muscular layer according to the severity of the lesion [52–55]. It is unclear why the vaginal mucosa is easily reached by the endometriotic process whereas the rectal mucosa is almost always spared. Differences in histological structure, receptor pattern, and lymphatic drainage may play a role. Unlike the rectum, the vagina has no submucosal layer separating the *tunica muscularis* and the mucosa. MRI and transrectal ultrasonography have been proposed to define the extension and degree of infiltration of these lesions [56]. In our opinion, the above techniques, although valid and helpful in specific circumstances, are not indispensable for routine preoperative assessment. In fact, endometriotic cul-de-sac plaques are easily reached by the gynecologist's examining fingers and a careful rectovaginal evaluation is usually informative enough [57–59]. It is important to determine whether the lesion is situated in the midline or if it extends laterally, involving the parametria. From a surgical point of view, the former situations are generally easier to handle, whereas the latter may be rendered problematic by proximity of the ureter as well as uterine and vaginal vessels. When lateral infiltration has occurred, the left side is more often affected than the right [42]. Different techniques have been suggested to excise deep cul-de-sac endometriotic plaques at laparotomy, laparoscopy, or by the vaginal route [3,52–55,60,61]. A safe and effective surgical approach should take into account the pathogenesis of these lesions. When the ureters are not involved, the major operative risk is rectal perforation. In this regard, endometriosis of the pouch of Douglas should usually be considered a contraindication to a vaginal approach. Moreover, because most of the patients are nulliparous, vaginal accessibility may be suboptimal, especially in operations at the apex at an unfavorable site. Finally, pelvic fibrosis may considerably reduce uterine mobility, which is important in excision of tissue located just behind the cervix. Consequently, we still adopt an abdominal approach at laparotomy in spite of the increase in laparoscopic alternatives, as in our experience it renders relatively easy, rapid and effective a procedure which otherwise might be rather cumbersome [3]. First, the upper, accessible portion of the pouch of Douglas is freed from any ovarian endometriomas. After exploration of what is the false bottom of the cul-de-sac and bilateral identification of the ureters, the surgeon inserts the index and middle fingers of the left hand in the vagina behind the cervix, pushing the posterior fornix upward. This results in optimal exposure of the operating field and enables the surgeon to detach the rectum from the posterior fornix with the scissors used with the right hand, directing the cuts towards the intravaginal fingertips. The juxtaposition of the left fingers and the tip of the scissors' blades handled by the right hand gives a precise and continuous feeling of the plane of dissection being progressively developed, minimizing the risk of bowel perforation. The fornix is then opened by cutting along the attachment of the vaginal cuff to the posterior part of the cervix. The incised posterior vaginal fornix is extended with delicate grasping forceps and a narrow-blade retractor is inserted between cervix and vagina, pushing the uterus towards the pubic symphysis. This allows direct inspection of the posterior vaginal wall and a precise estimate of the need for further rectal detachment. Once free margins are reached both laterally and caudally, the plaque is excised, usually with a "V" shaped incision which follows the original shape of the lower pouch of Douglas. The specimen removed is a sort of cast of the bottom of the cul-de-sac and usually involves part of the muscularis layer of the rectum. The vagina is reattached to the cervix by means of a "T" shaped suture and the anterior rectal wall is reinforced. With this procedure the cephalic portion of the rectovaginal septum is not dissected because it is generally not infiltrated by the endometriotic plaque. We agree with the authors who maintain that a low anterior rectal resection is almost never necessary [60,61], and strongly suggest that opening of the rectal lumen should be avoided if at all possible. The mucosal and submucosal bowel layers are very rarely affected, and the risk of secondary stenosis seems highly improbable.

*The right posterior hemipelvis*

In our experience, the right ovary is less frequently affected by an endometrioma then the left [34]. Furthermore, this side is generally easier to explore than the left side because the cecum, being cephalad, is usually not greatly involved in adhesions. Surgical treatment of an ovarian endometriotic cyst begins with gonadal mobilization. In fact, the ovary almost always adheres to a greater or lesser extent to the pelvic side wall [11,15,18]. This is in line with the pathogenetic theory of ovarian invagination around a superficial peritoneal implant. [35,36]. Mobilization allows complete and safe treatment of the pseudocysts, limiting the risk of ureteral damage. We perform this maneuver at laparoscopy with bipolar forceps and judicious application of a coagulating current to limit peritoneal bleeding which may be diffuse and disturbing [5]. Ovarian endometriomas usually open during adhesiolysis, spilling their chocolate content in the posterior pelvis. After aspiration and lavage, the collapsed gonad is grasped and mobilization is completed. The pseudocyst opening, generally located near the utero-ovarian ligament, is widened and used for inspection and as the site of initial excision. Some authors resect the pseudocyst wall, others spare it, treating its inner surface with lasers or electric current [11,15,36]. A comprehensive discussion of the pros and contras of the two modalities is outside the scope of the present chapter. We are not aware of formal comparisons that demonstrate definite advantages of any of the above techniques. Furthermore, it cannot be excluded that different types of cysts may exist [15,35,36,62,63]. Due to the high endometrioma recurrence rate observed by us after superficial coagulation, we are among those who prefer to excise the pseudocyst wall, although we admit that this probably does not fit the pathogenesis of most lesions [35,36] and that it may reduce the follicular reserve. Finding the correct plane to remove the pseudocyst wall, which is ovarian cortex [35,36], may be time-consuming but is important to limit bleeding and excessive damage to the remaining ovary. Opposite traction is applied to the cyst wall and the "healthy" ovary with two lateral grasping forceps while bipolar forceps are inserted though the median suprapubic port and used to facilitate progressive and complete cleavage. Intermittent coagulation is performed when bleeders are identified. Technical adaptations are needed when multiple cysts are encountered, but ovarian removal is rarely necessary at first-line surgery. However, anatomical conditions might contraindicate conservation when the woman has already undergone adnexal interventions. After inspection of the remaining ovary and of the pelvic side wall to complete hemostasis, the incised gonadal margins are carefully brought together. Suturing is not indispensable, but a surgical adhesion barrier may be applied at the very end of the entire procedure.

*The left posterior hemipelvis*

This anatomical region seems to be the preferential site of really severe endometriosis, i.e., infiltrative forms with involvement of retroperitoneal structures, and where dense, diffuse adhesions cause tenacious coalescence of several organs in spite of very limited visible active implants. The sigmoid may adhere to the tube, ovary and left broad ligament, burying the adnexa partially or completely [34]. In such cases, the rectum may also be involved, obliterating the pouch of Douglas and rendering recognition of the left uterosacral ligament difficult [3]. The sigmoid must be gently, progressively, and amply mobilized to expose the adnexal area. Hydrodissection is useful, but scissors may be needed. Sometimes the salpinx is stretched over and around an endometrioma, with the ampulla hidden under the ovary and fixed by dense adhesions. Adnexal mobilization must be especially careful because in these conditions anatomical landmarks may be altered. In particular, it may be difficult to recognize the ureter, which can be dislocated superiorly and attached to the ovary, or medially and adjacent to the uterosacral ligament. Moreover, ureteral involvement by endometriosis is more frequent here than on the right side [42]. When in doubt, it may be appropriate to adopt a retroperitoneal approach to identify the ureter clearly. This increases peritoneal trauma but may avoid inadvertent lesions which may become symptomatic during the postoperative period. Performance of laparoscopic uterosacral ligament resection by surgeons with limited endoscopic experience is not recommended when the pelvic anatomy is greatly altered [64]. When preoperative rectovaginal examination reveals severe endometriotic infiltration of the lateral parametria, an ultrasound scan of the urinary apparatus or an intravenous urography is opportune to recognize a ureteral stricture, schedule intraoperative urologic consultation [32,40,41,43], and avoid possible medicolegal disputes on whether the stenosis was caused by endometriosis or by surgical procedures.

**Adjuvant therapy**

The theoretical advantages of medical treatment before surgery are reduced inflammation and vascularization and shrinkage of implants. According to some authors, this may contribute to easier, quicker and less traumatic surgery, with more chance of complete eradication of the disease and a reduced risk of postoperative adnexal adhesions [64—70]. Practical advantages include avoidance of operating in the secretory phase with the disturbing presence of the corpus luteum and the possibility of hospital admission at any time [71]. This may be important in large, busy, public hospitals. Moreover, the carryover effect of most drugs used preoperatively prevents short-term ovulation in a recently traumatized gonad [71]. Finally, with preoperative treatment lasting a few months the differential diagnosis between endometriotic and luteal cysts can be easily made, avoiding an untimely intervention when a functional formation is present. On the other hand, under medical suppression small endometriotic foci may temporarily regress and thus escape laparoscopic recognition and ablation [72]. Moreover, delaying surgery may be inopportune in some circumstances, especially when the nature of the cysts is not completely defined and serum CA 125 and CA 19.9 levels are particularly elevated. Indisputable disadvantages are, obviously, the increase in the overall cost of treatment and drug-related side effects. Apart from general considerations, only limited data are available to evaluate the effect of preoperative medical treatments on both surgical aspects and long-term outcome. According to the extensive evaluations of preoperative medical therapies by Donnez et al. [69,73,74] a GnRH agonist in depot formulation is superior to progestins, danazol, gestrinone, and the same GnRH agonist given as nasal spray in terms of reduction of inflammation, vascularization, American Fertility Society score [75], mean endometrioma diameter, and mitotic index. In a randomized trial Donnez et al. [70] demonstrated that goserelin administration for 3 months after drainage of endometriomas partially prevented the regrowth to the original dimensions observed in the subjects who were not medically treated between first- and second-look laparoscopy. However, whether all the above factors contribute to easier, quicker, and more effective surgery remains debatable. In fact, when Muzii et al. [76] compared the intraoperative results of 20 patients undergoing laparoscopy after 3 months of GnRH agonist treatment with those of 21 women allocated to immediate surgery for unilateral ovarian endometriomas, no significant difference could be demonstrated in total operating time, cyst wall stripping time, and the time needed to obtain complete hemostasis. In the absence of convincing evidence of a treatment effect in terms of surgical advantages, pregnancy rate, and symptomatic relief, preoperative medical treatment seems unjustified if it means that the patient has to undergo two surgical procedures some months apart [77]. In these circumstances the increase in morbidity and costs seem to far outweigh the hypothetical benefits. However, several authors have demonstrated the good overall reliability of transvaginal ultrasonography in the diagnosis of ovarian endometriotic cysts [78]. Thus, a three-step diagnostic approach (laparoscopy-drug therapy-operative laparoscopy) is no longer indispensable to take advantage of preoperative medical treatment in advanced stages of the disease. A randomized controlled trial (RCT) in selected patients with ovarian endometriomas diagnosed at transvaginal ultrasonography could disentangle the uncertainties surrounding this issue.

Enthusiasm for adjuvant drug therapy after conservative interventions for endometriosis increased after publication of the retrospective findings of Wheeler and Malinak [79]. These authors reported a pregnancy rate of 79% (15/19) after combined surgery and postoperative danazol therapy compared with 30% (36/119) after surgery alone. The hypothetical advantages of postoperative medical treatment include resorption of residual visible lesions whose surgical removal was considered inopportune or not possible, "sterilization" of microscopic implants, and reduction in the risk of disease dissemination when endometriomas rupture during mobilization. This should increase the postoperative pregnancy rate and reduce the recurrence rate [65–68]. Unfortunately, the lesson learned with medical therapies when used alone obviously applies also to postoperative treatments, rendering the above considerations naive. Furthermore, medical treatment might prevent a pregnancy just when a conception may be most likely, i.e., in the immediate postoperative period. However, this last notion has never been confirmed formally.

The quality of the evidence supporting the use of medical treatment before conservative surgery for endometriosis is poor, coming only from noncomparative or small and nonrandomized trials, and no recommendations can be made based on the results of the published studies [77]. This schedule has inherent practical advantages but whether subsequent conception rates are better and pain recurrence rates are reduced is unproven. The effect of drug therapy after surgery can be better assessed as data from three true RCTs are available [80–82]. However, only one north-Italian multicenter study specifically included women with advanced endometriosis [81], whereas all stages were represented in another [80] and stages were not reported in the third [82]. In the first trial 75 women with unexplained infertility with or without pelvic pain who underwent conservative surgery for moderate or severe endometriosis were assigned to nasal nafarelin 400 mg/day (36 subjects) or placebo nasal spray (39 subjects) for 3 months [81]. Pelvic pain was assessed preoperatively and at a 12-month follow-up visit with a 10-point linear analog and a 7-point multidimensional verbal rating scale. Mean linear analog and verbal rating scale score reductions were 7.0 and 3.6 points, respectively, in women allocated nafarelin compared with 6.9 and 4.0, respectively, in those allocated placebo, the differences not being statistically significant. Within 1 year of randomization, 7/36 (19%) women in the experimental arm achieved a pregnancy compared with 7/39 (18%) in the control arm. The results of the above study do not support the notion that suppressing ovarian activity postoperatively increases the long-term pain relief and pregnancy rates.

**Conclusions**

Surgery for severe endometriosis may be as difficult as some gynecologic oncologic interventions, and procedures on the bowel, bladder, ureters, and retroperitoneal space may be needed [3,32,46,52,55,64,83–85]. Conversely, endometriosis is a nonmalignant disease which usually affects young women with high expectations in terms of conception and quality of life. In these circumstances intra- and postoperative complications are perceived and tolerated with difficulty, and invalidating pain recurrence or persistent infertility are particularly frustrating. Given this scenario, a thorough preoperative diagnostic investigation and careful, detailed counseling are of major importance. Whenever possible, involvement of the intestinal and urologic systems should be known in advance, to schedule intraoperative consultation if necessary and to inform the woman about the type of surgery required and its potential sequelae. This will also help to make patients and their families understand the clinical severity of the condition, balancing risks and benefits of the proposed treatments. In particular, as the chances of pregnancy after surgery may be limited, an alternative solution might be chosen, such as in vitro fertilization, adoption, or just expectant management. If the woman has already completed her family and disabling pain is the major problem, definitive surgery could be the best solution [86]. However, prolonged progestin administration may be preferred when hysterectomy or castration are psychologically intolerable [20]. Awareness of the real possibilities of different treatments [5,87,88] will enhance the patient's collaboration, facilitating acceptance of what may be revealed as a reasonable compromise but might otherwise

380

appear as a partial therapeutic failure.

Surgeons must understand that the first operation is usually crucial for the prognosis. Unduly traumatic or nonradical procedures greatly reduce the chance of spontaneous pregnancy and increase the risk of recurrence (or persistence). Second-line interventions for severe endometriosis cannot always or completely reverse previous iatrogenic damage [89—92]. When adequate endoscopic experience is not available locally to deal with all forms of severe endometriosis, the woman should be referred to tertiary-care, specialized centers [93,94]. If this is not feasible, it may be preferable for the "traditional" surgeon to perform a safe and effective intervention at laparotomy rather than operate incompletely at laparoscopy [5]. It has still not been demonstrated that the results obtained at laparoscopy for severe endometriosis are better than those at laparotomy in terms of postoperative pregnancy and pain recurrence rate (Figs. 1 and 2) [5,95—99]. In general, endometriotic lesions should not always be treated just because they are there. We have observed large deep cul-de-sac endometriotic plaques infiltrating the posterior vaginal fornix in completely asymptomatic women [100]. Follow-up evaluation demonstrated that these lesions are not necessarily progressive and may be managed without surgery, sometimes even without medical therapies.

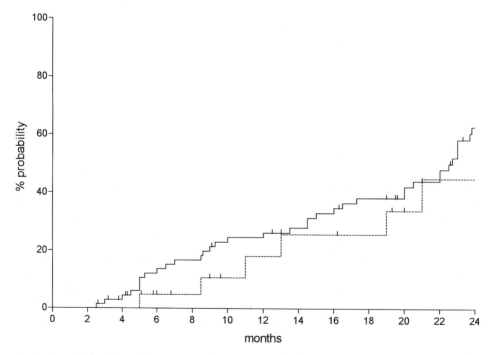

*Fig. 1.* Cumulative 24-month probability of becoming pregnant in 92 infertile women with severe endometriosis according to the conservative surgical treatment modality adopted: (- - -) surgery at laporoscopy (n = 22); (—) surgery at laporatomy (n = 70) (log rank test, $\chi^2_1 = 1.06$, p = 0.31). Vertical tick marks represent the censored observations. (Reproduced by permission from the American Society for Reproductive Medicine (Fertil Steril 1996;66:706—711).)

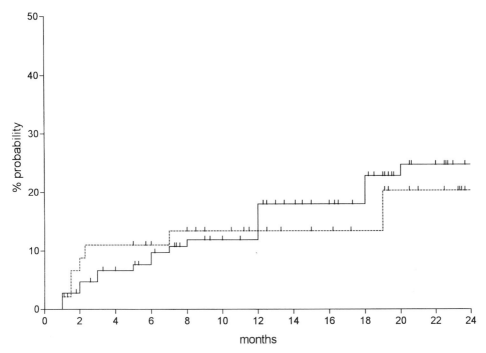

*Fig. 2.* Cumulative 24-month probability of recurrence of moderate or severe dysmenorrhea as assessed by the linear analogue scale in 155 symptomatic women with severe endometriosis according to the conservative surgical treatment modality adopted: (- - -) surgery at laporoscopy (n = 47); (—) surgery at laporatomy (n = 108) (log rank test, $\chi^2_1$ = 0.12, p = 0.74). Vertical tick marks represent the censored observations. (Reproduced by permission from the American Society for Reproductive Medicine (Fertil Steril 1996;66:706—711).)

Large ovarian cysts, or whose volume increases with time, or when the diagnosis is in doubt, as well as intestinal and ureteral foci causing progressive stenosis, constitute indisputable reasons for operating. Otherwise, surgery for asymptomatic endometriosis should not be considered mandatory in all cases. The results of treatment for a benign condition such as endometriosis are functional, and surgical indications should be based mainly on symptoms, especially pain and infertility. For the same reasons, the role of second-look laparoscopy should be reconsidered as pregnancy and long-term relief of pain are the outcomes of interest. Follow-up evaluation of adhesions and recurrent active lesions a few months after surgery increases morbidity and cost but appear to have limited predictive value and, more importantly, still undetermined clinical benefit.

## References

1. American Society for Reproductive Medicine. Revised American Society for Reproductive Medicine classification of endometriosis: 1996. Fertil Steril 1997;67:817—821.
2. Candiani GB, Vercellini P, Fedele L, Bianchi S, Vendola N, Candiani M. Conservative surgical

382

treatment for severe endometriosis in infertile women. Are we making progress? Obstet Gynecol Surv 1991;46:490–498.

3. Candiani GB, Vercellini P, Fedele L, Roviaro GC, Rebuffat C, Trespidi L. Conservative surgical treatment of rectovaginal septum endometriosis. J Gynecol Surg 1992;8:177–182.

4. Crosignani PG, Vercellini P. Conservative surgery for severe endometriosis: should laparotomy be abandoned definitively? Hum Reprod 1995;10:2412–2418.

5. Crosignani PG, Vercellini P, Biffignandi F, Costantini W, Cortesi I, Imparato E. Laparoscopy versus laparotomy in conservative surgical treatment for severe endometriosis. Fertil Steril 1996;66:706–711.

6. Guzick DS, Silliman NP, Adamson GD, Buttram VC, Canis M, Malinak RL, Schenken RS. Prediction of pregnancy in infertile women based on the American Society for Reproductive Medicine's revised classification of endometriosis. Fertil Steril 1997;67:822–829.

7. Olive DL. Classification of endometriosis. Infertil Reprod Med Clin N Am 1992;3:633–645.

8. Hoeger KM, Guzick DS. Classification of endometriosis. Obstet Gynecol Clin N Am 1997; 24:347–359.

9. Reich H, McGlynn F. Treatment of ovarian endometriomas using laparoscopic surgical techniques. J Reprod Med 1986;31:577–584.

10. Canis M, Mage G, Manhes H. Laparoscopic treatment of endometriosis. Acta Obstet Gynecol Scand 1989;15(Suppl):15–20.

11. Cook AS, Rock JA. The role of laparoscopy in the treatment of endometriosis. Fertil Steril 1991;55:663–680.

12. Adamson GD, Hurd SJ, Pasta DJ, Rodriguez BD. Laparoscopic endometriosis treatment: is it better? Fertil Steril 1993;59:35–44.

13. Adamson GD, Nelson HP. Surgical treatment of endometriosis. Obstet Gynecol Clin N Am 1997;24:375–409.

14. Garry R. Laparoscopic excision of endometriosis: the treatment of choice? Br J Obstet Gynaecol 1997;104:513–515.

15. Donnez J, Nisolle M, Gillet N, Smets M, Bassil S, Casanas F. Large ovarian endometriomas. Hum Reprod 1996;11:641–646.

16. Brosens IA, Verleyen A, Cornillie F. The morphologic effect of short-term medical therapy of endometriosis. Am J Obstet Gynecol 1987;157:1215–1221.

17. Nisolle-Pochet M, Casanas-Roux F, Donnez J. Histologic study of ovarian endometriosis after hormonal therapy. Fertil Steril 1988;49:423–426.

18. Vercellini P, Parazzini F, Bolis G, Carinelli S, Dindelli M, Vendola N, Luchini L, Crosignani PG. Endometriosis and ovarian cancer. Am J Obstet Gynecol 1993;169:181–182.

19. Vercellini P, Ventola N, Bocciolone L, Colombo A, Rognoni MT, Bolis G. Laparoscopic aspiration of ovarian endometriomas: effect with postoperative gonadotropin releasing hormone agonist treatment. J Reprod Med 1992;37:577–580.

20. Vercellini P, Cortesi I, Crosignani PG. Progestins for symptomatic endometriosis: a critical analysis of the evidence. Fertil Steril 1997;68:393–401.

21. Pickersgill A. GnRH agonists and add-back therapy: is there a perfect combination? Br J Obstet Gynaecol 1998;105:475–485.

22. Olive D, Haney AF. Endometriosis-associated infertility: a critical review of therapeutic approaches. Obstet Gynecol Surv 1986;41:538–555.

23. Shaw R. Treatment of endometriosis. Lancet 1992;340:1267–1271.

24. Hughes EG, Fedorkow DM, Collins JA. A quantitative overview of controlled trials in endometriosis-associated infertility. Fertil Steril 1993;59:963–970.

25. Vandekerckhove P, O'Donovan PA, Lilford RJ, Harada TW. Infertility treatment: from cookery to science. The epidemiology of randomised controlled trials. Br J Obstet Gynaecol 1993; 100:1005–1020.

26. The ESHRE Capri Workshop Infertility revisited: the state of the art today and tomorrow. Hum Reprod 1986;11:1779–1807.

27. Haney AF. The pathogenesis and aetiology of endometriosis. In: Thomas E, Rock J (eds) Modern Approaches to Endometriosis. Dordrecht, The Netherlands: Kluwer Academic Publishers, 1991;3—19.

28. Rock JA, Markham SM. Pathogenesis of endometriosis. Lancet 1992;340:1264—1267.

29. Olive D, Schwartz LB. Endometriosis. N Engl J Med 1993;24:1759—1769.

30. Vercellini P, De Giorgi O, Aimi G, Panazza S, Uglietti A. Crosignani PG. Menstrual characteristics in women with and without endometriosis. Obstet Gynecol 1997;90:264—268.

31. Jenkins S, Olive DL, Haney AF. Endometriosis: pathogenetic implications of the anatomic distribution. Obstet Gynecol 1986;67:335—338.

32. Vercellini P, Meschia M, De Giorgi O, Cortesi I, Panazza S, Crosignani PG. Bladder detrusor endometriosis: clinical and pathogenetic implications. J Urol 1996;155:84—85.

33. Vercellini P. Endometriosis: what a pain it is. Sem Reprod Endocrinol 1997;15:251—261.

34. Vercellini P, Aimi G, De Giorgi O, Maddalena S, Carinelli S, Crosignani PG. Is cystic ovarian endometriosis an asymmetric disease? Br J Obstet Gynaecol 1998;(In press).

35. Hughesdon PE. The structure of endometrial cysts of the ovary. Obstet Gynaecol Br J Emp 1957;44:69—84.

36. Brosens IA, Puttemans PJ, Deprest J. The endoscopic localization of endometrial implants in the ovarian chocolate cyst. Fertil Steril 1994;61:1034—1038.

37. Canis M, Pouly JL, Wattiez A, Manhes H, Mage G, Bruhat MA. Incidence of bilateral adnexal disease in severe endometriosis (revised American Fertility Society (AFS), stage IV): should a stage V be included in the AFS classification? Fertil Steril 1992;57:691—692.

38. Brosens IA, Puttemans P, Deprest J, Rombauts L. The endometriosis cycle and its derailments. Hum Reprod 1994;9:770—772.

39. Buka NJ. Vescical endometriosis after cesaerean section. Am J Obstet Gynecol 1988;158:1117—1118.

40. Shook TE, Nyberg LM. Endometriosis of the urinary tract. Urology 1988;31:1.

41. Schwartzwald D, Mooppan UM, Ohm HK, Kim H. Endometriosis of bladder. Urology 1992;39:219—222.

42. Markham SM, Carpenter SE, Rock JA. Extrapelvic endometriosis. Obstet Gynecol Clin N Am 1989;16:193—219.

43. Sircus SI, Sant GR, Ucci AA. Bladder detrusor endometriosis mimicking interstitial cystitis. Urology 1988;32:339—342.

44. Fedele L, Bianchi S, Raffaelli R, Portuese A. Preoperative assessment of bladder endometriosis. Hum Reprod 1997;12:2519—2522.

45. Foster RS, Rink RC, Mulcahy JJ. Vescical endometriosis: medical or surgical treatment. Urology 1987;29:64—65.

46. Nezhat CR, Nezhat FR. Laparoscopic segmental bladder resection for endometriosis: a report of two cases. Obstet Gynecol 1993;81:882—884.

47. Dubuisson JB, Chapron C, Aubriot FX, Osman M, Zerbib M. Pregnancy after laparoscopic partial cystectomy for bladder endometriosis. Hum Reprod 1994;9:730—732.

48. Koninckx PR, Martin DC. Deep endometriosis: a consequence of infiltration or retraction or possibly adenomyosis externa? Fertil Steril 1992;58:924—928.

49. Nisolle M, Donnez J. Peritoneal endometriosis, ovarian endometriosis, and adenomyotic nodules of the rectovaginal septum are three different entities. Fertil Steril 1995;68:585—596.

50. Kuhn RJP, Hollyock VE. Observation on the anatomy of the rectovaginal pouch and septum. Obstet Gynecol 1982;59:445—447.

51. Cornillie FJ, Oosterlynch D, Lauweryns JM, Koninckx PR. Deeply infiltrating pelvic endometriosis: histology and clinical significance. Fertil Steril 1990;53:978—982.

52. Martin DC. Laparoscopic and vaginal colpotomy for the excision of infiltrating cul-de-sac endometriosis. J Reprod Med 1988;33:806—808.

53. Reich H, Mc Glynn F, Salvat J. Laparoscopic treatment of cul-de-sac obliteration secondary to retrocervical deep fibrotic endometriosis. J Reprod Med 1991;36:516—522.

384

54. Redwine DB. Laparoscopic en bloc resection for treatment of the obliterated cul-de-sac in endometriosis. J Reprod Med 1992;37:695–698.
55. Nezhat C, Nezhat F, Pennington E. Laparoscopic treatment of infiltrative rectosigmoid colon and rectovaginal septum endometriosis by the technique of videolaparoscopy and the $CO_2$ laser. Br J Obstet Gynaecol 1992;99:664–667.
56. Fedele L, Bianchi S, Portuese A, Borruto F, Dorta M. Transrectal ultrasonography in the assessment of rectovaginal endometriosis. Obstet Gynecol 1998;91:444–448.
57. Martin DC, Hubert G, Levy B. Depth of infiltration endometriosis. J Gynecol Surg 1989; 55–59.
58. Ripps BA, Martin DC. Correlation of pelvic tenderness with implant dimension and stage of endometriosis. J Reprod Med 1990;37:620–624.
59. Ripps BA, Martin DC. Focal pelvic tenderness, pelvic pain and dysmenorrhea in endometriosis. J Reprod Med 1991;36:470–476.
60. Donnez J, Nissole M, Casanas F. Endoscopy surgery. Ballière's Clin Obstet Gynaecol 1993; 7:839–848.
61. Donnez J, Nisolle M, Casanas F, Bassil S, Anaf V. Rectovaginal septum, endometriosis or adenomyosis: laparoscopic management in a series of 231 patients. Hum Reprod 1995;10: 630–635.
62. Nezhat F, Nezhat C, Allan CJ, Metzger DA, Sears DL. A clinical and histological classification of endometriomas: implications for a mechanism of pathogenesis. J Reprod Med 1992;37: 771–776.
63. Nezhat C, Nezhat F, Nezhat C, Seidman DS. Improving the classification of endometriotic ovarian cysts. Hum Reprod Med 1994;9:2212–2213.
64. Chapron C, Dubuisson JB. Laparoscopic treatment of deep endometriosis located on the uterosacral ligaments. Hum Reprod 1996;11:868–873.
65. Kaplan RC, Schenken RS. Combination medical and surgical treatment. In: Schenken RS (Ed) Endometriosis: Contemporary Concepts in Clinical Management. Philadelphia, USA: JB Lippincott Company 1989;279–292.
66. Kettel LM, Murphy AA. Combination medical and surgical therapy for infertile patients with endometriosis. Obstet Gynecol Clin N Am 1989;16:167–177.
67. Malinak LR, Wheeler JM. Combination medical-surgical therapy for endometriosis. In: Shaw RW (Ed) Endometriosis. Carnforth: The Parthenon Publishing Group, 1990;85–91.
68. Thomas EJ. Combining medical and surgical treatment for endometriosis: the best of both worlds? Br J Obstet Gynaecol 1992;99:5–8.
69. Donnez J, Nisolle M, Clerckx F, Casanas F, Saussoy P, Gillert S. Advanced endoscopic techniques used in dysfunctional bleeding, fibroids and endometriosis, and the role of gonadotrophin-releasing hormone agonist treatment. Br J Obstet Gynaecol 1994;101:2–12.
70. Donnez J, Nisolle M, Gillerot S, Anaf V, Clerckx-Braun F, Casanas F. Ovarian endometrial cysts: the role of gonadotropin-realising hormone agonist and/or drainage. Fertil Steril 1994; 62:63–66.
71. Malinak LR. Surgical treatment and adjunct therapy of endometriosis. Int J Gynecol Obstet 1993;(Suppl):S43–S47.
72. Evers JLH. The second-look laparoscopy for evaluation of the result of medical treatment of endometriosis should not be performed during ovarian suppression. Fertil Steril 1987;47: 502–504.
73. Donnez J, Lemaire-Rubbers M, Karaman Y, Nisolle-Pochet M, Casanas F. Combined (hormonal and microsurgical) therapy in infertile women with endometriosis. Fertil Steril 1987;48: 239–242.
74. Donnez J, Nisolle M, Casanas F. Endometriosis-associated infertility: evaluation of preoperative use of danazol, gestrinone and buserelin. Int J Fertil 1990;35:297–301.
75. American Fertility Society. Revised American Fertility Society classification of endometriosis. Fertil Steril 1985;43:351–352.

76. Muzii L, Marana R, Caruana P, Mancuso S. The impact of preoperative gonadotropin-releasing hormone agonist treatment on laparoscopic excision of ovarian endometriotic cysts. Fertil Steril 1996;65:1235—1237.

77. Vercellini P, De Giorgi O, Pesole A, Zaina B, Pisacreta A, Crosignani PG. Endometriosis. Drugs and adjuvant therapy. In: Templeton A, Cooke I, O'Brien PMS (Eds) Evidence-based Fertility Treatment. London: Royal College of Obstetricians and Gynaecologists Press, 1998,(In press).

78. Guerriero S, Ajossa S, Paoletti AM, Mais V, Angiolucci M, Melis GB. Tumor markers and trans-vaginal ultrasonography in the diagnosis of endometrioma. Obstet Gynecol 1996;88:403—407.

79. Wheeler JM, Malinak LR. Postoperative danazol therapy in infertility patients with severe endometriosis. Fertil Steril 1981;36:460—463.

80. Telimaa S, Ronnberg L, Kauppila A. Placebo-controlled comparison of danazol and high-dose medroxyprogesterone acetate in the treatment of endometriosis after conservative surgery. Gynecol Endocrinol 1987;1:363—371.

81. Parazzini F, Fedele L, Busecca M, Falsetti L, Pellegrini S, Venturini PL, Stella M. Postsurgical medical treatment of advanced endometriosis: results of a randomized clinical trial. Am J Obstet Gynecol 1994;171:1205—1207.

82. Hornstein MD, Hemmings R, Yuzpe AA, Heinrichs WL. Use of nafarelin versus placebo after reductive laparoscopic surgery for endometriosis. Fertil Steril 1997;68:860—864.

83. Koninckx PR, Meuleman C, Demeyere S, Lesaffre E, Cornillie FJ. Suggestive evidence that pelvic endometriosis is a progressive disease whereas deeply infiltranting endometriosis is associated with pelvic pain. Fertil Steril 1991;55:759—765.

84. Koninckx PR, Timmermans B, Meuleman C, Penninckx F. Complications of $CO_2$-laser endoscopic excision of deep endometriosis. Hum Reprod 1996;11:2263—2268.

85. Nezhat C, Nezhat F, Nezhat C, Nasserbakht F, Rosati M, Seidman DS. Urinary tract endometriosis treated by laparoscopy. Fertil Steril 1996;66:920—924.

86. Magos A. Endometriosis: radical surgery. Baillière's Clin Obstet Gynaecol 1993;7:849—864.

87. Sutton CJG, Ewen SP, Whitelow N, Haines P. Prospective, randomized, double-blind controlled trial of laser laparoscopy in the treatment of pelvic pain associated with minimal, mild, and moderate endometriosis. Fertil Steril 1994;62:696—700.

88. Sutton CJG, Pooley AS, Ewen SP, Haines P. Follow-up report on a randomized controlled trial of laser laparoscopy in the treatment of pelvic pain associated with minimal to moderate endometriosis. Fertil Steril 1997;68:1070—1074.

89. Schenken RS, Malinak LR. Reoperation after initial treatment of endometriosis with conservative surgery. Am J Obstet Gynecol 1978;131:416—421.

90. Wheeler JM, Malinak LR. Recurrent endometriosis. Contrib Gynecol Obstet 1987;16:13—21.

91. Candiani GB, Fedele L, Vercellini P, Bianchi S, Di Nola G. Repetitive conservative surgery for recurrence of endometriosis. Obstet Gynecol 1991;77:421—424.

92. Redwine DB. Conservative laparoscopic excision of endometriosis by sharp dissection: life table analysis of reoperation and persistent or recurrent disease. Fertil Steril 1991;56:628—634.

93. Azziz R. Operative endoscopy: the pressing need for a structured training and credentialing process. Fertil Steril 1992;58:1100—1102.

94. Chapron C, Devroey P, Dubuisson JB, Pouly JL, Vercellini P. ESHRE guidelines for training, accreditation and monitoring in gynecological endoscopy. Hum Reprod 1997;12:867—868.

95. Adamson GD, Susak LL, Pasta DJ, Hurd SJ, von Franque O, Rodriguez BD. Comparison of $CO_2$ laser laparoscopy with laparotomy for treatment of endometriomata. Fertil Steril 1992;57:965—973.

96. Canis M, Mage G, Wattiez A, Chapron C, Pouly JL, Bassil S. Second-look laparoscopy after laparoscopic cystectomy of large ovarian endometriomas. Fertil Steril 1992;58:617—619.

97. Gantt NF. Infertility and endometriosis: comparison of pregnancy outcomes with laparotomy versus laparoscopic techniques. Am J Obstet Gynecol 1992;166:1072—1082.

98. Fayez JA, Dempsey RA. Short hospital stay for gynaecologic reconstructive surgery via laparotomy. Obstet Gynnecol 1992;81:598—600.

99. Adamson GD, Pasta DJ. Surgical treatment of endometriosis-associated infertility: Meta-analysis compared with survival analysis. Am J Obstet Gynecol 1994;171:1488—1505.
100. Vercellini P, Trespidi L, De Giorgi O, Cortesi I, Parazzini F, Crosignani PG. Endometriosis and pelvic pain: relation to disease stage and localization. Fertil Steril 1996;65:299—304.

# Endometriosis: prevention of recurrences

Johannes L.H. Evers[1], Gerard A.J. Dunselman[1], Jolande A. Land[1] and Peter X.J.M. Bouckaert[2]

[1]*Department of Obstetrics and Gynaecology, Academisch Ziekenhuis Maastricht, Maastricht; and* [2]*Department of Obstetrics and Gynaecology, Atrium Medical Center, Heerlen, Kerkrade, Brunssum, The Netherlands*

**Abstract.** Usually either pain or subfertility bring a patient with endometriosis to her doctor's office. The prevalence of active endometriosis in asymptomatic patients without fertility problems remains unknown. In many cases, however, endometriosis is a chance finding during surgery for another condition. The natural course of the disease is a mystery, and it is almost impossible to reach valid conclusions regarding the pathophysiologic development of the disease and its disappearance or recurrence after (or due to) therapy. Therefore, the time seems right to review the evidence we have today that endometriosis is a recurrent disease. It has been suggested that only in one-third of cases the disease is progressive, whereas in as much as 60% and more of cases the disease remains in a steady state, or eventually even resolves spontaneously with time. Only a few studies have been published that describe the evolution of the disease in a prospective way, without medical or surgical intervention. This survey of available evidence from the literature shows that treatment of recurrent endometriosis should be tailored to the patient and her chief complaint, i.e., pain and/or subfertility. Since probably most of the recurrent disease is reappearance of persistent microscopic disease, we conclude that treatment does not necessarily have to differ from that in patients with primary disease if pain is the patient's main problem. If subfertility is present, the results of reproductive (endoscopic) microsurgery should be compared to those of assisted reproduction.

**Keywords:** de novo formation, endometriosis, medical treatment, outcome, prevalence, recurrence, reoperation, surgical ablation.

## Introduction

Women were not meant to menstruate. Menstruation is a culturally determined phenomenon that a woman is exposed to nowadays at about 40 times the rate they were intended to be. This increase in exposure to ovulation and menstruation is reflected in a significant increase in menstrual-cycle-dependent disorders, one of which is endometriosis. The natural situation in the human female — which is the situation as it was 1,998 years ago — is to have menarche at the age of 18, to conceive for the first time in her first or second ovulatory cycle, and to do so only 10 or 20 more times during her reproductive life, i.e., for about 34 years, as the mean age of death 2,000 years ago was. During most of her reproductive life a woman was anovulatory, either due to (one of her six to 10) preg-

*Address for correspondence:* Prof Johannes L.H. Evers MD, Department of Obstetrics and Gynaecology, Academisch Ziekenhuis Maastricht, P.O. Box 5800, 6202 AZ Maastricht, The Netherlands. Tel.: +31-43-387-6764. Fax: +31-43-387-4765. E-mail: jev@sgyn.azm.nl

nancies or to the subsequent periods of lactation (2—3 years). Her peritoneal immune system was perfectly able to cope with the sparse periods of retrograde menstruation she experienced during her short life. Progress, however, always takes its toll: life expectancy increased, till well beyond the limits of reproductive life, and total lifetime exposure to menstrual reflux increased. Once women became emancipated, and cheap and reliable forms of contraception became widely available, the average number of pregnancies per woman decreased till well below two and the total lifetime number of menstrual periods increased even further. Apparently in some women, likely a growing number of women, this lifetime assault on the defense mechanisms in the peritoneal cavity led to an eventual defeat. The peritoneal clearing capacity fell short, and viable fragments of regurgitated menstrual debris were able to implant on the mesothelial lining and endometriosis developed.

### Prevalence and natural course of disease of endometriosis and endometriosis-related complaints

Usually either pain or subfertility bring a patient with endometriosis to her doctor's office. The prevalence of active endometriosis in asymptomatic patients without fertility problems remains unknown. In many cases, however, endometriosis is an incidental finding during surgery for another condition. The natural course of the disease is a mystery, and it is almost impossible to reach valid conclusions regarding the pathophysiologic development of the disease and its disappearance or recurrence after (or due to) therapy. Therefore the time seems right to review the evidence we have today that endometriosis is a recurrent disease.

It has been suggested that only in one-third of cases is the disease progressive, whereas in as much as 60% and more of cases the disease remains in a steady state, or eventually even resolves again spontaneously with time. Only a few studies have been published that describe the evolution of the disease in a prospective way, without medical or surgical intervention. A discussion of recurrence of the disease after various types of management needs at least some insight to the nature of the disease process, and the factors that allow or restrain its development. Whereas retrograde menstruation apparently occurs on an almost monthly basis in the vast majority of ovulating women, only a fraction of them come to our attention, either because of pain or subfertility. Perhaps only a disturbance of the delicate balance between the monthly peritoneal insult of retrograde menstruation and the defense mechanisms in the abdominal cavity will allow the disease to take root and develop. Thereafter, the disease may exist (and persist, in spite of medical or surgical therapy) as invisible, microscopic foci, which, depending on the circumstances, may progress into symptomatic disease. Although by surgical therapy one may remove all visible implants, and by medical therapy one may render all active implants inactive and hence invisible (due to the lack of sequelae: mucus, hemorrhage, inflammatory reaction), active microscopic foci may remain and progress again to active disease after varying periods of time.

Recurrence of disease therefore usually cannot be differentiated from expanding, previously microscopic, endometriotic implants.

A special — epidemiological — problem in judging the factual rate of recurrence is posed by the fact that the means which are applied to establish recurrence are in most studies predominantly patient- and doctor-dependent. Few studies report, for example, performance of a second look laparoscopy for documentation of follow-up results as part of a prospective study design. Others produce data based on recurrence of symptoms and confuse this with recurrence of disease.

**Recurrence of endometriosis: de novo formation or persistence?**

An intra-abdominal steady state exists in which defense mechanisms (including leukocytes, macrophages, inflammatory response, encapsulation and sequestration, fibrosis) are operative that keep peritoneal insult (by regurgitated menstrual sludge) at bay, and prevent, in most patients, the implantation of viable menstrual cells in crevices of the peritoneal and ovarian surfaces. If the defense is defective or the offense too overwhelming, regurgitated endometrial cells may implant and give rise to the development of a disease entity that is clinically recognized as endometriosis. The stage of development at which the disease may still be controlled by the peritoneal defense mechanisms is as yet unknown, but it may very well be that even after clinically recognizable implants have appeared the defense may regain the upper hand and abort the disease. On the other hand, if, after medical suppression of the disease, or after surgical destruction of all visible lesions, the defense mechanisms fail, the residual invisible but viable (microscopic) implants may become reactivated and start to develop into visible ones, especially after resumption of ovarian endocrine activity. Also, reseeding due to resumed menstruation may contribute to reappearance of the disease after discontinuing medical suppression of ovarian activity. Recurrent (or persistent) endometriosis will then be diagnosed.

**A self-limiting condition or a progressive disease?**

Thomas and Cooke's [1] is the first study reporting the natural evolution of the disease. They performed laparoscopies in a group of 17 untreated control patients, before and after 6 months of taking placebos as part of a randomized controlled study. In eight patients progress of the disease process was observed, in three of whom the deterioration included the appearance of adhesions. In nine patients the disease improved, or did not progress to such a degree that it became obvious in the 6-month interval between laparoscopies; it became completely invisible at second look laparoscopy in four of these nine patients. No factor, including the original severity score of endometriosis, the age of the patient, her parity, the Quetelet index, or the duration of subfertility, could accurately predict improvement or deterioration of the endometriosis in the placebo group.

Later studies (Table 1) confirmed these findings: one-third of endometriosis patients showed spontaneous improvement, one-third deterioration, and the remainder no change. Janssen and Russell [2] were the first to report on the natural course of disease of nonpigmented endometriosis. In their group of 77 patients they had the opportunity to relaparoscope six patients who did not receive any form of treatment. Nonpigmented lesions had progressed to typical pigmented endometriotic stigmas in these six patients within the course of 6 to 24 months between laparoscopies. In their opinion this confirmed the existence of a continuum between nonpigmented and pigmented endometriotic lesions.

Further corroboration of the presumption of endometriosis being a progressive disease came from the work of Redwine [3], who, in a cross-sectional study, found an age-related colour appearance of endometriotic lesions (Table 2). This would suggest a natural evolution from the fresh, clear, active and productive papules of early endometriosis to the old, black, fibrotic and inactive lesions that have always been described as powder-burn or tobacco-stained puckerings.

When studying recurrence of endometriosis one should always keep in mind that medical therapy most probably does not eradicate endometriosis, and that by surgery one can only destroy those lesions that are visible to the eye (with or without the magnification provided by the laparoscope). We [4] compared the number and the cumulative size of endometriotic implants before and after 6 months of treatment with danazol in two groups of patients. In both groups the first look laparoscopy was performed during the follicular phase of the cycle. In the first group the second-look laparoscopy (SLL) was performed at the end of the last treatment cycle, in the second group the SLL was performed in the follicular phase of the second spontaneous menstrual cycle after the end of treatment. A statistically significant reduction in the number and the cumulative size of the implants was found in the group with a SLL during ovarian suppression by danazol, but not in the group with a SLL after resumption of ovarian activity. It was concluded that medical therapy does not eradicate endometriosis. If suppression is discontinued, the endometriotic lesions will regenerate with time.

**Recurrence after surgical ablation**

Recurrence rates of endometriosis after conservative surgical treatment vary from

Table 1. Numbers of patients showing elimination, improvement, and deterioration of endometriosis in a placebo treatment group [1,34—36].

| Reference | Improvement | No change | Deterioration |
|---|---|---|---|
| Thomas and Cooke, 1987 | 4/17 | 5/17 | 8/17 |
| Telimaa, 1988 | 4/17 | 9/17 | 4/17 |
| Mahmood and Templeton, 1990 | 3/11 | 1/11 | 7/11 |
| Overton et al., 1994 | 8/15 | 3/15 | 4/15 |
| Accumulated results | 19/60 (32%) | 18/60 (30%) | 23/60 (38%) |

*Table 2.* Evolution of colour appearance of endometriosis with age (from [3]): mean age of patients with respective lesions.

| Colour appearance | Mean age in years |
| --- | --- |
| Clear papules only | 22 |
| Clear lesions only | 23 |
| Clear plus any others | 23 |
| Red lesions only | 26 |
| Red plus any others | 27 |
| All nonblack lesions | 28 |
| White plus any others | 28 |
| Black plus any others | 28 |
| White lesions only | 30 |
| Black lesions only | 32 |

7 to 66% [5–9]. Wheeler and Malinak [10] have determined long-term recurrence rates by means of a historical prospective study design coupled with life table analysis. The fact that their curve representing the cumulative recurrence rate does not (yet) show the typical asymptotic deflection one would expect from survival curves, makes one speculate whether endometriosis will eventually reappear in all patients who had their visible lesions removed at the initial surgery. After all, it is de facto impossible to remove all endometriotic lesions at the time of initial surgery. Even ablation of all the cul-de-sac peritoneum, as it has been reported in this era of laser surgery, will lead to recurrence. Microscopic endometriotic microfoci will remain [11–13]. These may subsequently develop into visible endometriotic implants and present, together with new implants from reseeded endometrial cells, a recurrence of disease, in these apparently endometriosis-prone patients. Ahmed and Barbieri have estimated the need for reoperation of recurrent ovarian endometriomas after surgical excision as low as 7% after 32 months of follow-up [14]. Laparoscopy and laparotomy seem equally effective techniques for the conservative surgical treatment of severe endometriosis [15].

## Recurrence after medical therapy

Recurrence figures after medical therapy of endometriosis vary from 29 to 51% [16–18]. The difference between the various recurrence rates reported may be explained by the difference in the length of follow up, and by the difference in the way recurrence is diagnosed, i.e., by recurrence of symptoms of endometriosis, by laparoscopy with or without histological confirmation, or by the clinical need to perform a repeat laparoscopy, for another reason. Also marker substances (e.g., antiendometrial antibodies, CA-125) have been used to document recurrence [19]. Although the sensitivity of most of the markers described is too low to allow their use as a screening tool, they may have a place in the follow-up of patients with proven (and treated) endometriosis.

## Recurrence or persistence?

In most studies on recurrence of endometriosis, it remains unclear whether the recurrence noted after cessation of therapy represents real recurrence, i.e., de novo formation, or rather persistence and reactivation of endometriotic lesions that had been rendered quiescent by medical suppression of ovarian hormonal activity. Biopsy specimens taken during SLL at the end of treatment repeatedly have shown occult inactive endometriosis [20] or active disease, even in the absence of laparoscopic (macroscopic) signs of endometriosis [12,21,22]. In a prospective study of 60 patients, Wheeler and Malinak [9] showed that in half of them so-called recurrence of endometriosis after conservative surgery actually represented persistence of disease and progression of previously invisible micro-foci to visible implants. Schweppe [23] showed that persistence of disease after 6 months of medical therapy was correlated with the histological differentiation of the endometriotic lesions at the initial diagnostic laparoscopy. Of the highly differentiated endometriotic lesions, two-thirds disappeared after 6 months of treatment, whereas of the poorly differentiated lesions three-quarters persisted. It has to be kept in mind, as stated before, that since in the past most of the SLL have been performed during ovarian suppression and not during normally cycling ovarian activity (as usually was the first look laparoscopy during which the diagnosis was made), the results of medical therapy may be overestimated: implants are suppressed, regardless of the type of drug administered, but most probably not eradicated [4,22,24,25]. This makes one wonder if most, if not all, of the recurrence should in fact better be defined as persistence of disease.

## Treatment problems

Several treatment options have been studied in the case of recurrent endometriosis after medical or surgical therapy. No essential difference exists between primary and recurrent endometriosis, as far as therapeutic options are concerned. Recurrent endometriosis is either de novo formation in a patient whose pelvic defense system allowed development of the disease in the first place, or it is progression of previously invisible microfoci into visible implants after surgical or medical therapy. Therefore, the choice of treatment in a patient with recurrent endometriosis will not be determined by the manifestation of the disease as such (be it primary or recurrent), but by the extent of the pelvic disturbances, especially the distortion of tubo-ovarian spatial relationships, and by the reason that made the patient return for medical help. In a patient who has a recurrence of endometriosis that interferes with her desire for fertility, repeat conservative surgery has a favorable prognosis for conception. We found a 27% crude pregnancy rate among our 11 patients undergoing repeat conservative surgery of endometriosis (Table 3). Seven of Wheeler and Malinak's 15 patients [10] (47%), and 29% of Ranney's patients [26] conceived after conservative reoperation. The average pregnancy rate of these series of reoperations is about 30%, a figure

*Table 3.* Conservative surgery for endometriosis in subfertility patients: results and recurrences in the Maastricht series.

|  | No. of patients |
| --- | --- |
| Conservative surgery I[a] | 76 |
|    Pregnant | 42 (55%) |
| Conservative surgery II | 11 |
|    Pregnant | 3 (27%) |
| Conservative surgery III | 2 |
|    Pregnant | 0 |

[a]I, II and III indicate first, second and third conservative operation performed in the same patient, respectively.

which should be compared with the pregnancy rate (per cycle) of one's local IVF center, and with the demands placed on the patient by surgery and IVF respectively.

### Assisted reproduction techniques (ART) and alternative treatment options

In patients in whom the pelvic disturbances — either due to endometriosis or to postoperative adhesion formation following previous surgery — do not appear to allow successful reoperation, assisted reproduction techniques should be considered. IVF or one of its many derivatives, possibly after prior medical suppression of endometriotic activity, may offer them a fair chance of pregnancy [27,28]. This chance should always be weighed against the chance that extensive pelvic invasive endometriosis, which requires protracted abdominovaginal surgical procedures, might provide resolution of symptoms, and even conception. Evidence is accumulating that the outcome of ART in endometriosis patients is unaffected by increasing severity of endometriosis [29].

In patients with symptomatic endometriosis not desiring future fertility, painkillers may bring relief. If not, long-term hormonal therapy is indicated, in the form of cyclic or continuous birth control pills, as uninterrupted progestogen medication, or as long-term GnRH agonist treatment, either alone or in combination with an estrogen-add-back regimen. The value of presacral neurectomy and of uterosacral nerve ablation in combatting endometriosis-related pain has yet to be determined.

If no wish for future fertility exists, and if medical and/or conservative surgical therapy have failed, definitive surgery may be indicated. It includes bilateral oophorectomy, resection of all endometriosis and/or hysterectomy. Hormone replacement therapy should be started in the premenopausal patient, although in severe cases some authors have advised to postpone treatment for an arbitrary period of at least 6 months. The risk of inciting regrowth of residual endometriosis seems negligible, however, even if hormone replacement therapy is started immediately after surgery [30]. Rare cases of aggressive recurrent endometriosis

394

in the postmenopause have been described. Aromatase inhibitors have been successfully applied in a 57-year-old woman with recurrent endometriosis after hysterectomy and bilateral salpingo-oophorectomy, who was refractory to standard drug regimes [31].

**Extrapelvic endometriosis**

Extrapelvic endometriosis occurs infrequently, except during the question and answer periods of endometriosis meetings. Most of the time it concerns implants of the disease in the abdominal wall, the inguinal canal, or surgical incisions, e.g., episiotomy. Adequate, wide excision should prevent recurrence in these cases [32]. Joseph and Sahn [33] reviewed the English language medical literature to determine demographics, clinical presentations, pathological findings, and the effectiveness of treatment in patients with the often- quoted thoracic endometriosis syndrome (TES). Their thorough search of the world literature revealed 110 of such cases. Pneumothorax was the most common presentation, occurring in 73% of these patients, followed by hemothorax (14%), hemoptysis (7%), and lung nodules (6%). The right half of the thorax was involved in over 90% of all manifestations except for nodules. The authors concluded that there is a significant association between pelvic endometriosis and TES, with the latter occurring approximately 5 years later. They conclude surgical pleural abrasion to be superior to hormonal treatment, which has a high-recurrence rate.

**Conclusions**

In conclusion, treatment of recurrent endometriosis should be tailored to the patient and her chief complaint, i.e., pain and/or subfertility. Since probably most of the recurrent disease is reappearance of persistent microscopic disease, treatment does not necessarily have to differ from that in patients with primary disease.

**References**

1. Thomas EJ, Cooke ID. Impact of gestrinone on the course of asymptomatic endometriosis. Br Med J 1987;294:272—274.
2. Janssen RPS, Russell P. Nonpigmented endometriosis: clinical laparoscopic and pathologic definition. Am J Obstet Gynecol 1987;155:1160—1163.
3. Redwine DB. Age-related evolution on color appearance of endometriosis. Fertil Steril 1987; 48:1062—1063.
4. Evers JLH. The second-look laparoscopy for evaluation of the result of medical treatment of endometriosis should not be performed during ovarian suppression. Fertil Steril 1987;47: 502—504.
5. Green TH. Conservative surgical treatment of endometriosis. Clin Obstet Gynecol 1966;9: 293—308.
6. Andrews WC, Larsen GD. Endometriosis: treatment with hormonal pseudopregnancy and/or operation. Am J Obstet Gynecol 1974;18:643—651.

7. Hammond CB, Rock JA, Parker RT. Conservative treatment of endometriosis: the effects of limited surgery and hormonal pseudopregnancy. Fertil Steril 1976;27:756–766.

8. Regidor PA, Regidor M, Kato K, Bier UW, Buhler K, Schindler AE. Long-term follow up on the treatment of endometriosis with the GnRH-agonist buserelin acetate. Eur J Obstet Gynaecol Reprod Biol 1997;73:153–160.

9. Wheeler JM, Malinak LR. Computer graphic pelvic mapping second look laparoscopy and the distinction of recurrent versus persistent endometriosis. Fertil Steril 1987:79 (Abstract 194): Program Suppl 43rd Ann Meeting.

10. Wheeler WC, Malinak LR. Recurrent endometriosis. Contrib Gynecol Obstet 1987;16:13–21.

11. Acosta AA, Buttram VC Jr, Besch PK, Malinak LR, Franklin RR, Vanderheyden JD. A proposed classification of pelvic endometriosis. Obstet Gynecol 1973;42:19–25.

12. Murphy AA, Green WR, Bobbie D, Cruz ZC de la, Rock JA. Unsuspected endometriosis documented by scanning electron microscopy in visually normal peritoneum. Fertil Steril 1986;46: 522–524.

13. Dmowski WP. Visual assessment of peritoneal implants for staging endometriosis: do number and cumulative size of lesions reflect the severity of a systemic disease? Fertil Steril 1987;47:382–384.

14. Ahmed MS, Barbieri RL. Reoperation rates for recurrent ovarian endometriomas after surgical excision. Gynecol Obstet Invest 1997;43:53–54.

15. Crosignani PG, Vercellini P, Biffignandi F, Costantini W, Cortesi I, Imparato E. Laparoscopy versus laparotomy in the conservative surgical treatment of severe endometriosis. Fertil Steril 1996;66:706–711.

16. Dmowski WP, Cohen MR. Antigonadotropin (danazol) in the treatment of endometriosis. Evaluation of posttreatment fertility and three-year follow-up data. Am J Obstet Gynecol 1978;130:41–48.

17. Greenblatt RB, Tzigounis V. Danazol treatment of endometriosis: long-term follow-up. Fertil Steril 1979;32:518–520.

18. Buttram VC Jr. Treatment of endometriosis with danazol: report of a 6-year prospective study. Fertil Steril 1985;43:353–360.

19. Kauppila A, Telimaa S, Ronnberg L, Vuori J. Placebo-controlled study on serum concentrations of CA-125 before and after treatment of endometriosis with danazol or high-dose medroxyprogesterone acetate or after surgery. Fertil Steril 1988;49:37–41.

20. Steingold KA, Cedars M, Lu JKH, Randle D, Judd HL, Meldrum DR. Treatment of endometriosis with a long-acting gonadotropin-releasing hormone agonist. Obstet Gynecol 1987;69: 403–411.

21. Dmowski WP, Cohen MR. Treatment of endometriosis with an antigonadotropin, danazol: a laparoscopic and histologic evaluation. Obstet Gynecol 1975;46:147–154.

22. Schweppe KW, Dmowski WP, Wynn RN. Ultrastructural changes in endometriotic tissue during danazol treatment. Fertil Steril 1981;36:20–26.

23. Schweppe KW. Morphologie und Klinik der Endometriose. Stuttgart and New York: FK Schattauer Verlag, 1984;198–207.

24. Cornillie FJ, Brosens IA, Vasquez G, Riphagen I. Histologic and ultrastructural changes in human endometriotic implants treated with the antiprogesterone steroid ethylnorgestrinone (Gestrinone) during 2 months. Int J Gynecol Path 1986;5:95–109.

25. Cornillie FJ, Puttemans P, Brosens IA. Histology and ultrastructure of human endometriotic tissues treated with dydrogesterone (Duphaston). Eur J Obstet Gynecol Reprod Biol 1987;26: 39–55.

26. Ranney B. Reoperation after initial treatment of endometriosis with conservative surgery (discussion). Am J Obstet Gynecol 1978;131:416–421.

27. Rosenwaks Z. IVF results in endometriosis patients. In: Buttram (ed) Proceedings 2nd international congress on endometriosis, Houston, USA: Parthenon Publishing, 1989.

28. Ruiz-Velasco V, Allende S. Goserelin followed by assisted reproduction: results in infertile

women with endometriosis. Int J Fertil Womens Med 1988;43:18—23.

29. Pal L, Shifren JL, Isaacson KB, Chang Y, Leykin L, Toth TL. Impact of varying stages of endometriosis on the outcome of in vitro fertilization-embryo transfer. J Assist Reprod Genet 1998; 15:27—31.

30. Hickman TN, Namnoum AB, Hinton EL, Zacur HA, Rock JA. Timing of estrogen replacement therapy following hysterectomy with oophorectomy for endometriosis. Obstet Gynecol 1998; 91:673—677.

31. Takayama K, Zeitoun K, Gunby RT, Sasano H, Carr BR, Bulun SE. Treatment of severe postmenopausal endometriosis with an aromatase inhibitor. Fertil Steril 1998;69:709—713.

32. Seydel AS, Sickel JZ, Warner ED, Sax HC. Extrapelvic endometriosis: diagnosis and treatment. Am J Surg 1996;171:239—243.

33. Joseph J, Sahn SA. Thoracic endometriosis syndrome: new observations from an analysis of 110 cases. Am J Med 1996;100:164—170.

34. Telimaa S. Danazol and medroxyprogesteron acetate inefficacious in the treatment of infertility in endometriosis. Fertil Steril 1988;50:872—875.

35. Mahmood TA, Templeton A. The impact of treatment on the natural history of endometriosis. Hum Reprod 1990;5:965—970.

36. Overton CE, Lindsay PC, Johal B, Collins SA, Siddle NC, Shaw RW, Barlow DH. A randomized, double-blind, placebo-controlled study of luteal phase dydrogesterone (Duphaston) in women with minimal to mild endometriosis. Fertil Steril 1994;62:701—707.

**Reproductive surgery in the male**

Fertility and Reproductive Medicine.
R.D. Kempers, J. Cohen, A.F. Haney and J.B. Younger, editors.

# Diagnosis and treatment of ejaculatory duct obstruction

Jonathan P. Jarow
*Brady Urological Institute, Johns Hopkins University School of Medicine, Baltimore, Maryland, USA*

**Abstract.** Ejaculatory duct obstruction is a rare but treatable cause of male infertility. The most common etiologies include congenital anomalies of the Wolffian and Müllerian ducts, trauma, and inflammation. The diagnosis of ejaculatory duct obstruction should be suspected in any azoospermic patient with low ejaculate volume. Transrectal ultrasonography is now the preferred imaging modality for these patients. Seminal vesicle aspiration documents the presence of obstruction, confirms the presence of intact spermatogenesis, and rules out more proximal obstruction. Seminal vesiculography provides important anatomic information that is helpful in deciding the best method of treatment and is a useful adjunct during transurethral resection of the ejaculatory ducts. Transurethral resection of the ejaculatory ducts is the standard method of treatment for ejaculatory duct obstruction but balloon dilation may be preferred in select patients with extraprostatic obstruction of the ejaculatory ducts. The exact criteria for the diagnosis of partial ejaculatory duct obstruction are still unclear and therapy for these patients should be considered investigational at this time.

**Keywords:** ejaculatory duct obstruction, infertility, male, transrectal ultrasonography.

## Introduction

Ejaculatory duct obstruction is a rare but treatable cause of male infertility. Patients with ejaculatory duct obstruction are usually asymptomatic except for their subfertility. Symptoms that have been associated with ejaculatory duct obstruction include hematospermia, perineal pain, and painful ejaculation [1]. The diagnosis and treatment of complete ejaculatory duct obstruction is well-established. In contrast, the diagnosis and management of partial ejaculatory duct obstruction remains controversial. Ejaculatory duct obstruction has not been shown to be associated with any long-term deleterious effects upon the prostate or male reproductive tract. Therefore, it is not necessary to treat asymptomatic patients with ejaculatory duct obstruction who do not complain of infertility. The etiology of ejaculatory duct obstruction is frequently unknown. Etiologic factors for ejaculatory duct obstruction include inflammatory diseases of the prostate, iatrogenic injury from urethral manipulation, and congenital anomalies [2]. A high degree of suspicion is necessary in order to diagnose ejaculatory duct obstruction because of the lack of clear etiologic events and the absence of significant symptoms in the majority of patients with this disorder.

*Address for correspondence:* Jonathan Peter Jarow MD, Department of Urology, Johns Hopkins Outpatient Center, 601 N. Caroline St, Baltimore, MD 21287-0850, USA. Tel.: +1-410-955-3617. Fax: +1-410-614-0789.

## Diagnosis

The human ejaculate is made up of fluid from the testis/epididymis, seminal vesicles, prostate and periurethral glands. The majority of human ejaculate volume is from the seminal vesicles. Patients with ejaculatory duct obstruction lack seminal vesicle secretions in their ejaculate in addition to testicular and epididymal secretions. Therefore, they will characteristically have low ejaculate volume in addition to azoospermia. Seminal vesicle fluid has an alkaline pH, contains fructose, and produces the seminal coagulum. The semen of patients with complete ejaculatory duct obstruction should be acidic, fructose negative, and fail to coagulate. The documentation of intact spermatogenesis, proximal patency of the male excurrent ductal system, and distal obstruction establishes the diagnosis of ejaculatory duct obstruction. The differential diagnosis for low ejaculate volume azoospermia includes bilateral congenital absence of the vas deferens, ejaculatory dysfunction, and hypogonadism in addition to ejaculatory duct obstruction [3].

The standard method used to diagnose complete ejaculatory duct obstruction is vasography [2,4–6]. Vasography is an invasive test which is frequently performed under anesthesia and introduces the risk of vasal injury with subsequent obstruction at a site distant from the original pathology. Therefore, it is imperative to rule out other causes of low ejaculate volume azoospermia before considering vasography. Bilateral congenital absence of the vas deferens is easily diagnosed upon routine physical examination by palpation of the spermatic cord. However, some patients with congenital anomalies have segmental atresia of the pelvic portion of the vas deferens, which is not detectable by routine physical examination [7]. The pelvic obstruction of the vas deferens in these patients may only be identified by vasography. The seminal vesicle and prostatic secretions are under androgenic endocrine control and, therefore, ejaculate volume is significantly reduced in hypogonadal patients. Hypogonadism is diagnosed by routine hormonal testing performed upon azoospermic patients. A serum testosterone and FSH level should be obtained in the evaluation of azoospermia and the testosterone level should be low in any patients with either primary and secondary hypogonadism [3]. Ejaculation disorders may also cause low ejaculate volume. The ejaculate is delivered to the posterior urethra by the process of seminal emission, which is under adrenergic control, by postganglionic neurons from the thoracolumbar spinal cord. A process of bladder neck closure and contraction of the pelvic musculature under combined sympathetic autonomic and somatic neural control then delivers the semen to the urethral meatus. Ejaculatory disorders may present as either failure of emission or retrograde ejaculation. However, low ejaculate volume azoospermia is not the typical presentation for either of these disorders. Patients with failure of emission usually have aspermia, which is complete absence of any ejaculate. Patients with retrograde ejaculation will usually have low ejaculate volume with sperm present in the antegrade specimen. The diagnosis of retrograde ejaculation is established by finding numerous sperm within a postejaculatory urine specimen. A patient's history will usually provide an indication that they have failure of emission. Factors such as prior bladder neck or retroperitoneal surgery, neurologic disorders, and diabetes mellitus are indicative of failure of emission. However, failure of emission represents a functional rather than anatomic obstruction of the ejaculatory ducts and may only be diagnosed by vasography in the rare patient in whom the diagnosis can not be established on the basis of historical findings.

The evaluation of a patient with low ejaculate volume azoospermia begins with a complete history and physical examination. Historical risk factors for ejaculatory duct obstruction and ejaculatory dysfunction may be identified. Physical examination should reveal normal-sized testes and a palpable vas deferens bilaterally. Rectal examination may reveal a mass within the prostate or enlarged seminal vesicles but is most often normal. The ejaculate volume is often less than 1 ml for patients with complete obstruction. A postejaculatory urinalysis and endocrine testing are performed to rule out retrograde ejaculation and hypogonadism, respectively. The next step in the traditional approach to patients who meet all of the clinical criteria for ejaculatory duct obstruction is testis biopsy and subsequent vasography if the biopsy reveals intact spermatogenesis [2]. However, transrectal ultrasonography is now replacing vasography as the standard diagnostic tool for the evaluation of patients with low ejaculate volume azoospermia [8–11].

Transrectal ultrasonography is a readily available, inexpensive, and minimally invasive imaging modality. Transrectal ultrasonography provides excellent imaging resolution to visualize the seminal vesicles, ampulla vas deferens, ejaculatory ducts and prostate deep within the male pelvis. The images obtained with transrectal ultrasonography are far superior to that obtained with either transabdominal ultrasonography or computerized axial tomography. Pelvic magnetic resonance imaging with or without an endorectal coil provides similar quality imaging but with a significantly increased cost [4]. The diagnosis of ejaculatory duct obstruction by transrectal ultrasonography is based upon the finding of dilation of structures located proximal to site of obstruction. Seminal vesicles that are unable to empty are likely to become dilated over time. In addition, sperm that are unable to travel through the ejaculatory duct will pool within the seminal vesicles. Therefore, one would expect to observe dilatation of the seminal vesicles in patients with ejaculatory duct obstruction. The normal size of the seminal vesicles in young fertile men is up to an anteroposterior width of 1.5 cm [12]. Therefore, ejaculatory duct obstruction is suspected in any patient with seminal vesicles wider than 1.5 cm on transverse imaging behind the bladder. Congenital absence of the vas deferens is frequently but not always associated with absence of the seminal vesicles [13]. The diagnosis of segmental atresia of the pelvic portion of the vas deferens should be suspected in any patient with a palpable scrotal vas deferens and absence of the seminal vesicle by transrectal ultrasonography. Unfortunately, not all patients with ejaculatory duct obstruction have dilated seminal vesicles and, conversely, not all patients with dilated seminal vesicles have ejaculatory duct obstruction. Therefore, seminal vesicle aspiration may be used in azoospermic patients to diagnose complete ejaculatory duct obstruction [14]. The finding of numerous sperm within the seminal vesicles of an azoospermic patient is diagnostic of ejaculatory duct obstruction. In addition, the finding of sperm within the seminal vesicles establishes the presence of active spermatogenesis and proximal ductal patency, obviating the need for testicular biopsy and vasography in these patients. Seminal vesicle aspiration is performed under transrectal ultrasonography guidance with an oocyte retrieval needle via either a transperineal or transrectal route. Patients undergoing seminal vesicle aspiration require a mechanical bowel and antibiotic preparation. This procedure can be performed without anesthesia and in an office setting.

The presence of sperm within the seminal vesicles does not rule out the possibility of a functional obstruction due to failure of emission since patients with failure of emission also have pooling of sperm within the seminal vesicles. In addition, seminal vesicle aspiration does not establish the exact site of ejaculatory duct obstruction. Seminal vesiculography may be performed at the time of seminal vesicle aspiration in order to determine the exact site of ejaculatory duct obstruction [14,15]. A mixture of nonionic contrast and colored dye may be injected through the oocyte retrieval needle into the seminal vesicle under fluoroscopic control in order to obtain radiographic imaging of the excurrent ductal system. Fluoroscopy is critical during seminal vesiculography in order to avoid reflux of contrast into the epididymis, which may cause epididymitis. Colored dye is added to the contrast for patients about to undergo transurethral resection of the ejaculatory ducts as an aid to the procedure.

It is logical to assume that patients may develop partial obstruction of the ejaculatory ducts since partial obstruction has been documented in other hollow organ systems. However, the diagnosis of partial ejaculatory duct obstruction is much more difficult to establish than complete obstruction. By definition, patients with partial ejaculatory duct obstruction will have sperm present in the ejaculate and vasography will reveal passage of contrast into the bladder. Therefore, the standard test for ejaculatory duct obstruction, vasography, is not diagnostic for patients with partial obstruction. A diagnostic test that establishes the normal flow parameters for the ejaculatory duct, analogous to a diuretic renogram for the ureter, does not exist. Therefore, the diagnosis of partial ejaculatory duct obstruction is currently based upon clinical findings alone. Partial obstruction is thought to lead to inefficient emptying of the seminal vesicles and vas deferens. Semen parameters suggestive of the diagnosis of partial obstruction include reduced ejaculate volume, oligospermia, and asthenospermia. Several clinical studies have used these clinical findings as criteria for further investigation in patients without any other obvious explanation for their abnormal semen parameters [8,16]. The next step in the evaluation of patients suspected of having partial ejaculatory duct obstruction is transrectal ultrasonography. As with the semen parameters, transrectal ultrasonography does not provide pathognomonic findings diagnostic of partial obstruction. Transrectal ultrasonographic findings suggestive of partial ejaculatory duct obstruction include seminal vesicle dilatation and abnormalities within the prostate in close proximity to the ejaculatory ducts [16]. These intraprostatic abnormalities include both Müllerian and Wolffian duct cysts as well as hyperechoic lesions within the prostate.

Investigation of young fertile volunteers has provided normative data for transrectal ultrasonography. Transrectal ultrasonography in 30 fertile volunteers was compared to 150 consecutive patients attending an infertility clinic in order to determine what is normal and the frequency of transrectal ultrasonographic abnormalities in the general infertile population [17]. The groups were similar in age and urologic history. Interestingly, the measurements of vas deferens, ejaculatory ducts, and seminal vesicles were the same for each group. This finding suggests, as anticipated, that the majority of infertile patients do not have an abnormality of the ejaculatory ducts. In addition, since the data displayed a normal distribution, normal measurements for these structures could be defined by using the criteria of the mean plus or minus two times the standard deviation. On this basis, the maximum normal size for the seminal vesicles of 1.5 cm was defined (Table 1). Other significant findings from this study include an increased incidence of both Müllerian duct cysts and ejaculatory duct diverticula in the infertile population. Both of these lesions may produce partial obstruction by extrinsic compression of the ejaculatory ducts. However, it must be kept in mind that the presence of a cyst alone does not connote obstruction. Finally, the incidence of hyperechoic lesions within the prostate gland was very common (40%) and equal in both groups. The location of these hyperechoic lesions was mapped in both groups and a significant difference was observed in the location of these lesions within the prostates of infertile men [18]. Hyperechoic lesions were most often seen in the verumontanum of fertile men and posterior to the urethra in the region of the ejaculatory ducts in the infertile patients. However, a significant number of fertile men also had hyperechoic lesions posterior to the urethra. Therefore, none of these ultrasonographic findings should be considered pathognomonic for partial ejaculatory duct obstruction.

The seminal vesicles join with the ampulla of the vas deferens to form the ejaculatory ducts and there is nothing to prevent sperm from entering the seminal vesicles at this location. However, the seminal vesicles do not normally serve as a sperm reservoir. Seminal vesicle aspiration is a potential test for the diagnosis of partial ejaculatory duct obstruction. Numerous sperm are found in the seminal vesicle aspirates of patients with complete ejaculatory duct obstruction and proxi-

*Table 1.* Normal transrectal ultrasonographic measurements based upon the mean plus and minus 2 times the standard deviation of 150 studies.

| Parameter | Lower limit of normal | Upper limit of normal |
|---|---|---|
| Ejaculatory duct diameter (mm) | 0 | 1.2 |
| Vas deferens diameter (mm) | 2 | 6 |
| Seminal vesicle width (cm) | 0.6 | 1.5 |
| Seminal vesicle length (cm) | 1.2 | 4.4 |

mal ductal patency. Patients with partial obstruction would be expected to have an increased number of sperm within the seminal vesicles due to inefficient emptying of the ductal system. However, the normal number of sperm within the seminal vesicles of fertile men is unknown. In a recent study, the number of sperm within the seminal vesicles of fertile men and the effect of duration of abstinence upon the results of seminal vesicle aspiration were assessed in 12 fertile volunteers. Only rare sperm were found in the seminal vesicle aspirates of men who had zero days of sexual abstinence. More sperm were seen in men who had abstained from sexual activity for 5 days. None of the patients with 0 days of abstinence had a positive seminal vesicle aspiration using three sperm per high-powered field as the criteria for a positive aspirate. In contrast, 33% of volunteers with 5 days abstinence had a positive aspirate. Therefore, the finding of significant numbers of sperm within the seminal vesicle immediately following ejaculation is an abnormal finding and is suggestive of the diagnosis of partial ejaculatory duct obstruction. In addition, the ratio of the number of sperm within the seminal vesicles to the ejaculate may be predictive of a patient's potential response to therapy. Patients who have a large number of sperm within the seminal vesicles may be more likely to benefit from therapy than those patients with lower quantities of sperm. Prospective studies using these diagnostic criteria are needed to determine whether they are predictive of clinical response to intervention and, therefore, useful in practice.

**Therapy**

There are two approaches to the management of patients with ejaculatory duct obstruction. The most common therapeutic modality employed for patients with ejaculatory duct obstruction is surgery. An alternative to surgery is assisted reproductive technology (intrauterine insemination or in vitro fertilization) using sperm harvested from the obstructed systems. Sperm may be harvested from the seminal vesicles, vas deferens, or epididymis in patients with ejaculatory duct obstruction and intact spermatogenesis. Anecdotal reports have been presented describing pregnancies initiated by either intrauterine insemination or in vitro fertilization using sperm harvested from the seminal vesicles of men with ejaculatory duct obstruction. However, a large enough experience with this technique has not been reported in order to provide the data needed to compare it with the results of surgical management.

The traditional surgical approach to the patient with ejaculatory duct obstruction is transurethral resection or incision of the ejaculatory ducts [19–22]. This procedure is performed under general or regional anesthesia with the patients in the lithotomy position and a small resectoscope sheath (24 French) is employed. An O'Conor drape allows digital manipulation of the prostate and seminal vesicles during the procedure, which greatly assists in the performance of transurethral resection of the ejaculatory ducts. The ejaculatory ducts normally open into the prostatic urethra on either side of the verumontanum. Their proximal course is just lateral to the midline and posterior to the bladder neck at the base of the prostate. Therefore, the incision or resection should be directed towards the region just posterior to the bladder neck rather than directly posterior towards the rectum. Simultaneous transrectal ultrasonography has been utilized as an adjunctive imaging modality to guide the depth and direction of the resection [23]. Incision with a Collings knife may be effective in patients with distal ejaculatory duct obstruction but resection with a resectoscope loop is the preferred technique in patients with a more proximal obstruction [24].

Seminal vesicle aspiration and seminal vesiculography are helpful adjuncts to transurethral resection of the ejaculatory ducts and can be performed in the operating room just prior to the resection. Cannulation of the seminal vesicle via either a transperineal or transrectal route provides useful diagnostic information. The presence of sperm within the seminal vesicle aspirate confirms the presence of active spermatogenesis and rules out the presence of a more proximal obstruction, such as an epididymal blowout [25]. In addition, seminal vesiculography may be performed just prior to resection. Seminal vesiculography provides anatomic information regarding the site of obstruction. Patients with extraprostatic ejaculatory duct obstruction are not good candidates for transurethral resection of the ejaculatory ducts because of an increased risk of rectal injury. The contrast utilized for seminal vesiculography may be mixed with colored dye such as indigo carmine. The adequacy of resection can be more easily determined if colored dye is seen flowing through the ejaculatory duct after digital massage of the seminal vesicles.

Potential complications from transurethral resection of the ejaculatory ducts include rectal injury, external sphincter injury, bladder neck resection resulting in retrograde ejaculation, and urine reflux into the ejaculatory ducts [26—28]. The close proximity of the rectum puts it at risk for injury if either the resection is inadvertently directed too far posteriorly or if the ejaculatory duct obstruction is located outside the prostate gland. The external sphincter may be damaged if the resection of the verumontanum is carried too far apically. Finally, the bladder neck is in close proximity to the proximal ejaculatory duct and is frequently undermined by the resection in patients with more proximal obstructions. The normal urethral orifice of the ejaculatory duct acts as a flap valve to prevent urine reflux into the ejaculatory duct and seminal vesicles during micturition. Resection of the ejaculatory duct destroys this normal antireflux mechanism and urine reflux is common following transurethral resection of the ejaculatory ducts. In fact, this urine reflux is often mistakenly interpreted as postoperative improvement of ejaculate volume.

An alternative approach to the management of ejaculatory duct obstruction is balloon dilation of the ejaculatory ducts. This minimally invasive technique has several advantages over transurethral resection of the ejaculatory ducts including less risk of rectal or sphincter injury and preservation of the normal ejaculatory duct orifice. Balloon dilation may be performed in either an antegrade or retrograde fashion. The ejaculatory duct orifice within the urethra is not easily cannulated and it is often impossible to pass a catheter or wire in a retrograde fashion through the ejaculatory ducts of obstructed patients. Some clinicians have resorted to a partial resection of the veru in order to gain access to the ejaculatory duct for subsequent balloon dilation. However, this partial resection obviates the main advantage of balloon dilation, which is preservation of the normal urethral orifice of the ejaculatory ducts. An alternative to retrograde cannulation is the antegrade transrectal approach via the seminal vesicles. Analogous to ureteral obstruction, it is frequently possible to pass a catheter through an obstruction in an antegrade direction when it was impossible to do so with a retrograde approach. This technique is performed under general or regional anesthesia with the patient in the lithotomy position. Transrectal ultrasonography is utilized to place a 17-gauge needle into the seminal vesicle. A Teflon-coated "J" wire is passed through the needle into the seminal vesicle. An angiographic catheter (5 French) is passed into the seminal vesicle over the guide wire, which is then exchanged for a straight 0.035-in. wire or glide wire. The wire and catheter are then manipulated under fluoroscopic control until the ejaculatory duct is cannulated. The wire is then retrieved from the urethra using a cystoscope. A 4-mm dilation balloon catheter is then passed over the wire in a retrograde fashion through the cystoscope and positioned within the ejaculatory duct using combined direct vision through the cystoscope and fluoroscopy. The wire and catheter are removed after adequate dilation has been achieved as demonstrated by disappearance of the waist in the inflated balloon. This technique has been successfully employed in a small number of patients with only short follow-up. Further study is needed to determine the overall success of this technique and the long-term patency since balloon dilation has not enjoyed high long-term success rates in other organ systems. The main advantage of the balloon dilation approach is the preservation of the normal urethral orifice, which prevents urine reflux. This technique is currently best reserved for patients with either partial ejaculatory duct obstruction or an extraprostatic site of obstruction.

**Results**

The overall success of transurethral resection of the ejaculatory ducts reported in the literature has been quite good. Ejaculatory duct obstruction is a relatively rare cause of male infertility and, therefore, there are very few large series of patients reported. Most reports of transurethral resection of the ejaculatory ducts in the literature describe a single case report and only two are made up of more than 10 patients (Table 2). The largest published series was by Pryor and Hendry and it described the findings and management of 87 patients with ejaculatory duct obstruction [2]. The vast majority of these patients (84) had complete obstruction and the remaining three had partial obstruction of the ejaculatory ducts. Only 31 of these patients underwent therapy to restore fertility and a variety of treatments were employed. Transurethral incision of a Müllerian duct cyst was performed in 12 men, of whom 10 (83%) experienced an undisclosed

*Table 2.* Results of transurethral resection of the ejaculatory ducts for ejaculatory duct obstruction.

| Author (year) | No. | Seminal improvement (%) | Pregnancy (%) |
|---|---|---|---|
| Weintraub (1980) | 4 | 2 (50%) | 2 (50%) |
| Siber (1980) | 4 | 1 (25%) | 0 (0%) |
| Amelar (1982) | 6 | 2 (33%) | 1 (17%) |
| Vicente (1983) | 9 | 3 (33%) | 1 (11%) |
| Carson (1984) | 4 | 3 (75%) | 1 (25%) |
| Pryor (1991) | 31 | 18 (58%) | 7 (23%) |
| Meacham (1993) | 24 | 12 (50%) | 7 (29%) |
| Weintraub (1993) | 5 | 3 (60%) | 2 (40%) |
| Total | 87 | 44 (51%) | 21 (24%) |

improvement in semen quality and five (42%) partners conceived. Epididymova-sostomy was performed in three patients with concomitant epididymal obstruction and only one was surgically patent. Nineteen patients underwent transurethral resection of the ejaculatory ducts for ejaculatory duct obstruction. The etiology of ejaculatory duct obstruction in the group undergoing transurethral resection of the ejaculatory ducts included congenital anomalies of the Wolffian duct, trauma, and infection. The results in this group were not as good as the group of patients with Müllerian duct cysts. Semen quality improved in eight patients (42%) and pregnancy was achieved in only four (21%).

The other large series reported by Meacham and associates was composed of almost an equal number of patients with partial and complete ejaculatory duct obstruction [8]. A total of 26 transurethral resections of the ejaculatory ducts was performed in 24 patients of whom 11 were thought to have partial obstruction based upon clinical findings and transrectal ultrasonography. Their diagnostic criteria for partial ejaculatory duct obstruction was described in a previous publication by Hellerstein and colleagues [16]. Patients with normal or reduced ejaculate volume, with or without abnormalities in sperm count or motility, were thought to have ejaculatory duct obstruction if their testis volume and serum FSH were normal and there was no other identifiable cause for their semen abnormalities, such as a varicocele. These patients underwent transrectal ultrasonography to detect any abnormality suggestive of ejaculatory duct obstruction. The transrectal ultrasonographic findings suspicious for obstruction included dilation of the seminal vesicles, prostatic cysts, and hyperechoic lesions within the prostate. Of the 13 patients with azoospermia due to complete ejaculatory duct obstruction, only three (27%) had sperm in the ejaculate postoperatively. In contrast, nine of the 11 (81%) patients with partial ejaculatory duct obstruction experienced improvement in semen quality postoperatively. Many patients had improvement in ejaculate volume postoperatively but this was most likely due to urine contamination of semen. Seven pregnancies were achieved and the vast majority (six) were in the group with partial obstruction preoperatively.

The compiled results from these two large series and other case reports reveal an overall rate of seminal improvement of approximately 60% and a pregnancy rate of approximately 20%. The results achieved in the limited number of patients with partial obstruction appear superior. All of the pregnancies following trans-urethral resection of the ejaculatory ducts for complete obstruction are likely to be treatment related but the number of treatment independent pregnancies following surgery in patients with partial obstruction is unknown without the use of appropriate controls. The most frequent complication following transurethral resection of the ejaculatory ducts is urine contamination of the semen [27,28]. This is not a major problem in most patients but can cause persistent infertility if the urine adversely affects sperm viability. Urine has an acidic pH and is often hypertonic. Patients with significant amounts of urine contamination may require alkalinization of the urine and hydration in an effort to preserve sperm viability. Patients who have concomitant epididymal obstruction secondary to chronic obstruction have a poor prognosis [25]. Epididymovasostomy may be performed in conjunction with the transurethral resection of the ejaculatory ducts or at a later date but should not be performed prior to transurethral resection of the ejaculatory ducts. The overall success in this small subgroup of patients has not been well reported but can be expected to be significantly lower than the routine patient without proximal obstruction.

## References

1. Littrup PJ, Lee F, McLeary RD, Wu D, Lee A, Kumasaka GH. Transrectal US of the seminal vesicles and ejaculatory ducts: clinical correlation. Radiology 1988;168:625.
2. Pryor JP, Hendry WF. Ejaculatory duct obstruction in subfertile males: analysis of 87 patients. Fertil Steril 1991;56:725.
3. Jarow JP, Espeland MA, Lipshultz LI. Evaluation of the azoospermic patient. J Urol 1989; 142:62.
4. Weintraub MP, De Mouy E, Hellstrom WJ. Newer modalities in the diagnosis and treatment of ejaculatory duct obstruction. J Urol 1993;150:1150.
5. Ford K, Carson CC, Dunnick NR, Osborne D, Paulson DF. The role of seminal vesiculography in the evaluation of male infertility. Fertil Steril 1982;37:552.
6. Nagler HM, Thomas AJ Jr. Testicular biopsy and vasography in the evaluation of male infertility. Urol Clin North Am 1987;14:167.
7. Hall S, Oates RD. Unilateral absence of the scrotal vas deferens associated with contralateral mesonephric duct anomalies resulting in infertility: laboratory, physical and radiographic findings, and therapeutic alternatives. J Urol 1993;150:1161.
8. Meacham RB, Hellerstein DK, Lipshultz LI. Evaluation and treatment of ejaculatory duct obstruction in the infertile male. Fertil Steril 1993;59:393.
9. Kuligowska E, Baker CE, Oates RD. Male infertility: role of transrectal US in diagnosis and management. Radiology 1992;185:353.
10. Belker AM, Steinbock GS. Transrectal prostate ultrasonography as a diagnostic and therapeutic aid for ejaculatory duct obstruction. J Urol 1990;144:356.
11. Patterson L, Jarow JP. Transrectal ultrasonography in the evaluation of the infertile man: a report of 3 cases. J Urol 1990;144:1469.
12. Carter SS, Shinohara K, Lipshultz LI. Transrectal ultrasonography in disorders of the seminal vesicles and ejaculatory ducts. Urol Clin North Am 1989;16:773.
13. Goldstein M, Schlossberg S. Men with congenital absence of the vas deferens often have seminal

vesicles. J Urol 1988;140:85.

14. Jarow JP. Seminal vesicle aspiration in the management of patients with ejaculatory duct obstruction. J Urol 1994;152:899.

15. Solivetti FM, D'Ascenzo R, Isidori A, Giovenco P, Montagna G, Valenti P. Transperineal vesiculodeferentography under ultrasound control: first experiences. Archiv Ital Urol Nefrol Androl 1992;64:133.

16. Hellerstein DK, Meacham RB, Lipshultz LI. Transrectal ultrasound and partial ejaculatory duct obstruction in male infertility. Urology 1992;39:449.

17. Jarow JP. Transrectal ultrasonography of infertile men. Fertil Steril 1993;60:1035.

18. Poore RE, Jarow JP. Distribution of intraprostatic hyperechoic lesions in infertile men. Urology 1995;45:467.

19. Weintraub CM. Transurethral drainage of the seminal tract for obstruction, infection and infertility. Br J Urol 1980;52:220.

20. Porch PP Jr. Aspermia owing to obstruction of distal ejaculatory duct and treatment by transurethral resection. J Urol 1978;119:141.

21. Vicente J, del Portillo L, Pomerol MM. Endoscopic surgery in distal obstruction of the ejaculatory ducts. Eur Urol 1983;9:338.

22. Carson CC. Transurethral resection for ejaculatory duct stenosis and oligospermia. Fertil Steril 1984;41:482.

23. Queralt JA, Gerscovich EO, Gould JE, Cronan MS. Intraoperative transrectal ultrasonography in the management of ejaculatory duct obstruction caused by midline prostatic cyst. J Clin Ultrasound 1993;21:293.

24. Sabanegh E Jr, Thomas A. Modified resectoscope loop for transurethral resection of the ejaculatory duct. Urology 1994;44:909.

25. Silber SJ. Ejaculatory duct obstruction. J Urol 1980;124:294.

26. Goluboff ET, Stifelman MD, Fisch H. Ejaculatory duct obstruction in the infertile male (Review). Urology 1995;45:925.

27. Goluboff ET, Kaplan SA, Fisch H. Seminal vesicle urinary reflux as a complication of transurethral resection of ejaculatory ducts. J Urol 1995;153:1234.

28. Vazquez-Levin MH, Dressler KP, Nagler HM. Urine contamination of seminal fluid after transurethral resection of the ejaculatory ducts. J Urol 1994;152:2049.

# Microsurgery for male ductal obstruction

J.M. Pomerol

*Fundacio Puigvert, Barcelona, Spain*

**Abstract.** The seminal duct can be partially or completed obstructed, at one or various levels, from either congenital or aquired causes. The work-up leading to the diagnosis of the seminal duct obstruction includes the history, physical examination, testicular biopsy and vasography.

The management of the epididymal and vas deferens obstruction requires the use of the operating microscope and microsurgical skills. Reconstructive surgery of the seminal duct allows sperm to enter the ejaculate and as many natural pregnancies as desired. During the reconstructive surgery, sperm may be aspirated and cryopreserved to be used in intracytoplasmatic sperm injection (ICSI) in the future in cases where surgery has failed. The two-layer vasovasostomy and the end-to-side vasoepididymostomy are the most frequent applied reconstructive techniques.

In cases where the female is older than 35 or reconstructive surgery is not possible or has failed, sperm may be aspirated from the epididymis or from the vas deferens to be used in ICSI. In these cases, the microsurgical techniques allow us to get sufficient sperm to be cryopreserved.

In cases of male ductal obstruction, the association of microsurgical reconstructive surgery, sperm aspiration/ICSI and sperm cryopreservation offers the couple the greatest possibility of success.

**Keywords:** aspiration, azoospermia, epididymal obstruction, microsurgical epididymal sperm aspiration (MESA), microsurgical vas deferens sperm vas deferens obstruction, vasoepididymostomy, vasovasostomy.

## Introduction

The basic indication of microsurgery in male infertility is the treatment of the obstructive pathology of the epididymis and of the vas deferens. In these cases, a suitable magnification and the use of microsurgical techniques make working on tubular structures with diameters between 0.1 and 0.5 mm easier, either with the intention of reconstruction or obtaining spermatozoa to be used in the intracytoplasmatic sperm injection (ICSI) technique.

Microsurgery can also be indicated in certain varicocele cases with veins of a small diameter. These veins can be tied easily, leaving the spermatic artery and the lymphatic vessels untouched [1].

The practice of microsurgery requires specialised training in training laboratories, where the students start by stitching inert material and practice on rats. Increasingly difficult tasks are performed, from anastomosis of the femoral artery and vein to complex organ transplants. Later, students are able to perform anastomosis of the epididymis and of the vas deferens. The latter can be carried

*Address for correspondence:* Dr Jose Pomerol, PJE Foraste 1—5 Atic 1A, Barcelona 08022, Spain.
Tel.: +34-3-4169732. Fax: +34-3-4169730.

out using sections of the human vas deferens removed following vasectomy. When sufficient microsurgical skill has been acquired in the training laboratory, clinical practice can follow under the supervision of expert surgeons. In this clinical area, the most adequate technique is microsurgical tying of spermatic veins in certain cases of varicocele. Since microsurgery requires constant training, it is advisable that it be performed on a frequent basis solely by those surgeons who have the opportunity of operating on patients for this kind of surgery.

## Obstruction of the seminal duct

The seminal tract can be partially or completely obstructed, at one or various levels, from either congenital or acquired causes. The most frequently observed obstruction in infertility clinics is the complete type and at the same level, bilaterally producing azoospermia. The obstruction might be intraductal (e.g., inflammation) or secondary to an external compression (e.g., cyst) as well as to a complete or partial section of the seminal duct (e.g., herniorrhaphy).

The epididymis is the segment of the seminal tract that is most frequently obstructed. The causes can be congenital, with or without the presence of vas deferens; inflammatory, generally from a local prostatic infection; genetic (e.g., cystic fibrosis) [2]; associated with a respiratory pathology (Young syndrome) [3—5]; secondary to more distal obstructions of the seminal duct (vas deferens, ejaculatory duct); traumatic; iatrogenic (e.g., epididymal cystectomy); secondary to cysts; or idiopathic (Table 1).

The epididymal obstruction is diagnosed when encountering azoospermia with a normal seminal volume and when preserved spermatogenesis is established by means of a testicular biopsy.

When faced with any epididymal obstruction, it is essential to perform urine and sperm cultures with the aim of ruling out the presence of an infectious process, and an immunologic study with the purposes of ruling out the presence of the antispermatic antibodies. In those patients with congenital bilateral absence of vas deferens who choose spermatic recovery techniques and ICSI, a genetic study must be carried out to determine the presence of the cystic fibrosis gene, which is found in over 70% of cases [6—9].

*Table 1.* Causes of epididymal obstruction.

— Idiopathic
— Congenital
— Inflammatory
— Secondary to a more distal obstruction of the seminal duct
— Genetic (cystic fibrosis, Young syndrome)
— Iatrogenic
— Traumatic
— Secondary to cysts
— Neoplastic

The vas deferens is obstructed infrequently, and the main causes are iatrogenic in the course of herniorrhaphies [10,11], orchiopexies, varicocelectomies or other inguinoscrotal surgery. Vasectomy with contraceptive aims is the most frequent cause of vas deferens obstructions. The most infrequent one is inflammatory pathology (Table 2).

In cases other than vasectomy, the diagnosis is established by the presence of azoospermia with a normal seminal volume, preserved spermatogenesis and significant surgical history (e.g., herniorrhaphy). The vasography, normally made during the testicular biopsy, confirms the diagnosis and discloses the level of the obstruction. The immunologic study is important to rule out the presence of anti-spermatic antibodies.

### Reconstructive surgery vs. sperm retrieval techniques and ICSI

Facing the epididymal obstruction treatment, it is important to choose one of the following alternatives: reconstructive surgery, sperm retrieval techniques and ICSI or both methodologies at the same time. The following factors have to be considered: evolution time and type of infertility, female age, possible female pathology as a cause of infertility, etiology of the seminal duct obstruction, and availability of the couple to undergo the different therapeutic alternatives.

Reconstructive surgery is a relatively complex procedure when performed by the expert microsurgeon. It can be done under local anesthesia on an outpatient basis with few complications. In reconstructive surgery, the female need not have to be involved in the procedure and when the result is successful, this allows us to achieve the pregnancy as many times as desired without the necessity of new surgical interventions. During the reconstructive surgery, sperm may be aspirated and cryopreserved to be used in ICSI in the future in cases where surgery has failed. When, after surgery, there is a low concentration or quality of sperm, these may be utilized in ICSI, without performing new surgical procedures. In addition, reconstructive surgery is more efficient and less costly than ICSI. Because of everything mentioned, we prefer to perform reconstructive surgery as a first step in the treatment of seminal duct obstruction. However, if the female age is over 35 or if she has some pathology in which reproductive techniques are indicated, we proceed with sperm retrieval techniques and ICSI with the possibility of performing reconstructive surgery. In cases of reconstructive

*Table 2.* Causes of vas deferens obstruction.

— Vasectomy
— Iatrogenic
— Inflammatory
— Traumatic
— Congenital
— Neoplasic
— Idiopathic

surgery failure, where ICSI with cryopreserved sperm is not possible or has also failed, we proceed with new reconstructive surgery and fresh sperm retrieval/ ICSI at the same time. Following this protocol (Fig. 1), we are able to offer the couple the greatest possibilities of success.

### Reconstructive surgery

*Epididymal obstruction surgery*

With the purpose of establishing the continuity between the healthy preobstructive epididymal tube and the vas deferens, the most advisable and most widely practiced surgery is now the terminolateral vasoepididymostomy (VE) [12–14]. Below we describe the surgical technique we prefer, including the basic details acquired from experience.

Since VE is a comparatively lengthy surgical technique — and the epididymis a considerably sensitive organ — it is advisable to perform it under general anesthesia. However, if indicated, it can also be done under local anesthesia and con-

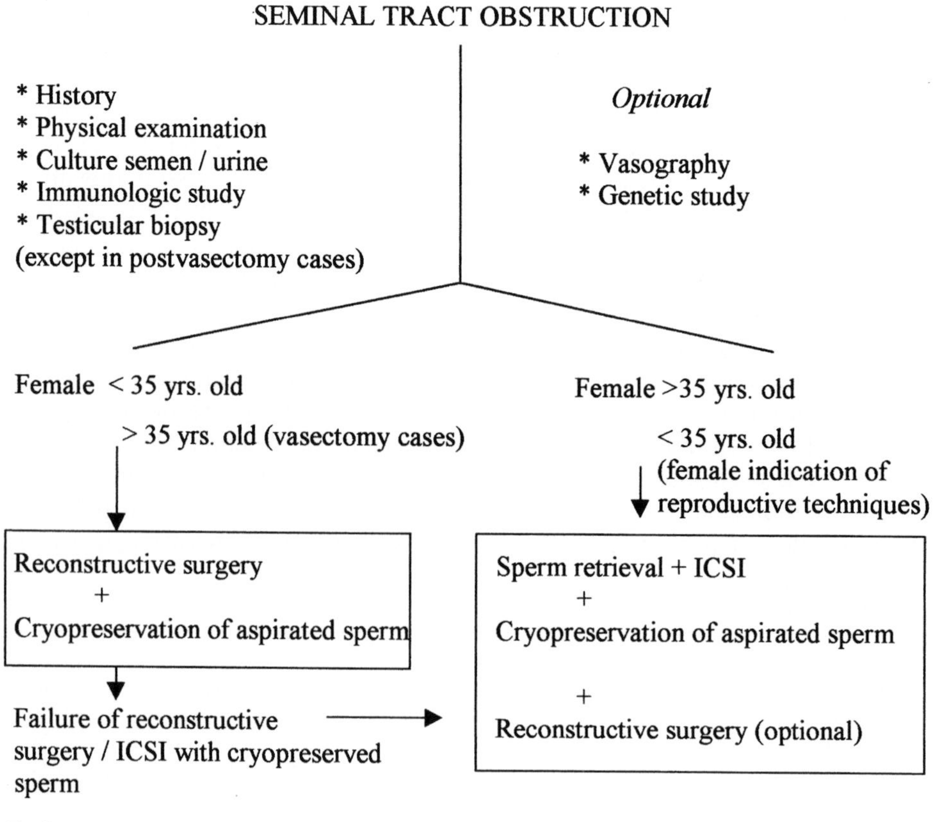

**SEMINAL TRACT OBSTRUCTION**

* History
* Physical examination
* Culture semen / urine
* Immunologic study
* Testicular biopsy
(except in postvasectomy cases)

*Optional*

* Vasography
* Genetic study

Female < 35 yrs. old
> 35 yrs. old (vasectomy cases)

Female > 35 yrs. old
< 35 yrs. old
(female indication of
reproductive techniques)

Reconstructive surgery
+
Cryopreservation of aspirated sperm

Sperm retrieval + ICSI
+
Cryopreservation of aspirated sperm

+

Reconstructive surgery (optional)

Failure of reconstructive surgery / ICSI with cryopreserved sperm

*Fig. 1.*

cious sedation.

A 3- to 4-cm incision is made at the upper part or root of the scrotum on its anterior part. The first step consists in releasing the vas deferens at the point where the straight portion starts. A cross hemisection is made in the front part, under the operating microscope, until the lumen is seen. The shield of a No. 24 abbocat is introduced through this incision in distal direction, and the distal deferential permeability is verified by injecting saline solution (Fig. 2A). This technique prevents the epididymal tube from opening in those infrequent cases where a distal seminal duct obstruction had not been previously diagnosed.

The vas deferens is completely sectioned at the point where the hemisection was made, and widely released as it must reach the epididymis with no stretching whatsoever, as this would make both the execution and the success of the anastomosis difficult. The lumen at the proximal deferential end is obstructed by means of electrocoagulation.

The most distal epididymal area showing tubular dilatation is identified under the operating microscope, or, when the tubular dilatation is not evident, the

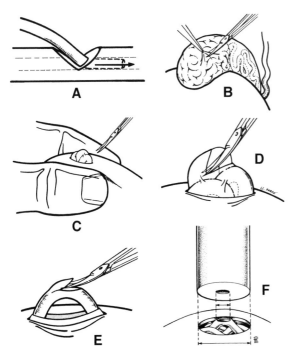

*Fig. 2.* Terminolateral vasoepididymostomy. **A:** Introduction of a No. 24 abbocat shield through the distal hemisectioned vas deferens. The injection of saline solution enables the distal vas deferens permeability to be checked. **B:** Circular opening of the epididymal tunic. **C:** Compression of the epididymis between the thumb and the forefinger. **D:** Section of the peritubular connective tissue. **E:** Opening of the epididymal tube. **F:** The diameters of the incisions of the epididymal tunic and tube must be similar to the diameters of the vas deferens and its lumen, respectively.

most distal part of the cauda. The epididymal tunic is raised with forceps and a circular opening made in it with scissors, with a diameter approximately the same as that of the vas deferens (Fig. 2B,F). The compression of the epididymis between the thumb and the forefinger favours the protrusion of the tubular loops (Fig. 2C). One of these is chosen and the peritubular connective tissue is released with very thin blade scissors (Fig. 2D). At this point, Marmar proposes to place one 11-0 nylon monothread stitch in the anterior wall of the tubule to allow its traction [15].

After the tubular section has been correctly identified, an opening is made with scissors or a microknife at the level of maximum convexity (Fig. 2E), of a diameter similar to that of the deferens lumen (Fig. 2F). A microscope slide is passed through the tubular opening while the macroscopic characteristics of the outgoing fluid are noted. This fluid may be absent, abundant or scarce, and it may be either fluid or thick and its color yellow, white or transparent.

The microscope slide is observed in the operating theatre itself under the light microscope, and the number of spermatozoa per × 40 field is assessed, together with their motility and morphology. Table 3 shows the graduation guideline proposed by the Vasovasostomy Study Group of USA [16]. If no spermatozoa are observed in the first sample, other samples should be assessed after thorough squeezing of the testicle and of the epididymis proximal to the opening. If no spermatozoa are found, or if these are not complete (cutoff heads and tails), other more proximal tubular openings must be made, even including to the efferent ducti [17,18] until complete spermatozoa are found, independently from their being or not motile. The presence of incomplete spermatozoa might indicate a more proximal secondary epididymal obstruction. In time, the spermatozoa trapped between two obstructive areas lose their tails [19].

When complete spermatozoa are found, they can either be aspirated to be used in ICSI techniques or else be frozen for latter application of this method. Meticulous attention is paid to the attainment of perfect hemostasis with a fine tipped bipolar coagulation forcep. The vas deferens is brought close to the epididymal tube and three or four stitches are placed with 9-0 nylon monothread between the epididymal tunic and the rear muscular deferens wall (Fig. 3A). The needle is passed from the outside to inside the tunic and from the inside to outside the deferential wall to ensure that the knots stay at the back of the anastomosis. Two or three stitches with 10-0 nylon monothread are made using the same technique

*Table 3.* Vas fluid sperm quality.

| Grade | |
|---|---|
| 1 | Mainly motile normal sperm |
| 2 | Mainly nonmotile normal sperm |
| 3 | Mainly sperm heads along with some normal sperm |
| 4 | Only sperm heads |
| 5 | No sperm |

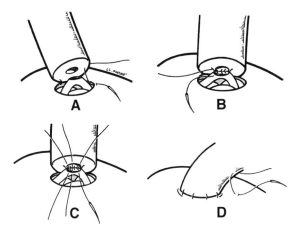

*Fig. 3.* Terminolateral vasoepididymostomy. **A:** 9-0 nylon monothread stitches between the epididymal tunic and the rear muscular vas deferens wall. **B:** 10-0 nylon monothread stitches between the rear wall of the epididymal tube and the rear mucous layer of the vas deferens lumen. **C:** 10-0 nylon monothread stitches between the vas deferens mucous layer and the front wall of the epididymal tube. **D:** 9-0 nylon monothread stitches between the front muscular vas deferens wall and the epididymal tunic.

between the rear wall of the epididymal tube and the rear mucous layer of the vas deferens lumen (Fig. 3B). To facilitate the correct observation of both tubular lumens, the first threads, which should be left very short, are not knotted until the last one is placed. In order to better observe the epididymal lumen, some authors find it useful to define it with a drop of methylene blue [15,20]. Once the posterior anastomosis has been completed, two or three stitches are placed between the deferens mucosa and the front wall of the epididymal tube (Fig. 3C). The anastomosis is considered as complete after making several stitches with 9-0 nylon monothread between the front muscular deferens wall and the epididymal tunic (Fig. 3D). This technique ensures suitable continuity between both tubular structures, as well as the impermeability of the anastomosis. The same procedure is applied in the contralateral hemiscrotum.

When we first started to apply the microsurgical techniques to perform the VE, the terminoterminal technique described by Silber [19] was done on many patients. In this technique, the epididymis is transversely sectioned and the patent tubule is terminoterminal anastomosed to the vas deferens lumen. In our opinion, the lateroterminal VE is less aggressive and the localization of the patent tubule is easier. However, Schlegel does not find any significant difference, in terms of pregnancy, between the lateroterminal and the terminoterminal techniques [12].

The first semen analysis is performed 1 month after surgery and then repeated every month for the first 6 months, and every 2 months until completing 1 year.

Many times, the spermatozoa do not appear at ejaculation until 4—8 months after surgery. Matthews, in 100 VE, reported a mean time to observe spermato-

418

zoa in the ejaculate of 3.6 months, however, 12 months were necessary to complete the permeability process [21]. In the series reported by Jarrow, the mean time to observe spermatozoa in the ejaculate was 6 months [22]. According to our experience, in some cases the spermatozoa appear only after 1 year post-surgery. The reasons for this are difficult to identify, although there seems to be a connection with postsurgical edema and a little precise anastomosis. In the latter case, the pressure exercised by the spermatozoa and the spermatic fluid would facilitate the passage through the weakest area, that is the anastomotic area. The presence of antispermatic antibodies might also play a role in the VE failure.

Because of other mechanisms also difficult to understand, in a considerable number of cases the spermatozoa obtained at ejaculation are scarce and/or of deficient quality, spontaneous pregnancies thereby not being achieved. In these cases it may be suitable to turn to any of the various assisted reproduction techniques, depending on the characteristics of the sperm. In other cases, the spermatozoa are never seen in the ejaculate. Depending upon the characteristics of the sperm as observed during surgery, these patients might be advised to undergo another VE and, at the same time, to undergo spermatozoa microaspiration to be used in the ICSI technique.

The best VE prognosis is seen in those patients who have abundant and motile spermatozoa, for whom a correct surgical technique has been applied, and in whom the obstruction of the epididymis is acquired, has had a short development time, and is located at the distal part of the organ [23,24].

Table 4 shows the VE results of the most important published series. Many of them were done in postvasectomy cases, which have a better prognosis. In others, the cause of the epididymal obstruction was not identified. The patency rates vary between 39 and 86% and the pregnancy rates between 13 and 42% [13,15,21–23,25–30]. In 47 cases of acquired etiology, usually inflammatory or

Table 4. Vasoepididymostomy. Results of the most important published series.

| Author/year | No. | Technique | Permeability (%) | Pregnancy (%) |
| --- | --- | --- | --- | --- |
| Silber 1978 [19] | 14 | TT | 86 | — |
| McLoughlin 1982 [28] | 23 | — | — | 39 |
| Dubin 1984 [25] | 46 | TT | 39 | 13 |
| Wagenknecht 1985 [30] | 50 | LT | — | 23 |
| Fogdestam 1986 [26] | 41 | LT | 85.3 | 36.6 |
| Thomas 1986 [13] | 50 | LT | 66 | 41.9 |
| Niederberger 1993 [29] | 22 | LT | 48 | 18 |
| Matsuda 1994 [23] | 26 | TT/LT | 80.8 | 41.7 |
| Marmar 1995 [15] | 19 | LT | 73.6 | 42 |
| Matthews 1995 [21] | 100 | TT/LT | 65 | 21 |
| Jarow 1995 [22] | 89 | LT | 56 | — |
| Lee 1987 [27] | 158 | TT | 37 | 20 |

TT: terminoterminal; LT: lateroterminal.

secondary to a more distal obstruction, we obtained 58% patency and 32% pregnancies. When the cause was either idiopathic or congenital (127 cases), the percentage of patency was 34 and that of pregnancies 9.

*Vas deferens obstruction surgery*

When dealing with obstruction of the vas deferens, it is essential to establish the difference between the obstruction settled after the performance of a vasectomy and that elicited by other causes, usually of the iatrogenic kind. In the latter, the development period is usually long (e.g., herniorrhaphy in childhood), there is the possibility of a secondary obstruction appearing at the level of the epididymis and the absence of extended sections of the vas deferens or the retraction of the distal end is frequently observed. The latter of these features makes it difficult, in most cases, to locate the distal end of the vas deferens when performing the anastomosis.

*Postvasectomy vas deferens obstruction*
Some 1—3% of vasectomized men ask about the possibility of recovering their fertility. The causes, in order of frequency, are: change of partner, death of children, wish for a new child with the same partner, vasectomy performed before having had any children and a psychological intolerance of sterilization. The main prognostic factors for the success of the vasovasostomy (VV) depend upon the level at which the vasectomy was performed and whether the proximal deferens end was occluded. The ideal conditions are: a vasectomy made as distally as possible in the straight section of the vas deferens, no occlusion with arising from any method, of the proximal deferential lumen. This obviates the effect of hyperpressure and secondary breakage of the epididymal tube.

The most advisable VV technique is the one carried out at two levels (mucosal and muscular) [31,32]. Under local anesthesia, a 2—3 cm incision is made at the root of the scrotum. The portion where the vasectomy was made is released extravaginally. The vas deferens distal from the obstruction is cross-sectioned with straight scissors and widely released. The shield of a 24 abbocat is introduced through this light and the distal deferens permeability is verified by saline solution injection. Then, the preobstructive deferens end is cross-sectioned and the macroscopic features of the fluid (quantity, colour and thickness) are assessed. Immediately following this, a microscope slide is glided on its surface and the concentration and quality of the sperm is assessed in the operation theatre itself, and scored according to the graduations referred to in Table 4. Independently from the presence or absence of spermatozoa, the anastomosis is then made.

If the proximal lumen was occluded in the course of the vasectomy, a great difference in diameter is appraised between the proximal lumen (0.5—0.8 mm) and the distal lumen (0.3 mm). Both deferens ends are placed on an approximating clamp. A piece of colored plastic is placed as a background, which enables easy isolation of the elements of the surgical field and the handling of the stitching materials. Three stitches of 10-0 nylon monothread are made in the mucosal layer of both front deferential sides under microscopic vision. When the front mucosal anastomosis is completed, the clamp is turned over and the same procedure is carried out in the rear part. Finally, four to six stitches of 9-0 nylon monothread are made between the back and front muscular walls (Fig. 4). The same procedure is applied to the contralateral scrotum.

VV can also be performed on one layer according to the triangular technique to place the stitches described by Schmidt [33]. Other proposed VV techniques use a laser [34—36] or fibrine glue [37]. The first semen analysis is made 1 month after surgery. Differently from what was stated concerning the VE, rapid appearance of the spermatozoa is verified in the VV; initially they may be scarce and of low quality but the situation will improve at every ensuing semen analysis. Most pregnancies are generally achieved after 6—12 months following surgery. In those cases where no spermatozoa were seen in the course of surgery, and still do not appear at ejaculation after the VV, the possibility of a secondary epididymal obstruction should be envisaged, so a VE should be carried out. According to the results reported by the US Vasovasostomy Study Group [16], which are superimposable to our own results, in those cases where no spermatozoa are observed in the course of the VV, 60% repermeabilizations and 31% pregnancies have been verified. These results are the ones presently directing the protocol that advises initial VV under local anesthesia.

Sperm can be present in the ejaculate but its concentration or quality is altered. In these cases, if antispermatic antibodies are present, they might have a spermatic adverse effect [38] and a treatment with corticoesteroids might be indicated. However, antispermatic antibodies are present in more than 50% of patients with vas deferens obstruction [39,40]. After VV, Thomas does not find any significant difference, in terms of pregnancy, when comparing patients with

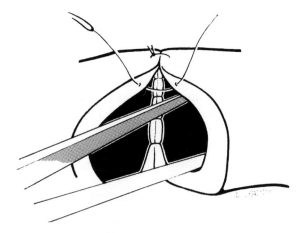

*Fig. 4.* Vasovasostomy in two layers.

and without antispermatic antibodies. In cases of oligozoospermia post-VV, a partial obstruction of the vas deferens might be the cause. When there are alterations of the sperm concentration and/or quality, assisted reproductive techniques can be applied.

Table 5 shows the VV results of the most important published series [16,21,41–46]. The percentage of patency varies between 75 and 99 and the percentage of pregnancy between 46 and 82. The Vasovasostomy Group of the USA published the most important series [16]. Out of 1,247 VV, patency and pregnancy were achieved in 86 and 52%, respectively.

In our series of 102 patients with a mean age of 37 years (range 25–54 years) who consulted for vasectomy reversal, the causes for this were: new partner (53%), desire to have more children with the same partner (26.4%), death of children (7.8%) and vasectomy performed without having children (7.8%). During surgery the sperm quality was grade 1 in 22%, 2 in 32%, 3 in 17%, 4 in 11% and 5 in 18%. Out of all patients, only 71.5% were available for follow-up. Patency was achieved in 93.2% of patients and pregnancy in 40%.

## Sperm recovery and ICSI

When reconstructive surgery of the seminal duct is either not possible or a failure, spermatozoa can be obtained from the epididymis, the vas deferens or the testicle to be used in ICSI. This technique has enabled the remarkable improvement of the results that formerly were achieved by means of the classic in vitro fertilization (IVF) technique [47,48].

### Microsurgical epididymal sperm aspiration

The basic indications of microsurgical epididymal sperm aspiration (MESA) are the absence of the vas deferens, and the epididymal obstruction from other causes where reconstructive surgery has failed. Once ovulation has been stimulated and the follicles have been punctured according to the customary IVF method, MESA is carried out.

*Table 5.* Vasovasostomy. Results of the most important published series.

| Author/year | No. | Permeability (%) | Pregnancy (%) |
|---|---|---|---|
| Fenster 1981 [42] | 26 | 96 | 54 |
| Cos 1983 [41] | 87 | 75 | 46 |
| Owen 1984 [44] | 475 | 93 | 82 |
| Soonawala 1984 [46] | 339 | 89 | 63 |
| Lee 1986 [43] | 185 | 91 | 52 |
| Silber 1989 [45] | 282 | 91 | 81 |
| Belker 1991 [16] | 1247 | 86 | 52 |
| Matthews 1995 [21] | 100 | 99 | 52 |

The epididymal tube is exposed and cut using the same method as described for VE. When tube fluid flows, the presence of spermatozoa is verified immediately. If spermatozoa are either absent or immotile, more proximal tubular openings are made. In most cases the best quality spermatozoa are located at the epididymal head level. The reason for this is that, contrary to what happens in the normal epididymis, in the obstructed one the spermatozoa that are closest to the occluded area have long ago reached said area, and there they have aged, lost motility and degenerated; it is also possible to find incomplete spermatozoa. Those that are closest to the testicle are newly formed spermatozoa that have had sufficient time to mature and gain motility; these properties are essentially acquired over time [49—51].

Once the tube containing the best-quality spermatozoa has been found — even though this quality is never excellent — a careful bipolar hemostasis is performed to avoid, as far as possible, the presence of erythrocytes in the field. The maximum possible quantity of fluid is then aspirated. To this purpose, our team has designed a mechanism which permits the continuous aspiration of spermatozoa by means of the introduction of a micropipette into the tubular opening (Fig. 5) [52]. This pipette is connected, by means of a silicon tube, to a Falcon tube containing the culture medium and this, in turn, is connected to a 50-ml syringe which constitutes the aspirating mechanism of the system. The culture medium used (Ham F-10, Hepes, Earle's, Flushing, etc.) depends upon the experience and the preferences of the working team. Different tubes are sent to the IVF

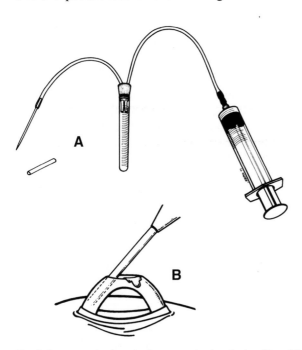

*Fig. 5.* Sperm aspiration. **A:** Sperm aspirating device; **B:** epididymal tube sperm aspiration.

laboratory to be processed in two or more layers by a gradient separation technique. This enables selection of the best quality spermatozoa and, at the same time, their separation from the erythrocytes and other kinds of cells, and from detritus.

In cases where no spermatozoa are found at the epididymal level, including the efferent ducti, which could indicate an intratesticular obstruction, it is advisable to remove one or several fragments of testicular tissue. These fragments are squeezed over a plate containing culture medium, with the aim of releasing the spermatozoa [53].

Depending upon the number of spermatozoa obtained at any of the levels, as per the IVF laboratory report, the contralateral side is operated or not. The larger the portion of intact epididymis is preserved, the higher the possibility of repeating the method.

Some authors support the possibility of aspirating spermatozoa from the epididymis or the testicle by means of trans-scrotum puncture [54]. In our opinion this technique could be exceedingly damaging, particularly in the case of the epididymal tube, and cause the appearance of granulomas and hematomas that are difficult to control. Moreover, the number of spermatozoa obtained is very small, which makes their cryopreservation for future use impossible.

As in any IVF technique, once the ovum fertilization is achieved, a maximum of three embryos are transferred either to the uterine cavity or to the tubes, according to each working team's experience. The remaining embryos are cryopreserved for eventual future transfer.

The pregnancy rates for MESA varied between 5 and 15% when classical IVF techniques were applied [47,48]. With ICSI, oocyte fertilization rates between 50 and 80% and pregnancy rates between 20 and 35% were achieved [47,55—61]. Using testicle spermatozoa, fertilization rates between 34 and 62% and pregnancy rates between 19 and 43% were obtained [60,62—68]. ICSI has also allowed the achievement of pregnancy with cryopreserved spermatozoa extracted from the epididymis [55,69] and from the testicle [70].

It may be deduced from these results that ICSI is essential in the sperm recovery method, independently from the level of the seminal duct where it is performed.

*Vas deferens sperm aspiration*

Several clinical circumstances exist in which spermatogenesis and epididymal patency are preserved, and in which for different reasons spermatozoa cannot be ejaculated. Among them are distal obstruction of the vas deferens and of the ejaculatory duct, where reconstructive surgery either cannot be performed or else has failed, retrograde ejaculation where no high quality spermatozoa can be recovered from the postorgasmic urine, and an ejaculation of an organic or a psychogenic origin where the methods tested (electrovibration, electrostimulation) have failed. In these cases, it is possible to aspirate spermatozoa from the

424

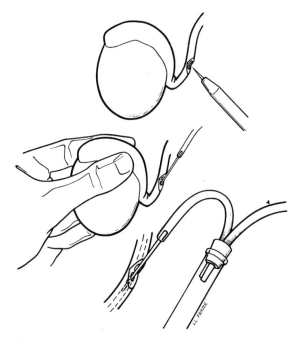

*Fig. 6.* Vas deferens sperm aspiration.

vas deferens to be used in IVF techniques [71,72]. The vas deferens is released under local anesthesia and a cross-hemisection is made until the lumen is perceived. The micropipette belonging to the already described aspirating mechanism is introduced in the proximal deferential end while performing the compression of the testicle and the epididymis (Fig. 6).

Depending upon spermatozoa number and quality, which is usually better than that of the spermatozoa obtained from the epididymis, either the classical IVF or the ICSI technique may be applied. In the cases of deferential sperm aspiration, the percentage of fertilizations varies between 60 and 80. The percentage of pregnancies is not assessable as most studies base their conclusions on isolated cases.

### References

1. Goldstein M, Gilbert BR, Dicker AP, Dwosh J, Gnecco C. Microsurgical inguinal varicocelectomy with delivery of the testis: an artery and lymphatic sparing technique. J Urol 1992; 148:1808.
2. Stern RC, Boat TF, Doershuk CF. Obstructive azoospermia as a diagnostic criterion for the cystic fibrosis syndrome. Lancet 1982;i:1401–1404.
3. Hughes TM, Judah L, Skolnick Y, Belker A. Young's syndrome: an often unrecognized correctable cause of obstructive azoospermia. J Urol 1987;137:1238–1240.
4. Neville E, Brewis R, Yeates WK, Burridge A. Respiratory tract disease and obstructive azoospermia. Thorax 1983;38:929–933.

5. Young D. Surgical treatment of male infertility. J Reprod Fertil 1970;23:541−542.
6. Anguiano A, Oates RD, Amos JA, Dean M, Gerrard B, Stewart C, Maher TA, White MB, Milunsky A. Congenital bilateral absence of the vas deferens. A primarily genital form of cystic fibrosis. JAMA 1992;267:1794−1797.
7. Casals T, Bassas L, Ruiz-Romero J, Chillon M, Gimenez J, Ramos MD, Tapia G, Narvaez H, Numes V, Estivill V. Extensive analysis of 40 infertile patients with congenital absence of the vas deferens: in 50% of cases only one CFTR allele could be detected. Hum Genet 1995;95:205−211.
8. Oates RD, Amos JA. Congenital bilateral absence of the vas deferens and cystic fibrosis. A genetic commonality. World J Urol 1993;11:82−88.
9. Patrizio P, Asch R, Handelin B, Silber SJ. Aetiology of congenital absence of vas deferens: genetic study of three generations. Hum Reprod 1993;8:215−220.
10. Matsuda T, Horii Y, Muguruma K, Komatz Y, Yoshida O. Unilateral obstruction of the vas deferens caused by childhood inguinal herniorrhaphy in male infertility patients. Fertil Steril 1992;58:609−613.
11. Parkhouse H, Hendry WF. Vasal injuries during childhood and their effect on subsequent fertility. Br J Urol 1991;67:91−95.
12. Schlegel P, Berkeley AS, Goldstein M et al. Microsurgical vasoepididymostomy: refinaments and results. J Urol 1993;150:1165−1168.
13. Thomas AJ Jr. Vasoepididymostomy. Urol Clin N Am 1987;14:527.
14. Wagenknecht LV, Klosterhalfen H, Schirren C. Microsurgery in andrologic urology. I. Refertilization. J Microsurg 1980;1:470.
15. Marmar JL. Management of the epididymal tubule during an end-to-side vasoepididymostomy. J Urol 1995;154:93−96.
16. Belker A, Thomas AJ Jr, Fuchs EF, Konnak JW, Sharlip ID. Results of 1469 microsurgical vasectomy reversals by the vasovasostomy study group. J Urol 1991;145:505−511.
17. Silber SJ. Pregnancy caused by sperm from vasa efferentia. Fertil Steril 1988;49:373−375.
18. Weiske W-H. Pregnancy caused by sperm from vasa efferentia. Fertil Steril 1994;62:642−643.
19. Silber SJ. Microscopic vasoepididymostomy: specific microanastomosis to the epididymal tubule. Fertil Steril 1978;30:565−571.
20. Belker AM. Vasography and techniques for epididymal microsurgery. Urol Times 1994;22:8.
21. Matthews GJ, Schlegel PN, Goldstein M. Patency following microsurgical vasoepididymostomy and vasovasostomy: temporal considerations. J Urol 1995;154:2070−2073.
22. Jarrow JP, Sigman M, Buch JP, Oates RD. Delayed appearance of sperm after end-to-side vasoepididymostomy. J Urol 1995;153:1156−1158.
23. Matsuda T, Horii Y, Yoshida O, Komatz Y. Microsurgical epididymovasostomy for obstructive azoospermia: factors affecting postoperative fertility. Eur Urol 1994;26:322−326.
24. Pontonnier F, Mansat A, Mieusset R. Le facteur de pronostic épididymaire de l'anastomose épididymo-déférentielle. J d'Urol 1986;2:105−110.
25. Dubin L, Amelar RD. Magnified surgery for epididymostomy. Urology 1984;23:525−528.
26. Fogdestam I, Fall M, Nilsson S. Microsurgical epididymovasostomy in the treatment of occlusive azoospermia. Fertil Steril 1986;46:925.
27. Lee HY. A 20-year experience with epididymovasostomy for pathologic epididymal obstruction. Fertil Steril 1987;47:487−491.
28. McLoughlin MG. Vasoepididymostomy: the role of the microscope. Can J Surg 1982;25:41.
29. Niederberger C, Ross LS. Microsurgical epididymovasostomy: predictors of success. J Urol 1993;149:1364−1367.
30. Wagenknecht LV. Ten years experience with microsurgical epididymostomy: results and proposition of a new technique. J Androl 1985;6:26.
31. Goldstein M. Vasectomy and vasectomy reversal. Curr Ther Endocrinol Metab 1986; 1985−1986:180−185.
32. Silber SJ. Vasectomy and vasectomy reversal. Fertil Steril 1978;29:125−140.

426

33. Schmidt SS. Vasovasostomy. Urol Clin North Am 1978;5:585.
34. Rosenberg SK, Elson L, Nathan LE Jr. Carbon dioxide laser microsurgical vasovasostomy. Urology 1985;25:53.
35. Rosenberg SK. Further clinical experience with $CO_2$ laser in microsurgical vasovasostomy. Urology 1988;32:225—227.
36. Shanberg A, Tansey L, Baghdassarian R, Sawyer D, Lynn CH. Laser-assisted vasectomy reversal: experience in 32 patients. J Urol 1990;143:528—530.
37. Silverstein JI, Mellinger BC. Fibrine glue vasal anastomosis compared to conventional sutured vasovasostomy in the rat. J Urol 1991;145:1288—1291.
38. Linnet L. Association between failure to impregnate after vasovasostomy and sperm agglutinins in semen. Lancet 1981;1:117.
39. Alexander NJ, Anderson DJ. Vasectomy: consequences of autoimmunity to sperm antigens. Fertil Steril 1979;32:253.
40. Meinertz H, Linnet L, Fogh P, Hjort T. Antisperm antibodies and fertility after vasovasostomy: a follow-up study of 216 men. Fertil Steril 1990;54:315—321.
41. Cos LR, Valvo JR, Davis RS, Cockett ATK. Vasovasostomy: current state of the art. Urology 1983;22:567—575.
42. Fenster H, McLoughlin MG. Vasovasostomy: Is the microscope necessary? Urology 1981;28: 60—64.
43. Lee HY. Twenty year's experience with vasovasostomy. J Urol 1986;136:413—415.
44. Owen E, Kapila H. Vasectomy reversal: Review of 475 microsurgical vasovasostomies. Med J Aust 1984;140:398—400.
45. Silber SJ. Pregnancy after vasovasostomy for vasectomy reversal: a study of factors affecting long-term return of fertility in 282 patients followed for 10 years. Hum Reprod 1989;4:318—322.
46. Soonawalla FB, Lal SS. Microsurgery in vasovasostomy. Indian J Urol 1984;1:104—108.
47. Silber SJ, Nagy ZP, Liu J, Godoy H, Devroey P, Van Steirteghem AC. Conventional in-vitro fertilization versus intracytoplasmatic sperm injection for patients requiring microsurgical sperm aspiration. Hum Reprod 1994;9:1705—1709.
48. The Sperm Microaspiration Retrieval Techniques Study Group: Results in the United States with sperm microaspiration retrieval techniques and assisted reproductive technologies. J Urol 1994;151:1255—1259.
49. Cooper TG. In defense of a function for the human epididymis. Fertil Steril 1990;54:965—975.
50. Schoysman RJ, Bedford JM. The role of the human epididymis in sperm maturation and sperm storage as reflected in the consequences of epididymovasostomy. Fertil Steril 46:293—299.
51. Silber SJ. Role of epididymis in sperm maturation. Urology 1989;33:47—51.
52. Ruiz-Romero J, Sarquella J, Pomerol JM. A new device for microsurgical sperm aspiration. Andrologia 1993;26:119—120.
53. Jow WW, Steckel J, Schlegel PN, Magid MS, Goldstein M. Motile sperm in human testis biopsy specimens. J Androl 1993;14:194—198.
54. Craft IL, Khalifa Y, Boulos A, Pelekanos M, Foster C, Tsirigotis M. Factors influencing the outcome of in-vitro fertilization with percutaneous aspirated epididymal spermatozoa and intracytoplasmatic sperm injection in azoospermic men. Hum Reprod 1995;10:1791.
55. Nagy Z, Liu J, Cecile J, Silber S, Devroey P, Van Steirteghem A. Using ejaculated, fresh, and frozen-thawed epididymal and testicular spermatozoa gives rise to comparable results after ICSI. Fertil Steril 1995;63:808—815.
56. Olar TT, La Nasa J, Dickey RP, Taylor SN, Curole DN. Fertilization of human oocytes by microinjection of human sperm aspirated from the caput epididymidis of an individual with obstructive azoospermia. J In Vitro Fertil Embryo Transfer 1990;7:160—164.
57. Schlegel PN, Berkeley AS, Goldstein M, Cohen J, Alikani M, Adler A, Gilbert BR, Rosenwaks Z. Epididymal micropuncture with in vitro fertilization and oocyte micromanipulation for the treatment of unreconstructable obstructive azoospermia. Fertil Steril 1994;61:895—901.
58. Silber SJ, Ord T, Borrero C, Balmaceda J, Asch R. New treatment for infertility due to congeni-

tal absence of vas deferens. Lancet 1987;2:850—851.

59. Tournaye H, Devroey P, Liu J, Nagy Z, Lissens W, Van Steirteghem A. Microsurgical epididymal sperm aspiration and intracytoplasmatic sperm injection: a new effective approach to infertility as a result of congenital bilateral absence of the vas deferens. Fertil Steril 1994;61:1045—1051.

60. Tucker MJ, Morton PC, Witt MA, Wright G. Intracytoplasmatic injection of testicular and epididymal spermatozoa for treatment of obstructive azoospermia. Hum Reprod 1995;10:486.

61. Van Der Zwalmen P, Nÿs M, Segal-Bertin G, Segal L, Schoysman R. Epididymal sperm aspiration for in vitro fertilization. In: Schoysman R (ed) Microsurgery of Male Infertility. Fondazione Per Gli Studi Sulla Riproduzione Umana, 1994;229—248.

62. Craft I, Bennet V, Nicholson N. Fertilizing ability of testicular spermatozoa (letter). Lancet 1993;342:864.

63. Devroey P, Liu J, Nagy Z, Tournaye H, Silber SJ, Van Steirteghem AC. Normal fertilization of human oocytes after testicular sperm extraction and intracytoplasmatic sperm injection. Fertil Steril 1994;62:639—661.

64. Gil-Salom M, Mínguez Y, Rubio C, de los Santos MJ, Remohi J, Pellicer A. Efficacy of intracytoplasmatic sperm injection using testicular spermatozoa. Hum Reprod 1995;10:3166—3170.

65. Hirsh A, Montgomery J, Mohan P, Mills C, Bekir J, Tan SL. Fertilization by testicular sperm with standard IVF techniques (letter). Lancet 1993;342:1237—1238.

66. Schoysman R, Vanderzwalmen P, Nijs M, Segal L, Segal-Bertin G, Geerts L, Van Roosendaal E, Schoysman R. Pregnancy after fertilization with human testicular spermatozoa (Letter, Comment). Lancet 1993;342:1237.

67. Schoysman R, Vanderzwalmen P, Nijs M, Segal-Bertin G, van de Casseye M. Successful fertilization by testicular spermatozoa in an in-vitro fertilization programme. Hum Reprod 1993;8:1339—1340.

68. Silber SJ, Van Steirteghem AC, Liu J, Nagy Z, Tournaye H, Devroey P. High fertilization and pregnancy rate after intracytoplasmatic sperm injection with spermatozoa obtained from testicle biopsy. Hum Reprod 1995;10:148—152.

69. Oates RD, Lobel SM, Harris DH, Pang S, Burgess CM, Carson RS. Efficacy of intracytoplasmatic sperm injection using intentionally cryopreserved epididymal spermatozoa. Hum Reprod 1996;11:133—138.

70. Gil-Salom M, Romero J, Mínguez Y, Rubio C, de los Santos MJ, Remohi J, Pellicer A. Pregnancies after intracytoplasmatic sperm injection with cryopreserved testicular spermatozoa. Hum Reprod 1996;11:1309—1313.

71. Bustillo M, Rajfer J. Pregnancy following insemination with sperm aspirated directly from vas deferens. Fertil Steril 1986;46:144—146.

72. Hovatta O, von Smitten K. Sperm aspiration from vas deferens and in-vitro fertilization in cases of non tratable anejaculation. Hum Reprod 1993;8:1689—1691.

# ICSI and the biological sperm reservoir

Michael A. Witt

*Reproductive Biology Associates, Atlanta, Georgia, USA*

## Introduction

My discussion can be broadly categorized as follows:
1) What are the various sperm retrieval techniques?
2) When should each technique be employed?
3) How is each technique performed?
4) How often can these procedures be performed?
5) How and who should process the specimens?
6) When can and how should specimens be cryopreserved?
7) What are the results with each type of specimen?

## Options

The various techniques for sperm retrieval are defined by the type of surgical approach used and reservoir accessed. The surgical approaches are defined as either open or percutaneous. Open procedures involve direct visual inspection of the reservoir during which excisional or aspiration techniques are employed. Percutaneous techniques utilize aspiration techniques combined with palpation or ultrasonographic imaging. The primary reservoirs used for sperm retrieval are the epididymis and testicle. The terms most commonly used to describe these procedures are:

MESA  microsurgical epididymal sperm aspiration
PESA  percutaneous epididymal sperm aspiration
TESE  testicular sperm extraction
TESA  testicular sperm aspiration

## Indications

The type of procedure performed depends upon the reservoir availability, the indications for the use of a particular procedure, the cost of the procedure, the

*Address for correspondence:* Michael A. Witt MD, 5505 Peachtree-Dunworthy Road, Suite 550, Atlanta, GA 30342, USA. Tel.: +1-404-256-6987. Fax: +1-404-256-8376.
E-mail: ewittmd@mindspring.com

experience of the laboratory personnel handling the specimen,the importance of cryopreservation to the patient and the potential for success.

The type of reservoirs available will be largely dependent upon the indications for the use of a procedure and where sperm can be found. Identical diagnoses do not produce the same available sperm reservoirs. In cases of nonobstructive azoospermia (i.e., maturation arrest or Sertoli cell only syndrome) the testicle, via open biopsy, is the only available reservoir. In structural or functional obstructive (i.e., neurologic) azoospermia the testicle and the epididymis are available reservoirs. The epididymis provides the greatest numbers of motile sperm. The testicle provides the cleanest specimen at the lowest cost. For these reasons the epididymal specimen will be the easiest to handle while providing the best potential for multivial cryopreservation. The epididymis can be accessed with an open or percutaneous technique. I prefer the open technique because it reliably provides the cleanest and greatest number of motile sperm. If the epididymis is not available, then the testicle becomes my next choice. The testicle can be accessed either percutaneously or with an open excisional biopsy. I prefer percutaneous techniques in obstructive azoospermia because it is equally reliable in comparison to the open technique and provides a cleaner specimen for the laboratory at a lower cost and lesser degree of invasion for the patient. The vas deferens can also be used in men with a functional obstruction. This is most frequently encountered in psychogenic, traumatic or neurologic anejaculation.

For nonobstructive azoospermia, nonobstructive severe oligospermia or nonobstructive necrospermia the best reservoir is the testicle and the best method is the open excisional approach. Although the seminal vesicle, vas deferens and epididymis are available in these instances the success of retrieval tends to be less reliable.

## Surgical technique

The principle qualifications for the surgeon performing sperm retrieval is the ability to perform all of the various techniques. This is because the goal of these procedures is to obtain sperm and not to reconstruct. It is not uncommon for me to modify the original procedure because I do not find sperm where I originally thought they would be. The secondary requirement for performing these procedures is the necessity of having a skilled andrology laboratory that can inspect and process these specimens. It is the laboratory that will tell me when I have enough sperm and if these sperm can be used in the designated assisted reproductive technique (ART). The laboratory will also be in charge of any processing or sperm cryopreservation. It is important to remember that the criteria for a successful procedure is the placement of sperm in the reproductive tract or oocyte. The fact that sperm have been found and procured during a diagnostic or therapeutic procedure does not necessarily mean the retrieval procedure is complete. The procurement procedure is complete when the laboratory reports that a usable specimen has been obtained.

The open surgical techniques involve exposing the vas deferens, epididymis or testicle and retrieving sperm from various sites of the dissection. For optimal results optical magnification is recommended and when possible an operating microscope should be utilized. The vas deferens is handled in the same way as an open vasotomy. The irrigation of the testicular and abdominal end of the vasotomy is necessary in order to flush sperm out of the lumenal compartment. The effluent is collected, inspected and processed.

The epididymis is approached by visually identifying the tubules that have the potential to produce sperm of good quality. The ideal tubule is one that is dilated and possesses a pearl gray appearance as opposed to a yellow or white appearance. The tubule is opened or punctured and the fluid is extracted and inspected. As many tubules as necessary are entered. Meticulous hemostasis is critical for securing an uncontaminated specimen. I recommend closing the parietal tunica vaginalis with a 7-0 prolene in order to avoid this site at the time of future aspirations.

The testicle is approached in the exact same fashion as a diagnostic testicular biopsy. The ideal site is in the midline on the antiepididymal side of the testicle. I prefer to take only one specimen from this site weighing between 0.2 and 0.5 g. The reason for selecting and using only one site is that the data seem to indicate that the distribution of sperm in the nonobstructed azoospermic testicle is diffusely homogeneous as opposed to being located in isolated pockets. Thus, the use of one site will typically yield sperm with the lowest risk of testicular devascularization. The tissue is then handed to the laboratory for processing. Since most of my open testicular cases are for nonobstructive azoospermia, I either know that sperm are present on the basis of a previous diagnostic sperm retrieval or because the couple have donor sperm as a back up. Therefore, I do not wait to for a report from the laboratory in order to determine if more tissue should be taken. This is because it can take our laboratory upwards of 2 h to find sperm.

The percutaneous techniques involve placing a fine needle into the intended reservoir and aspirating its contents in the hope of obtaining sperm. These procedures have the advantages of being less expensive and invasive but the disadvantages of being less reliable and lower in yield. The seminal vesicle is punctured under ultrasonographic guidance with an 18-g needle and aspirated. This was developed as a diagnostic technique for identifying complete or partial ejaculatory duct obstruction. The epididymis can be entered percutaneously after being localized and isolated with palpation. A 21- to 23-g needle is used with aspiration. Multiple passes are required and slow placement is critical in order to successfully withdraw fluid. Percutaneous testicular aspiration or nonsurgical sperm aspiration involves making multiple passes with a 2- to 3-in. 21 gauge needle under high negative pressure. The pressure must be released very slowly back to equilibrium in order to avoid the loss of the aspirated contents. Typically, fragments of seminiferous tubules become trapped in the tip of the needle. This is where the sperm are found.

## Frequency

Multiple procedures can be performed in any reservoir as long as previous retrievals have not completely eliminated the compartment from which the sperm were obtained. Percutaneous retrieval of sperm from the testicle in the case of obstructive azoospermia has almost unlimited application. Repeat percutaneous aspiration of sperm from the epididymis is fraught with more difficulty because the initial uncontrolled access to the tubules obliterates most of the remaining tubules. This is in contrast to an open epididymal aspiration in which controlled access and anatomical restoration of the tubule and tunica allow for repeat procedures. Open testicular sperm retrieval can be readily repeated. It is recommended to wait at least 3 months between attempts in order to allow for a better delineation of viable and nonviable segments of the seminiferous tubules and the full recovery of the germinal epithelium from the initial insult. In general, repeat open retrievals of the epididymis and testicle are more difficult than the initial attempt due to the inevitable formation of scar tissue.

## Specimen processing

I cannot stress how important the laboratory function is in guaranteeing a successful retrieval and outcome. The laboratory is solely responsible for the processing and manipulation of the specimen. It is important the laboratory personnel be motivated in the handling of these specimens because it can be a tedious and painstaking process. The laboratory must be flexible with the processing techniques it uses. Our laboratory currently employs microdissection, vortexing and homogenization. It is also essential that good communication be established between the urologist and the laboratory. Feedback is critical in modifying procedures intraoperatively, planning for future retrievals and reviewing past successes and failures in order to improve outcomes. The limitations of the laboratory also need to be defined because not all of the described procedures can be performed by all laboratories.

## Cryopreservation

The cryopreservation of vasal, epididymal and testicular specimens has provided patients with the capacity to perform multiple cycles of assisted reproduction from one retrieval procedure. This has significantly reduced the total cost of establishing a pregnancy, subjected the patient to fewer invasive procedures and allowed for greater predictability in the scheduling of the initial sperm retrieval.

I have found that quite a few misconceptions exist about the cryopreservation of vasal, epididymal and testicular specimens. It is presumptive to think that all specimens and all sperm can be successfully cryopreserved. Just as ejaculated specimens vary in their postthaw survivability, so do pre-ejaculated specimens. This survivability rate determines the critical number of sperm needed before freezing in order to end up with a usable specimen after thawing. Even when good numbers of sperm survive upon thawing, identifying viable nonmotile sperm is still not an exact science. Until this identification process is more refined the mere fact that you can freeze the sperm does not mean that it is usable. This fact is particularly critical in the age of intracytoplasmic sperm injection because a single sperm is matched with a single oocyte. A general rule to follow is that the better the specimen you begin with the greater the likelihood that a usable fraction will be obtained when the specimen is finally thawed. In addition, it is imperative to determine how well your laboratory can freeze and thaw these specimens and to find what their fertilization and pregnancy rates with these cryopreserved specimens are like. I have found that not all specimens can be frozen. I cryopreserve all open epididymal specimens. I currently attempt to obtain at least 20 million motile sperm before the procedure is terminated. For this reason I intentionally retrieve and cryopreserve all specimens from patients undergoing MESA for obstructive azoospermia. Our laboratory has found that pregnancy rates with testicular sperm in the nonobstructive patient to be lower in comparison to the pregnancy rates with fresh testicular sperm. For that reason I still retrieve sperm from nonobstructive azoospermic patients on the same day as the wife's egg retrieval. I also recommend to all patients with good frozen epididymal sperm to be prepared for a retrieval procedure on the day of their wife's ovulation in the event that the frozen specimen thaws poorly.

## Results

In general fresh epididymal or testicular specimens from men with obstructive azoospermia will generate fertilization rates between 50 and 70% with an associated pregnancy rate between 35 and 50% when used in combination with intracytoplasmic sperm injection. Fresh testicular specimens from men with nonobstructive azoospermia will generate fertilization rates between 40 and 60% with associated pregnancy rates between 35 and 55% when used in combination with intracytoplasmic sperm injection. I do not think epididymal sperm behave differently to testicular sperm. Testicular sperm do present some additional challenges to the laboratory in that the numbers of sperm obtained are significantly less and the specimen is predominately nonmotile. Another factor which can also affect these rates is the age of the wife. As maternal age exceeds 37 the fertilization and pregnancy rates drop significantly.

## Conclusion

Sperm retrieval from the genital tract has provided couples previously considered terminally infertile with a means of initiating a pregnancy in which both partners contribute genetically to the offspring. As these techniques have developed they have created a bigger role for the expertise of the urologist in performing the procedure and managing the couple. Contrary to some predictions that intracyto-

434

plasmic sperm injection has eliminated the need for someone with the skill to evaluate and treat the male. I think it has accomplished just the opposite.

## References

1.  Belker AM et al. Pregnancy with microsurgical vas sperm aspiration from patient with neuro-logic ejaculatory dysfunction. J Androl 1994;15:6S.
2.  Devroey P et al. Ongoing pregnancies and birth after intracytoplasmic sperm injection with fro-zen-thawed epididymal spermatozoa. Hum Reprod 1995;10:903.
3.  Craft IL et al. Factors influencing the outcome of in vitro fertilization with percutaneous aspi-rated epididymal spermatozoa and intracytoplasmic sperm injection in azoospermic men. Hum Reprod 1995;10:1791.
4.  Mulhall P et al. Presence of mature sperm in testicular parenchyma of men with non obstructive azoospermia: prevalence and predictive factors. Urology 1997;49:91.
5.  Schlegel PN et al. Testicular sperm extraction with intracytoplasmic sperm injection for non obstructive azoospermia. Urology 1997;49:435.
6.  Lisek EW, Levine LA. Percutaneous technique for aspiration of sperm from the epididymis and testicle. Techniques in Urology 1997;3:81.

# Psychological approach and medical management of male sexual dysfunction

Fertility and Reproductive Medicine.
R.D. Kempers, J. Cohen, A.F. Haney and J.B. Younger, editors.

# Psychogenic impotence: assessment and counselling

Caroline M. Harrison

*Human Assisted Reproduction Unit, Rotunda Hospital, Dublin, Ireland*

**Abstract.** *Background.* The assessment and treatment of psychogenic impotence in the male is discussed in detail in the context of the sex and relationship service at the Human Assisted Reproduction Unit Rotunda Hospital Dublin.

*Methods.* A psychodynamic and behavioural approach is utilized, both with individual men and with couples where partnerships exist.

*Results.* Men with primary psychogenic impotence are younger than those with secondary. Their problems appear more deep-rooted but the number of sessions needed to overcome the problem was the same in both groups. Success was achieved in 63% in each of the two groups.

*Conclusions.* Successful therapy requires cooperation and belief from the couple and demands enthusiasm and expertise of the therapist.

**Keywords:** impotence, male, outcome, psychodynamic behaviour approach, psychogenic.

## Introduction

"Impotence is defined as the persistent failure to develop erections of sufficient rigidity for penetrative intercourse" [1]. However, in recent times there has been a move away from the word impotence because it has such negative connotations. Those working in the area of sex therapy now use the term "erectile dysfunction". Psychogenic implies that the cause of the erectile dysfunction is psychologic in nature and therefore it is hoped that the problem will respond favourably to psychotherapy.

The basic principle of the phenomenon "erection" has been known since the pioneering work of Kolliker, Eckhard and Langley in the 19th Century [2]. However, Freud was extremely influential in attributing all erectile dysfunctions to psychological causes. But since the 1960s a much more liberal approach has developed. This is largely due to new diagnostic techniques and the increase in research in this area expanding the concept of erectile dysfunction to include arteriogenic, venogenic, endocrinologic and myopathic (cavernous smooth muscle dysfunction) factors [2].

The male sexual response cycle has been divided into four phases by Masters and Johnson [3]. Firstly excitement leads to erection. Second is a plateau where lubrication and glandular secretion takes place. Orgasm with emission and ejaculation occurring follows and lastly there is resolution leading to detumescence

*Address for correspondence:* Caroline M. Harrison, Sex and Relationship Therapist, Human Assisted Reproduction Unit, Rotunda Hospital, Dublin I, Ireland.

and the refractory period. Where there is an erectile dysfunction this process will be impaired in some way.

The psychological diagnosis and the evaluation of erectile dysfunction is extremely important within the multidisciplinary examination of this condition. Many men now expect an instant solution to the problem of erectile dysfunction with the increasing use of intracavernous self-injections and the recent approval of the oral therapy Sildentafil Citrate (Viagra, Pfizer, USA) which works by improving blood flow to the penis [4]. Since long-term complications cannot be ruled out, and judging by the high dropout rates when using intracavernous self-injections patient acceptance levels are not what they were thought they would be and although it is early days the oral therapy has been shown to have side effects which may be unacceptable to many. It therefore remains necessary to maintain a broad and critical point of view.

The inappropriate and pointless controversy concerning whether the cause of the erectile dysfunction is organic or psychogenic achieves nothing and needs to be replaced by a broader more encompassing view point. The psychogenic approach will continue to be appropriate for many situations. We know that men suffering from this condition represent an extremely heterogeneous group of patients. "The inability to achieve or maintain erections during intercourse is the end result of a variety of possible etiological patterns" [5].

There is sometimes an unclear divide between psychological and physical causes, one may lead to the other, one may be caused by the other. A multidisciplinary approach is required to adequately treat the patient experiencing erectile dysfunctions. A successful outcome requires more tolerance from both the psychological and medical viewpoints and a withdrawal from deeply entrenched attitudes regarding this issue.

## Methods

The psychological evaluation of erectile dysfunction is best carried out by the diagnostic interview or assessment. This would be favoured by those working in the field as it allows for a significant amount of information gathering and can be personalised to meet the needs of the individual patient. Before commencing a diagnostic interview by a sex therapist it is necessary that the patient has had a full medical evaluation regarding the erectile problem to establish that the cause is not physical or not full physical. It is also necessary to check whether the condition is brought about by medication. Many drugs are associated with erectile dysfunction [6].

In the past traditional psychoanalytic theories saw any sexual dysfunction as the symptomatic expression of an underlying neurotic conflict. However, the majority of those working in the area today support the works of Masters and Johnson [3] who criticized that this is not necessarily so. Those of us working in the area witness that the causes of sexual dysfunctions can be quite superficial at times. In some cases one stressful or traumatic episode can precipitate the onset of the dysfunction. Even if the initial cause of the dysfunction is removed or no longer exists the problem can persist and become chronic in nature. This is due to the learned part of the behaviour — the behaviour becomes reinforced — the cycle of causation and aggravation takes place.

Having experienced the dysfunction maybe once or on a few occasions, fear of failure and performance anxiety can occur leading to avoidance behaviour. Sometimes lack of sexual knowledge or exaggerated expectations regarding sexual performance can compound the problem. It is also now widely accepted that psychosexual problems not only affect the individuals but constitute a partnership problem as well. For this reason it is very important that the female partner is included in the evaluation and treatment of erectile dysfunction.

According to the etiological concept of Kaplan [7] regarding psychogenic erectile dysfunction the determinants operate on different layers of causation ranging from rather superficial factors to problems deeply rooted in the personal history. My own findings would support this viewpoint. Performance anxiety and fear of failure are instrumental in all sexual dysfunctions but deeper individual problems and relationship problems may also be present.

Kaplan would argue that if defences against performance anxiety breakdown at an early stage no erection will occur. If the anxiety occurs at a later stage, loss of the existing erection will result.

*The assessment*

In the Department of Human Assisted Reproduction at the Rotunda Hospital Dublin all the men who are referred with erectile dysfunction are seen by a sex and marital therapist. The majority of the men would have already been seen by the medical staff to establish whether the cause of the dysfunction is physical or not. Where the man is either married or in a long-term significant relationship his partner is requested to attend with him. At the initial session there are certain issues that need to be examined in detail.

Firstly the current sexual problem — the erectile dysfunction and its history needs to be explored. The duration and chronicity, whether it is primary — has always been there or secondary — occurred at a later date, or is phasing — occurs on occasions or situational — in specific situations, needs to be discerned. Can the man achieve erections during masturbation or spontaneously, does he experience nocturnal or morning erections?

It is necessary to ask about the strength of the erection, look at the level of desire, has this changed? It is important to ask about the expectations of the man and his partner regarding his sexual functioning and explore any myths [8] that might be believed by the couple. It is important at this stage to establish whether there is a partner-related sexual disorder such as vaginismus present on the female side. These factors would all be explored at the initial interview.

A detailed history then needs to be taken from both partners. This will take several sessions, one of which where the man and woman are seen separately so that they both have the opportunity to disclose any "secrets they may wish to keep from one another".

The history taking is extremely important. It may identify some hidden causes of the erectile dysfunction if they exist. The patient may not himself be aware of these. It will also reveal the attitudes and values of the man and his partner. This may also uncover and explain deep-rooted causes of the dysfunction if they exist. As previously mentioned not all sexual dysfunctions have deep-rooted intrapsychic causes. But patients are not always aware of traumatic experiences in their past. These may have been buried very deeply or blocked completely to avoid the pain of living with the related feelings. Cultural and educational indoctrination can also produce dysfunction which acts as a defence against sometimes unconscious fears brought about by sexual behaviour.

Having taken an in-depth history it is then necessary to move on to the present relationship if one exists. Firstly take a history of the relationship to examine the "fit" between the couple. Even if it is the man solely who has the problem the causes can be partner-related. How is the woman involved in this problem? Couples can and often do collude to maintain the problem. Their very choice of partner may have been influenced by the dysfunction or potential dysfunction. Treatment can be easily sabotaged by the partner or by collusion between the couple. It is also very important to remember that even if the male has the dysfunction both partners are affected. What are the woman's feelings in this respect?

If there is a lot of conflict in the relationship itself it is not, in my opinion, appropriate to work with the erectile dysfunction at this stage. Relationship counselling would be the primary necessity. If and when the relationship is good then the couple could progress to sex therapy if it were still necessary.

The next stage in the process of assessment is to establish whether there is alcoholism, drug addiction, or any psychiatric symptoms present such as depressive disorders, anxiety and panic attacks and personality disorders. The psychiatric illness may be the cause of the dysfunction or it may be secondary, but if it is severe it would need to be addressed first.

When examining these areas, the history, the relationship and the psychiatric status, it is important to establish that it is an erectile dysfunction that is present and that the man is not actually suffering from a disorder of desire where his loss of interest in being sexual is actually creating the erectile problem. If this were the case the approach to treatment would be different. If "loss of desire" is not detected at the start of the assessment it should become apparent by the time the assessment is completed. The two disorders can present in similar ways initially.

The final important factors to remember in carrying out an assessment is that organic factors can subtly intertwine in the pathogenesis. Diabetes would be a very good example of this. It is accompanied by erectile dysfunction in 30–50% of all male patients [9]. An interplay arises between the physical and psychological factors. Apart from the neurological or vascular causes psychological problems such as fear of future complications, the role of the chronically sick person with the implied restrictions, poor body image and fatigue will all affect their sexual functioning.

*Counselling*

After the initial diagnostic interview takes place and the goals of therapy are determined by the therapist and the individual or couple, the therapy becomes two-pronged in approach. As the history of the patient and his partner unfolds a psychodynamic approach is used to address any problems or causes that are revealed. It is hoped that some level of understanding and acceptance will come about. Sometimes it is necessary to work through difficult blocks or resistance that have been built up over years. A lot of permission giving may also be necessary. There are times when no clearly defined cause can be identified.

In conjunction with this and at the same time behavioural therapy also commences providing the sexual dysfunction has been clearly identified. The form of behavioural therapy used was originally developed in the late 1950s by Masters and Johnson [3]. It has since been updated considerably and varies to some extent according to the individual therapist's own professional orientation and the client's needs [10].

The behavioural therapy used for erectile dysfunction would vary depending on whether the condition is primary, secondary or situational. In the case of primary erectile dysfunction one would start with a self-focus programme for the male. A ban is put on the couple attempting intercourse to break through the rigid sexual patterns and to prevent disappointment and a sense of failure. Using relaxation and fantasy the man is encouraged through exercises carried out at home on his own to become comfortable with his own body and to gain and maintain an erection and eventually to ejaculate. At the same time he commences sensate-focus exercises with his partner. These are intended to encourage the couple to enjoy each others bodies using all senses in a relaxed and erotic way. These exercises progress from being sensual to being sexual and gradually the man is encouraged to show his partner how to help him masturbate provided he has been successful at this stage on his own.

The aim of the exercises starting in such a nonthreatening way is to detach sensuality and sexuality from an atmosphere of inhibition, guilt and performance anxiety and to remove the pressures that the couple have been under. It is important that the woman's sexual needs are being met at the same time.

Once the man knows he can obtain an erection and can ejaculate, when an erection does occur the female assumes a position astride her partner, stimulating him to maintain the erection and then lowering herself onto his penis. The man lies still on his back and does not strive for an orgasm. This exercise is slowly expanded until successful intercourse is reached. Finally the goal of therapy is reached simply by initially distracting all attention from it.

Where the therapist is working with a man who is not in a relationship the goal of therapy necessarily has to be that the man can obtain an erection and ejaculate using self-stimulation. This goal would have been set at the onset of treatment at the assessment interview.

**Clinical results and analysis**

It is difficult to compare results of such an approach to assessment and counselling for psychogenic impotence from unit to unit. Personnel, a highly significant factor in terms of end prognosis will have methodological variations which although based on the core approach preclude comparisons to be made. End-point goals and follow-up time may differ and culture differences in and between the various populations being treated in different parts of the world will also have a high degree of influence on outcome. However, data from the Human Assisted Reproduction Unit Dublin which deals almost exclusively with a stable population domiciled in Ireland can be used to illustrate what can be achieved.

Between August 1989 and February 1998, 71 referrals were seen by the sex and marital therapist (the author) for male sexual dysfunctions. Twenty-two of these were erectile dysfunctions, 23 were ejaculatory dysfunctions, six masturbatory inhibitions and eight men had inhibited sexual desire. There were also 12 men with problems related to sexual preference or orientation some of whom needed sex therapy. These referrals were from the hospital setting and outside referrals from other hospitals, general practitioners and other agencies.

The mean age of all 22 patients with erectile dysfunction was 41 years (range 27–60). As Table 1 shows, 11 had always had the problem, in seven the onset had been at a later date, and in four the problem only occurred in specific situations. It can also be seen that those with a secondary constant problem were considerably older. The age of the situational group reflects the fact that all four were under considerable pressure to have intercourse at specific times of the month in an attempt to overcome an infertility problem. The number of therapeutic sessions needed in both the primary and secondary group and the number who attained positive outcome was almost identical.

Two of the men with primary erectile dysfunction attended without partners as did two with constant secondary erectile dysfunction. One man from each of these two groups had a successful outcome to his therapy.

*Table 1.* Erectile dysfunction, n = 22 (means and ranges).

| | Primary | Secondary | |
| --- | --- | --- | --- |
| | | Constant | Situational |
| Number | 11 | 7 | 4 |
| Age (years) | 35 (28–43) | 53 (45–60) | 37 (27–51) |
| Therapy sessions | 13 (7–20) | 12 (6–20) | 12.5 (11–22) |
| Positive outcome | 7 | 5 | 2 |

As treatment progressed in the group of 11 men with primary erectile dysfunction it became apparent that two of the female partners suffered from vaginismus. This was treated alongside the erectile dysfunction. Both couples were successful in their outcome. One woman amongst the secondary group was known already to have vaginismus at the onset of treatment. They were unsuccessful. Indeed perhaps the secondary male dysfunction was related to the previous vaginismus. Finally two of the situational erectile dysfunction patients partners had had vaginismus in the past. Both these couples were successfully treated.

At the completion of treatment successful outcome was measured in the men with a partner by the ability to obtain and maintain an erection of sufficient strength for full penetrative intercourse to take place. The men who attended without partners who were successful could all obtain strong erections through masturbation and ejaculate. The efficacy of therapy was further checked by a follow-up visit 6 weeks afterwards. In all cases the successful outcome was being maintained.

## Discussion and Conclusions

When a man presents with erectile dysfunction he is often experiencing a deep sense of failure. His general sense of wellbeing is affected profoundly. The problem is self-perpetuating. Each failure increases the anxiety associated with subsequent attempts at erection. He is often embarrassed and ashamed of his condition and it requires a great deal of courage to request help.

When evaluating whether the cause of the condition is psychogenic there are a few important factors to bear in mind. We know from recent research that it is necessary to consider the interaction of at least three components [5]:
1. A constitutionally predetermined vulnerability of the sexual response system.
2. The effect of certain risk factors arising from the sexual biography, the partnership and also organic pathologies.
3. The individual coping strategies.
In other words some men could experience certain upbringing, certain traumatic experiences and not be affected sexually whereas others would. Their level of vulnerability and their coping mechanisms are important indicators as to how they have experienced these life events. Others who present as having had a stable background and are in warm loving relationships may after one negative experience suffer erectile dysfunction.

An erectile dysfunction that is cured spontaneously or by sex therapy strongly points to psychological etiology. There is a definite distinction when treating this condition between those who are affected by factors from their early childhood and family or origin or those whose causes are more immediate. The latter are usually easier to treat and respond more immediately. It is also necessary to look for couples that maintain the disorder.

Factors that indicate a poor outcome of treatment are where the patient or his partner are uncooperative, where the man has and always had a low sex drive, homosexual inclinations, major interpersonal problems with their sexual partner, psychosis or major mood disorder and finally failure of previous psychosexual treatment [9].

Psychogenic erectile dysfunction classically begins suddenly but there is no loss of nocturnal and early morning erections. By contrast organic erectile dysfunction has a gradual onset and is associated with loss of nocturnal and early morning erection. The disorder is strongly related to age with an overall estimated prevalence of 2% at the age of 40 rising to 25—30% by the age of 65 [9]. Therefore the age of the man presenting with the problem is highly significant. While psychogenic erectile dysfunction is the most common cause of intermittent erectile failure in younger men it is more likely to be secondary to some organic dysfunction or drug therapy in elderly men.

It is interesting to note that in the Dublin patients, while the overall mean age was 41, that of the men with primary psychogenic impotence was 35 compared with a mean age of 53 for those presenting with a constant secondary problem. This perhaps illustrates that while primary and secondary psychogenic impotence both manifest as the same dysfunction they may be very different in etiology. Primary is more likely to be deep-rooted and entrenched whereas the onset of the constant secondary can occur at any age as the precipitating factors (often life events rather than infertility-related) are likely to be more immediate. The age of the situational secondary group is typical of that of infertile male patients presenting to the clinic [11]. However, it should be noted that the mean number of sessions needed to treat primary, constant and situational secondary was the same as was the final outcome.

Psychosexual counselling aims at decreasing performance anxiety by increasing the range of sexual activities that do not require an erection of sufficient rigidity for penetrative intercourse. This intervention is paradoxical in nature. By initially removing the desired outcome of therapy from the equation the patient relaxes and this frees him up so that erections can occur spontaneously. Once the man experiences this the psychological "blocks" can be overcome. While in some cases a more pharmacological approach such as oral therapy [4] or intracavernous injections [12] may be useful in breaking the psychogenic circle this will not always work. More mechanistic approaches such as the implantation of prostheses or vacuum devices [12] will fail in patients whose problem is known to be psychogenic in nature. These methods do not reverse the potency problem itself or address the psychological factors underlying the symptoms. They can lead to a dependency on the intervention for all sexual functioning.

In order for treatment to be successful the cooperation of both the patient and his partner is required. An important factor in the choice of treatment is what they want. Their belief in the chosen method of treatment will come to a large extent from the enthusiasm and expertise of the therapist. With this in place as the data from Dublin shows, over 60% of those males presenting with psychogenic impotence will be cured even in that often intractable group of patients with primary erectile dysfunction.

# References

1. Kirby RS. Impotence: diagnosis and management of male erectile dysfunction. Br Med J 1994; 308:957—961.
2. Jonas U, Thon WF, Stief CG (eds). Erectile Dysfunction. The Preface. Berlin: Springer-Verlag, 1991.
3. Masters WH, Johnson VE. Human Sexual Response. Boston: Little Brown and Co., 1966.
4. Charatan F. First pill for male impotence approved in US. Br Med J 1998;316:1112.
5. Hartmann U. Psychological evaluation and psychometry. In: Jonas U, Thon WF, Stief CG (eds) Erectile Dysfunction. Berlin: Springer-Verlag, 1991;93—103.
6. Cotter E. GP treatment of erectile dysfunction. Ir Med News 1998;Feb.21.
7. Kaplan HS. The New Sex Therapy. New York: Binner/Mazel, 1974.
8. Zilbergeld B. Men & Sex. Boston: Little Brown and Co., 1979.
9. Hengeveld MW. Erectile disorders: a psychosexiological review. In: Jonas U, Thon WF, Stief CG (eds) Erectile Dysfunction. Berlin: Springer-Verlag, 1991;207—220.
10. Harrison CM. Vaginismus. In: Hedon B, Bringer J, Maras P (eds) Fertility and Sterility: A Current Overview. Carnforth: Parthenon, 1995;173—179.
11. Harrison RF, Barry-Kinsella C, Drudy L, Gordon A, Hannon K, Hennelly B, Keogh I, Kondaveeti U, Nargund G, Verso J. An Irish out-patient based in-vitro fertilisation service. Ir Med J 1992;85(2):63-65.
12. Dawson C, Whitfield H. Subfertility and male sexual dysfunction. Br Med J 1996;312:902—905.

# Psychological approach and medical management of male sexual dysfunction. New drug delivery systems: the patch, urethral suppositories, and the pill

Edward D. Kim and Larry I. Lipshultz
*Scott Department of Urology, Baylor College of Medicine, Houston, Texas, USA*

**Abstract.** Over the last decade the treatment of organic erectile dysfunction has witnessed significant changes in practice patterns as a result of numerous advances in drug delivery systems and the basic science of erectile physiology. Included in this overview are discussions on the newer, non-surgical, first-line treatment options such as transdermal testosterone delivery systems, intraurethral MUSE® (medicated urethral system for erections; Vivus, Melo Park, CA), and sildenafil citrate (Viagra). Other present primary therapies include penile prosthesis placement and intracavernous injection therapy.

Testosterone replacement therapies are appropriate for men with clearly documented hypogonadism resulting in decreased libido, and for carefully selected men with hypogonadism and decreased quality of erections. While the most traditional method of delivery is intramuscular injection, transdermal application is now highly efficacious in restoring testosterone levels to physiologically normal levels. While series vary in terms of treatment efficacy of testosterone for restoring erectile function, these transdermal systems are well-accepted and promising for the delivery of future pharmacologic agents to the penis.

MUSE® is an intraurethral suppository of alprostadil, synthetic prostaglandin E-1. Introduced in 1997, MUSE® works by causing penile smooth muscle relaxation, which eventually leads to increased arterial inflow and an erection. While this treatment can result in erections usable for intercourse in up to 49% of men, a limitation has been its inability to consistently produce full rigidity of the penis. In contrast, sildenafil citrate or Viagra™, does not cause an erection, but improves the quality of a naturally stimulated erection by its mechanism as a selective type V phosphodiesterase inhibitor. Viagra™, the first effective oral agent for the treatment of erectile dysfunction was approved by the US F.D.A. in March 1998 and results in improved erections in up to 80% of men. Enjoying tremendous popularity because of its efficacy and route of administration, Viagra™ has stimulated tremendous interest in other "pills" for impotence therapy.

**Keywords:** alprostadil, apomorphine, erectile dysfunction, hypogonadism, phentolamine, phosphodiesterase inhibitor, prostaglandin, sildenafil, testosterone, urethral suppository.

## Introduction

Because of significant advances in drug delivery systems and the basic science of erectile physiology, the treatment of erectile dysfunction has witnessed major changes over the last decade. As recently as the mid-1980s, the only dependable treatment for impotent men whose problems were not hormonally related was

---

*Address for correspondence:* Larry I. Lipshultz MD, 6560 Fannin, Suite 2100, Houston, TX 77030, USA. Tel.: +1-713-798-6163. Fax: +1-713-798-6007.

the implantation of a penile prosthesis. By the early 1990s, noninvasive therapies such as vacuum constriction devices and intracavernous injections utilizing vasoactive agents gained in popularity and relegated the penile prosthesis to essentially a "second-line" form of therapy.

Continuing the trend of noninvasive therapies, the intraurethral suppository MUSE® (medicated urethral system for erections; Vivus, Melo Park, CA) was introduced in January 1997. Because of MUSE's ability to produce an erection sufficient for intercourse, this suppository joined vacuum devices and intracavernous injections as a first-line form of therapy. However, by the spring of 1998, these forms of therapy were quickly supplanted by the oral pill known as Viagra™ (sildenafil citrate). Tremendous interest by the media, physicians, industry, and patients has brought this once-hidden problem of impotence to the immediate attention of health care professionals. Interestingly, this attention to male sexual dysfunction has stimulated study in female sexual dysfunction, a field clearly in its infancy.

The success of a erectogenic medication is dependent on its ability to reach an appropriate concentration in its target organ. Target organs can be classified as *peripheral* or *central* [1]. While the penis is a peripheral organ, the central nervous system is, as its name implies, central in its action. In general, the action of a medication can be classified as an *initiator* or *enhancer*. An initiator produces an erection, while an enhancer augments the quality of an exsisting erection. With this background in mind, medications used with intracavernous injections and MUSE are considered peripheral initiators, while sildenafil is a peripheral conditioner. In contrast, apomorphine, a medication presently in phase III testing is a central initiator. The intent of this article is to review the recent developments in erectile dysfunction treatments such as MUSE® and Viagra™, with a vision to promising agents for the future.

## Testosterone patches

Parenteral testosterone supplementation has been used extensively in the recent past for the treatment of erectile dysfunction. However, proper patient selection is quite important for obtaining the best results. Frequently, secondary hypogonadism and impotence are two common and independently distributed conditions of older men [2], and a causal relationship between hypogonadism and erectile dysfunction is not always clear [3]. Although variable, hypogonadism is found in about 1.7–35% of men with erectile dysfunction [4–7], with many series reporting a prevalence of around 8–16%. In general, testosterone replacement therapies are most appropriate for men with clearly documented hypogonadism resulting in decreased libido, and for carefully selected men with hypogonadism and decreased quality of erections [4,8–11]. According to the National Institutes of Health consensus development panel on impotence, "for some patients with hypogonadism androgen replacement therapy may sometimes be effective in improving erectile function" [12].

While the most traditional method of delivery is intramuscular injection, androgens may be delivered orally or transdermally. Intramuscular injections of esterified testosterone are advantageous because administration is required only several times a month, in general. The limitations are the need for injection, which patients may find uncomfortable, and the peaks and troughs in testosterone levels after administration. They remain a popular route of administration in our practice.

The use of oral androgens, especially unmodified testosterone, has been limited by their extensive first-pass metabolism in the liver prior to reaching the systemic circulation. Taken on a daily basis, examples of commercially available oral androgens include Testred® and Android® (both from ICN Pharmaceuticals; Costa Mesa, CA). These preparations are modified 17-$\alpha$ alkyltestosterones, which include methyltestosterone and fluoxymesterone. Doses of 10—50 mg daily are required. Morales et al. studied the effect of two different commercial preparations of methyltestosterone for a 1-month course in 22 hypogonadal men and found complete recovery of sexual function in only 9% [13]. Because the positive responses were found in men with the most profound testosterone deficiency, they concluded that oral androgens have limited efficacy in treating men with hypogonadal impotence, unless profound hypogonadism is present. Men on oral therapies are especially prone to the development of adverse hepatic effects.

Transdermal application systems are highly effective in restoring testosterone levels to physiologically normal levels that imitate normal circadian patterns. Applied on a daily basis, examples of commercially available topical testosterone preparations include Testoderm® TTS (Testosterone Transdermal System; Alza Pharmaceuticals; Palo Alto, CA) and Androderm® (SmithKline Beecham; Philadelphia, PA). Doses of 2.5—6.0 mg daily, which approximates the usual male production of 4—7 mg per day, are typically required. As of July 1998, a 1 month supply of Testoderm® TTS costs approximately US$98.10, compared to US$132.30 for Androderm®.

Testoderm® was the first transdermal system and was clinically introduced in the early 1990s, but had the limitation of requiring scrotal application, which many men found inconvenient because of the need for skin shaving and use of a hair dryer for optimal adhesion. The scrotum was initially selected because of its excellent absorptive properties. The Testoderm® TTS provided the advantage of application to the arm, back, or upper buttocks, because of the added presence of a skin permeation enhancer. It is supplied as a transparent 60-cm$^2$ patch. While the testosterone is gelled with hydroxypropyl cellulose, its time release is controlled by their propietary PIB (polyisobutylene) adhesion technology. Androderm® is available in two strengths providing either 2.5 or 5.0 mg of testosterone daily. Like Testoderm® TTS, it is applied in similar locations on the body once daily, thus providing a continuous 24-h release. The 5-mg patch has a total contact surface area of 44 cm$^2$ with a band-aid color backing.

In clinical studies, 94% of men using Testoderm® TTS were able to achieve average serum concentrations of testosterone, free testosterone, estradiol, and dihydrotestosterone within the normal range [14]. Androderm® has a similar efficacy in restoring normal serum testosterone levels. McClure et al. studied the effect of Testoderm® applied scrotally for 3—26 months in four men with hypogonadal impotence [15]. This study demonstrated that this system promptly increased serum testosterone and dihydrotestosterone (DHT) to physiologic levels, restoring normal erectile activity with an increased frequency of ejaculation and a positive effect on both mood and energy. Similar results using a testosterone transdermal system in improving nocturnal erectjons and patient assessments of sexual desire and weekly number of erections were reported by Arver [16].

Androgens should be administered with caution to men with voiding symptoms secondary to benign prostatic hyperplasia, although the data do not suggest a worsening of symptoms or increase in prostate size [17,18]. Obtaining a serum-prostate-specific antigen level and performing a digital rectal exam are also prudent to exclude abnormalities suggestive of prostate cancer. Men on chronic therapy should be warned that the true relationship between prostate cancer and androgen supplemention and testosterone levels is unknown [19,20], hepatic adverse effects may be seen, and that gynecomastia may develop.

Side effects of Testoderm® TTS are relatively minimal with transient itching (12%), moderate—severe erythema (3%), and headache (5%) most commonly noted. Androderm® may cause skin reactions such as burn-like blister reactions, moderate erythema, and allergic contact dermatitis in up to 53% of patients, but only 9% had to discontinue treatment in clinical trials (SmithKline Beecham information on file). When these reactions occur, treatment and later pretreatment with a triamcinolone acetonide 0.1% cream has been shown to reduce the severity and incidence of skin irritation [21].

In summary, topical administration of androgens is highly effective in restoring serum testosterone levels to normal. The technology of application has progressed from scrotal administration to more comfortable alternatives on other parts of the body as a result of skin permeation enhancers. The difficult part of prescribing androgens remains the prediction of which impotent patients will respond to their satisfaction.

## MUSE

MUSE® has been available for the treatment for erectile dysfunction since January 1997. This form of therapy is novel because the active medication, alprostadil (synthetic prostaglandin E1), a potent vasodilator, is admininstered and absorbed intraurethrally. In contrast, Caverject® (Upjohn-Pharmacia, Kalamazoo, MI) represents the same medication at a much lower dose injected directly into the corporal bodies. The US patent for MUSE refers to its unique application system for intraurethral delivery. This intraurethral route of therapy was first described in 1993 [22]. MUSE is available in four doses: 125, 250, 500, and 1,000 µg, which cost approximately US$20—25 per application. As of July 1998, MUSE accounts for about < 1% of prescriptions written for the treatment of erectile dysfunction.

The application of MUSE, a peripheral initiator of erections, is simple and straightforward (Fig. 1). After the patient urinates to lubricate the urethra, he places the stem end of the applicator approximately 3.2 cm in the urethra. To disperse the 3—6 mm alprostadil pellet, he depresses the applicator button and gently rolls the penis. Men who do not achieve good rigidity of the penis with prior applications may find that the ACTIS$^{TM}$ band applied around the shaft of the penis may help augment the subsequent erection. The alprostadil pellet is rapidly absorbed by the corpus spongiosum within 10 min of application and then disseminated to the corpora cavernosa by vascular communications between these distinct compartments of the penis. The alprostadil functions as a corporal and arterial smooth muscle relaxant, leading to an increased arterial inflow into the sinusoidal spaces of the cavernous bodies and a compression of the trabecular smooth muscle against the emissary veins. This mechanism results

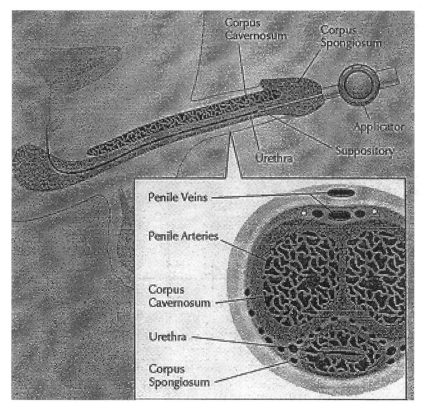

*Fig. 1.* MUSE$^{®}$: The 3.2-cm-long applicator is inserted into the urethra after the patient urinates. After depressing the applicator button and applying a gentle rocking motion, the patient rolls his penis to facilitate dispersion of the alprostadil. The absorption is within several minutes. The medication exerts vasodilatory effects based on venous communications between the corpus spongiosum and the corpora cavernosa.

in a decreased venous outflow and the maintenance of the rigidity of an erection.

Clinically, the rapid absorption of alprostadil is evidenced by the onset to erection in 7 min. Erections typically are maximal about 22—24 min after administration, then completely detumesce by 64—79 min after application. With a half-life of several minutes and extensive pulmonary metabolism, clearance is rapid and plasma levels are nearly undetectable.

In a multicenter, placebo-controlled study sponsored by Vivus and involving 996 men, 65.9% had grade 4—5 erections judged to be "sufficient" for intercourse during inoffice testing [23]. Of those men who responded in the clinic, 64.9% were able to have intercourse at least once during home application. Erections were scored on the erection assessment scale which ranges from 0—5, with 4 = erection sufficient for intercourse (i.e., "stuffable") and 5 = full ridigity (i.e., "stickable"). Regardless of the cause of erectile dysfunction and the age of the patient, MUSE was significantly more efficacious than placebo. Hellstrom et al. reported similar findings [24].

When examining the responses per dose administered, however, only 48.8% of men using the highest dose of 1,000 μg had a grade 4 or 5 erection [23] (Fig. 2). Of men using the 125-μg dose, 12.3% were able to develop similar quality erections. Werthman and Rajfer using an erection scale of rigid, full, and poor had more disappointing results, reporting that only 7% of men had well-sustained, rigid erections [25]. Another 30% had erections, but with only partial rigidity. These same men developed rigid and full erections using intracavernous injections 49 and 40% of the time, respectively. Another comparative study by Porst concluded that due to superior efficacy and lower side effects, self-injection therapy with alprostadil remains the "gold standard" in the management of male impotence, and that MUSE should be reserved for a subset of patients suffering from erectile dysfunction [26]. Only 10% of men had rigid erections with MUSE in this study.

In contrast, a subgroup of 95 men for whom intracavernous injections were "not effective" stated that MUSE resulted in an erection sufficient for intercourse [27]. Fifty-eight percent of these "not effective" men had an erection sufficient for intercourse after MUSE application in the clinic, and 47% of these men

| | Dose of alprostadil | | | |
|---|---|---|---|---|
| | 125 μg | 250 μg | 500 μg | 1000 μg |
| # men | 1490 | 1492 | 1117 | 1140 |
| % with score of 4 or 5 | 12.3 | 16.6 | 39.6 | 48.8 |
| Mean time to onset of response (min) | 7 | 7 | 7 | 7 |
| Mean time to maximal response (min) | 21 | 22 | 23 | 24 |
| Mean time to nonerect state (min) | 67 | 70 | 74 | 79 |

*Fig. 2.* Medical therapy: Muse. (Reproduced from Padma-Nathan et al.: NEJM 1997;336:1.)

reported successful intercourse after home administration. Such studies suggest that men should not be discouraged or excluded from trying MUSE if intracavernous injections, which are considered more potent, fail. The efficacy of MUSE was consistent regardless of a number of factors including duration and cause of erectile dysfunction, age of the patient, and history of previous therapy.

Adverse effects include penile and perineal discomfort, minor urethral trauma, and hypotension (Table 2). Local pain in the penis (36%), urethra (13%), and testes (5%) was typically mild and self-limited. This discomfort, seen with PGE-1 intracavernous injections also, is likely an inherent effect of PGE-1 because of its pain-sensitizing activity. The pain is manifested as a delayed aching, beginning 5–10 min after application and often lasting up to several hours. Because of the small, but significant risk of hypotension (3.3%), MUSE should be initially tested in the office. Priapism, defined as a rigid erection lasting $\geq 6$ h, was reported in only 0.1% of applications. Only 7% of men discontinued MUSE because of adverse events. The efficacy and safety studies led to its FDA approval for the treatment of erectile dysfunction in December 1997.

We do not advocate the use of MUSE in men trying to help establish a pregnancy, although alprostadil does not appear to have any effect on in vitro sperm motility, viability, or membrane integrity [28]. While the concentration of PGE-1 in the semen is slightly higher after MUSE administration, this increase was not significant. The effects of the PGE-1 did, however, cause vaginal burning or itching in 5.8% of female partners vs. 0.8% in the placebo group.

Dosing of MUSE should be guided by the results in Table 3. The significant increase in efficacy appears at the 500-µg dose. With in-office testing, we have been starting men with spinal cord injury at 125 µg; psychogenic impotence of men < 50 years of age with no identifiable cause at 250 µg; and clearly evident organic dysfunction, postradical prostatectomy, and men > 50 years of age at 500 µg.

In summary, MUSE remains a first-line therapy for erectile dysfunction treatment. The main advantages of MUSE are the avoidance of needles and the ease of application. By avoiding needles as with intracavernous injections, the risk of penile fibrosis, generally in the range of 3–7%, but as high as 23%, may be minimized [29]. The drawbacks include its cost of US$20–$25 per application and relative lack of efficacy in producing rigid hard erections.

**Viagra**

Few medications ever have created as much interest among patients, physicians, the media, and the general population on a worldwide basis as sildenafil citrate (Viagra™; Pfizer, New York, NY) has since its clinical introduction in April 1998. Viagra™ is the first effective oral pill for the treatment of erectile dysfunction and functions as a selective inhibitor of cyclic guanosine monophosphate (GMP)-specific phosphodiesterase type 5. Clinically, Viagra™ enhances an erection, but does not itself produce an erection. Sexual excitation and stimulation

454

must be present for Viagra™ to have an effect.

During sexual activity, erotic stimulation results in the release of nitric oxide (NO) from terminal branches of the S2-S4 derived cavernous nerves (nonadrenergic, noncholinergic-NANC) [30] (Fig. 3). Acting within the extensive smooth muscle network of the corpus cavernosum, NO activates guanylate cyclase, which in turn increases levels of cyclic guanosine monophosphate (cGMP). This increased level of cGMP results in smooth muscle relaxation, allowing for the inflow of blood within the penis and a resultant erection.

Type 5-phosphodiesterase (PDE) is an enzyme which is found predominantly in the smooth muscle of the penis, blood vessels and circulating platelets. It is responsible for the degradation of cGMP to GMP, resulting in smooth muscle contraction and loss of erection. By inhibiting type 5-PDE, Viagra™ causes increased smooth muscle relaxation, inflow of blood into the corpus cavernosum, and thus improved erections.

While the first published account was by Boolell et al. [31], the first large-scale, multicenter trials of oral sildenafil were reported by Goldstein et al. in May 1998 [32]. They presented two sequential double-blind studies of men with predominantly organic erectile dysfunction. The first study was a 24-week dose-response study of 532 men, and the second was a flexible dose-escalation study of 329 men. The primary measure of efficacy was the validated questionnaire called the International Index of Erectile Function (IIEF) [33].

Overall, 56, 77 and 84% of men taking the 25-, 50-, and 100-mg doses, respectively, had improved erections, compared to 25% of men on placebo [32]. In the final 4 weeks of testing, 72, 80 and 85% of men using the same doses were able to achieve an erection hard enough for intercourse, as compared with 50% for placebo. When the rigidity of erections was examined, over half the erections men obtained were completely hard, not just hard enough for penetration. Men using Viagra™ also had a significantly increased number of sexual intercourse encounters and successful attempts.

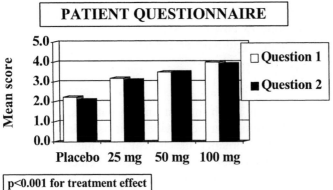

*Fig. 3.* Viagra: erectile function.

During the course of study, men were asked the following questions: 1) when you attempted sexual intercourse, how often were you able to penetrate your partner?, and 2) during sexual intercourse, how often were you able to maintain your erection after you had penetrated your partner?

The scoring system was as follows:

0 = No sexual activity
1 = Almost never or never
2 = A few times
3 = Sometimes
4 = Most times
5 = Almost always or always

Men on Viagra™ scored significantly higher with regard to these questions in comparison to the placebo group (Fig. 4). The mean scores of men on Viagra™ approached, but did not exceed, those from normal potent men in the same age group.

When the IIEF questionnaire was examined according to various domains, men using Viagra™ had significant increases in erectile function, orgasmic function, intercourse satisfaction, and overall satisfaction. The only domain that did not increase was sexual desire, which would be expected based on its mode of action. Improvement in erectile function was demonstrated across a wide variety of patient types. However, the best results were seen in those men with a psychogenic etiology. When examining results based on the severity of erectile dysfunction, while Viagra™ without question has good efficacy in those men with mild to moderate organic erectile dysfunction, results in men with severe organic dysfunction were less pronounced.

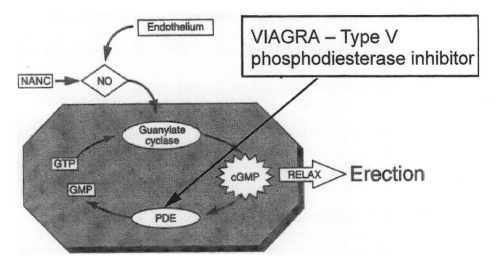

*Fig. 4.* Mechanism of action of sildenafil citrate: by inhibiting action of type-5-phosphodiesterase, sildenafil minimizes the breakdown of cGMP. The net result is increased corporal smooth muscle relaxation, leading to an enhanced erection.

Viagra$^{TM}$ has been shown to be effective in men with a wide range of etiologies for erectile dysfunction including the following: hypertension, coronary artery disease, diabetes mellitus, depression, peripheral vascular disease, psychogenic, radical prostatectomy, and spinal cord injury. Results in men with Peyronie's disease, corporal veno-occlusive dysfunction, and other specific anatomic/physiologic defects of penile function have not yet been determined.

The major contraindication to the use of Viagra$^{TM}$ is the concomitant use of medications containing nitrates, e.g., nitroglycerin, pentaerythritol, isosorbide [34]. Because Viagra$^{TM}$ can potentiate the hypotensive effects of nitrates, a potentially dangerous situation may arise if prescribed inappropriately. Unpublished studies indicate that the use of both medications in healthy young volunteers can result in a decrease of the systolic blood pressure by up to 50 mmHg. Retinitis pigmentosa is an uncommon, heriditary, degenerative condition of the retina. Because of some mild crossover effects with the type 6-PDE in the retina, Viagra$^{TM}$ should not be used in patients with this condition.

Viagra$^{TM}$ should be used with caution in men with cardiac disease, because increased sexual activity may increase the aerobic requirements of the myocardium. For men with suspected cardiac disease who wish to initiate or resume sexual activity, Drory et al. have demonstrated that an exercise stress test can accurately predict which men would experience angina during intercourse [35]. Viagra$^{TM}$ should also be started at a lower dose in patients with significant hepatic impairment, severe renal impairment (creatinine clearance < 30 ml/min), or age > 65 years.

Possessing a half-life of 4 h, the side effects tend to be short-lived and generally mild. The most common side effects include mild headache, dyspepsia, and flushing, which are seen in 7–16% of men in a dose-dependent fashion. The overall incidence of mild to moderate side effects is 9%. In a series of 225 men participating in a 32-week open-label extension study, only 2% discontinued the use of Viagra$^{TM}$ because of side effects [32]. At the end of the trial, 92% were still participating. There have been no reported cases of priapism.

An unusual side effect evidenced in about 3% of men is a several hour change in color or brightness perception. Specifically, affected men reported a transient and reversible decreased ability to discriminate between blue and green, or a blue haze and increased brightness. Night driving, visual acuity, and ocular pressures are not affected. This side effect is a result of PDE-6, which is present in the human retina. Sildenafil has some effect on PDE-6, although it is 10 times more selective for PDE-5 than PDE-6. In phase III testing, ophthalmologists did not identify any long-lasting effects.

Viagra$^{TM}$ is available in 25-, 50- and 100-mg tablets. In a flexible dose-escalation study, 74% of men preferred the 100-mg dose and 23% the 50-mg dose [32]. For this reason, we start men at 50 mg and encourage them to increase to 100 mg if the initial doses are not successful. Sildenafil has been tried at 200 mg without significant improvements in efficacy. Rather, the incidence of side effects increased. Doses of 800 mg have been used without significant side effects.

The patient should be instructed to take Viagra<sup>TM</sup> about 1—2 h prior to sexual activity for peak effect. The maximum plasma concentration is reached in less than 60 min, but may be delayed if a large meal or one high in fat is ingested. It is recommended that only one dose a day be taken. The approximate cost is US$8—11 per pill regardless of the dose.

Although Viagra<sup>TM</sup> was developed for male erectile dysfunction, a considerable amount of interest has become apparent for its use in women. While not an approved indication, numerous women have claimed an enhanced sexual response in a variety of weekly magazines and talk shows. This field of female sexual dysfunction treatment will be of considerable interest with active research for the next several years.

**On the horizon**

The search for effective and noninvasive forms of treatment for erectile dysfunction is presently an area of intense investigation. Because the intracorporal and intraurethral routes of application are not readily acceptable by many men, the greatest interest has centered around oral therapies. The challenge is to find medications which are effective and specific for the penis, but have few systemic side effects. While a comprehensive summary of ongoing reseach is beyond the scope of this chapter, we will highlight recent important advances.

Apomorphine is presently in phase III testing by TAP Pharmaceuticals (Deerfield, IL). A dopaminergic agonist, apomorphine functions as a central initiator of erections. After sublingual adminstration, an erection becomes evident 9—11 min later. In a multicenter, double-blind study of men with medical erectile dysfunction in the absence of any major organic component, 59.6% of men using the 6 mg, vs. 34.2% of the placebo group ($p < 0.001$) dose were able to obtain an erection sufficient for intercourse [36]. The most common side effect was nausia of mild to moderate severity in 39% of men.

Oral phentolamine, an $\alpha$-adrenergic antagonist, has been in later phases of clinical testing by Zonagen (The Woodlands, TX). Having a trade name of Vasomax<sup>TM</sup>, improvement in erections were identified in 45% of 159 men using the highest dose tested of 80 mg, compared to 16% of the placebo group, in two multicenter US trials [37]. These men had mild-to-moderate dysfunction. Side effects, seen in < 10% using a 40-mg dose, included headaches, facial flushing, and nasal congestion. Becker had similar efficacy and side effect profiles in a smaller European series [38].

The topical route has been tried with a number of vasodilatory medications, but with disappointing results. The basic problem is one of absorption. When agents are applied to the shaft of the penis, they must pass through the stratified keratinous layer of skin and the thick tunica albuginea of the corporal bodies, a formidable obstacle. When applied to the glans penis, absorption must still pass through the skin, into the corpus spongiosum, then into the corporal bodies through vascular communications of variable integrity [39]. While the scrotum is an excellent absorptive surface, direct local passage of the medication to the corporal bodies does not follow any well-described anatomic pathways.

Minoxidil, nitroglycerine, papaverine, and prostaglandin E1 have all been tried topically with mixed results in investigations conducted in the late 1980s and early 1990s [40–43]. More recently, a variety of skin enhancers have been used in an attempt to facilitate absorption, but still with less than satisfactory results. At the 1998 American Urological Association (AUA) Meeting in San Diego, CA, McVary et al. presented a phase I study with PGE-1 compounded with 5% SEPA (2-n-nonyl-1, 3-dioxolane), a transdermal permeation enhancer developed by Macrochem Corporation (Lexington, MA) [44]. While modest erectile responses of a 70–90° were clinically noted in about 70% of men, transient penile erythema and pain suggest the need for improvements in this particular delivery system. Also presented at the AUA Meeting was a formulation of 4% PGE-1 with NexAct$^{TM}$ technology enhancer (NexMed, Inc.; Commerce, CA) [45]. This formulation, tested in 10 men after radical prostatectomy, resulted in significant increases in penile blood flow as measured by duplex ultrasonography. However, clinical responses were not noted, and moderate erythema of the glans was observed.

The intraurethral route of absorption is presently being tested with combinations of medications. Vivus reported that a combination of PGE-1 and prazosin had a slightly better result than PGE-1 alone [46]. A dose of 500 μg PGE-1 and 2,000 μg prazosin produced full enlargement or rigidity in 58.9% of doses.

Jet injection devices (M injector; MADA International; Miami, FL) delivering 100 μl of fluid at a pressure of 1,400 psi have been tested in animal models [47]. These type of injections have been used in humans for local anaesthesia, insulin injection, and immunization and have the advantages of minimal pain, ease of use, absence of needles, and direct delivery of small quantities of medications. This particular study by Seyam et al. demonstrated that jet injection is effective for the delivery of medications intracavernously through the thick tunica albuginea.

Advances in drug delivery systems will undoubtedly be tested in the near future with erectogenic medications. For example, studies by Pfizer (New York, NY) are being performed with Viagra$^{TM}$ as a sublingual agent, in codevelopment with R.P. Scherer (New York, NY). The advantage is for men who are not able to use pills. Another potential advantage may be quicker delivery to the systemic circulation by avoiding gastrointestinal absorption. Active investigations with inhalational agents may be a future venue for drug delivery, and is already in phase III testing with insulin. Finally, advances in the basic sciences may ultimately enable the use of gene therapy strategies for improving erections. Clearly, the future is bright for the treatment of erectile dysfunction.

## Conclusions

The treatment of erectile dysfunction has experienced significant developments in a relatively short period of time. Advances in drug delivery systems and the understanding of the basic science of erectile physiology have enabled and facilitated these changes. At present, tremendous interest exists for the first effective oral agent, sildenafil citrate, for the treatment of erectile dysfunction. Safe and effective, sildenafil is easy to use and well-accepted by patients. However, because sildenafil does not work in satisfactory fashion for 20−30% of men, newer oral agents such as apomorphine and phentolamine are being developed. Intraurethral MUSE remains a first-line form of therapy because of its ability to restore erections suitable for intercourse and its safety. Its relative inability to produce rigid erections, however, has stimulated interest in forms of combination intraurethral therapy. Testosterone patches have also been a recent development over the last decade for the treatment of the hypogonadal male. Interest in this topical route of drug delivery has led to trials of direct erectogenic medications applied to the penis and scrotum. However, results have been modest at best.

A constantly evolving field always generating considerable interest, the treatment of erectile dysfunction promises considerable efficacy for most men. Involving a combination of developments in drug delivery, newer agents, and combination therapies, more significant advances undoubtedly will be made over the next decade.

## References

1. Heaton JPW. Neural and pharmacological determinants of erection. Int J Impot Res 1998; 10(Suppl 2):S34−39.
2. Korenman SG, Morley JE, Mooradian AD, Davis SS, Kaiser FE, Silver AJ, Viosca SP, Garza D. Secondary hypogonadism in older men: its relation to impotence. J Clin Endocrinol Metab 1990;71:963−969.
3. Carani C, Zini D, Baldini A, Della Casa L, Ghizzani A, Marrama P. Effects of androgen treatment in impotent men with normal and low levels of free testosterone. Arch Sex Behav 1990; 19:223−234.
4. Buvat J, Lemaire A. Endocrine screening in 1,022 men with erectile dysfunction: clinical significance and cost-effective strategy. J Urol 1997;158(5):1764−1767.
5. Govier FE, McClure RD, Kramer-Levien D. Endocrine screening for sexual dysfunction using free testosterone determinations. J Urol 1996;156(2 Pt 1):405−408.
6. Nickel JC, Morales A, Condra M, Fenemore J, Surridge DH. Endocrine dysfunction in impotence: incidence, significance and cost-effective screening. J Urol 1984;132(1):40−43.
7. Johnson AR III, Jarow JP. Is routine endocrine testing of impotent men necessary? J Urol 1992;147:1542−1543.
8. Guay AT, Bansal S, Heatley GJ. Effect of raising endogenous testosterone levels in impotent men with secondary hypogonadism: double blind placebo-controlled trial with clomiphene citrate. J Clin Endocrinol Metab 1995;80:3546−3552.
9. Zonszein J. Diagnosis and management of endocrine disorders of erectile dysfunction. Urol Clin N Am 1995;22:789−802.
10. Kropman RF, Verdijk RM, Lycklama A, Nijeholt AAB, Roelfsema F. Routine endocrine screening in impotence: significance and cost-effectiveness. Int J Impot Res 1991;3:87−91.
11. van Basten JP, van Driel MF, Jonker-Pool G, Sleijfer DT, Schraffordt Koops H, van de Wiel HB, Hoekstra HJ. Sexual functioning in testosterone-supplemented patients treated for bilateral testicular cancer. Br J Urol 1997;79(3):461−467.

460

12. NIH Consensus Development Panel on Impotence. Impotence. JAMA 1993;270:83—90.
13. Morales A, Johnston B, Heaton JW, Clark A. Oral androgens in the treatment of hypogonadal impotent men. J Urol 1994;152(4):1115—1118.
14. Matsumoto AM. Hormonal therapy of male hypogonadism. Endocrinol Metab Clin N Am 1994;23:857—875.
15. McClure RD, Oses R, Ernest ML. Hypogonadal impotence treated by transdermal testosterone. Urology 1991;37(3):224—228.
16. Arver S, Dobs AS, Meikle AW, Allen RP, Sanders SW, Mazer NA. Improvement of sexual function in testosterone deficient men treated for 1 year with a permeation enhanced testosterone transdermal system. J Urol 1996;155(5):1604—1608.
17. Tenover TS. Effect of testosterone supplementation in the aging male. J Clin Endocrinol Metab 1992;75:1092—1098.
18. Franchi F, Luisi M, Kicovic PM. Long term effect of testosterone undecanoate in hypogonadal males. Int J Androl 1978;1:270—275.
19. Svetec DA, Canby ED, Thompson IM, Sabanegh ES Jr. The effect of parenteral testosterone replacement on prostate specific antigen in hypogonadal men with erectile dysfunction. J Urol 1997;158(5):1775—1777.
20. Morgentaler A, Bruning CO III, DeWolf WC. Occult prostate cancer in men with low serum testosterone levels. JAMA 1996;276(23):1904—1906.
21. Wilson DE, Kaidbey K, Boike SC et al. Use of topical corticosteroiod cream in the pretreatment of skin reactions associated with Androderm Testosterone Transdermal System. Program and Abstracts of the 79th Annual Meeting of the Endocrine Society, June 1997, Minneapolis, MN. Abstract PI—323.
22. Wolfson B, Pickett S, Scott NE, deKernion JB, Rajfer J. Intraurethral prostaglandin E-2 cream: a possible alternative treatment for erectile dysfunction. Urology 1993;42:73—75.
23. Padma-Nathan H, Hellstrom WJG, Kaiser FE, et al. Treatment of men with erectile dysfunction with transurethral alprostadil. N Engl J Med 1997;336(1):1—7.
24. Hellstrom WJ, Bennett AH, Gesundheit N, Kaiser FE, Lue TF, Padma-Nathan H, Peterson CA, Tam PY, Todd LK, Varady JC et al. A double-blind, placebo-controlled evaluation of the erectile response to transurethral alprostadil. Urology 1997;48:851—856.
25. Werthman P, Rajfer J. MUSE therapy: preliminary clinical observations. Urology 1997;50(5): 809—811.
26. Porst H. Transurethral alprostadil with MUSE (medicated urethral system for erection) vs intracavernous alprostadil — a comparative study in 103 patients with erectile dysfunction. Int J Impot Res 1997;9(4):187—192.
27. Engel JD, McVary KT. Transurethral alprostadil as therapy for patients who withdrew from or failed prior intracavernous injection therapy. Urology 1998;51:687—692.
28. Peterson CA, Cowley C, Dzerk AM et al. The medicated urethral system for erections: does transurethral alprostadil affect the concentration of prostaglandins in human ejaculate or the viability and motility of human sperm? Presented at the 12th Congress of the European Association of Urology, September 1—4 1996, Paris, France.
29. Chew KK, Stuckey BG, Earle CM, Dhaliwal SS, Keogh EJ. Penile fibrosis in intracavernosal prostaglandin E1 injection therapy for erectile dysfunction. Int J Impot Res 1997;9(4):225—229.
30. Burnett AL. Role of nitric oxide in the physiology of erection. Biol Reprod 1995;52(3): 485—489.
31. Boolell M, Gepi-Attee S, Gingell JC, Allen MJ. Sildenafil, a novel effective oral therapy for male erectile dysfunction. Br J Urol 1996;78:257—261.
32. Goldstein I, Lue TF, Padma-Nathan H, Rosen RC, Steers WD, Wicker PA et al. Oral sildenafil in the treatment of erectile dysfunction. N Engl J Med 1998;338:1397—1404.
33. Rosen RC, Riley A, Wagner G, Osterloh IH, Kirkpatrick J, Mishra A. The International Index of Erectile Function (IIEF): a multi-dimensional scale for assessment of erectile dysfunction. Urology 1997;49:822—830.

34. Morales A, Gingell C, Collins M, Wicker PA, Osterloh IH. Clinical safety of oral sildenafil citrate (Viagra$^{TM}$) in the treatment of erectile dysfunction. Int J Impot Res 1998;10:69—74.

35. Drory Y, Shapira I, Fisman EZ, Pines A. Myocardial ischemia during sexual activity in patients with coronary artery disease. Am J Cardiol 1995;75(12):835—837.

36. Padma-Nathan H, Fromm-Freeck S, Ruff DD, McMurray JG, Rosen RC, Apomorphine SL Study Group. Efficacy and safety of apomorphine SL vs. placebo for male erectile dysfunction (MED). J Urol 1998;159:241. Abstract 920.

37. Goldstein I, Vasomax Study Group. Efficacy and safety of oral phentolamine (Vasomax) for the treatment of minimal erectile dysfunction. J Urol 1998;159:240 (Abstract 919).

38. Becker AJ, Stief CG, Machtens S, Schultheiss D, Hartmann U, Truss MC, Jonas U. Oral phento-lamine as treatment for erectile dysfunction. J Urol 1998;159:1214—1216.

39. Vardi Y, Saenz de Tejada I. Functional and radiologic evidence of vascular communication between the spongiosal and cavernosal compartments of the penis. Urology 1997;49;749—752.

40. Owen JA, Saunders F, Harris C, Fenemore J, Reid K, Surridge D, Condra M, Morales A. Topi-cal nitroglycerin: a potential treatment for impotence. J Urol 1989;141:546—548.

41. Cavallini G. Minoxidil versus nitroglycerine: a prospective double-blind controlled trial in transcutaneous erection facilitation of organic impotence. J Urol 1991;146:50—53.

42. Kim ED, McVary KT. Papaverine topical gel for treatment of erectile dysfunction. J Urol 1995;153:361—365.

43. Kim ED, El-Rashidy R, McVary KT. Topical prostaglandin E-1 for the treatment of erectile dys-function. J Urol 1995;153:1828—1830.

44. McVary KT, Polepalle S, Riggi S, Pelham RW. Topical Septa/PGE-1 gel for the treatment of erectile dysfunction. J Urol 1998;159:239. Abstract 914.

45. Becher E, Borghi M, Momesso A, Montes de Oca L. Penile hemodynamics findings with a new topical formulation of alprostadil. J Urol 1998;159:239. Abstract 915.

46. Peterson CA, Bennett AH, Hellstrom WJG, Kaiser FE, Morley JE, Nemo KJ, Padma-Nathan H, Place VA, Prendergast JJ et al. Erectile response to transurethral alprostadil, prazosin and alprostadil-prazosin combinations. J Urol 1998;159:1523—1528.

47. Seyam RM, Begin LR, Tu LM, Dion SB, Merlin SL, Brock GB. Evaluation of a no-needle penile penetration and its hemodynamic consequences in the rat. Urology 1997;50:994—998.

# Challenges in reproduction

# Predicting treatment success for male infertility

Thinus F. Kruger and Kevin Coetzee
*Reproductive Biology Unit, Tygerberg Hospital/University of Stellenbosch, Tygerberg, South Africa*

**Abstract.** The basic semen analysis is still the cornerstone of evaluation of the male. In a structured review discussed in this section, it was clearly shown that sperm morphology is the most reliable semen parameter to predict the outcome of fertilization in vitro. It is also highlighted that the use of automated sperm morphology analyzer instruments (ASMA) are valuable predictors of both fertilization and pregnancy outcome. In a prospective study using an ASMA instrument (IVOS, Hamilton Thorne Research), the pregnancy outcome in gamete intrafallopian transfer (GIFT) was studied. The pregnancy rate in the P pattern group (0–4% normal) was 15.4% compared to 35.6% in the group above 5% normal morphology (p < 0.01). Futhermore, comparisons between a number of sperm functional tests and sperm morphology were made. Excellent correlation is reported between most of these tests and sperm morphology. It is concluded that sperm morphology evaluated by strict criteria is a valuable tool to make sound clinical decisions.

**Keywords:** automated sperm morphology analysis (ASMA), semen analysis, sperm morphology, sperm functional tests.

## Introduction

In assisted reproductive programs it is common practice to make decisions on the choice of treatment technique after evaluation of the male factor. In spite of extensive research in this field, the field of diagnostic andrology, most clinics make pragmatic decisions using only a few tests of which perhaps the basic semen analysis is still the most important. In a recent review, Coetzee [1] looked carefully at all articles dealing with sperm morphology and its impact on fertilization vitro. It was concluded that sperm morphology is the most valuable parameter when using the basic semen analysis [1].

### Is there any value in establishing fertility thresholds for sperm morphology?

In a previous publication [2] it was shown that the fertilization rate in the morphology group 0–4% was only 7.6% compared to 63% in patients with morphology 5–14% normal forms. It was also shown that in the group with sperm morphology > 14% the fertilization rate was > 80% [3]. These thresholds were studied by numerous workers and accurately covered in the review by Coetzee [1].

It is of utmost importance to obtain good quality control in a laboratory evaluating sperm morphology. The adherence to these principles have helped to estab-

---

*Address for correspondence:* Thinus F. Kruger, Reproductive Biology Unit, Tygerberg Hospital/University of Stellenbosch, Tygerberg 7505, South Africa.

lish the strict criteria as a dependable diagnostic tool. While the strict morphology classification system has been refined with time (P pattern $\leqslant 4\%$, G pattern $5-14\%$ and N pattern $> 14\%$) [2], the physiological-based criteria [4] and clinically based threshold [3] have remained constant since 1986. The classification system has now been adopted and used successfully by authors worldwide. The majority of the studies [5–8] have confirmed the predictive value of normal sperm morphology within the established thresholds. In comparison, the World Health Organization (WHO) guidelines [9,10], another of the major classification system's in use worldwide, have changed dramatically since 1980, becoming stricter with each revision. The result has been a high level of subjectivity and a lack of consensus, especially with regards its clinical value and corresponding fertility thresholds [1]. On the other hand, a consistent trend was shown by most groups regarding the use of strict criteria, especially at the 5% threshold.

### Why is the basic semen analysis still the cornerstone of evaluation of the male in predicting in vitro fertilization (IVF) outcome?

In the structured literature review by Coetzee et al. [1] the impact of sperm morphology was studied on fertilization and pregnancy rates in in vitro fertilization (IVF). 216 articles were sourced of which 49 dealt with sperm morphology. The majority of articles (82%; 36/44) concluded that normal sperm morphology plays a role in the diagnosis of male fertility potential [1].

To be able to study the thresholds and IVF outcome, and to calculate confidence intervals and odds ratios, the raw data was necessary. In the WHO group, three articles were available with thresholds that vary widely [1]. In the strict group using a 5% threshold, 10 studies provided data that could be analysed for the prediction of fertilization and 11 studies for the prediction of pregnancy. All the studies showed a positive predictive value for fertilization, with only one [11] (OR = 1.42; CI: 0.90–2.25), not reaching significance. In the prediction of pregnancy (per cycle), nine studies obtained a positive predictive value with predictive value association. The studies of Oehninger et al. [5], Enginsu et al. [12] and Grow et al. [13] reached significance. Using a 14% threshold (strict criteria), five studies provided data that could be analysed for the prediction of fertilization and eight for the prediction of pregnancy. Similarly, all the studies analysed showed positive and significant predictive value with regard to fertilization. In the prediction of pregnancy, two studies [11,14] did not obtain a positive predictive value while the studies of Oehninger [5] and Kruger [15] were both positive and significant.

When combining all the data in the 5% (strict criteria) threshold analysis, the zero transfer rate was 24.0% (86/359) in the $\leqslant 4\%$ group compared to 7.4% (80/1088) in the $> 4\%$ group. Today one can reason that with the help of intracytoplasmic sperm injection (ICSI) the chances of no transfer can be limited if one is familiar in using the strict criteria and thus be able to identify the poor prognosis group.

## What about automated sperm morphology analyzers?

*How do computer morphology analyzers work?*

Automated sperm morphology analysis (ASMA) instruments work much like current versions of computer-aided sperm analyses instruments for motion, except that no movement information is required [16–21]. The system consists of a microscope, a video camera, a computer frame grabber and morphology software. The video camera delivers the image to the computer's frame grabber which stores it for analysis [16,18,20]. The image is evaluated by the morphology software to determine whether sperm are present. Sperm recognition is based on software specifications for size, shape, colour intensity and other characteristics. Once sperm have been recognised and segregated from debris and other objects, metric measurements are performed on the head, midpiece, acrosome and other cytological features. These measurements are the basis for sperm morphologic classification. The accuracy and precision of ASMA instruments depend on: 1) the microscope optics, magnification, and focusing capabilities, 2) video camera quality, 3) array size of the frame grabber, 4) image processing techniques, 5) definitions of metric measurements [16,18,19], and 6) staining methods used [18,22,23].

*How do the automated sperm morphology analyzer (ASMA) instruments compare to the human?*

In a study dealing with this topic, the computer's ability to classify normal morphology per slide was reported to be promising, especially in the group where sperm morphology was < 20% normal forms [19]. The computer gives excellent repeatability on normal and abnormal cells. Based on results obtained, it was postulated that this system can be of clinical value both in IVF units and andrology laboratories [24].

*Are there clinical studies available correlating ASMA instruments with assisted reproduction outcome?*

In our initial work the computer evaluation was also compared with the manual evaluation in a clinical study using fertilization rate as an end point. The computerized system identified the < 14% of normal forms very well and showed a significant difference in fertilization rate in the groups with ≤ 14% and > 14% normal forms. It was concluded that this new development holds promise for clinical practice [18].

The IVOS system's ability was evaluated to predict fertilization in vitro in a prospective study [25]. Eighty patients from the Tygerberg gamete intrafallopian transfer (GIFT) program were evaluated in a prospective manner. Only patients with more than two oocytes available after GIFT was performed were allowed into the study. In all cases an insemination concentration of 500,000 spermatozoa per oocyte was used where normal morphology was 14% or lower. Logistic regression analysis was used to study predictors of fertilization in vitro on excess oocytes. 338 oocytes were obtained from the 80 patients of which 239 fertilized.

The logistic regression analysis of the manual method (% normal morphology) and computer morphology evaluation (IVOS, dimensions) indicated that both were predictors of fertilization. It was shown that in patients where 10 million or less sperm per ml were obtained, the role of morphology (evaluated by IVOS) as well as the number of oocytes were significant predictors of fertilization [25].

By using a more simplistic approach on the same data set it was noted that the overall fertilization rate for IVOS in the group 0–4% normal forms (P pattern) was 45.6% (37/81); 5–9% normal morphology group, 72.5% (87/120); 10–14% normal morphology group, 82.1% (46/56) and in the group >14%, 85.2% (69/81) ($p < 0.0001$ for P pattern vs. other groups) [25].

The computer can thus be of great help to identify the poor prognosis group as far as fertilization is concerned [25].

Recently Coetzee reported on 206 GIFT cycles where sperm morphology was prospectively analysed by computer (IVOS) (unpublished). The pregnancy rate per cycle in the group <5% normal forms was 15.4% (4/26), compared to 35.6% (64/180) pregnancy rate in the morphology group ⩾5%. Bearing in mind that the ICSI pregnancy rate in our unit was 31% per cycle for 1997 (unpublished), the computer can be used as a screening method to select patients for this procedure.

It is thus obvious from the above-mentioned data that the computer can become a helpful clinical tool in andrology laboratories and in vitro fertilization (IVF) centres. If adhering to careful slide preparation the computerized morphology evaluation can bring more objectivity in morphology evaluation worldwide [22,26,27]. More research in this field in the next few years is, however, mandatory to give final answers.

**Sperm functional tests and sperm morphology. Can sperm morphology be considered as a functional test?**

Sperm morphology is used as a predictor of fertilization in vitro. This was clearly outlined by the Tygerberg and other groups [1,5–7,12]. All these authors indicated a lower fertilization rate (significantly so <5% normal forms) and based on the consistent significant trend according to the meta-analysis done by Coetzee, it can be decided on the data that, yes, sperm morphology can be used as a predictor of fertilization thus reflecting function.

## Correlation of sperm morphology with functional tests

*The hemizona assay (HZA)*

Zona binding and subsequent fertilization in vitro are known to be impaired among men with teratozoospermia [28]. In an article by Franken et al. [29] it was clearly shown that teratozoospermic men do not bind at the same level as those with normozoospermia. In a group of patients studied with no fertilization in vitro compared to a control group showing good fertilization in vitro, the hemizona assay (HZA) in the group with fertilization was 36 ± 7, and in the group with no fertilization the HZA (tightly bound sperm per hemizona) was 10 ± 3. It was also shown that by increasing the number of spermatozoa each teratozoospermic man revealed a specific sperm concentration necessary to achieve to zona binding parity compared to the number of bound sperm to the control sample (normozoospermic men). This observation in the HZA model fits the observation by Oehninger et al. [5] where increased fertilization rate per oocyte was observed in men with severe teratozoospermia when the insemination concentration was increased from 50,000 sperm/ml to 500,000 sperm/ml.

In a study by Oehninger [30] where a meta-analysis was performed in 10 selected studies, excellent correlation was observed between the hemizona assay and IVF results. From this analysis it can be concluded that the results of sperm-zona pellucida binding tests (expressed as hemizona index and sperm-zona-binding ratio) and fertilization rate are significantly correlated and that the best estimate of the correlation based on the largest set of homogeneous studies is about 0.64.

*Acrosome reaction (AR)*

Acrosome reaction (AR) is an exocytotic process involving fusion of sperm plasma membrane and outer acrosomal membrane. Only acrosome-reacted spermatozoa can penetrate the zona pellucida [31]. Oehninger et al. [32] studied the acrosome reaction and its prerequisite, a calcium influx, in spermatozoa of infertile men with a high incidence of abnormal sperm forms. They concluded that infertile patients with a high incidence of abnormal sperm forms as diagnosed by strict criteria have a low incidence of spontaneous AR and a diminished progesterone-stimulated AR, whereas the nonspecific response to a calcium ionophore is conserved. Parallel abnormalities of $(Ca^{2+})i$ were observed in these patients with teratozoospermia, suggesting that these sperm populations may have a defective nongenomic progesterone sperm receptor and/or abnormalities of other membrane transduction system.

In a study by Bastiaan [33] sperm samples from 29 men randomly selected from the andrology laboratory were used to evaluate the acrosome reaction response to solubalized human zona pellucida. Three basic groups were identified, namely, fertile donors, teratozoospermic (normal sperm morphology

5—14%, G pattern; n = 25), and severely teratozoospermic (normal sperm morphology $\leqslant$ to 4%; n = 4) groups. Results were analysed and expressed as correlations between sperm morphology and acrosomal response to solubalized zona pellucida, spontaneous and calcium ionophore-induced acrosome reactions. Sperm morphology evaluated by strict criteria correlated positively and highly significantly with the responsiveness of the acrosome reaction (r = 0.91; p = 0.0001). At a morphology cutoff value of 4%, the ROC curve analysis showed sperm morphology to be highly predictive of ZP-induced acrosome responsiveness. Of importance was the observation that spontaneous and calcium ionophore induced acrosome reactions revealed no correlation with sperm morphology. It was concluded that: 1) morphological features of human spermatozoa are indicative of specific functional characteristics, and 2) ZP induction of the acrosome is superior as a predictor of sperm morphology compared to calcium ionophore-induced and spontaneous acrosome reactions. This observation can lead to the development of a valuable diagnostic functional test.

It is well known that calcium ionophore A23187 can induce acrosome reaction at a high rate [34,35]. The drawback with this reagent is that it bypasses the receptor activation/signal transduction elements of the stimulation process. The use of progesterone or recombinant ZP3 [36,37] overcomes the problem of the calcium ionophore (A23187), and in the case of the former has been shown to induce results that correlate with IVF outcome [37,38].

*Zona-free hamster oocyte penetration assay [34]*

To quote Aitken and Irvine directly [34]: "This bioassay examines the ability of human spermatozoa to capacitate, undergo the acrosome reaction and fuse with the vitelline membrane of the oocyte. From a clinical perspective, it generates results that correlate well with the outcome of both human IVF [39] and the achievement of spontaneous pregnancy [40—43]. However, this bioassay is labour-intensive, technically demanding and extremely difficult to standardize. Nevertheless, as a research tool it is one of the most sensitive measures of sperm function available and provides invaluable information on the ability of acrosome reacted human spermatozoa to initiate sperm-oocyte fusion. It should also be recognized that the outcome of this bioassay correlates closely with the motility of the spermatozoa. This contrasts with assessments of the acrosome reaction which are dependent on sperm viability, but not motility. Thus, if the acrosome reaction is used as a means of monitoring sperm function, it should be accompanied by measurements of sperm movement in order to obtain an accurate assessment of the fertilizing potential of a given sperm population."

*Creatine kinase*

A cellular marker of sperm quality, creatine kinase, has been found to be a key enzyme in synthesis of energy transport factors. Higher levels seem to indicate a defect in sperm cytoplasmic extrusions [44]. Motile sperm fractions from oligo-zoospermic samples enriched by the swim-up method were found to have lower creatine kinase levels than the original samples. Furthermore, when IVF was performed in oligozoospermic men, the group that proved to be fertile could be predicted on the basis of their sperm creatine kinase activity. However, more work is necessary to make this observation valuable for routine clinical use.

Huszar et al. [45] found that mature sperm selectively bind to the zona pellucida using immunocytochemistry for creatine kinase. Spermatozoa with immature creatine kinase-staining patterns seem to be deficient in ooctye recognition and binding capabilities. This corroborates the report of Menkveld et al. [45] that morphologically superior sperm have a higher binding capacity than abnormally shaped sperm forms. Furthermore, a good relationship has been found between the sperm biochemical parameters of creatine kinase concentration, lipid peroxidation and abnormal sperm morphology [46].

*Reactive oxygen species (ROS)* [34]

Aitken [34] recently stated that: "Another example of a biochemical lesion involved in the etiology of defective sperm function is perioxidative damage to spermatozoa created by the excessive generation of reactive oxygen species (ROS) [47—49]. Produced at low, physiological levels, molecules such as hydrogen peroxide are extremely important to spermatozoa in fuelling the capacitation process. However, when produced in excessive amounts, ROS disrupts sperm function by inducing peroxidative damage to the sperm plasma membrane and generating strand breaks in the spermatozoa's DNA. Spermatozoa are particularly susceptible to such damage because the cytoplasmic antioxidant enzymes that protect most cell types (superoxide dismutase, catalase, glutathione peroxidase) are in limited supply, while the substrates for oxidative damage (unsaturated fatty acids and DNA) are relatively abundant. As a consequence, assays of ROS generation by the washed ejaculate have been shown to exhibit a negative correlation with fertilization rates in vivo and in vitro." [40,50]. Correlation with morphology and ROS has not been done so far by our group.

*Sperm receptors (SR)*

Sperm receptors (SR), i.e., wheat germ agglutinin receptors, on the sperm head is an interesting development in the field of diagnostic andrology [51]. Gabriel indicated a correlation between wheat germ agglutinin receptors at the equatorial region with semen parameters and, specifically, morphology. Potentially, this observation can be of clinical value as well as part of the evaluation of the male. He observed the percentage wheat germ agglutinin receptor localization on human sperm membrane domain in P and G patterns and normal semen samples. In the P pattern group 6.46 ± 14% was observed compared to 32.91 ± 21% in the normal group.

472

Based on the correlation between the sperm functional tests (e.g., HZA, SPA, AR and SR) and sperm morphology, as well as the data on fertilizing in vitro, one can make the assumption that sperm morphology reflects function and can thus be considered as a sperm functional test.

## Conclusion

Although there is excellent correlation between semen parameters, and especially sperm morphology and certain sperm functional tests, one would like to see in published literature analysis of more than one semen parameter and functional tests working in concert to improve the predictive ability helping the clinician to make sound decisions. It is of importance to distinguish the patient requiring ICSI from those who will benefit from normal IVF, GIFT or intrauterine insemination (IUI).

It is our view that with careful planning in IVF clinics by doing a battery of tests based on the sequential analysis principle, one will move closer to a more refined approach. I am convinced that by continuing research on the sperm functional tests, the basic semen analysis and correlation with IVF using multiple regression analysis, we should be able to achieve a workable formula to make sound scientific decisions in the very near future.

## References

1. Coetzee K, Kruger TF, Lombard CJ. Predictive value of normal sperm morphology: a structured literature review. Hum Reprod Update 1998;4:73–82.
2. Kruger TF, Acosta AA, Simmons KF, Swanson RJ, Matta JF, Oehninger S. Predictive value of abnormal sperm morphology in in vitro fertilization. Fertil Steril 1988;49:112–117.
3. Kruger TF, Menkveld R, Stander FSH et al. Sperm morphologic features as a prognostic factor in in vitro fertilization. Fertil Steril 1986;46:1118–1123.
4. Menkveld R, Stander FSH, Kotze JvW, Kruger TF, Van Zyl JA. The evaluation of morphological characteristics of human spermatozoa according to the stricter criteria. Hum Reprod 1990;5: 586–592.
5. Oehninger S, Acosta AA, Morshedi M, Veeck L, Swanson RJ, Simmons K, Rosenwaks Z. Corrective measures and pregnancy outcome in in vitro fertilization in patients with severe sperm morphology abnormalities. Fertil Steril 1988; 50:283–287.
6. Enginsu ME, Dumoulin JCM, Pieters MHEC et al. Comparison between the hypoosmotic swelling test and morphology evaluation using strict criteria in predicting in vitro fertilization. J Ass Reprod Genetics 1992b;9:259–264.
7. Ombelet W, Fourie F le R, Vandeput H et al. Teratozoospermia and in-vitro fertilization: a randomized prospective study. Hum Reprod 1994;9:1479–1484.
8. Hernandez M, Molina R, Coetzee K, Olmedo J, Brugo Olmedo S, Estofan D. Prognostic value of the strict criteria: an Argentinian experience. Arch Androl 1996;37:85–87.
9. World Health Organization. WHO Laboratory Manual for the Examination of Human Semen and Semen-Cervical Mucus Interaction, 2nd edn. Cambridge: Cambridge University Press, 1987.
10. World Health Organization. WHO Laboratory Manual for the Examination of Human Semen and Sperm-Cervical Mucus Interaction. Cambridge: Cambridge University Press, 1992.
11. Figueiredo H, Tavares A, Farras L et al. Isolated teratozoospermia and *in vitro* fertilization. J

Ass Reprod Genetics 1996;13:64—68.

12. Enginsu ME, Pieters MHEC, Dumoulin JCM et al. Male factor as determinant of in-vitro fertilization outcome. Hum Reprod 1992a;7:1136—1140.

13. Grow DR, Oehninger S, Seltman HJ et al. Sperm morphology as diagnosed by strict criteria: probing the impact of teratozoospermia on fertilization rate and pregnancy outcome in a large in vitro fertilization population. Fertil Steril 1994;62:559—565.

14. Yue Z, Meng FJ, Jorgensen N et al. Sperm morphology using strict criteria after Percoll density separation: influence on cleavage and pregnancy rates after in-vitro fertilization. Hum Reprod 1995;10:1781—1785.

15. Kruger TF, Acosta AA, Simmons KF, Swanson RJ, Matta JF, Veeck LL, Morshedi M, Brugo S. New method of evaluating sperm morphology with predictive value for human in vitro fertilization. Urology 1987;3:248—251.

16. Wang C, Leung A, Tsoi W-L et al. Computer-assisted assessment of human sperm morphology: usefullness in predicting fertilizing capacity of human spermatozoa. Fertil Steril 1991a;55: 989—993.

17. Wang C, Leung A, Tsoi W-L at al. Computer-assisted assessment of human sperm morphology: comparison with visual assessment. Fertil Steril 1991b;55:983—988.

18. Kruger TF, Du Toit TC, Franken DR, Acosta AA, Oehninger SC, Menkveld R, Lombard CJ. A new computerized method of reading sperm morphology (strict criteria) is as efficient as technician reading. Fertil Steril 1993;59:202—209.

19. Kruger TF, Du Toit TC, Franken DR, Menkveld R, Lombard CJ. Sperm morphology: assessing the agreement between the manual method (strict criteria) and the sperm morphology analyser IVOS. Fertil Steril 1995;63:134—142.

20. Davis RO, Gravance CG. Standardization of specimen preparation, staining, and sampling methods improves automated sperm-head morphometry analysis. Fertil Steril 1993;59: 412—417.

21. Garrett C, Baker HWG. A new fully automated system for the morphometric analysis of human sperm heads. Fertil Steril 1995;63:1306—1317.

22. Lacquet FA, Kruger TF, Du Toit TC, Lombard CJ, Sanchez Sarmiento CA, De Villiers A, Coetzee K. Slide preparation and staining procedures for reliable results using computerized morphology (IVOS). Arch Androl 1996;36:133—138.

23. Menkveld R, Kruger TF. Advantages of strict (Tygerberg) criteria for evaluation of sperm morphology. Int J Androl 1995;(Suppl 2):36—42.

24. Coetzee K, Kruger TF. Automated sperm morphology analysis: quo vadis. Ass Reprod Rev 1997;7:109—113.

25. Kruger TF, Lacquet FA, Sanchez Sarmiento CA et al. A prospective study on the predictive value of normal sperm morphology as evaluated by computer (IVOS). Fertil Steril 1996; 66:285—291.

26. Coetzee K, Kruger TF, Vandendael A, De Villiers A, Lombard CJ. Comparison of two staining and evaluation methods used for computerized human sperm morphology evaluations. Andrologia 1997;29:133—135.

27. Menkveld R, Lacquet FA, Kruger TF, Lombard CJ, Sanchez Sarmiento CA, De Villiers A. Effects of different staining and washing procedures on the results of human sperm morphology evaluation by manual and computerised methods. Andrologia 1997;29:1—7.

28. Franken DR, Oehninger S, Kaskar K et al. Sperm-zona pellucida binding and penetration assays. In: Acosta AA, Kruger TF (eds) Human Spermatozoa in Assisted Reproduction. New York: Parthenon Publishing Company, 1996;237.

29. Franken DR, Kruger TF, Menkveld R et al. Hemizona assay and teratozoospermia: increasing sperm insemination concentrations to enhance zona pellucida binding. Fertil Steril 1990;54: 497—503.

30. Oehninger S, Sayed E, Kolm P. Role of sperm morphology tests in subfertility treatment strategies. In: Ombelet W, Bosmans E, Vandeput H, Vereecken A, Renier M, Hoomans E (eds) Mod-

ern ART in the 2000s. New York: Parthenon Publishing Group, 1998(8);25—36.

31. Koehler JK, De Curtis I, Stechener MA et al. Interaction of human sperm with zona free hamster eggs. A freeze fracture study. Gamete Res 1982;6:371—386.

32. Oehninger S, Blackmore P, Morshedi M et al. Defective calcium influx and acrosome reaction (spontaneous and progesterone-induced) in spermatozoa of infertile men with severe teratozoospermia. Fertil Steril 1994;61:349—354.

33. Bastiaan H. Physiological factors influencing the human acrosome reaction. M.Sc. Dissertation (Medical Science), Department of Anatomical Pathology (Cytology), University of Stellenbosch, South Africa, November, 1997;1—132.

34. Aitken RJ, Irvine DS. Reliability of methods for assessing the fertilizing capacity of human spermatozoa. In: Ombelet W, Bosmans E, Vandeput H, Vereecken A, Renier M, Hoomans E (eds) Modern ART in the 2000s. New York: Parthenon Publishing Group, 1998(8);179—189.

35. Blackmore PF, Beeve SJ, Danford DR et al. Progesterone and 17-hydroxy-progesterone: novel stimulators of calcium influx in human sperm. J Biol Chem 1990;265:1376—1380.

36. Van Duin M, Polman JEM, De Breet ITM et al. Production, purification and biological activity of recombinant human zona pellucida protein, ZP3. Biol Reprod 1994;51:607—617.

37. Liu DY, Bourne H, Baker HWG. High fertilization and pregnancy rates after intracytoplasmic sperm injection in patients with disordered zona pellucida-induced acrosome reaction. Fertil Steril 1997;67:955—958.

38. Krausz C, Bonaccorsi L, Maggio P et al. Two functional assays of sperm responsiveness to progesterone and their predictive values in *in-vitro* fertilization. Hum Reprod 1996;11:1661—1667.

39. Aitken RJ, Thatcher S, Glasier AF et al. Relative ability of modified versions of the hamster oocyte penetration test, incorporating hyperosmotic medium or the ionophore A23187, to predict IVF outcome. Hum Reprod 1987;2:227—231.

40. Aitken RJ, Irvine DS, Wu FC. Prospective analysis of sperm-oocyte fusion and reactive oxygen species generation as criteria for the diagnosis of infertility. Am J Obstet Gynecol 1991;164:542—551.

41. Irvine DS, Aitken RJ. Predictive value of *in-vitro* sperm function tests in the context of an AID service. Hum Reprod 1986;8:539—545.

42. Irvine DS, Aitken RJ. Clinical evaluation of the zona-free hamster egg penetration test in the management of the infertile couple: prospective and retrospective studies. Int J Androl Suppl 1986;6:97—112.

43. Aitken RJ. The future of the hamster oocyte penetration assay. Fertil Steril 1994;62:17—19.

44. Huszar G, Vigue L, Corrales M. Sperm creatine kinase activity in fertile and infertile oligospermic men. J Androl 1990;61:136—142.

45. Huszar G, Vigue L, Oehninger S. Creatine kinase immunocytochemistry of human sperm-hemizona complexes: selective binding of sperm with mature creatine kinase-staining pattern. Fertil Steril 1994;61:136—142.

46. Huszar G, Vigue L. Correlation between the rate of lipid peroxidation and cellular maturity as measured by creatine kinase activity in human spermatozoa. J Androl 1994;15:71—77.

47. Aitken RJ, Clarkson JS. Cellular basis of detective sperm function and its association with the genesis of reactive oxygen species by human spermatozoa. J Reprod Fertil 1987;81:459—469.

48. Aitken RJ, Fisher H. Reactive oxygen species generation and human spermatozoa: the balance of benefit and risk. Bioessays 1994;16:259—267.

49. Sharma RK, Agarwal A. Role of reactive oxygen species in male infertility. Urology 1996;48:835—850.

50. Krausz C, Mills C, Rogers S et al. Stimulation of oxidant generation by human sperm suspensions using phorbol esters and formyl peptides: relationship with motility and fertilization *in vitro*. Fertil Steril 1994;62:599—605.

51. Gabriel LK, Franken DR, Van der Horst G et al. Wheat germ agglutinin receptors on human sperm membranes and sperm morphology. Andrologia 1994;26:5—8.

# Intracytoplasmic sperm injection in nonmale factor patients

Mohamed A. Aboulghar[1,2], Ragaa T. Mansour[1] and Gamal I. Serour[1]

[1] The Egyptian IVF-ET Center, Maadi, Cairo; and [2] Department of Obstetrics and Gynecology, Faculty of Medicine, Cairo University, Cairo, Egypt

**Abstract.** *Background.* The improved therapeutic power of intracytoplasmic sperm injection (ICSI) for treatment of male factor infertility has been consistently reported in world literature. Following these reports, it was suggested that ICSI should be performed for all patients irrespective of semen parameters.

*Methods.* The literature was searched for studies that investigated the role of ICSI in the treatment of nonmale factor infertility including tubal factor with normal semen parameters, patients with unexplained infertility and patients with borderline semen parameters.

*Results.* In tubal-factor infertility with normal semen, a prospective randomized study showed that there was no significant difference in the implantation or pregnancy rates between IVF and ICSI. In patients with borderline semen parameters, IVF and ICSI were tried on sibling oocytes and complete failure of fertilization occurred in 49% of patients following conventional IVF, while fertilization was successful in all patients in ICSI oocytes. In cases of unexplained infertility, when ICSI and IVF were performed on sibling oocytes total failure of fertilization occurred after conventional IVF in 27% of patients and fertilization occurred in all cases after ICSI.

*Conclusions.* ICSI does not offer a higher pregnancy rate over conventional IVF in the treatment of tubal-factor infertility with normal semen. IVF and ICSI should be performed on sibling oocytes in patients with unexplained infertility or borderline semen.

**Keywords:** IVF, ICSI, nonmale factor, sibling oocytes, tubal factor.

## Introduction

In vitro fertilization has become a standard procedure for the treatment of tubal-factor infertility. It has also been used to treat couples with male factor infertility for over a decade with relatively disappointing results [1].

The first successful pregnancy after intracytoplasmic sperm injection (ICSI) in humans was reported by Palermo et al. [2]. In a large series, Van Steirteghem et al. [3] reported a high success rate using ICSI in male factor infertility. After publication of this report, ICSI became a standard treatment of male factor infertility irrespective of the severity of the condition [4]. The improved therapeutic power of ICSI for treatment of male factor infertility compared with conventional IVF performed during the same period of time in couples with tubal infertility, using the same batches of culture media and identical criteria and laboratory methods, has been reported [1].

It has even been suggested that ICSI should completely replace conventional

*Address for correspondence:* Prof Mohamed Aboulghar MD, The Egyptian IVF-ET Center, 3 B Street 161 Hadaek El-Maadi, Maadi, Cairo 11431, Egypt. Fax: +20-2-525-3532.

IVF in the future, as even better pregnancy rates might be expected if normal'
spermatozoa are injected [5]. To some extent, Hamberger et al. [5] explored this
possibility in their IVF program in which IVF and ICSI were performed on a
1:1 ratio in cases of failed fertilization in earlier conventional IVF trials. In one-
third of these cases (14/42), no fertilization occurred with conventional IVF in
the second trial, whereas, in two-thirds (28/42) of the cases, fertilization and
pregnancy rates were similar with both techniques. They concluded that, until
more knowledge is gained concerning the outcome of pregnancies, most centers ·
have taken the attitude that ICSI should be applied only when conventional IVF
fails.

A growing number of programs are reporting success rates for male factor
patients equal or greater than those reported for tubal-factor patients [3,6]. The
same findings were also observed in our program, and this was surprising
because it was previously reported that embryos resulting from poor-quality
semen in conventional IVF are of lesser quality and are associated with a low
pregnancy rate [7]. One possible explanation is that the embryos resulting from
regular IVF are usually surrounded by many of sperm embedded by the heads
in the zona pellucida and the tails are outside. It has been demonstrated that the
sperm tails' fibrous sheath contains multiple antigens that appear late during
spermatogenesis [8]. Therefore, it is likely in some cases that those antigens might
include antibody reactions at the site of implantation. Another possible explanation is that ICSI embryos may have been assisted indirectly to hatch through the
procedure of the injection itself, despite the small size of the puncture. And it
has been shown that assisted hatching improves the implantation rate when used
in clinical IVF [9].

Because of the excellent results of ICSI reported by different people, several
centers started performing ICSI for all their patients irrespective of the semen
parameters. They achieved high fertilization and pregnancy rates and the scope
of ICSI widened to include patients with acrosomeless spermatozoa [10], unexplained infertility [11], borderline semen [12], immunological infertility [13], and
previous failure of fertilization in conventional IVF [6]. Different sperm sources
having different sperm parameters representing various etiologic conditions
were used for ICSI procedures.

The aim of this review is to evaluate the possible value of ICSI in the treatment
of nonmale factor infertility patients.

**Intracytoplasmic sperm injection for treatment of tubal-factor infertility with
normal semen**

This concept was not studied in a prospective manner until we published our
first study on this subject [14]. The objective of the study was to compare the
results of IVF and ICSI in tubal-factor infertility with normal semen parameters.

The study group included 116 tubal-factor infertility patients. All male partners had normal semen according to World Health Organization criteria, 1992 [15]. All patients were counseled about the details of the study and they gave informed consent. The protocol was approved by our institutional ethics committee. Patients were divided randomly on an alternate basis into two groups: group A (58 patients) were allocated to our conventional IVF protocol [16] and group B (58 patients) were allocated to our standard ICSI protocol [17]. Ovulation induction was the same in both groups using a GnRH agonist long protocol.

Embryo transfer was carried out on day 2 after the pick-up, using the Wallace catheter or the labotect catheter if the Wallace catheter could not be introduced. Luteal phase support was given routinely in the form of 2,500 IU of hCG (human chorionic gonadotropin) every 4th day. Cases that were considered at high risk of developing ovarian hyperstimulation syndrome were given a daily P injection (100 mg, progesterone). Clinical pregnancy was diagnosed by the presence of a gestational sac with fetal echoes. All patients in this study reached the ET stage.

There was no statistically significant difference between the age, period of infertility, E2 level on day of hCG, and the number of oocytes retrieved between both groups.

Also, there was no statistically significant difference in the implantation or pregnancy rates between IVF and ICSI. Both groups had no significant difference in the clinical parameters, patient characteristics, and stimulation protocols. Culture conditions and laboratory methods were also the same in both groups. The fertilization rate per retrieved oocyte was significantly higher in conventional IVF compared with ICSI, resulting in more fertilized oocytes in group A. In ICSI, the oocytes are denuded from the granulosa cells and only metaphase II oocytes are injected. In conventional IVF, the oocytes are left in culture for normal fertilization and it is possible that a percentage of metaphase I oocytes would mature to metaphase II in vitro and become fertilized. In ICSI, this subgroup of metaphase I oocytes does not have the same chance of maturation. This may be a possible explanation for the lower fertilization rate per retrieved oocyte in ICSI compared with conventional IVF.

The difference in the age between ICSI patients for male factor and conventional IVF for tubal factor in several programs could be one of the reasons for the excellent results of ICSI. Patients with male factor infertility tend to come for treatment at a younger age. This may be because tubal-factor patients spend a number of years trying different conservative and surgical modalities of treatment. Another explanation is that ICSI patients are usually healthy females with no pelvic pathology. It was also reported previously that the presence of extensive adhesions reduces the pregnancy rate in conventional IVF [18]. There is also growing evidence that the presence of a hydrosalpinx reduces the chances of pregnancy in IVF [19].

The results of the present work have shown that ICSI does not offer a higher pregnancy rate over conventional IVF in the treatment of tubal-factor infertility with normal semen. Intracytoplasmic sperm injection is a more expensive technique that is time consuming and requires more equipment and extra skill. In addition to the invasive nature of the procedure, it is not superior to conventional IVF in this group of patients. We do not recommend using it for the treatment of tubal-factor patients with normal semen.

## Intracytoplasmic sperm injection in patients with borderline semen

Controlled ovarian stimulation and intrauterine insemination [20] or conventional IVF [21] are often used as a first line of treatment for patients with borderline semen parameters. A group of 53 patients in this category underwent treatment. The semen parameters in this group showed variable results in different tests. The semen counts were $10-20 \times 10^6$ per ml, motility was $30-35\%$ and abnormal forms were $> 50\%$. All patients were counseled for treatment with IVF and were informed that because of the possibility of total failure of fertilization, ICSI and IVF would be performed on sibling oocytes [22].

In this group, the oocytes were randomly divided between IVF and ICSI; a total of 560 oocytes were recovered and 361 were allocated for ICSI and 199 oocytes for conventional IVF. The fertilization rate in ICSI oocytes was 60%, while in conventionally inseminated oocytes, it was 18% ($p < 0.001$). There was complete failure of fertilization in the conventional IVF of oocytes in 26 patients (49%). In the remaining 27 patients, fertilization was successful in both ICSI and conventional IVF and cryopreservation was carried out on all the fertilized oocytes in the conventional IVF group.

In this group, 49% of patients would have completely lost the chance of pregnancy because of total failure of fertilization if ICSI had not been performed on sibling oocytes in that cycle. There were no specific criteria in the semen of these patients which could predict the occurrence of fertilization with conventional IVF. None of these patients had extremely poor semen quality.

Payne et al. [23] treated 18 patients with a normal semen count but with $< 20\%$ normal morphology using both ICSI and conventional IVF on sibling oocytes, and the fertilization rate was significantly higher: 76% in the ICSI group in comparison with 15% in the control group. They recommended the use of ICSI for all forms of demonstrated or suspected male factor infertility.

Clark and Sherins [24] reported that parameters of semen quality can only be used to assign patients to broad clinical categories. Overstreet et al. [25] divided the semen parameters into normal, abnormal and marginal. We believe that the fertilization potential of patients with borderline semen is difficult to assess based on the examination of semen parameters only.

## Intracytoplasmic sperm injection in the treatment of unexplained infertility

Different methods of assisted reproduction such as controlled ovarian hyperstimulation (COH) with intrauterine insemination (IUI) [26] and gamete intrafallopian transfer (GIFT) [27] have been used for the treatment of unexplained infertility. In vitro fertilization is usually resorted to after failure of these lines of treatment. It was reported previously that there was a significantly lower fertilization rate in patients with unexplained infertility compared to patients with tubal-factor infertility [28, 29]. Kahn et al. [30] reported total failure of fertilization in 30% of cases of unexplained infertility which were subjected to IVF after failure of COH and IUI. Audibert et al. [29] reported that in cases of unexplained infertility with previously normal semen, several abnormalities in sperm analysis were reported, affecting at least one parameter on the day of retrieval. Their results suggested that there was a small proportion in the unexplained infertility group with undiscovered male abnormalities, which behaved in IVF like patients with male factor infertility. Atiken et al. [31] reported the weakness of conventional criteria in semen analysis, with a finding of 20% of sperm abnormalities in a second check-up following normal evaluation in a group of infertility patients.

We published a study on 22 patients with unexplained infertility treated by ICSI [32]. Investigation of the female partners showed normal findings. All patients showed normal semen parameters. All patients were counseled for treatment by IVF and were informed that because of the possibility of total failure of fertilization, ICSI and IVF would be performed on sibling oocytes.

Out of 160 oocytes randomly selected for ICSI, the procedure was performed on 128 metaphase II oocytes and fertilization occurred in 80 oocytes (63%), and out of 138 oocytes for which conventional IVF was performed, fertilization occurred in 70 oocytes (50.7%). There was no statistically significant difference in the fertilization rate per oocyte between ICSI and conventional IVF, however, there was total failure of fertilization after conventional IVF in five of the 22 patients and fertilization occurred in all cases after ICSI.

Performing ICSI and conventional IVF for sibling oocytes in patients with unexplained infertility resulted in a significantly higher fertilization rate in the ICSI oocytes. It saved 34.8% of the patients from canceling embryo transfer due to total failure of fertilization with conventional IVF. It was also an excellent test for the sperm fertilizing ability to be used as a guideline for management of possible future cycles.

## Conclusion

It is believed that ICSI should not be performed for tubal-factor patients with normal semen and indications of ICSI should include, in addition to male factor infertility, patients with borderline semen parameters and unexplained infertility.

## References

1. Palermo GD, Cohen J, Alikani M, Alder A, Rosenwaks Z. Intracytoplasmic sperm injection: a novel treatment for all forms of male factor infertility. Fertil Steril 1995;63:1231–1240.
2. Palermo G. Joris H, Devroey P, Can Steirteghem AC. Pregnancies after intracytoplasmic injection of single spermatozoon into an oocyte. Lancet 1992;340:17–18.

480

3. Van Steirteghem AC, Nagy Z, Joris H, Liu J, Staessen C, Smitz J et al. High fertilization and implantation rates after intracytoplasmic sperm injection. Hum Reprod 1993;8:1061—1066.

4. Mansour R. Gamete micromanipulation and assisted fertilization. Middle East Fertil Soc J 1996;1:91—100.

5. Hamberger L, Sjogren A, Lundin K, Soderlind, B, Nilsson L, Bergh C et al. Microfertilization techniques — the Swedish experience. Reprod Fertil Dev 1995;7:263—268.

6. Cohen J, Alikani M, Santiago M, Palermo G. Micromanipulation in clinical management of fertility disorders. Sem Reprod Endocrinol 1994;12:151—168.

7. Parinaud J, Mieusset R, Vieitez G, Labal B, Richoilley G. Influence of sperm parameters on embryo quality. Fertil Steril 1993;60:888—892.

8. Jassin A, Chen YL. AJ-FSI monoclonal antibody detects a novel group of nonglycosylated antigens within the human sperm tail fibroid sheath. Hum Reprod 1994;9:1459—1465.

9. Cohen J, Elsner C, Kort H, Malter H, Massey J, Mayer MP et al. Impairment of the hatching process following IVF in the human improvement of implantation by assisting hatching using micromanipulation. Hum Reprod 1990;5:7—13.

10. Lundin K. Sjorgren A, Nilsson L, Hamberger L. Fertilization and pregnancy after intracytoplasmic microinjection of acrosomeless spermatozoa. Fertil Steril 1994;62:1266—1267.

11. Aboulghar MA, Mansour RT, Serour GI, Sattar MA, Amin Y. Intracytoplasmic sperm injection and conventional in vitro fertilization for sibling oocytes in cases of unexplained infertility and borderline semen. J Ass Reprod Genet 1995;13:38—42.

12. Aboulghar MA, Mansour RT, Serour GI, Amin Y. The role of intracytoplasmic sperm injection (ICSI) in the treatment of patients with borderline semen. Hum Reprod 1995;10:2829—2830.

13. Nagy ZP, Verheyen G, Liu J, Joris H, Janssenswillen C, Wisanto A et al. Results of 55 intracytoplasmic sperm injection cycles in the treatment of male-immunological infertility. Hum Reprod 1995;10:1775—1780.

14. Aboulghar M A, Mansour RT, Serour GI, Amin YA, Kamal A. Prospective controlled randomized study of in vitro fertilization versus intracytoplasmic sperm injection in the treatment of tubal factor infertility with normal semen parameters. Fertil Steril 1996;66:753—756.

15. World Health Organization. Laboratory Manual for the Examination of Human Semen and Semen-cervical Mucus Interaction. 3rd edn. New York: Cambridge University Press, 1992.

16. Aboulghar MA, Mansour RT, Serour GI, Amin YM. The prognostic value of successful in vitro fertilization in subsequent trials. Hum Reprod 1994;9:1932—1934.

17. Mansour RT, Aboulghar MA, Serour GI, Amin YM, Ramzi AM. The effect of sperm parameters on the outcome of intracytoplasmic sperm injection. Fertil. Steril. 1995;64:982—986.

18. Molloy O, Martin M, Speirs A, Lopata A, Clark G, MaBain J et al. Performance of patients with a "frozen pelvis" in an in vitro fertilization program. Fertil Steril 1987;47:450—455.

19. Blazar AS, Hogan JW, Seifer DB, Frishman GN, Wheeler CA, Haning RV. The impact of hydrosalpinx on successful pregnancy in tubal factor infertility treated by in vitro fertilization. Fertil Steril 1997;67:517—520.

20. Mansour RT, Serour GI, Aboulghar MA. Intrauterine insemination with washed capacitated sperm cells in the treatment of male factor, cervical factor and unexplained infertility. Asia-Oceania J Obstet Gynecol 1989;15:151—154.

21. Cohen J, Edwards R, Fehilly C et al. In vitro fertilization: a treatment for male infertility. Fertil Steril 1985;43:422—432.

22. Aboulghar M A, Mansour RT, Serour GI, Amin YA. The role of intracytoplasmic sperm injection (ICSI) in the treatment of patients with borderline semen. Hum Reprod 1995;10: 2829—2830.

23. Payne D, Flaherty SP, Jeffrey R, Warners GM, Matthews CD. Successful treatment of severe male factor infertility in 100 consecutive cycles using intracytoplasmic sperm injection. Hum Reprod 1994;9:2051—2057.

24. Clark RV, Sherins RJ. Use of semen analysis in the evaluation of the infertile couple. In: Santen RJ, Swerdloff RS (eds) Male Reproductive Dysfunction. New York: Marcel Dekker, 1986;253.

25. Overstreet JW, Davis RO, Katz DF. Semen evaluation. In: Overstreet JW (ed) Infertility and Reproductive Medicine: Clinics of North America. Philadelphia: WB Saundres Company, 1992; 329.

26. Aboulghar MA, Mansour RT, Serour GI, Amin Y, Abbas AM, Salah IM. Ovarian superstimulation and intrauterine insemination for the treatment of unexplained infertility. Fertil Steril 1993;60:303—306.

27. Asch RH, Balmaceda JP, Ellsworth LR, Wong PC. Preliminary experience with gamete intrafallopian transfer (GIFT). Fertil Steril 1986;45:366.

28. Navot D, Muasher SJ, Oehninger S, Liu H-C, Veeck LL, Kreiner D, Rosenwaks Z. The value of in vitro fertilization for the treatment of unexplained infertility. Fertil Steril 1988;49:854—857.

29. Audibert F, Hedon B, Arnal F, Humeau C, Badoc E, Virenque V, Boulot P, Mares P, Laffargue F, Viala J L. Results of IVF attempts in patients with unexplained infertility. Hum Reprod 1989; 4:766—771.

30. Kahn JA, Sunde A, During V, Sordal T, Molne K. Treatment of unexplained infertility. Fallopian tube sperm perfusion (FSP). Acta Obstet Gynecol Scand 1993;72:193—199.

31. Atiken J, Best F, Richardson DW, Djahanbakhch O, Mortimer D, Templeton A, Less M. An analysis of sperm function in cases of unexplained infertility: conventional criteria movement characteristics and fertilization capacity. Fertil Steril 1982;38:212—221.

32. Aboulghar M A, Mansour RT, Serour GI, Sattar MA, Amin YA. Intracytoplasmic sperm injection and conventional in vitro fertilization for sibling oocytes in cases of unexplained infertility and borderline semen. J Assist Reprod Genet 1996;13:38—42.

# Failure to fertilize

Shuetu Suzuki[1], Yasuhisa Araki[2], Mitsuhiro Motoyama[2], Midori Yoshizawa[3], Osamu Kato[4], Koji Yano[5], Ryutaro Tojo[5], Masaru Fukuda[6], Hirokatsu Kitai[7] and Shigeaki Kurasawa[8]

[1]Tojo Womens Hospital; [2]Institute of Advanced Medical Technology Central Clinic; [3]Utsunomiya University; [4]Kato Ladies Clinic; [5]Yano Obstetrics and Gynecology; [6]Fukuda Womens Clinic; [7]Saitama Insurance Central Hospital; and [8]Sebo Hospital, Japan

**Abstract.** Fertilization failure is an important problem in infertile patients even in the age of IVF. However, the precise mechanism has not yet been proved.

We will discuss this topic from the points of zona thickness and unfertilized ICSI cases.

**Keywords:** fertilization failure, ICSI, spermatozoa, zona pellucida.

The natural fertilization process in the fallopian tube in the human is not yet completely understood. However, the recent advances in the area of assisted reproductive technology have opened a window to the understanding of normal fertilization and some mechanism(s) of fertilization failure.

Successful fertilization is a complicated process of gamete interaction. At the first step of this phenomenon, the sperm works more actively than the ovum. The sperm need to be transported through the female reproductive tract before binding and penetration into the zona pellucida. The penetrated sperm work thereafter as a trigger of signal transduction and exocytosis.

Complete failure to fertilize is quite a frustrating experience for IVF couples. The rate of fertilization failure is estimated to be approximately 10—20% of all IVF cycles. However, little is known about the mechanism of fertilization failure during these cycles.

The causes of fertilization failure in IVF could be categorized as follows (numbered sites as shown in Fig. 1.):
1) sperm in the cumulus cells;
2) acrosome reaction, attachment and binding to the zona pellucida;
3) penetration into the zona pellucida;
4) signal transduction; and
5) pronuclei formation and fusion.
Araki et al. examined 412 unfertilized oocytes after conventional IVF by nuclear staining of the ooplasma. They found that in 76.4% (282/378) of unfertilized

*Address for correspondence:* Shuetu Suzuki MD, WHO, Human Reproduction Program, Scientific and Technical Adviser, 1-5-2 Higashitamagawa, Setagaya-ku, Tokyo 158, Japan. Tel.: +81-3-3727-9702. Fax: +81-3-3726-4715.

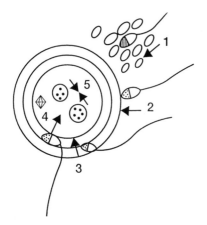

*Fig. 1.*

oocytes, sperm could not be recognized in ooplasma and in 20.7% (78/378) they could demonstrate sperm penetration. However, in 7.7% (29/378) no sperm head was enlarged and in 11.4% (43/378) the pronuclei were not fused. Polyspermy was found in 1.6% (6/378). Araki et al. then carried out second IVF and first ICSI for groups of fertilization failure recognized after the first conventional IVF. As a result they confirmed the fertilization rate in 8.4% (13/457) after the repeated conventional IVF and in 40.4% (70/173) after ICSI.

The zona thickness was identified as a barrier for sperm penetration resulting fertilization failure. We measured the thickness of human zona pellucida using video monitoring.

Biologically, fertilization failure can be an important cause for unexplained infertility. IVF has been accepted for treatment of this disease and, in fact, many infertile couples with unexplained infertility have been pregnant by IVF, especially by ICSI. However, we need to learn more regarding the mechanisms of fertilization failure for greater understanding of natural human fertility.

# Infection and reproduction

# Management of fertile and infertile HIV positive patients wanting to become parents

Pierre Jouannet[1], Emmanuel Dulioust[1], Jean-Marie Kunstmann[1], Anne Tachet[4], Isabelle Heard[2], Dominique Salmon[3], Marta de Almeida[1], Laurent Finkielsztejn[3], Didier Sicard[3], Laurent Mandelbrot[2] and Christine Rouzioux[4]

[1]Laboratoire de Biologie de la Reproduction — CECOS, [2]Service de Gynécologie Obstétrique, and [3]Service de Médecine Interne, Groupe Hospitalier Cochin Port-Royal, Université Paris, Paris; and [4]Laboratoire de Virologie, Groupe Hospitalier Necker Enfants Malades, Université Paris, France

**Abstract.** Soon after the beginning of the AIDS epidemic, the desire for fertility in human immunodeficiency virus (HIV)-infected people became a matter of concern for medical teams. For many years, the questions raised by such a wish received little attention. Most frequently, a negative response was given to the couples who needed or asked for medical assistance to procreate. Recently, several factors have profoundly modified the situation. The number of people living with HIV infection who want to become parents is continuously increasing. Recent advances in antiretroviral therapies allow them to hope for a much longer life expectancy than before. Finally, new scientific data provide a better understanding of the factors influencing horizontal and vertical contamination, and help to design procedures to greatly reduce the risk of virus transmission, either through conception or during pregnancy. The present state of knowledge in this field is discussed and perspectives are proposed for the management of procreation in HIV-infected persons.

**Keywords:** AIDS, assisted procreation, donor insemination, semen, virus.

## Introduction

As soon as epidemiological evidence of human immunodeficiency virus (HIV) sexual transmission and the presence of the virus in human semen was demonstrated, the infertility clinics were confronted with the risk of transmitting the virus through medically assisted procreation. The contamination of several women by donor insemination led rapidly to recommend systematic screening of gamete donors for HIV antibodies and to use a 6-month quarantine before transferring donated gametes and/or embryos. No contamination was reported when these recommendations were applied. The same precautions were taken for the use of serum or other products of human origin, e.g., albumin in culture media for assisted reproductive technologies (ART).

Besides these problems concerning the security of medical treatment, the physicians involved in infertility management have had to face more difficult questions raised by HIV-infected patients who either requested ART because

*Address for correspondence:* P. Jouannet, Laboratoire de Biologie de la Reproduction, Hôpital Cochin, 123 boulevard de Port Royal, 75014 Paris, France. Tel.: +33-1-42-34-50-29. Fax: 33-1-42-34-50-28. E-mail: pierre.jouannet@cch.ap-hop-paris.fr

they were infertile or who wanted to become parents with no or lower risk of virus transmission. Such demands raised critical questions on the vertical transmission of the virus and the future health of the child, the potential death of the future parents, the risk of transmission to other patients and to the medical staff, and the liability of the staff refusing a treatment. There were many ethical, legal, medical and personal issues to resolve.

For a long time these important questions were not clearly addressed, probably because the number of people concerned was very low. However, the situation is rapidly changing. The number of HIV-infected patients of reproductive age is increasing rapidly and many of them, women or men, live with a serodifferent partner. Also, more efficient treatments have sufficiently modified the evolution of the infection to strikingly change social and effective life of many infected people, allowing them to wish to become parents. However, most of them are greatly concerned with the risk of horizontal and/or vertical transmission of HIV and strongly demand means able to reduce or suppress it.

We discuss various aspects of this problem, considering first the case of the seropositive woman and then the case of the seropositive man.

*The HIV-positive partner is the woman*

The rate of mother-to-child HIV transmission is about 20% in the absence of treatment. Since the important probability of death of the infected woman and child it has usually been recommended to avoid pregnancies in HIV-infected women. In recent years several studies have brought important information which have modified the clinical management of pregnant women and the prognosis of mother and child.

In 1994, results from a randomized trial showed that zidovudine administered to a group of HIV-infected women during pregnancy and labor and to the newborn reduced the risk of transmission from 25.5 to 8.3% [1]. Since then, zidovudine treatment of pregnant women has been widely used, at least in industrialized countries. As a consequence, HIV testing in pregnancy was recommended in several countries, e.g., France, and the epidemiology of mother-to-child transmission was modified [2]. Furthermore, alternative therapeutic strategies became available with the development of new antiretroviral association [3]. However, the possible adverse maternal and neonatal effects of the various treatments have to be precise.

Could a greatly reduced risk of transmission allow the treatment of infertility in HIV-infected women? There are no clear guidelines in this field. In 1991 the British Medical Journal published a debate considering the legal, ethical and medical issues of infertility management in HIV-positive patients [4]. Most of the opinions were negative taking into account "the welfare of any child who may result, including the need of such a child for a father", "the rights of any resultant offspring to be free of disease", "the right of the attendant medical and laboratory staff to maintain their own health" or claiming that "we have no positive duty to accede to an infertile couple's request for help. If procedures to make this couple pregnant cannot be justified as being in their or the future child's best medical interests then it is wrong to administer them".

The debate raised again in human reproduction in 1996–1997 when Olaitan et al. suggested that "the ethical issues associated with the management of this problem demand urgent attention, and guidelines should be drawn up, so that doctors can have a clear idea of what is appropriate to offer such couples and a consistent approach can be adopted by all treatment centres" [5]. Once again the opinions expressed were negative. Rizk and Dill concluded "it is premature and unethical to treat HIV-infected women for infertility at this time" [6].

Similarly, the American Society for Reproductive Medicine stated in 1994 that HIV infection is a serious contraindication to treatment and the FIGO (Federation of International Gynecology and Obstetrics) Committee for the Study of Ethical aspects of human reproduction published guidelines concluding that "to protect interests of those at risk of unwanted exposure to HIV including the potential child, only seronegative individuals should be allowed to participate" in assisted reproductive technology [7].

The great majority of gynecologists and biologists involved in infertility treatment are also unwilling to treat HIV-infected infertile patients. In a recent survey conducted in France, only 2% of ART practitioners answered that they would be willing to perform an in vitro fertilization (IVF) when the woman is HIV-infected [8]. Three out of 58 HFEA licensed fertility centers would do the same in the UK [9].

However, new progress in the reduction of HIV-vertical transmission has been achieved recently, when it was demonstrated that an elective cesarean delivery performed prior to labor or membrane rupture in women receiving zidovudine therapy could reduce the HIV-transmission rate to the child to only 0.8% compared to 11.4% in the case of emergent cesarean and 6.6% after vaginal delivery [10]. If this result is confirmed and if the efficiency and innocuity of antiretroviral therapies could be improved, new clinical attitudes could be defined to help HIV-infected infertile mothers to have children.

In the case where the infertility treatment of the HIV-infected woman could necessitate IVF, the risk of transmission of the virus to other patients and to the members of the medical and laboratory staff during the different phases of the treatment should be considered. The blood collected together with the oocyte and the follicular fluid could contain viral particles. Therefore, it should be necessary to follow very strict precautions in the management of gametes and embryos.

*The HIV-positive partner is the man*

While unprotected sexual intercourse is, overall, the major route of HIV transmission, the probability of infection through one sexual contact appears to be low, when compared to that resulting from exposure to blood [11]. Although the virus has already been detected in 1984 by culture in the semen of HIV-infected men [12], research to understand the factors influencing the infectivity of semen has not been greatly developed until recent years.

Viral culture, HIV PCR assays have been used to detect the virus in the cellular compartments of semen. Results of viral culture were positive in 9 [13] to 55% [14] of seminal cells samples. The proviral form of HIV has been detected by PCR with similar rates on unselected seminal cells [15,16], and more frequently in lymphocyte-monocyte-enriched fractions [17]. Using electromicroscopy, some authors have reported the detection of virus in germ cells and spermatozoa of infected men [18,19], but these results remain controversial. HIV-RNA can be quantified by RT-PCR in seminal plasma (SP); it is usually detected in a large majority of HIV-positive men [20].

The large differences in the rate of positive-published results may be explained by various factors, such as the number of men included in the study, their origin, their clinical status, the association with infectious genital diseases, and the treatments received. The differences can also be linked to technical factors influencing the sensitivity of viral detection. Human SP contains inhibitors of PCR which may often hamper the detection and quantification of HIV-RNA ([21] — Tachet et al., submitted).

Some temporary conclusions were drawn in 1996 by Mostad and Krebs in a review of the most important published data [20]: detection of HIV-1 in semen could be associated with seminal leucocytosis, ureteral inflammation and gonococcal ureteritis, as well as with CD4 lymphocyte depletion in blood, advanced HIV-1 disease, and inversely associated with antiretroviral therapy. However, in the perspective of medically assisted procreation using spermatozoa of HIV-infected men to reduce the risk of virus transmission, many questions have still to be answered: what are the origin and the localization of the virus in semen? What amount of virus is required to make the transmission effective? What are the respective roles of free viral particles and cell-associated virus in contamination? What are the phenotypic characteristics of the transmitted viral strains? Can the quantification of HIV in blood predict the risk of transmission by semen?

Several recent publications gave important information on this last question, by providing evidence for a compartmentalization of viral populations between blood and semen. Coombs et al. found a lack of association between positive-virus culture in semen and HIV-RNA load in blood, discordant distribution of viral phenotypes, discordant viral RNA levels, a weak correlation between RNA level in semen and CD4 cell count, differences in the variability of viral RNA levels and differences in the response of RNA load to antiretroviral therapy [21]. Kiessling et al. reported that the ratio of infected to uninfected leucocytes in ejaculated semen specimens was highly discordant with that found in paired blood samples, suggesting that these leucocytes derived from distinct populations of infected cells. In addition, they found significant divergence in the protease gene sequence of HIV clones isolated from semen cells and from peripheral blood cells [22].

Assessing HIV burden in both acellular and cellular fractions of semen in 52 HIV-1 seropositive men, Tachet et al. (submitted) found that SP HIV-RNA load was significantly correlated with HIV-RNA load in blood plasma and CD4 count, but two groups of men could be distinguished: a group of men who had HIV-RNA levels in SP significantly lower than in blood plasma, and another group where HIV-RNA loads in SP were equal to or higher than in blood plasma. In this last group, HIV was detected in 100% of the seminal cells, either non-spermatozoal cells and/or spermatozoa. In contrast, HIV was detected in only 44% of the cellular fractions from the men of the first group (Table 1). These results suggest that some men may have a high potential for sexually transmitting HIV which could be related to an independent production of virus in the genital tract. Such results, if they are confirmed, would be of great importance in counselling and treating serodiscordant couples who want to have a child.

*What would be the benefits and risks of assisted procreation in these situations?*

When the HIV-infected partner is a fertile woman, there is no reason for discussing assisted procreation in order to reduce the risk of vertical transmission, since this risk is mainly related to the perinatal period and parturition. The only issues to consider are those raised by a pregnancy in an HIV-infected woman. Intraconjugal artificial insemination could be discussed to avoid horizontal transmission during sexual intercourse. However, the artificial insemination could be done by the seronegative husband himself [23].

More questions are raised by serodifferent couples in which the man is infected by HIV and not the woman. It has been shown that sperm from infected men could transfer HIV-like particles to human oocyte in vitro [24], but to our knowledge there has not been any report of direct vertical transmission of HIV from an infected man to his child. In all cases of children infected at birth, the mother was infected. Therefore, the main purpose is to avoid an horizontal transmission from the infected man to his partner during conception.

When unprotected intercourse is strictly limited to the fertile period, the risk of HIV transmission through natural conception is very low. In a series of 104 con-

*Table 1.* Detection of HIV in semen fractions of seropositive men according to the difference between HIV-RNA load in blood and SP.

|  | Mean HIV-RNA load in SP (log/ml) | Positive HIV detection in NSC (PCR or culture) | Positive HIV-RNA detection in sperma-tozoa |
|---|---|---|---|
| G1 (n = 35) | 3.3 | 16/35 | 1/28 |
| G2 (n = 16) | 4.6 | 13/15 | 5/12 |

G1 = men with at least 0.3 log less HIV-RNA copies in SP than in BP; G2 = men with similar or higher numbers of HIV-RNA copies in SP than in BP; SP = seminal plasma; NSC = nonspermatozoal cells.

secutive pregnancies, among which 17 occurred after a single intercourse, no seroconversions were observed within the first 3 months following conception [25]. Before conception, genital infections were diagnosed and treated, and a basic fertility work up was offered where appropriate and couples were advised to pinpoint ovulation in order to reduce possible exposure. Seroconversion was observed in two women at 7 months of pregnancy and two others after birth. These seroconversions were not related to the fertilizing coitus but to inconsistent use of condom. The main inconvenience of this approach is that the impression is given to some couples that they may be less strict in protecting their sexual contact. It is often said that such approach should not be recommended by medical doctors. However, if a couple has decided to choose it, very strict counselling should be given.

Artificial insemination of sperm populations isolated from SP has been proposed by Semprini et al. [26]. In 29 couples, 17 pregnancies were obtained after 59 inseminations of motile spermatozoa selected by gradient centrifugation and swim-up. No maternal or children seroconversion were observed. More recently, the same group reported similar results after 1,461 inseminations made in 443 women which led to 216 pregnancies [27]. Another group used the same sperm preparation for 101 inseminations from which 31 pregnancies could be obtained in 63 couples without detected contamination in the mothers or the children [28]. In this study, the presence of HIV-RNA and DNA were assessed in the fraction of motile spermatozoa obtained after washing. The detection was positive in six cases and insemination was cancelled. These results show the importance of a very accurate detection of the virus in the sperm population to be used for ART. Safety of the inseminated sperm population can be dependent on the sensitivity of the method used to detect the virus. In the work of Semprini et al., the detection threshold was 800 copies/ml (personal communication). In the work of Marina et al., it was 200 copies/ml. Lower detection thresholds would be needed. Since there could be a variability of virus detection from one sample to another, and also because the amount of virus present in semen can be largely reduced by treatments [29,30], it could be recommended to select a virus-free sperm sample from the infected man after an appropriate treatment, and to freeze it for assisted conception.

In every case, it will not be possible to be sure that virus particles are absent in the sperm population because of limitations in the sensitivity of the laboratory assays. Furthermore, intrauterine insemination needs several million motile spermatozoa to be deposited in the uterus cavity. In the Spanish study, the mean number of inseminated spermatozoa was $13.2 \pm 17.9/10^6$ [28]. Some bleeding may be induced by the catheter during such insemination. Therefore, it is of concern whether artificial insemination is the safest technique using spermatozoa at risk, even if it is very low.

Intracytoplasmic injection of spermatozoa into the oocyte needs only one spermatozoon and suppression of any contact between the sperm and the female genital tract. It should dramatically reduce the risk of transferring viral particles together with the spermatozoa. Since the quantity of virus present in semen is seriously reduced after only 1 month of treatment including antiprotease [29,30], such a strategy could also be discussed if it can be demonstrated that it has no deleterious influence on sperm quality, embryo development and if it does not impair future treatment of the man when it will be needed.

When the couples want to avoid any risk of HIV transmission, the use of the husband's sperm for ART should not be recommended. The first serodiscordant couple with an HIV-infected man requesting donor insemination (AID) came to the CECOS Bicêtre-Cochin in 1986. This kind of demand induced a large debate among the CECOS in France. The main question was: are we allowed to help conceive a child with a donor semen knowing that the health prognostic of his father is very bad and his life expectancy very short?

In the early 1990s, a protocol was set up in order to determine whether the couples in the donor insemination program should be included [31]. Strict attention was accorded to the health status and the prognosis of the man, the protection taken by the couple to avoid HIV transmission in his sexual life, to the attitude towards a parenthood with a donor gamete and towards the risk of the father's death. Evaluation and counselling were undertaken by a multidisciplinary approach including internists, psychiatrists, gynecologists and physicians of the CECOS. At the end of 1996, more than 200 serodifferent couples requested AID in this center. Nearly 20% of the couples were not included in the program mainly for health reasons. In recent years this proportion decreased because of the progress of antiviral therapies. About 30% of couples changed their mind or were lost to follow up. Nearly 50% of couples were included in the program but not all of them started insemination. In some cases the treatment had to be stopped because of health deterioration of the man. More than 40 couples had a child and in only one case the father died when his child was 3 years old.

## Conclusion

Until recently, most of the expressed opinions were that HIV infection was a serious contraindication to infertility treatments. Several recent developments could change the approach of fertility centres to treat infertile and fertile couples in which one or both partners are infected with HIV.

Increasingly, the number of HIV-positive patients are men and women in their reproductive years, and they may wish to become parents. The efficiency of antiviral treatments reduces the risk of rapid death of HIV-infected future parents. A better management of HIV-infected pregnant women could limit seriously the risk of vertical-HIV transmission. Improved laboratory assays for the detection on the virus in the different seminal compartments with a better understanding of the factors influencing the infectivity of HIV-1 seropositive men and with appropriate use of sperm freezing and assisted reproductive technologies could dramatically decrease the risk of HIV transmission between partners of serodifferent couples.

If it seems acceptable to use assisted reproductive technologies to help serodifferent couples to become parents, clear guidelines should be defined in order to avoid the risk of HIV transmission to other patients and to medical and biological staff during the in vitro treatments of gametes and embryos. Of course precautions are necessary for treatments of all patients, whether or not they are HIV-infected, but it should be useful to define specific requirements for this new and at high-risk situation. Specific and careful information and counselling should be also offered to the patients knowing that in most cases it will not be possible to guarantee a complete suppression if HIV transmission is a risk. The respective responsibilities of the demanding patients and the medical staff should be clearly defined and accepted by all participants, including public authorities.

## Acknowledgements

The research work made by our group in this field was supported by the Agence Nationale de Recherches sur le SIDA (ANRS 90V88, EP6 and EP12).

## References

1. Connor EM, Sperling RS, Gelber R, Kiselev P, Scott G, O'Sullivan MJ et al. Reduction of maternal-infant transmission of human immunodeficiency virus type 1 with Zidovudine treatment. N Engl J Med 1994;331:1173—1180.
2. Mayaux MJ, Teglas JP, Mandelbrot R, Berrebi A, Gallais H, Matheron S et al. Acceptability and impact of Zidovudine for prevention of mother-to-child human immunodeficiency virus 1 transmission in France. J Pediatr 1997;131:857—862.
3. Minkoff H, Augenbaum M. Antiretroviral therapy for pregnant women. Am J Obstet Gynecol 1997;176:478—489.
4. Smith JR, Forster GE, Kitchen VS, Hooi YS, Munday PE, Paintin DB et al. Infertility management in HIV positive couples: a dilemma. Br Med J 1991;302:1447—1450.
5. Olaitan A, Reid W, Mocroft A, McCarthy K, Madge S, Johnson M. Infertility among human immunodeficiency virus-positive women: incidence and treatment dilemnas. Hum Reprod 1996;12:793—796.
6. Rizk B, Dill SR. Counselling HIV patients pursuing infertility investigation and treatment. Hum Reprod 1997;12:415—416.
7. Schenker JG. FIGO Committee for the Study of Ethical Aspects of Human Reproduction: guidelines on the subject of AIDS and human reproduction. Hum Reprod 1997;12:1619.
8. Hamamah S, Isnard V, Hubert B. Assistance médicale à la procréation et risques infectieux: enquête sur les risques des centres Français en 1997. Contr Fertil Sex 1998;26:49—52.
9. Balet R, Lower AM, Wilson C, Anderson J, Grodzinskas JG. Attitude towards routine human immunodeficiency virus (HIV) screening and fertility treatment in HIV positive patient — a UK survey. Hum Reprod 1998;13:1085—1087.
10. Mandelbrot L, Le Chenadec J, Berresi A, Bongain A, Benifla JL, Delfraissy JL et al. Perinatal HIV-1 transmission. Interaction between zidovudine prophylaxis and mode of delivery in the French perinatal cohort. JAMA 1998;280:55—60.
11. De Vincenzi I. Longitudinal study of human immunodeficiency virus transmission by heterosexual partners. N Engl J Med 1994;331:341—346.
12. Zagury D, Bernard J, Leibowitch J, Groopman JE, Feldman M, Gallo RC. HTLV III in cells cultured from semen of two patients with AIDS. Science 1984;226:449—451.

13. Anderson DJ, O'Brien TR, Politch JA, Martinez A, Seage III GR, Padian N et al. Effect of disease stage and zidovudine therapy on the detection of human immunodeficiency virus type 1 in semen. JAMA 1992;267:2769—2774.

14. Vernazza PL, Eron JJ, Fiscus SA. Sensitive method for the detection of infection HIV in semen of seropositive individuals. J Virol Meth 1996;56:33—40.

15. Van Vorhis BJ, Martinez A, Mayer K, Anderson DJ. Detection of human immunodeficiency virus type 1 in semen from seropositive men using culture and polymerase chain reaction deoxyribonucleic acid amplification technique. Fertil Steril 1991;55:588—594.

16. Xu C, Politch JA, Tucker L, Mayer KH, Seage JR III, Anderson D. Factors associated with increased levels of human immunodeficiency virus type 1 DNA in semen. J Infect Dis 1997; 176:941—947.

17. Mermin JH, Holodnig M, Katzenstein DA, Merigan TC. Detection of human immunodeficiency virus DNA and RNA in semen by polymerase chain reaction. J Infect Dis 1991;164: 769—772.

18. Dussaix E, Guetard D, Dauguet C, De Almeida M, Auer J, Ellrodt A et al. Spermatozoa as potential carriers of HIV. Res Virol 1993;144:187—195.

19. Nuovo GJ, Becker J, Simsir A, Margiotta M, Khalife G, Shevchuk M. HIV nucleic acid localize to the spermatogonia and their progeny. A study bu polymerase chain reaction in situ hybridization. Am J Pathol 1994;144:1142—1148.

20. Rostad SB, Kreiss JK Shedding of HIV-1 in the genital tract. AIDS 1996;10:1305—1315.

21. Coombs RW, Speck CE, Hughes JP, Lee W, Sampoleo R, Ross SO et al. Association between culturable human immunodeficiency virus type 1 (HIV-1) in semen and HIV-1 levels in semen and blood. Evidence for compartmentalization of HIV-1 between semen and blood. J Infect Dis 1998;177:320—330.

22. Kiessling AA, Fitzgerald LM, Zhang D, Chay H, Brettler D, Eyre RC et al. Human immunodeficiency virus in semen arises from a genetically distinct virus reservoir. AIDS research and human retroviruses 1998;14(Suppl 1):533—541.

23. Smith JR, Reginald PW, Forster SM. Safe sex and conception: a dilemna. Lancet 1990;335:359.

24. Baccetti B, Benedetto A, Burrini AG, Collodel G, Costantino Ceccarini E, Crisa N et al. HIV particles in spermatozoa of patients in the AIDS and their transfer into the oocyte. J Cell Biol 1994;127:903—914.

25. Mandelbrot L, Heard I, Henrion-Gean E, Henrion R. National conception in HIV-negative women with HIV-infected partners. Lancet 1997;349:850—851.

26. Semprini AE, Levy-Setti P, Bozzo M, Ravizza M, Tglioretti A, Sulpizio P et al. Insemination of HIV-negative-women with processed semen of HIV positive partners. Lancet 1992;340: 1317—1319.

27. Semprini AE, Fiore S, Oneta M, Castagna C, Savasi V, Giuntelli S et al. Assisted reproduction in HIV discordant couples. Hum Reprod 1998;13:0—176(Abstract 14th ESHRE Meeting).

28. Marina S, Marina F, Alcolea R, Exposito R, Huguet J, Nadal J et al. Healthy children born using IUI in HIV-1-serodiscordant couples. Fertil Steril 1998;(In press).

29. Politch JA, Mayer KH, Abbott AF, Anderson DJ. The effects of disease progression and zidovudine therapy on semen quality in human immunodeficiency virus type 1 seropositive men. Fertil Steril 1994;61:922—928.

30. Dulioust E, Tachet A, Finkielsztejn L, Salmon-Ceron D, Rouzioux C, Sicard D. HIV RNA Load in Blood and seminal plasma of Patients Receiving Antiretroviral Therapy with Protease Inhibitors. 12th World AIDS Conference 1998 (Abstract).

31. Jouannet P, Kunstmann JM. Donor insemination and fatherhood of HIV infected men. In: Gillet JY (ed) SIDA et Reproduction. Sauramp Medical 1994;267—268.

# *Chlamydia trachomatis* infection — from diagnosis to treatment and prevention

Jorma Paavonen

*Department of Obstetrics and Gynecology, University of Helsinki, Helsinki, Finland*

**Abstract.** *Chlamydia trachomatis* infections are the most prevalent bacterial sexually transmitted infections recognized throughout the world. According to the WHO, 90 million chlamydial infections are annually detected worldwide. *C. trachomatis* is a common cause of urethritis and cervicitis, and sequelae include pelvic inflammatory disease (PID), ectopic pregnancy, tubal factor infertility, epididymitis, proctitis and reactive arthritis. Chlamydial infections cause major medical, social and economic problems. Chlamydial infections, like sexually transmitted infections in general, are primarily a woman's health care issue since the manifestations and consequences are more damaging to the reproductive health in women than in men. Worldwide, the magnitude of morbidity associated with sexually transmitted chlamydial infections is enormous. The sharp worldwide increase in the incidence of PID during the past two decades has led to the secondary epidemics of tubal factor infertility and ectopic pregnancy. Chlamydial PID is the most important preventable cause of infertility and adverse pregnancy outcome. Immunopathogenesis of *C. trachomatis* infection is the focus of current chlamydia research. Nucleic acid amplification tests are the tests of choice for diagnosing *C. trachomatis* infection. These tests for the first time provide diagnostic tests for *C. trachomatis* that are more sensitive than culture or antigen tests. Azithromycin prescribed as a single oral dose is equivalent to the traditional 7-day regimen of doxycycline for treating uncomplicated genital chlamydial infections. Chlamydial infection fills the general prerequisites for disease prevention by screening, i.e., chlamydial infections are highly prevalent, usually asymptomatic, are associated with significant morbidity, can be reliably diagnosed and are treatable. Screening programs for *C. trachomatis* will be of paramount importance in the prevention of long-term sequelae. Emerging cost-benefit studies demonstrate that the cost of screening is only a fraction of the health care costs incurred due to the short-term and long-term complications resulting from undiagnosed and untreated chlamydial infections.

**Keywords:** *Chlamydia trachomatis* infection.

## Introduction

*Chlamydia trachomatis* infections are the most prevalent bacterial sexually transmitted infections recognized throughout the world. According to the WHO, 90 million chlamydial infections are annually detected worldwide [1]. *C. trachomatis* is a common cause of urethritis and cervicitis, and sequelae include pelvic inflammatory disease (PID), ectopic pregnancy, tubal factor infertility, epididymitis, proctitis and reactive arthritis [2]. Chlamydial infections cause major medi-

*Address for correspondence:* Prof Jorma Paavonen MD, Department of Obstetrics and Gynecology, University of Helsinki, 00290 Helsinki, Finland. Tel.: +358-9-4712807. Fax: +358-9-4714902.
E-mail: jorma.paavonen@huch.fi

cal, social and economic problems. Chlamydial infections, like sexually transmitted infections (STI) in general, are primarily a woman's health care issue since the manifestations and consequences are more damaging to the reproductive health in women than in men. Worldwide, the magnitude of morbidity associated with sexually transmitted chlamydial infections is enormous.

## Cell biology of *C. trachomatis*

Chlamydiae are small intracellular bacteria that need living cells to multiply. The chlamydial chromosome consists of approximately 1 million base pairs and has a capacity to encode for up to 600 proteins. There are 18 distinct serotypes of *C. trachomatis* currently identified. Serotypes D−K cause sexually transmitted genital infections and neonatal infections (Table 1). There is no strong evidence that specific genital syndromes or clinical manifestations, such as PID, are serotype-specific. The cell cycle of chlamydiae is distinct from all other bacteria. Endocytosis leads to the formation of membrane-bound intracellular inclusions. The ability of chlamydia to convert from resting to replicating infectious forms within host cells creates increasing difficulties in eliminating this microbe. However, much is not yet understood about specific mechanisms in the membrane events, attachment and endocytosis, multiplication of the organism in the cell, transformation from metabolically inactive elementary body (EB) into metabolically active replicative reticulate body (RB), and expression of different chlamydial antigens during the cell cycle. The amount of new information on the cell biology of chlamydia infection recently emerged has been enormous. Richard S. Stephens and his colleagues from Stanford have recently sequenced the first chlamydia genome (R.S. Stephens, S. Kalman, C. Fenner, R. Davis, "Chlamydia Genome Project" at http://chlamydia-www.berkeley.edu:4231/.). This information has already revolutionized approaches to study these unique obligate intracellular bacteria.

Chlamydial infection begins by contact of infectious EB with the epithelial apical surface of a target cell. The specific interaction triggers a series of early events which helps program the chlamydia and prime the host cell for productive infec-

*Table 1.* Spectrum of human diseases caused by *Chlamydia trachomatis.*

| Species | Acute diseases | Sequelae/chronic diseases |
| --- | --- | --- |
| *C. trachomatis* | | |
| Serovars A−C | Conjunctivitis | Trachoma |
| Serovars D−K | Urethritis | Proctitis, epididymitis, Reiter syndrome |
| | Cervicitis | Pelvic inflammatory disease, ectopic pregnancy, tubal infertility |
| | Ophthalmia neonatorum | |
| | Neonatal pneumonia | |
| LGV serovars | Lymphogranuloma venerum | |

tion [3]. Proposed mechanisms of chlamydia uptake are parasite-specified phago-cytosis, receptor-mediated endocytosis and pinocytosis. Chlamydia primes the host cell early for its obligate intracellular growth and inclusion development. Early intracellular fate and early chlamydial gene expression results in vacuole modification to ensure trafficking of EB to the exocytic pathway. Chlamydia goes through a development cycle involving transition of EB to RB, RB to RB via binary fission, maturation of RB to EB, and the release of infectious EB. *C. trachomatis* develops a single inclusion in which the glycogen is retained. Glyco-gen may provide an extra energy source within the *C. trachomatis* inclusion, since it is devoid of associated mitochondria.

## Clinical manifestation of chlamydial infection in women

*C. trachomatis* is the major cause of mucopurulent cervicitis (MPC) [4] and pel-vic inflammatory disease (PID) in women [5]. Urethritis or acute urethral syn-drome is often associated with chlamydial cervicitis [6]. MPC is the ignored counterpart in women of urethritis in men. Chlamydial MPC can lead to at least three types of complications:

1) ascending intraluminal spread of organisms from the cervix, producing pelvic inflammatory disease (PID) [7];
2) ascending infection during pregnancy resulting in premature rupture of the membranes, chorionamnionitis, premature delivery and puerperal and neona-tal infections [8]; and
3) the development of cervical neoplasia. Although oncogenic types of human papillomavirus clearly cause most, if not all, cervical carcinomas, *C. tracho-matis* seems to play an important cofactor role [9].

Although simple objective criteria have been developed for the presumptive diag-nosis of MPC, most cases of chlamydial cervicitis are asymptomatic or mini-mally symptomatic, and show no specific clinical signs. Approximately half of all women with chlamydial infection have the infection both in the cervix and the urethra, one-third in the cervix only and approximately 15—25% in the ure-thra only. Specific colposcopic, cytological and histopathological manifestations of chlamydial cervicitis have been described [10—12]. Histopathological findings associated with chlamydial cervicitis include plasma cell infiltrations of cervical stroma, intraepithelial and intraluminal inflammation, and well-formed lym-phoid follicles comprising transformed lymphocytes.

Pelvic inflammatory disease (PID) refers to infection of the uterus, fallopian tubes and the adjacent pelvic structures that is not associated with surgery or pregnancy [7]. *C. trachomatis* is the major cause of PID. The clinical spectrum of chlamydial PID ranges from subclinical endometritis to frank salpingitis, tubo-ovarian abscess, pelvic peritonitis, periappendicitis and perihepatitis. Most studies of chlamydial PID have focused on inpatients with acute symptoms and severe disease. However, such cases may represent only the tip of the iceberg of all chlamydial infections of the upper genital tract. The relative role of *C. tracho-*

*matis* in PID has increased since the gonorrhoea rates have recently dramatically decreased in many countries [13]. An increasing proportion of cases with chlamydial PID are atypical or silent. Simultaneously there has been a dramatic drop in the incidence of inpatient PID. Hospitalizations of women with PID have rapidly decreased which is probably due to a change in the clinical manifestations of PID [14]. However, this does not necessarily mean that the overall incidence of PID has decreased. In fact, minimally symptomatic patients usually delay in seeking medical care, which may further increase the risk for tubal damage and long-term sequelae [15].

Demonstrations of plasma cell endometritis by endometrial biopsy in women with MPC in the absence of symptoms or signs of PID has focused attention on silent chlamydial infection of the upper genital tract [16]. Studies have shown that not just clinical PID but also silent PID is associated with permanent tubal damage [17]. Thus, symptomatic PID is not a prerequisite for the eventual development of tubal damage.

**Sequelae of chlamydial infection of the upper genital tract**

The sharp worldwide increase in the incidence of PID during the past two decades has led to the secondary epidemics of infertility and ectopic pregnancy. Chlamydial PID is the most important preventable cause of infertility and adverse pregnancy outcome. The proportion of tubal factor infertility of all infertility ranges from less than 40% in developed countries to up to 85% in developing countries [18]. After a single episode of PID the relative risk for tubal factor infertility is approximately 10%. Each repeat episode of PID doubles the risk so that it is approximately 20% after two episodes, and almost 40% after three or more episodes [19,20]. Results of both epidemiological studies and animal model studies are consistent with the hypothesis that both symptomatic and asymptomatic *C. trachomatis* infection of the female genital tract can induce reproductive tract damage. Seroepidemiological studies also support the concept of silent chlamydial PID demonstrating a strong link between serum antibodies to *C. trachomatis* and tubal factor infertility or ectopic pregnancy, both in women with and without self-reported history of PID [21]. Not surprisingly, most women who have tubal factor infertility have never been diagnosed as having chlamydial infection or PID.

Tubal factor infertility remains the most common indication for in vitro fertilization (IVF). Worldwide, huge amounts of money are spent on PID sequelae. For instance, the cost of IVF, most often performed for post-PID tubal factor infertility, is extremely high [22].

Adverse pregnancy outcome is another major complication of chlamydial infection. Ectopic pregnancy is the main cause of maternal mortality in the first trimester of pregnancy in developing countries. In the USA, ectopic pregnancy related deaths account for 9% of all pregnancy related deaths. Women with a history of PID have a 7- to 10-fold increased risk of tubal pregnancy compared to women with no history of PID [19,23]. The incidence of ectopic pregnancy has been increasing during the past two decades. Ectopic pregnancy is also a marker of subsequent repeat ectopic pregnancy and infertility. The recurrence rate of ectopic pregnancy is approximately 20%.

In addition to infertility and ectopic pregnancy, other morbidity is also associated with a history of PID, such as chronic pelvic pain caused by extraluminal scarring. Chronic pelvic pain following PID occurs in 24—75% of women. In one study, women with a diagnosis of PID were 10 times more likely to be admitted for abdominal pain, 4 times more likely to be admitted for gynaecological pain, and 6 times more likely to be admitted for ectopic pregnancy [24]. A substantially higher risk of hysterectomy after PID was found. Hysterectomy rates were approximately 8 times higher in cases of PID than in the controls. Women with a history of hospitalization for PID had greatly increased rates of subsequent hospital admission for a variety of other conditions. Thus, women with PID suffer substantial long-term gynecological morbidity later in their lives.

There is some evidence that *C. trachomatis* may also contribute to other pregnancy complications than ectopic pregnancy, including premature rupture of membranes, preterm birth, low birth weight and stillbirth [8]. Early pregnancy loss may be induced by asymptomatic *C. trachomatis* infection through the operation of immune mechanisms [25,26].

## Immunopathogenesis of *C. trachomatis* infection

*C. trachomatis* is a strong immunogen which stimulates both humoral and cell-mediated immune responses [27]. In addition to the immunogenetic antigens, the outcome of *C. trachomatis* infection depends on interaction and balance of cytokines secreted by the activated lymphocytes. IFN-$\gamma$, a typical product of Th1 cells, has been described as a single most important factor in host defense against chlamydia while disease susceptibility has been linked with enhanced expression of IL-10, a marker of Th2 cell activation [28,29]. Immune system perturbations induced by *C. trachomatis* may in fact assist its own survival in the infected host and induce persistent infections. Several previous clinical or epidemiological observations suggest that there is an intimate relationship between chlamydia and the host immune system. Such observations suggest that a single acute episode of chlamydial infection per se cannot account for all the striking pathology associated with chlamydial disease. Persistent inflammation after proper curative therapy for chlamydial infection has been a puzzling phenomenon in many clinical studies. For instance, persistent inflammation of the cervix not explained by relapse or reinfection was still present 3 months after proper curative therapy in one-third of women treated for chlamydial MPC [30]. Similarly, not only adhesion formation and tubal occlusions but also persistent striking inflammation of the fallopian tubes was frequently seen during second-look laparoscopy which was performed 4—6 months after the index episode of PID [31]. Experimental studies on the monkey "pocket" model support the role of T cell response to HSP60 in the pathogenesis of chlamydial salpingitis [32]. Pig-tailed monkeys were sensitised by inoculation of live *C. trachomatis* organisms into subcutaneous pockets containing salpingeal autotransplants. When recombinant chlamydial HSP60 was injected into such pockets, either previously sensitised or not sensitised in the same monkey, a typical delayed hypersensitivity reaction was observed. However, much less is known of the cell-mediated immune response to HSPs in humans. A positive lymphocyte proliferation response of peripheral blood mononuclear cells to recombinant HSP60 was more common in women with PID than women without PID, or in controls [33]. Most of those with a positive response had a history of PID or ectopic pregnancy, suggesting that the duration of exposure plays an important role in the chlamydia-specific T cell response. Induction of Th1- or Th2-type T helper cell response may be an important determinant of chlamydial disease pathogenesis. Th1 response induces IFN-$\gamma$ which turns on the efferent arm of the cell-mediated immunity. High levels of IFN-$\gamma$ have been detected in endocervical secretions of patients with chlamydial cervicitis and in sera of patients with chlamydial PID (for a review see [34,35]). Many in vitro studies have shown that treatment of infected cells with IFN-$\gamma$ limits the replication of chlamydiae. Interestingly, IFN-$\gamma$ mediates the development of atypical chlamydial forms in vitro [28]. These atypical forms display reduced levels of chlamydial major outer membrane protein (MOMP) and lipopolysaccharide (LPS) antigens, but continued high production of chlamydial heat shock protein, HSP60. In vivo, such persistently infected cells could serve as accumulations of HSP60 antigen capable of inducing chronic inflammation.

**The role of chlamydial heat shock proteins in the immunopathogenesis**

Heat shock proteins (HSPs) serve as important antigens of infectious agents, and are among the most conserved molecules in phylogeny. HSPs are important in a variety of cellular functions and are highly conserved between mammalian and bacterial species. Among the most studied HSPs is the HSP60 family which includes, for instance, groEL of *Escherichia coli*, HSP65 of mycobacteria, and mitochondrial P1, the mammalian cognate of bacterial HSP60. One current hypothesis is that chronic sequelae of chlamydial infection are caused by a delayed hypersensitivity reaction to chlamydial HSPs, particularly the 57-kDa HSP which belongs to the HSP60 family [36]. The amino acid homology between microbial and human HSP counterparts is high [37]. The HSP60 is the major chlamydial protein produced during chronic, silent or nonproductive infections.

Many studies have already looked at the antibody responses to intact chlamydial HSP60, and generally found a good correlation between the serum antibodies HSP60 and PID, tubal factor infertility or ectopic pregnancy. In women with a prior history of chlamydial PID, laparoscopically observed tubal obstruction, laparoscopically observed degree of tubal inflammation, and the presence of moderate to severe adhesions were all associated with serum antibodies to

HSP60 [38]. Thus, serum antibodies to intact chlamydial HSP60 seem to predict reproductive tract damage better than serum antibodies to chlamydial MOMP antigen.

Although the antigenic structure of HSP60 has been analysed in detail by monoclonal antibodies and polyclonal antisera, data on specific B cell epitopes or T cell epitopes of chlamydial HSP60 recognised by human sera are still limited. However, antibody response to specific B cell epitopes of *C. trachomatis* HSP60 have been described in infants with chlamydial infection [39] in women with PID [40].

The high molecular mimicry of human and chlamydial HSPs may also induce an autoimmune response. Chlamydial and human HSP60 are candidate targets to autoimmune T cells, although so far not much is known of possible cross-reactive T cell epitopes. Local accumulation of chlamydial HSPs and cross-reactive immune response can generate an autoimmune reaction that explains part of the inflammatory reaction and pathology seen after chlamydial PID. However, although autoimmune reactions may play some role in the chronic sequelae of chlamydial infections, delayed hypersensitivity response to chlamydial HSP60 associated with persistent or recurrent infections probably plays a more important role.

Future studies should characterize the relevant T helper cell epitopes of *C. trachomatis* HSP60 with particular attention to epitopes associated with the delayed type hypersensitivity (DTH) reaction, and the nature of chlamydial DTH reaction in women. The working hypothesis is that Th1 and Th2 type cells discriminate between specific peptides, that CD8+ cells suppress the Th1 type response, and that these findings show a significant correlation with the histopathological severity of upper tract infection and immune perturbations subsequently leading to long-term sequelae. Future studies showed also investigate the regulation of T cell subset differentiation (Th1 and Th2 cells) by different antigen presenting cells (macrophages, B cells, and Langerhans cells).

**Diagnosis of *C. trachomatis* infections**

Nucleic acid amplification tests (NAAT) must be considered the tests of choice for diagnosing *C. trachomatis* infection [41–43]. The NAATs for the first time provide diagnostic tests for *C. trachomatis* that are more sensitive than culture or antigen tests. This holds true for all three of the currently available commercial tests: the polymerase chain reaction (PCR) (Roche Molecular Systems, Branchburg, NJ), the ligase chain reaction (LCR) (Abbott Laboratories, Abbott Park, IL), and transcription mediated amplification (TMA) (Gen-Probe, Inc, La Jolla, CA). PCR and LCR each target nucleotide sequences in the chlamydial cryptic plasmid. The plasmid is present in approximately seven to 10 copies per elementary body, thus giving a sensitivity advantage over a chromosomal DNA target. It appears that the NAATs each provide sensitivities over 90% [44]. NAATs have very few false-positive results and the specificities approach 100%. It has become clear that the older literature underestimated the true prevalence of chlamydial infection.

The nucleic acid amplification tests have another major advantage in that they can be used with first void urine (FVU) specimens and with vaginal or vulvar swabs. The absolute number of positive results with the urine specimens approaches that obtained with cervical swabs. If a women is having a pelvic examination, a specimen should be collected from the cervix. However, if a pelvic examination is not being performed, a urine specimen may be tested with the reasonable assurance of getting an accurate result.

Although the nucleic acid amplification tests are more expensive than the antigen tests, they still should be considered the tests of choice because they will detect many more infected individuals. It is cost-effective to use the more expensive test because the management of complications of chlamydial infections is very expensive. Detecting and treating the maximal number of infections is the goal of chlamydia screening programs. The use of noninvasive specimen collection, with no requirement for a physical examination for specimen collection to diagnose chlamydial infection will have a major impact on chlamydia control programs in the near future. The bottom line is that the prevalence of *C. trachomatis* infection in more than enough to justify the broad-based use of screening using NAATs.

**Treatment of *C. trachomatis* infections**

New guidelines for the treatment of patients with sexually transmitted chlamydial infection have been recently published [45]. Azithromycin prescribed as a single oral 1-g dose is equivalent to the traditional 7-day regimen of doxycycline (100 mg twice daily) for treating ocular and uncomplicated genital chlamydial infections [46]. Compared with conventional therapy, azithromycin has excellent pharmacokinetic characteristics, such as bioavailability; lower incidence of gastrointestinal tract side effects, and increased concentration in mucus, macrophages and tissues with a half-life of 5–7 days. These characteristics allow for single dosing, which alleviates the problem of patient noncompliance with multiday regimens. With single-dose therapy, the potential for reinfection due to earlier resumption of sexual activity is a concern. At present, there are limited data on the use of single-dose therapy in adolescents, during pregnancy, and for syndromes such as PID. Studies are needed to determine if these regimens achieve clinical and microbiologic cures while preserving fertility and preventing further tissue damage to the upper genital tract. Although the higher cost of azithromycin may be prohibitive for its use in resource-limited settings, selective use in persons at high risk or in those with a history of noncompliance may prove cost-effective. The cost of retreatment as a result of noncompliance and the additional cost of contact tracing can make single-dose azithromycin more cost-effective than doxycycline.

Alternative treatment regimens include erythromycin base 500 mg four times daily for 7 days, erythromycin ethyl succinate 800 mg three times daily for 7 days, and ofloxacin 300 mg twice daily for 7 days.

## Prevention of *C. trachomatis* infections

The control of STDs is a public-health priority and one that has become of even higher priority with the HIV epidemic. Since STDs and HIV share many behavioral risk factors, efforts to encourage individuals to modify sexual behaviors and adopt safer sexual practices will have a beneficial impact on both. Screening for *C. trachomatis* is of paramount importance in the prevention of long-term sequelae associated with PID. Chlamydia control programs should include the development of diagnostic services with proper quality control, guidelines for clinicians in the clinical diagnosis and management of cervicitis and PID, screening to identify asymptomatic carriers of *C. trachomatis*, the establishment of surveillance systems, training of health care workers, periodic monitoring and evaluation of control measures, routine evaluation of sex partners, and effective patient education in behavioral aspects and contraception.

Disease prevention can be primary, secondary or tertiary. Primary and secondary prevention programmes need to be strengthened and integrated into health care systems, and must be accessible to all. Tertiary prevention of acute and chronic chlamydial infections of the upper genital tract has largely failed because substantial tubal damage has already occurred by the time symptoms develop. Delay of care is another critical factor predicting permanent tubal damage. Although patients respond to antimicrobial therapy, the risk of developing tubal factor infertility or ectopic pregnancy may still be high.

Primary prevention involves preventing both exposure to and acquisition of chlamydial infection through lifestyle counselling and health education. Clinicians play an important role in the primary prevention by asking questions about high-risk sexual behavior, by encouraging screening tests for those at risk, by ensuring that male sex partners are evaluated and treated, and by counseling about safe sex practices. Primary prevention by health education has not proven to be very effective so far. However, studies of the efficacy of primary prevention are slow and extremely complicated to conduct. Clearly, more emphasis should be directed to primary prevention. Effective health education programmes should be implemented among adolescents.

Secondary prevention by universal screening is likely to play a critical role in the prevention of PID and long-term sequelae. Chlamydial infection fills the general prerequisites for disease prevention by screening, since chlamydial infections are highly prevalent, are associated with significant morbidity, can be diagnosed, and are treatable. Secondary prevention means early detection of asymptomatic disease by screening in order to prevent lower genital tract infection from becoming upper genital tract infection. One recent randomized controlled trial has provided strong evidence that intervention with selective screening for chlamydial infections effectively reduces the incidence of PID (Table 2) [47]. Recent techno-

*Table 2.* Randomized intervention trial: selective screening for *C. trachomatis* reduces the incidence of pelvic inflammatory disease (PID) in patients (n = 380,000) at the Group Health Cooperative of Puget Sound (see [46]). Both the intervention group and control group were followed for 12 months.

| Group | Incidence and rate of PID | | |
|---|---|---|---|
| | No. | Rate[a] | RR |
| Intervention group[b] | 9 | 8 | 0.44 (0.2—0.9) |
| Control group | 33 | 18 | refer |

[a]Rate per 10,000 woman-months; [b]comprised 2,607 (13%) of 20,836 eligible women.

logical advances should further enhance efforts to prevent chlamydial infection. These include single-dose therapy using azithromycin, use of nucleic acid amplification tests and the use of first-void urine specimens for the diagnosis. However, it still remains to be seen whether such intervention will also have a significant effect on the incidence of ectopic pregnancy and tubal factor infertility.

More research will also be required to increase our knowledge of the distribution of these infections in different populations, and to understand the link between chlamydial infection and reproductive health in women.

### Cost-benefit analysis of first-void urine *C. trachomatis* screening program

Cost analyses are still rare among trials that compare pharmacological or procedural health care interventions. Socioeconomic studies linking secondary prevention of *C. trachomatis* infection and infertility and adverse pregnancy outcome are needed to convince public health authorities of the need for and benefit of such programs. Rates of *C. trachomatis* infection still remain high both in developed and in developing countries which suggests that the traditional STD control programs are not effective against *C. trachomatis*. The current practice of detection of *C. trachomatis* infection in most clinical settings is presumptive and expectant, and screening programs have not been implemented extensively.

Screening through first-void urine testing may contribute to the early detection of chlamydial infections because most infections are asymptomatic or minimally symptomatic. It is likely that the cost of screening is only a fraction of the health care costs incurred due to short-term and long-term complications resulting from undiagnosed and untreated chlamydial infection. In a recent study, a decision tree was developed to conduct a cost-benefit analysis of screening compared to nonscreening situation [48]. Selected variables based on assumptions were subjected to sensitivity analyses in order to make the model accurate and defensible. Screening for chlamydial infections using the first void urine PCR test was shown to be cost-effective even in low-prevalence populations. Compared with a symptom-driven nonscreening situation, a universal *C. trachomatis* screening program using the PCR test would save money, in terms of direct costs, when the baseline prevalence of *C. trachomatis* infection exceeds 3.9%. In addition to cost savings,

*Table 3.* The health-related outcomes of *C. trachomatis*-infected patients predicted by the decision tree model (see [46]).

| Outcomes | Nonscreening (%) | Screening (%) | Health benefits of screening (%) |
|---|---|---|---|
| Cured | 44.6 | 71.6 | +62.3 |
| Infertility | 11.0[a] | 5.6[b] | −50.9 |
| Tubal pregnancy | 13.8 | 7.0 | −50.7 |
| Pain | 30.3 | 15.5 | −51.2 |
| Laparotomy | 0.3 | 0.2 | −66.7 |

[a]8.3% will have ⩾1 IVF (96 IVF attempts per 10,000 individuals); [b]4.2% will have ⩾1 IVF (49 IVF attempts per 10,000 individuals).

the screening situation also produced considerable health benefits compared with nonscreening situation. In the screening situation, the proportion of cured patients increased by approximately 62% and approximately 50% fewer had long-term complications (Table 3). This model can of course be developed further. From a practical point of view, an important question is whether specific subpopulations of women (i.e., high-risk groups) could be selected for screening. If the selection criteria are practical (i.e., a smaller population with a higher prevalence of infection is studied), the screening would cost less and save even more money. The most effective strategy would likely be to target only women less than 25 years of age. Since repeat screening would further lower the baseline prevalence of *C. trachomatis* infection, universal screening would become less favorable over time, and more targeted screening approaches then would be required to maintain an acceptable cost-benefit.

## References

1. Gerbase AC, Rowley JT, Mertens TE. Global epidemiology of sexually transmitted diseases. Lancet 1998;351(Suppl III) S2–S4.
2. Schachter J. Chlamydial infections (in three parts). N Engl J Med 1978;298:428–435; 490–495; 540–549.
3. Wyrick PB. Cell biology of chlamydial infection: a journey in the host epithelial cell by the ultimate cellular microbiologist. In: Stephens RS, Byrne GI, Christiansen G et al. (eds) Proceedings of the Ninth International Symposium on Human Chlamydial Infection. 1998;69–78.
4. Brunham RC, Paavonen J, Stevens C et al. Mucopurulent cervicitis — the ignored counterpart of urethritis in men. N Engl J Med 1984;158:510–517.
5. Mårdh PA, Ripa KT, Svensson L et al. *C. trachomatis* infection in patients with acute salpingitis. N Engl J Med 1977;296:1377–1379.
6. Stamm WE, Wagner KF, Amsel R, Alexander ER, Turck M, Counts GW, Holmes KK. Causes of the acute urehral syndrome in women. N Engl J Med 1980;303:409–415.
7. McCormack WM. Pelvic inflammatory disease. N Engl J Med 1994;330:115–119.
8. Gravett MG, Nelson HP, DeRouen T, Critchlow C, Eschenbach DA, Holmes KK. Independent associations of bacterial vaginosis and chlamydia trachomatis infection with adverse pregnancy outcome. JAMA 1986;256:1899–1903.

508

9. Paavonen J, Anttila T, Koskela P, Lehtinen M, and the Nordic Serum Bank Study Group. Chlamydia trachomatis and cervical cancer. In: Stephens RS, Byrne GI, Christiansen G et al. (eds) Proceedings of the Ninth International Symposium on Human Chlamydial Infection. 1998;39—42.

10. Paavonen J, Kiviat N, Wölner-Hanssen P, Stevens CE, Critchlow CW, DeRouen T, Koutsky L, Stamm WE, Corey L, Holmes KK. Colposcopic manifestation of cervical and vaginal infections. Obstet Gynecol Surv 1988;43:373—381.

11. Kiviat N, Paavonen J, Brockway J, Critchlow C, Brunham RC, Stevens CE, Stamm WE, Kuo C-C, DeRouen T, Holmes KK. Cytologic manifestation of cervical and vaginal infections. 1. Epithelial and inflammatory cellular changes. JAMA 1985;253:989—996.

12. Kiviat N, Paavonen J, Wolner-Hanssen P et al. Histopathology of endocervical infection caused by C. trachomatis, herpes simplex virus, trichomonas vaginalis, and neisseria gonorrhoeae. Hum Pathol 1990;21:831—837.

13. Hiltunen-Back E, Rostila T, Kautiainen H, Paavonen J, Reunala T. Rapid decrease of epidemic gonorrhea in Finland. Sex Transm Dis 1998;25:181—186.

14. Kamwendo F, Forslin L, Bodin L, Danielsson D. Programmed to reduce pelvic inflammatory disease — the Swedish experience. Lancet 1998;351(Suppl III):S25—S28.

15. Hillis SD, Joesoef R, Marchbanks PA et al. Delayed care of pelvic inflammatory disease as a risk factor of impaired fertility. Am J Obstet Gynecol 1993;168:1503—1509.

16. Paavonen J, Kiviat N, Brunham RC et al. Prevalence and manifestations of endometritis among women with cervicitis. Am J Obstet Gynecol 1985;152:280—286.

17. Patton DL, Moore DE, Spadoni LR et al. A comparison of the fallopian tubes response to overt silent salpingitis. Obstet Gynecol 1989;73:622—630.

18. World Health Organization. Infections, pregnancies and infertility: perspectives on prevention. Fertil Steril 1987;47:964—968.

19. Weström L. Incidence, prevalence and trends of acute pelvic inflammatory disease and its consequences in industrial countries. Am J Obstet Gynecol 1980;138:880—892.

20. Weström LV. Sexually transmitted diseases and infertility. Sex Transm Dis 1994;21:32—37.

21. Cates W, Wasserheit JN. Genital chlamydial infections: epidemiology and reproductive sequelae. Am J Obstet Gynecol 1991;164:1771—1781.

22. Neumann PJ, Gharib SD, Weinstein MC. The cost of a successful delivery in vitro fertilization. N Engl J Med 1994;331:239—243.

23. Weström L, Bengtsson LP, Mårdh PA. Incidence, trends and risks of ectopic pregnancy in a population of women. BMJ 1981;82:15—18.

24. Buchan H, Vessey M, Goldacre M et al. Morbidity following pelvic inflammatory disease. Br J Obstet Gynaecol 1993;100:558—562.

25. Witkin SS. Immune pathogenesis of asymptomatic chlamydia trachomatis infections in the female genital tract. Infect Dis Obstet Gynecol 1995;3:169—174.

26. Witkin SS, Ledger WJ. Antibodies to chlamydia trachomatis in sera of women with recurrent spontaneous abortion. Am J Obstet Gynecol 1992;167:135—139.

27. Peeling RW, Brunham RC. Chlamydia as pathogens: new species and new issues. Emerg Infect Dis 1996;2:1—7

28. Beatty WL, Byrne GI, Morrison RP. Morphologic and antigenic characterization of interferon γ-mediated persistent chlamydia trachomatis infection in vitro. Proc Natl Acad Sci 1993;90:3998—4002.

29. Yang X, HayGlass KT, Brunham RC. Genetically determined differences in IL-10 and IFNγ responses correlate with clearance of chlamydia trachomatis mouse pneumonitis infection. J Immunol 1997;156:4338—4344.

30. Paavonen J, Roberts PL, Stevens CE, Stamm WE, Kuo CC, Wölner-Hanssen P, Brunham RC, Hillier S, DeRouen T, Holmes KK, Eschenbach DA. Randomized treatment of mucopurulent cervicitis with doxycycline or amoxicillin. Am J Obstet Gynecol 1989;161:128—135.

31. Teisala K, Heinonen PK, Aine R, Punonen R, Paavonen J. Second laparoscopy after treatment

of acute pelvic inflammatory disease. Obstet Gynecol 1987;69:343—346.

32. Patton DL, Cosgrowe Sweeney YT, Kuo CC. Demonstration of delayed hypersensitivity in chlamydia trachomatis salpingitis in monkeys: a pathogenic mechanism of tubal damage. J Infect Dis 1994;69:680—-683.

33. Witkin SS, Jeremias J, Toth M et al. Proliferative response to conserved epitopes of the C. trachomatis and human 60-kilodalton heat-shock proteins by lymphocytes from women with salpingitis. Am J Obstet Gynecol 1994;171:455—460.

34. Paavonen J, Lehtinen M. Chlamydial pelvic inflammatory disease. Hum Reprod Update 1996; 2:519—529.

35. Paavonen J. Chlamydia trachomatis infection and host response. In: Templeton A (ed) The Prevention of Pelvic Infection. Proceedings of the 31th Study Group of the Royal College of Obstetrics and Gynecology. London: RCOG Press, 1996;107—120.

36. Morrison RP, Beland RP, Lyng K et al. Chlamydia disease pathogenesis. The 57-kDa chlamydial hypersinsitivity is stress response protein. J Exp Med 1989;169:663—675.

37. Paavonen J, Lehtinen M. Immunopathogenesis of chlamydial pelvic inflammatory disease — the role of heat-shock proteins. Infect Dis Obstet Gynecol 1994;2:105—110.

38. Eckert LO, Hawes SE, Wölner-Hanssen P, Money DM, Peeling RW, Brunham RC, Stevens CE, Eshenbach DA, Stamm WE. Prevalence and correlates of antibody chlamydial heat shock protein in women attending sexually transmitted disease clinics and women with confirmed pelvic inflammatory disease. J Infect Dis 1997;175:1453—1458.

39. Paavonen J, Lähdeaho ML, Puolakkainen M, Mäki M, Parkkonen P, Lehtinen M. Antibody response to B cell epitopes of chlamydia trachomatis 60-kDa heat-shock protein and corresponding mycobacterial and human peptides in infants with chlamydial pneumonitis. J Infect Dis 1994;169:908—911.

40. Domeika M, Domeika K, Paavonen J, Måardh PA, Witkin SS. Humoral immune response to conserved epitopes of chlamydia trachomatis and human 60-kDa heat-shock protein in women with pelvic inflammatory disease. J Infect Dis 1998;177:714—719.

41. Black CM. Current methods of laboratory diagnosis of chlamydia trachomatis infection. Clin Microbiol Rev 1997;10:160—184.

42. Lee HH, Chernesky MA, Schachter J et al. Diagnosis of C. trachomatis genitourinary infection in women by ligase chain reaction of urine. Lancet 1995;345:213—216.

43. Schachter J, Moncada J, Whidden R, Shaw H, Bolan G, Burczak JD, Lee HH. Noninvasive tests for diagnosis of chlamydia trachomatis infection: application of ligase chain reaction to first-catch urine specimens of women. J Infect Dis 1995;172:1411—1444.

44. Puolakkainen M, Hiltunen-Back E, Reunala T, Suhonen S, Lähteenmäki P, Lehtinen M, Paavonen J. Comparison of performances of two commercially available tests, a PCR assay and a ligace chain reaction test, in detection of urogenital chlamydia trachomatis infection. J Clin Microbiol 1998;36:1489—1493.

45. Centers for Disease Control and Prevention. 1998 guidelines for treatment of sexually transmitted diseases. MMWR 1998;47:1—111.

46. Martin DH, Mroczkowski TF, Dalu ZA et al. A controlled trial of a single dose of azithromycin for the treatment of chlamydial urethritis and cervicitis. N Engl J Med 1992;327:921—925.

47. Scholes D, Stergachis A, Heidrich FE et al. Prevention of pelvic inflammatory disease by screening for cervical chlamydial infection. N Engl J Med 1996;334:1362—1366.

48. Paavonen J, Puolakkainen M, Paukku M et al. Cost-benefit analysis of universal C. trachomatis screening program. Obstet Gynecol 1998;(In press).

©1998 Elsevier Science B.V. All rights reserved.
Fertility and Reproductive Medicine.
R.D. Kempers, J. Cohen, A.F. Haney and J.B. Younger, editors.

# The impact of contaminant genital tract microorganisms on the results of ART

E. Cottell and R.F. Harrison
*Department of Obstetrics and Gynaecology, Royal College of Surgeons in Ireland, at the Rotunda Hospital, Dublin, Ireland*

**Abstract.** *Background.* Contamination of the IVF/ET culture system by potentially infective microorganisms, usually commensals, can be detrimental to outcome.

*Methods.* This paper reviews in the context of present clinical practice the three main sources of potential contamination, environment, semen and vagina.

*Results.* Good laboratory practice and assiduous preparation should eliminate environmental causes. Both seminal fluid and the vagina may be significant reservoirs. Washing with culture medium containing minimum levels of antibiotics, however, appears effective in eliminating contaminating microbes from the culture system and preserving the in vitro fertilisation process except in certain circumstances where there is a heavy presence of pathogens.

*Conclusions.* Bacterial contamination of the culture system is a potential hazard which deserves attention. It may be detrimental to outcome. Present techniques for elimination taken from the veterinary field, while unproven, appear effective. The overall effect of microorganism presence on outcome is perhaps being underestimated.

**Keywords:** antibiotics, IVF culture system, microorganisms, semen, vagina.

## Introduction

When microorganisms become involved in any reproductive process this may lead to suboptimal results. This is particularly true with in vitro conception where the normal built-in eliminatory bodily defence mechanisms cannot come into play [1]. The result may be equally catastrophic whether the invasion is caused by pathogen contamination or local commensals becoming opportunistic pathogens in situ.

The need to recognise and combat this invasion was first recognised 50 years ago [2]. It was found that the quality and fertility potential of bulls' semen was improved when the antibiotics penicillin and streptomycin were added prior to insemination [3]. The concentration of antibiotics used was, however, minimal, adequate perhaps to cope only with commensal contamination rather than a heavy growth of pathogens.

This practice has been continued in human-assisted conception, where the need to provide a sterile closed culture system has been recognised from the

*Address for correspondence:* Robert F. Harrison MD, Academic Department of Obstetrics and Gynecology, Royal College of Surgeons, Rotunda Hospital, Rotunda Hospital, Dublin 1, Ireland. Tel.: +3531-8730140. Fax: +3531-8727831.

start. While contamination by microorganisms is not synonymous with clinical infection [4] their presence can have a negative influence even through to the embryonic stage [4,5]. The main sources are commensal microbes present in the bodily fluid and genital tracts although the work environment may also be implicated.

## Sources

There are three possible ways in which microorganisms may enter and contaminate the IVF/ET process. The first source is from the environment and the laboratory-related equipment [6]. The second is from seminal fluid [7] and the third the vagina [8].

### Environmental and IVF equipment and instruments

This includes the glassware, culture dishes, media, incubators, air conditioning and operatives. Fully sterile operating theatre conditions for oocyte recovery and ET practice are not essential. There is little evidence to suggest that sterilised disposable ware is advantageous or that commercial medium is better than that self-made on site. A high-grade, pyrogen-free water system for all processes carried out in association with IVF is, however, essential as are a regular cleaning schedule for the laminar air flow system and incubators.

These preventative measures are the province of good laboratory and clinical practice [6]. Contamination from these sources should be totally preventable. When such an occurrence is, however, suspected, full infection control measures to detect it and treat the source must be employed immediately.

### Seminal fluid

When tested, up to 90% of seminal fluid may contain bacteria (Table 1) [9]. In vivo the female genital tract appears to have perfectly adequate defence mechanisms to cope with this [10]. The organisms may be resident in the male genital tract, particularly in the prostatic area, but many are surface contaminants from the skin. They enter the equation as a result of poor hygiene at masturbation. This appears to be a problem even when strict instructions are given [11].

The high prevalence of bacteriospermia in men of both proven fertile and infertile relationships [12] does not seem to influence reproductive outcome in vivo but, in addition to a potentially detrimental effect on the spermatozoa themselves, in the situation where natural female defence mechanisms are compromised, such as with antibiotic therapy or bypassed as in intrauterine insemination (IUI) or GIFT or, removed altogether as in IVF/ICSI microbes could well have a negative influence on conception on gaining access to the culture system. This might lead to impaired fertilising capacity of spermatozoa or an affect on embryonic development [1,5] or through a possible influence at endometrial level [13].

Table 1. % Types of aerobic and anerobic bacteria found and their incidence in males attending a Dublin infertility clinic. n = 464 [9] ($10^3$/ml organisms grown counted as positive).

| | |
|---|---|
| Nil | 9.9 |
| Staph. Coag. Neg. | 71.6 |
| Diptheroids | 40.5 |
| Strep. viridans | 9.5 |
| Strep. fecalis | 8.6 |
| Lactobacilli | 6.5 |
| Pneumococci | 4.3 |
| Strep Gp B. | 3.4 |
| E. coli | 2.1 |
| Anerobic Strep | 2.1 |
| Neisseria catarrhalis | 1.4 |
| Haemophillus vaginalis | 0.9 |
| Candida species | 0.4 |
| Klebsiella pneum. | 0.4 |
| Meningococci | 0.4 |
| Micrococci | 0.4 |

A number of approaches have been utilised to eliminate this potential problem. Culturing all semen as a routine has been practised [1,4,5,14]. Confirmed positives are treated with relevant antibiotics in an attempt to produce a less contaminated specimen pre-IVF. Other workers give prophylactic antibiotics to all [4]. However, these approaches are costly, not always effective [14] and cannot possibly cover all potential organisms [9]. Chlamydia, for instance, cannot be cultured from semen [15]. Indeed the treatment often seems to result in nothing more than a change of one dominant identified organism to another [16]. It may also disturb the microbial ecosystem of the genital tract allowing selection of resistant organisms [17].

The alternative approach involves accepting the semen sample as produced and treating it thereafter. Some [4,14,18,19] but not all [20] have found a wash and swim-up technique to be most effective. Earles balanced salts, supplemented with pyruvic acid, 10% heat inactivated maternal serum and penicillin and streptomycin solution to final concentrations of 56 and 100 mg/ml, respectively, may be used and is of proven value as shown in Table 2 [19]. Alternatives include fall-down [20] and density gradient centrifugation [21,22].

Whatever method is used to attempt decontamination, proven efficacy is important. There is no doubt that semen has the potential to contaminate a woman's reproductive tract and destroy the function of an IVF culture system. Fertilisation [1,14] and zygote development [4] may be affected. The addition of the prophylactic antibiotics penicillin and streptomycin to the semen preparation medium [5] used pre-IUI, GIFT or IVF therefore appears wise. Although differing antibiotics and concentrations may need to be considered in some circumstances [23] and, although not fully proven in the human, in our experience such treatment will eliminate almost all organisms (Table 3), both aerobic and anaerobic from the processed sample [19].

Table 2. Microorganisms isolated from 140 semen and corresponding swim-up samples prior to IVF in Dublin [19].

| Aerobes | Semen | | Swim-up | | Anaerobes | Semen | | Swim-up | | Mycoplasmas | Semen | | Swim-up | |
|---|---|---|---|---|---|---|---|---|---|---|---|---|---|---|
| | n | % | n | % | | n | % | n | % | | n | % | n | % |
| Non-haemolytic streptococci | 42 | 30.0 | 1 | 0.7 | Mixed anaerobes | 4 | 2.8 | — | — | M. hominis and U. urealyticum | 5 | 3.6 | — | — |
| Staphylococcus epidermidis | 40 | 28.6 | 3 | 2.2 | Eikenella species | 4 | 2.8 | — | — | U. urealyticum | 19 | 13.6 | — | — |
| Diphtheroids | 20 | 14.3 | — | — | Anaerobic streptococci | 1 | 0.7 | — | — | | | | | |
| β-haemolytic streptococci | 17 | 12.1 | 1 | 0.7 | Unidentified anaerobe | 1 | 0.7 | — | — | | | | | |
| Streptococcus viridans group | 14 | 10.0 | 3 | 2.2 | | | | | | | | | | |
| Escherichia coli | 9 | 6.4 | 2 | 1.4 | | | | | | | | | | |
| Proteus species | 6 | 4.3 | — | — | | | | | | | | | | |
| Acinetobacter species | 2 | 1.2 | 1 | 0.7 | | | | | | | | | | |
| Klebsiella pneumonia | 1 | 0.7 | 1 | 0.7 | | | | | | | | | | |
| Gram-negative bacilli | 1 | 0.7 | — | — | | | | | | | | | | |
| Branhamella catarrhalis | 1 | 0.7 | — | — | | | | | | | | | | |

*Table 3.* Microorganisms isolated and their colony counts in samples found to be culture positive both before and after processing prior to IVF in Dublin [19].

| Case | Semen (preprocessing) | Colony count (organisms/ml) | Swim-up (postprocessing) | Colony count (organisms/ml) |
|---|---|---|---|---|
| 1 | *Staphylococcus epidermidis* | 25,000 | *Staphylococcus epidermidis* | 4,000 |
|  | β-haemolytic streptococcus (nongroupable) | 6,000 |  |  |
|  | Gram-negative bacilli (CDC Group IV C-2) | 54,000 |  |  |
| 2 | *Escherichia coli* | > 100,000[a] | *Escherichia coli* | > 100,000[a] |
|  | *Acinetobacter* species |  | *Acinetobacter* species |  |
| 3 | *Staphylococcus epidermidis* | 40,000 | *Streptococcus viridans* group | 2,000 |
|  | *Streptococcus viridans* group | 25,000 |  |  |
|  | *Eikenella corrodens* | 40,000 |  |  |
| 4 | Diphtheroids | 7,000 | *Streptococcus viridans* group | 2,000 |
|  |  |  | *Staphylococcus epidermidis* | 6,000 |
| 5 | *Streptococcus viridans* group | > 100,000 | *Streptococcus viridans* group | 1,000 |
| 6 | β-haemolytic streptococcus (Group D) | > 100,000[a] | β-haemolytic streptococcus (D) | > 100,000[a] |
|  | *Escherichia coli* |  | *Escherichia coli* |  |
|  |  |  | *Staphylococcus epidermidis* |  |
| 7 | *Streptococcus viridans* group | > 100,000[a] | *Klebsiella pneumonia* | 2,000 |
|  | *Klebsiella pneumonia* |  | Nonhaemolytic streptococcus | 6,000 |
|  | Nonhaemolytic streptococcus |  |  |  |

[a]Total colony counts are reported as counts for individual organisms cannot be determined accurately when cultures had in excess of $10^5$ organisms/ml.

## The vagina

The vagina has long been known to harbour organisms. Many are commensals (Table 4) [8] themselves part of the body's protective mechanisms [10]. In the vagina they are usually of little or no pathological importance. But, if transported and deposited elsewhere in the genital tract or to an IVF culture system they may become opportunistic pathogens.

It is easy to visualise organisms being carried via a needle tip from the vagina, a penetrated viscus such as bowel or a contaminated area in the peritoneum into the follicular fluid during oocyte harvesting. Not only can this give rise to pelvic inflammatory disease, a known complication of IVF, it will provide the microbes with access to the culture system through the follicular fluid along with the oocyte. In this manner both aerobic and anaerobic organisms have been shown to gain entry [23].

Preoperative swabbing of the vaginal wall, full aseptic handling technique by operatives and embryologist will not eliminate the microorganisms. Indeed it is

*Table 4.* Normal aerobic and anaerobic flora of the midvagina in 100 normal premenopausal women (positive more than 10 colonies per ml). (After Pfau and Sacks [8].)

| Organisms | Positive culture | Minimum No. colonies/ml |
|---|---|---|
| Nil | 29 | |
| Lactobacilli | 44 | $10^5$ |
| *Staphlyococcus aureus* and *epidermidis* | 27 | $10^2$ |
| Diphtheroids | 12 | $10^2$ |
| *Streptococcus* species | 11 | $10^2$ |
| *Micrococcus* species | 4 | $10^2$ |
| Gram-negative enterobacteria | | |
|     *E. coli* | 4 | 10 |
|     *Klebsiella* sp. | 1 | 10 |
|     *Citrobacter diversus* | 1 | 10 |

[a]Mycoplasma and ureaplasma species not sought.

also noteworthy that they can be found in up to 50% of cases at various stages in the process (Table 5) [23] despite the presence of antibiotics in the washing fluid and immediate transfer of any identified oocyte to a dish containing Earles balanced salts culture medium with 5% serum and antibiotics penicillin and streptomycin to respective concentrations of 56 and 100 µg/ml.

We found microbes in 27% of needle washes after oocyte collection, in 40 and 32% of follicular fluids from left and right ovaries, respectively, and in 2 culture media from the egg sperm preparations at 20 h after insemination. However, by the time the process had moved on to the stage of zygote transfer at 46 h, as Table 5 shows further testing revealed that the contaminating microbes had all been eliminated from the system. This reassuring result is likely due to a combination of the antibiotic-rich culture medium, daily change of incubation media and assiduous attention to cleanliness of operatives and their working environment.

## Conclusions

In addition to the potential they have to initiate or reactivate pelvic inflammatory disease, both the semen and the vagina almost invariably contain a reservoir of microbes with the potential to contaminate and infect an IVF culture system to its detriment. Indeed the pathogenic effect thus created could even infect the host female upper genital tract at transfer [20]. The agents usually found are commensal organisms, normally regarded as innocuous, and not worthy of treatment in their usual environment. While presence does not necessarily imply infection, nevertheless if optimum conception results are to be achieved an awareness of the potential to cause a problem is important and all suitable prophylactic hygienic measures need to be taken.

The methodology used and the reason for its use has not been totally proven beyond all doubt. The presence of bacteria does not necessarily mean infection.

*Table 5.* Microorganisms isolated from various loci analysed during 30 IVF-ET cycles in Dublin [23].[a]

| Case No.[a] | Semen sample | Postoocyte retrieval needle wash | First follicular fluid Right ovary | First follicular fluid Left ovary | 10% culture medium | 15% culture medium | Outcome |
|---|---|---|---|---|---|---|---|
| 1a | — | — | — | Diphtheroids (23 × 10³) | — | — | Nonpregnant |
| 3 | — | β-haem. strep. (Group B) (5 × 10³) | β-haem. strep. (group B) (10 × 10³) | β-haem. strep. (group B) (20 × 10³) | — | — | Nonpregnant |
| 4 | — | Staph. epidermidis (13 × 10³) | — | Staph. epidermidis (42 × 10³) | — | — | Nonpregnant |
| 5 | — | — | Lactobacilli sp. (90 × 10³) Diphtheroids (3 × 10³) | Lactobacilli sp. (90 × 10³) Diphtheroids (3 × 10³) | — | — | Nonpregnant |
| 6 | — | — | Nonhaem. strep (10 × 10³) | — | Nonhaem. strep. (3 × 10³) | — | Nonpregnant |
| 7 | M. hominis | M. hominis | M. hominis | — | — | — | Pregnant |
| 9 | — | Staph. epidermidis (10 × 10³) | Staph. epidermidis (2 × 10³) | Staph. epidermidis (4 × 10³) | — | — | Nonpregnant |
| 11 | — | — | U. urealyticum | — | — | — | Nonpregnant |
| 15a | E. coli (10 × 10³) | M. hominis | — | M. hominis | M. hominis | — | Nonpregnant |
| 15b | — | — | M. hominis | M. hominis Gardnerella vaginalis (9 × 10³) | — | — | Pregnant |
| 16 | — | β-haem. strep. (group C) (> 100 × 10³) | β-haem. strep. (group C) (> 100 × 10³) | β-haem. strep. (group C) (10 × 10³) | — | — | Nonpregnant |
| 18 | — | — | Viridans strep. (10 × 10³) Nonhaem. strep. (99 × 10³) | — | — | — | Nonpregnant |
| 22 | M. hominis | M. hominis | M. hominis | M. hominis | — | — | Nonpregnant |
| 23 | — | — | Viridans strep. (6 × 10³) | — | — | — | Nonpregnant |
| 28 | An. Strep. (70—10³) Veillonella sp. (30 × 10³) | Diphtheroids (11 × 10³) | Diphtheroids (50 × 10³) | Diphtheroids (100 × 10³) | — | — | Pregnant |

[a]Cases 1b, 2, 8, 10, 12—14, 17, 19, 20, 21, and 24—27: No growth of microorganisms in any fluid cultured. Colony counts are reported for aerobic and anaerobic bacteria only.

518

This is particularly true in semen. If the microorganisms are low in concentration they do not appear to effect the outcome of IVF [5,24]. This conclusion was, however, reached using semen processed as described and this fact coupled with the data from oocyte harvesting showing contamination can occur does make it appear wise to process spermatozoa and oocytes to be used in all ART in a dynamic bacteriostatic environment. This appears effective in managing the commensal contamination that can occur. Complacency as to efficacy of the present measures is, however, possibly misplaced. Indeed the potential inefficiencies have provoked much comment in the literature cited in this paper. It may yet be another reason why IVF results are not as good as originally anticipated. Research on better methodology is needed. This must, however, also include looking at measures to treat the very rare case [25] where a heavy microbial growth of pathogens occurs or when antibiotic-resistant microorganisms become established. In this situation the present system of therapy of washing with culture media with containing minimal concentrations of antibiotics becomes overwhelmed and demonstrably inadequate to cope.

### References

1. Hewitt J, Cohen J, Fehilly CB, Rowland G, Steptoe P, Webster J et al. Seminal bacterial pathogens and in vitro fertilization. J In Vitro Fertil Embryo Transf 1985;2:105—107.
2. Almquist JO. The effect of penicillin upon the fertility of semen from relatively infertile bulls. J Diary Sci 1949;32:950—954.
3. Foote RH, Bratton RW. The fertility of bovine semen in extenders containing sulphanilamide, penicillin, streptomycin and polymyxin. J Diary Sci 1950;33:544—547.
4. Guillet-Rosso F, Fari A, Taylor S, Forman R, Belaisch-Allart J, Testart J et al. Systematic semen culture and its influence on IVF management. Br J Obstet Gynecol 1987;94:543—547.
5. Forman R, Guillet-Rosso F, Fari A, Volante M, Frydman R, Testart J. Importance of semen preparation in avoidance of reduced in vitro fertilization results attributable to bacteria. Fertil Steril 1987;47:527—530.
6. Collins CH. Lab-Acquired Infection. Host, Incidence, Causes and Prevention. London: Butterworth, 1988.
7. Toth A, Lesser ML. Asymptomatic bacteriospermia in fertile and infertile men. Fertil Steril 1981;36:88—91.
8. Pfau A, Sacks T. The bacterial flora of the vaginal vestibule, urethra and vagina in the normal premenopausal woman. J Urol 1977;188:292—295.
9. Harrison RF, Hannon K, Butler M. Aerobic and anerobic culture of human semen and the relationship to characteristics in the spermiogram. In: Schirren C, Holstein AF (eds) Diagnostic Aspects in Andrology. Berlin: Grosse-Verlag; 1983;8:46—54.
10. Larzen B. Host defence mechanisms in obstetrics and gynaecology. In: Charles D (ed) Clinics in Obstetrics and Gynaecology. London: Saunders, 1983;10:37—64.
11. World Health Organisation. WHO Laboratory Manual for the Examination of Human Semen and Semen-Cervical Mucus Interaction. New York: The Press Syndicate of the University of Cambridge, 1992.
12. Megory E, Zuckerman H, Shoham SZ, Lunenfeld B. Infections and male fertility. Obstet Gynecol Surv 1987;42:283—290.
13. Montagut JM, Lepretre S, Degoy J, Rousseau M. Ureaplasma in semen and IVF. Hum Reprod 1991;6:727—729.

14. Huyser C, Fourie le RF, Oosthuizen M, Neethling A. Microbial flora in semen during in vitro fertilisation. J In Vitro Fertil Embryo Transf 1991;8:260—264.

15. Busolo F, Zanchetta R, Lanzone E, Cusinato R. Microbial flora in semen of asymptomatic infertile men. Andrologia 1984;16:269—275.

16. Stiver HG, Forward KR, Tyrrell DL, Krip G, Livingstone RA, Fugere P et al. Comparative cervical microflora shifts after cefoxitin or cefazolin prophylaxis against infection following cesarean section. Am J Obstet Gynecol 1984;149:718—721.

17. Eggert-Kruse W, Hofmann H, Gerhard I, Biklke A, Runnebaum B, Petzoldt D. Effect of antimicrobial therapy on sperm-mucus interaction. Hum Reprod 1988;3:861—869.

18. Wong PC, Balmaceda JP, Blanco JD, Gibbs RS, Asch RH. Sperm washing and swim-up technique using antibiotics removes microbes from human semen. Fertil Steril 1986;45:97—100.

19. Cottell E, Lennon B, McMorrow J, Barry-Kinsella C, Harrison RF. Processing of semen in an antibiotic-rich culture medium to minimise microbial presence during in vitro fertilization. Fertil Steril 1996;67(1):98—103.

20. Sun L-S, Gastaldi C, Peterson EM, de la Maza LM, Stone SC. Comparison of techniques for the selection of bacteria-free sperm preparations. Fertil Steril 1987;48:659—663.

21. Hyne RV, Stojanoff A, Clarke GN, Lopata A, Johnston WIH. Pregnancy from in vitro fertilization of human eggs after separation of motile spermatozoa by density gradient centrifugation. Fertil Steril 1986;45:93—96.

22. Bolton VN, Warren RE, Braude PR. Removal of bacterial contaminants from semen for in vitro fertilisation or artificial insemination by the use of buoyant density centrifugation. Fertil Steril 1986;46:1128—1132.

23. Cottell E, McMorrow J, Lennon B, Fawsy M, Cafferkey M, Harrisőn RF. Microbial contamination in an in vitro fertilization-embryo transfer system. Fertil Steril 1996;66(5):776—780.

24. Stovall DW, Bailey LE, Talbert LM. The role of aerobic and anerobic semen cultures in asymptomatic couples undergoing in vitro fertilization: Effect on fertilization and pregnancy rates. Fertil Steril 1993;59:197—201.

25. Cottell E. The Association of Non-Specific Genital Tract Infection and Male Infertility. PhD. Thesis. National University of Ireland, 1997.

# Ovulation induction

# Induction of monofolliculogenesis with pulsatile gonadotropin-releasing hormone

M. Filicori, G. Gessa, G.E. Cognigni, C. Taraborelli, P. Pocognoli, D. Spettoli,
P. Casadio, W. Ciampaglia, B. Cantelli, S. Taraborelli and F. Ferlini
*Reproductive Endocrinology Center, University of Bologna, Bologna, Italy*

**Abstract.** Pulsatile gonadotropin-releasing hormone (GnRH) is used to induce monofolliculogenesis in hypogonadotropic hypogonadism (HH); however, its application in the polycystic ovary syndrome (PCOS) is more controversial. Treatment of anovulation with pulsatile GnRH in HH yields up to 90% ovulatory rates and 25—30% pregnancy rates; frank ovarian hyperstimulation is nonexistent and the occurrence of multiple pregnancy is unusual and mostly limited to low-order gestations. Conversely, pulsatile GnRH alone in PCOS results in less than 50% ovulatory rates and no more than 10% pregnancy rates; PCOS patients who ovulate on pulsatile GnRH have elevated LH, FSH, and $E_2$ levels and brisk folliculogenesis, suggesting that the deranged PCOS endocrine profile can be overridden by pulsatile GnRH but at the risk of multiple folliculogenesis. Approaches used to enhance response to pulsatile GnRH in PCOS include combining it with clomiphene citrate and hMG, pretreating these patients with GnRH. This latter regimen virtually normalizes hormone levels, improves ovulatory and pregnancy rates to over 75 and 18%, respectively, permits the avoidance of ovarian hyperstimulation and multiple pregnancy, and reduces abortion rates to about 23%. While excessive body weight does not affect pulsatile GnRH outcome in HH, it is associated with worse results in PCOS. Thus, pulsatile GnRH is the most physiologic and safe method to induce monofolliculogenesis in ovulatory disorders. Nevertheless, drug and device distribution difficulties have so far severely hindered the use of this treatment modality.

**Keywords:** amenorrhea, folliculogenesis, gonadorelin, ovulation induction, polycystic ovary, pulsatile.

## Introduction

Several biological features render pulsatile GnRH unique among the different methods of ovulation induction. The clinical peculiarities of hMG and pulsate GnRH can be easily explained if the endocrine characteristics of the major ovulation induction method are appreciated. When menotropins are given to anovulatory subjects FSH levels are elevated throughout the follicular phase and peak before ovulation. This pattern is in stark contrast to the endocrine events of the normal menstrual cycle when elevated FSH levels are present only in the perimenstrual transition (late luteal and early follicular phase) and decline thereafter until just before the preovulatory surge. Although LH levels progressively

*Address for correspondence:* Dr Marco Filicori, Reproductive Endocrinology Center, Department of Obstetrics and Gynecology, Via Massarenti 13, 40138 Bologna, Italy. Tel.: +39-051-342820. Fax: +39-051-397350. E-mail: filicori@med.unibo.it

increase across the follicular phase of the spontaneous menstrual cycle, LH is usually low in the hMG-induced follicular phase. This dynamic interplay between LH and FSH levels in spontaneous cycles provides an optimal stimulus for follicular recruitment at first and for the selection of the dominant follicle later; conversely, the tonically elevated FSH levels typical of the menotropin-induced follicular phase predispose patients to develop multiple folliculogenesis and conception, and ovarian hyperstimulation.

A remarkable characteristic of pulsatile GnRH administration is that during treatment the pituitary retains its ability to modify gonadotropin output in response to negative and positive feedback stimuli. When the gonadotropin secretory pattern of the GnRH-induced menstrual cycle is analyzed, several similarities with the normal menstrual cycle become evident [1]. As in spontaneous cycles, FSH concentrations are elevated only in the early follicular phase and decline thereafter, whereas LH levels progressively increase until ovulation. Thus, the physiological events leading to the maturation and ovulation of a single dominant follicle are preserved. The endocrine dynamics of the midcycle preovulatory surge in GnRH cycles are also noteworthy. Preovulatory $E_2$ levels peak at 300–450 pg/ml, thus indirectly confirming that a single ovarian follicle has achieved maturity. The midcycle LH surge occurs spontaneously after the estrogen peak and a modest increment of P concentrations. These endocrine events faithfully recapitulate the preovulatory dynamics of the normal menstrual cycle and assure that the ovulation signal occurs when optimal follicular maturity is achieved and not at a time artificially chosen by the physician. Furthermore, the existence of a spontaneous gonadotropin surge enables withholding the preovulatory administration of hCG. This factor contributes to the safety of GnRH-induced cycles, considering that hCG administration precipitates clinical ovarian hyperstimulation when excessive dosages of hMG are given.

**Treatment of hypogonadotropic hypogonadism**

In most anovulatory patients pulsatile GnRH is administered at a dose of 5 µg GnRH per bolus at intervals of 60–90 min at least until ovulation [1]; thereafter, pulsatile GnRH can be continued until menstruation or a positive βhCG determination or replaced by two to three administrations of 1–2,000 IU of hCG at 2- to 3-day intervals. Pulsatile GnRH can be given subcutaneously (s.c.) or intravenously (i.v.); the s.c. route appears to be slightly less effective and requires a greater GnRH dosage (about 15 µg per bolus) and the longer interpulse interval of every 90 min. In our center we prefer the i.v. administration route that in our hands is not associated with significant septic complications. Greater GnRH dosages (usually 20 µg/bolus, i.v.) can be applied to obese and/or poorly responding patients.

Patients with HH present absent or reduced endogenous GnRH secretion; primary pituitary disorders are rare, and normal gonadotropin secretion is restored by the administration of exogenous pulsatile GnRH in the majority of cases. We

reported the treatment of 73 patients with primary hypogonadotropic amenorrhea for a total of 161 cycles [2]; the ovulatory rate in response to pulsatile
GnRH was high (83 per treatment cycle), and pregnancy ensued in 31 subjects.
Pulsatile GnRH administration in these patients resulted in an almost perfect
restoration of the endocrine and morphological features of the normal menstrual
cycle. The uterus and ovaries were small at baseline but rapidly grew and
achieved normal size; thus, E pretreatment to increase uterine volume is not
required. It had been suggested that patients which such a profound form of
hypogonadism may be resistant to pulsatile GnRH administration and that high
GnRH doses (> 15 µg/bolus) would be required. However, in our hands [3] a
dose/bolus as low as 2.5 µg is fully adequate to restore normal reproductive hormone secretion and ovulation in these patients. Finally, the occurrence of multiple pregnancy is rare in these patients, probably in relation to the lack of pituitary
gonadotroph priming at the outset of treatment.

Less severe forms of hypogonadotropic menstrual disorders (secondary amenorrhea, oligomenorrhea) are associated with decrements in the frequency and/or
amplitude of LH peaks. In some patients, menstrual derangements may be present in spite of normal mean gonadotropin levels; nevertheless, pulsatile LH
release is usually altered. Thus, it is not surprising that in most of these patients
restoration of a physiological pattern of pulsatile LH secretion with exogenous
GnRH results in the resumption of ovulation. Pulsatile GnRH is highly effective
in inducing ovulation in these subjects [2]. In our experience (107 cycles in 57
patients) the overall ovulatory rate per cycle was 79%, whereas pregnancy was
achieved in 22% of treatment cycles; other studies have confirmed that good
clinical results and low rates of complications can be obtained in these disorders.
However, greater levels of gonadotropin secretion are elicited by pulsatile GnRH
in patients with less severe forms of HH and this may cause the maturation of
more than a single dominant ovarian follicle; thus, the occurrence of multiple
pregnancy is highest among this group of HH patients [1].

**Treatment of PCOS**

The ultrasonographic identification of polycystic ovaries is common in anovulatory women. Ovulation induction is often resorted to in these patients when infertility is also present. Unfortunately in many PCOS patients traditional ovulation
induction methods are associated with either a high rate of treatment failures or
with an elevated occurrence of major complications such as the ovarian hyperstimulation syndrome (OHSS) and multiple conception.

When administered alone to PCOS patients, pulsatile GnRH elicits an exaggerated LH (and sometimes FSH) response [4]. Nevertheless, once gonadotropin
levels decline, no progression of estrogen levels is often seen and about half of
the patients remains anovulatory despite continuation of treatment for up to 30
days. In other subjects, however, folliculogenesis may progress, albeit dysfunc-
tionally. In 1986 [5] we described the endocrine pattern of one such patient who

developed a triplet pregnancy.

To overcome the limitations associated with the use of pulsatile GnRH in PCOS several steps can be taken:

- Patient selection: obese/overweight PCOS (but not HH) patients are known to respond worse to pulsatile GnRH. Use of pulsatile GnRH in normal weight PCOS subjects (unfortunately a minority in this disorder) is associated with a reasonably good response rate [6].
- Route of administration: as previously indicated the i.v. route is marginally more effective over the s.c. route.
- Use of unconventional drug regimens: association of pulsatile GnRH to CC, gonadotropins, or GnRH agonists has been shown to offset reduced responsiveness encountered in PCOS.

**Unconventional ovulation induction drug regimens in PCOS**

Use of supplemental CC (100 mg/day for 5 days) in pulsatile GnRH ovulation induction has been advocated by Homburg et al. [7] since 1989 in PCOS patients resistant to pulsatile GnRH alone. Remorgida and his group [8,9] reported good clinical results in few patients treated with the association of pulsatile GnRH (20 µg i.v. every 60 min) and two ampoules of purified FSH per day on cycle days 5, 7, and 9. It appears that optimal results are obtained when FSH administration is preceded by pulsatile GnRH while follicle luteinization may occur when FSH is given early in the cycle. More recently Tan et al. [10] reported in a large study the combined use of pulsatile GnRH with CC (100 mg/day for 5 days) or hMG/FSH (1 ampoule/day for 5—7 days). Pulsatile GnRH alone resulted in ovulatory and pregnancy rates of 50 and 11.5%, respectively, while CC supplementation in resistant patients gave ovulatory rates of 66% and pregnancy rates of 11.3%. Supplementation with hMG/FSH fared better as the ovulatory rate was 70% and the pregnancy rate was 20.3%; however, in this last group a multiple pregnancy rate of 14% was reported.

In 1988 we proposed a different approach to the management of anovulation in PCOS patients [11]. We pretreated our PCOS subjects with a short-acting GnRH agonist (e.g., Buserelin 300 µg, s.c., every 12 h) for a period of 4—6 weeks; immediately thereafter pulsatile GnRH was begun (5 µg, i.v. every 60 min) and continued at least until ovulation. The rationale of this approach is to reduce pituitary gonadotropin sensitivity and ovarian androgen production, and thus temporarily reproduce the endocrine milieu of hypogonadotropic hypogonadism, the condition that responds best to pulsatile GnRH. Intraovarian testosterone production appears to be highly relevant in this context as in a study we conducted with a GnRH agonist and exogenous gonadotropins we found elevated intrafollicular testosterone to be associated with reduced folliculogenesis [12].

We showed that the combination of GnRH agonists and pulsatile GnRH resulted in a markedly improved endocrine profile in PCOS patients, as follicular phase LH and testosterone were markedly reduced and ovulation and pregnancy was achieved in previously unresponsive patients [4]. While an earlier study by Surrey et al. [13] did not confirm our finding, two other later investigations done with this combined regimen [14,15] achieved OR and PR of 82—83 and 17%, respectively. In a recently updated series of over 200 ovulation induction cycles in PCOS patients we confirmed our previously published data [2] and found that this regimen yielded an ovulatory rate of 77% per treatment cycle (vs. 44% in non-GnRH agonist pretreated patients; $p < 0.05$) and a pregnancy rate of 18% (vs. 6%; $p < 0.05$). This approach appears to specifically affect anovulation caused by LH-dependent hyperandrogenism as the same regimen applied to hypogonadotropic hypogonadism or to patients with non-LH-dependent hyperandrogenism did not significantly affect ovulatory rates.

**Conclusions**

Pulsatile GnRH is an effective ovulation induction method in most ovulatory disorders with preserved ovarian function. While optimal results can be achieved in HH, management of PCOS patients with pulsatile GnRH combined with GnRH agonists or menotropins can be also effective and associated with a reduced rate of complications such as overt OHSS and multiple conception. These positive results are related to the physiologic stimulation of pituitary and ovarian function achieved by pulsatile GnRH which causes the development of a single dominant follicle in most treatment cycles. Finally, pulsatile GnRH reduces monitoring needs and lowers the overall cost of ovulation induction when monitoring and complication-related charges are considered. Thus, it is unfortunate that this ovulation induction method has not raised more interest among pharmaceutical companies, something that has resulted in limited availability of drug and infusion devices. Hopefully, future developments in drug delivery systems may renew industry interest in this treatment option and provide greater physician access to pulsatile GnRH.

**References**

1.  Filicori M, Flamigni C, Meriggiola MC, Cognigni G, Valdiserri A, Ferrari P et al. Ovulation induction with pulsatile gonadotropin-releasing hormone: technical modalities and clinical perspectives. Fertil Steril 1991;56:1—13.
2.  Filicori M, Flamigni C, Dellai P, Cognigni G, Michelacci L, Arnone R et al. Treatment of anovulation with pulsatile gonadotropin-releasing hormone: prognostic factors and clinical results in 600 cycles. J Clin Endocrinol Metab 1994;79:1215—1220.
3.  Filicori M, Flamigni C, Campaniello E, Ferrari P, Meriggiola MC, Michelacci L et al. Evidence for a specific role of GnRH pulse frequency in the control of the human menstrual cycle. Am J Physiol 1989;257:E930—E936.
4.  Filicori M, Flamigni C, Campaniello E, Valdiserri A, Ferrari P, Meriggiola MC et al. The abnormal response of polycystic ovarian disease patients to exogenous pulsatile gonadotropin-releasing hormone: characterization and management. J Clin Endocrinol Metab 1989;69:825—831.
5.  Filicori M, Michelacci L, Ferrari P, Campaniello E, Pareschi A, Flamigni C. Triplet pregnancy after low-dose pulsatile gonadotropin- releasing hormone in polycystic ovarian disease. Am J

528

Obstet Gynecol 1986;155:768—769.

6. Filicori M, Flamigni C, Meriggiola MC, Ferrari P, Michelacci L, Campaniello E et al. Endocrine response determines the clinical outcome of pulsatile gonadotropin-releasing hormone ovulation induction in different ovulatory disorders. J Clin Endocrinol Metab 1991;72: 965—972.

7. Homburg R, Eshel A, Armar NA, Tucker M, Mason PW, Adams J et al. One hundred pregnancies after treatment with pulsatile luteinising hormone releasing hormone to induce ovulation. Br Med J 1989;298:809—812.

8. Remorgida V, Venturini PL, Anserini P, Salerno E, de Cecco L. Use of combined exogenous gonadotropins and pulsatile gonadotropin-releasing hormone in patients with polycystic ovarian disease (published erratum appears in Fertil Steril 1991 Jun;55(6):1213). Fertil Steril 1991; 55:61—65.

9. Venturini PL, Remorgida V, Anserini P, de Cecco L. Use of combined exogenous gonadotropins and pulsatile gonadotropin-releasing hormone in patients with polycystic ovarian disease: a new approach to induction of ovulation. Gynecol Endocrinol 1988;2:205—213.

10. Tan SL, Farhi J, Homburg R, Jacobs HS. Induction of ovulation in clomiphene-resistant polycystic ovary syndrome with pulsatile GnRH. Obstet Gynecol 1996;88:221—226.

11. Filicori M, Campaniello E, Michelacci L, Pareschi A, Ferrari P, Bolelli G et al. Gonadotropin-releasing hormone (GnRH) analog suppression renders polycystic ovarian disease patients more susceptible to ovulation induction with pulsatile GnRH. J Clin Endocrinol Metab 1988;66:327—333.

12. Filicori M, Flamigni C, Cognigni GE, Falbo A, Arnone R, Capelli M et al. Different gonadotropin and leuprorelin ovulation induction regimens markedly affect follicular fluid hormone levels and folliculogenesis. Fertil Steril 1996;65:387—393.

13. Surrey ES, de Ziegler D, Lu JHK, Chang RJ, Judd HL. Effects of gonadotropin-releasing hormone (GnRH) agonist on pituitary and ovarian responses to pulsatile GnRH therapy in polycystic ovarian disease. Fertil Steril 1989;52:547—552.

14. Gerhard I, Matthes J, Runnebaum B. The induction of ovulation with pulsatile gonadotrophin-releasing hormone (GnRH) administration in hyperandrogenic women after down-regulation with buserelin or suppression with an oral contraceptive. Hum Reprod 1993;8:2033—2038.

15. Scheele F, Hompes PG, van der Meer M, Schoute E, Schoemaker J. Pulsatile gonadotrophin releasing hormone stimulation after medium-term pituitary suppression in polycystic ovary syndrome. Hum Reprod 1993;8(Suppl 2):197—199.

# Ovulation induction: step-up and step-down regimens

Nicholas S. Macklon and Bart C.J.M. Fauser
*Division of Reproductive Medicine, Department of Obstetrics and Gynecology, University Hospital Rotterdam, Rotterdam, The Netherlands*

**Abstract.** Gonadotropins are effective in achieving monofollicular development and subsequent ovulation in anovulatory infertile women. The application of recently obtained knowledge relating to normal follicular development may enhance the efficacy and safety of gonadotropin regimes. The concept of an FSH "threshold", above which follicular development may proceed, forms the basis of the widely employed low-dose step-up regimen. The FSH "window" concept stresses the significance of the duration of FSH elevation above the threshold level in allowing for single dominant follicle selection. The step-down protocol applies this concept in a therapeutic context. In this article these theoretical concepts are discussed, and the application of the low-dose step-up and step-down regimens for ovulation induction are described. The effect of different gonadotropin preparations is considered and outcomes for the two treatment regimens are discussed.

**Keywords:** FSH threshold, FSH window, hyperstimulation, monofollicular.

## Introduction

The goal of ovulation induction is to induce monofollicular development and subsequent ovulation in anovulatory infertile women. In most centers, clomiphene citrate (CC) constitutes the first line of treatment since it is simple to administer, leads to cumulative ovulation rates of over 70% [1] and has a low complication rate [2]. It is uncertain as to whether women who remain anovulatory following CC constitute a different subgroup from those who do ovulate but do not conceive. In practice, however, anovulatory women who do not respond to CC may be successfully treated with gonadotropin therapy. Since their introduction into clinical practice in 1961, gonadotropins have assumed a central role in ovulation induction. Refinement of the initially crude preparation procedure resulted in the availability of purified and highly purified urinary FSH. Since 1996, recombinant human FSH (rFSH, > 99% purity) has been available in the clinic [3]. The improvement in our understanding of the physiology and endocrinology of normal monofollicular development has enabled the development of effective and safe treatment regimens for anovulatory infertility.

*Address for correspondence:* Dr Nicholas S. Macklon, Division of Reproductive Medicine, Department of Obstetrics and Gynecology, University Hospital Rotterdam, Rotterdam, The Netherlands. Tel.: +31-10-463-9222. Fax: +31-01-463-3381.

## Theoretical basis for gonadotropin ovulation induction

The concept of the FSH "threshold" proposed by Brown [4] postulated that FSH concentrations must exceed a certain level before follicular development will proceed. Once this level is reached, normal follicular growth requires only a minor further increase above this threshold. Excessive FSH production may lead to excessive follicular development. The FSH threshold is surpassed in the normal cycle during the luteal follicular transition [5] (Fig. 1) and occurs as a result of reduced estrogen secretion from the corpus luteum [6].

The duration of this period in which the threshold is exceeded is limited in the normal cycle by a decrease in FSH which occurs in the early to mid follicular phase [7] secondary to a negative feedback exerted by rising inhibin levels [8] and/or estradiol production by developing follicles. Should this period be extended, the recruited cohort of follicles will be increased and more follicles will continue development. In the normal cycle, only one follicle continues developing despite falling FSH levels because of an increased sensitivity to FSH [9]. Remaining follicles respond to falling FSH levels by undergoing atresia. The duration of elevated FSH may play a crucial role in determining the number of follicles, which will undergo further development. The concept of the FSH "window" has been proposed, stressing the significance of the duration of FSH elevation above the threshold level, rather than the level of elevation of FSH for single dominant selection [10]. The aim of ovulation induction with gonadotropins, as with CC, is the formation of a single dominant follicle. In order to achieve development of a single dominant follicle with exogenous gonadotropin, specific treatment and monitoring protocols are needed. While several approaches to ovulation induction with gonadotropins have been described, the two most frequently

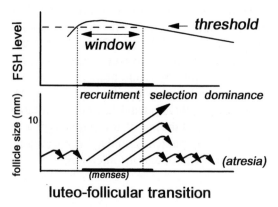

*Fig. 1.* Follicular phase of the normal menstrual cycle. The intercycle rise in serum follicle stimulating hormone (FSH) concentrations exceeds the threshold for recruitment of a cohort of follicles for further development. The number of follicles recruited is determined by the time ("window") in which the serum FSH is above the threshold at which recruitment occurs. (Adapted form [10].)

encountered in the literature and in clinical practice are the low-dose step-up protocol and, more recently, the step-down protocol.

## Low-dose regimens

### Step-up regimen

The conventional "standard" step-up protocol has a starting dose of FSH 150 IU/day. However, this regimen is associated with a high complication rate. A multiple pregnancy rate of up to 36% has been reported, and ovarian hyperstimulation may occur in up to 14% of treatment cycles [10]. As a result, many centers have abandoned this protocol in favor of a low-dose, step-up protocol designed to allow the FSH threshold to be reached gradually, minimizing excessive stimulation and therefore the risk of development of multiple preovulatory follicles. In this protocol, the initial subcutaneous or intramuscular dose of FSH is 37.5–75 IU/day; the dose is only increased if, after 14 days, no response is documented on ultrasonography (and serum estradiol monitoring). Increments of 37.5 IU are then given at weekly intervals up to a maximum of 225 IU/day. In patients with a high FSH threshold stimulation sufficient to achieve an ovarian response may take many weeks. The detection of an ovarian response (either an increase in follicle diameter as assessed by ultrasound or increasing serum E2 levels) is an indication to continue the current dose until human chorionic gonadotropin (hCG) can be given to stimulate ovulation, as described below (Fig. 2).

### Step-down regimen

The step-down protocol of ovulation induction mimics more closely the physiol-

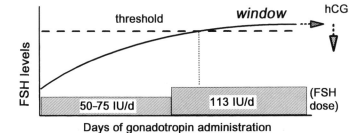

*Fig. 2.* Schematic representation of the low-dose, step-up protocol of gonadotropin administration for ovulation induction. The initial subcutaneous or intramuscular dose of follicle-stimulating hormone (FSH) is 37.5–75 IU/day; the dose is increased only if, after 14 days, no response is documented on ultrasonography and serum estradiol monitroing. Increments of 37.5 IU are then given at weekly intervals up to a maximum of 225 IU/day. Detection of an ovarian response is an indication to continue the current dose until human chorionic gonadotropin (hCG) can be given to stimulate ovulation. (Adapted from [28].)

532

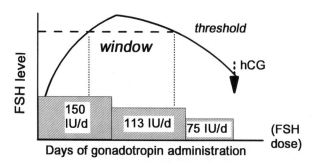

*Fig. 3.* Schematic representation of the step-down protocol of gonadotropin administration which is designed to bring about monofollicular development. This regimen mimics more closely the physiology of normal cycles. Therapy with follicle-stimulating hormone (FSH) at 150 IU/day is started shortly after a spontaneous or progesterone-induced bleed and continued until a dominant follicle ⩾ 10 mm) is seen on transvaginal ultrasonography. The dose is then decreased to 112.5 IU/day followed by a further decrease to 75 IU/day, which is continued until human chronionic gonadotropin (hCG) is administered to induce ovulation. (Adapted from [28].)

ogy of normal cycles (Figs. 1 and 3) [11]. The underlying FSH window theory emphasizes the significance of decremental serum FSH levels for single dominant follicle development [12]. Therapy with 150 IU FSH/day is started shortly after a spontaneous or progesterone-induced bleed and continued until a dominant follicle (⩾ 10 mm) is seen on transvaginal ultrasonography. From a diameter of 10 mm onwards, the dominant follicles can be identified during the normal menstrual cycle [13,14]. The dose is then decreased to 112.5 IU per day followed by a further decrease to 75 IU/day 3 days later, which is continued until hCG is administered to induce ovulation (Fig. 3). For some patients an initial dose of 2 ampoules/day may be too high, reflecting major individual differences in the FSH threshold. The appropriate starting dose may be determined by using the low-dose step-up regimen for the first treatment cycle (van Santbrink et al., in preparation). Patients who demonstrate good follicular growth with a starting dose of 1 ampoule/day, the "good responders" who might have been at risk of OHSS (ovarian hyperstimulation syndrome) with the normal starting dose of the step-down regimen, can thus be identified. Conversely, those who do not respond with ongoing follicle growth to the initial dose should have the daily dosage increased. The second cycle is then initiated as a step-down regimen with a starting dose one-half ampoule above the effective dose in the preceding low-dose step-up cycle. This approach is currently under investigation.

## Monitoring

Ovarian response to gonadotropin therapy is monitored using transvaginal ultrasonography to measure follicular diameter. The scans, usually performed every 2 or 4 days during step-down regimens, should be focused on identifying follicles of intermediate size. hCG (5,000—10,000 IU intramuscularly) is given on the day that at least one follicle measures > 18 mm. If more than three follicles larger than 16 mm are present, stimulation should be stopped, hCG withheld, and use of a barrier contraceptive advised in order to prevent multiple pregnancies and ovarian hyperstimulation. Measurements of serum estradiol may also be useful in patients at risk of ovarian hyperstimulation. Preovulatory concentrations far above the normal range (14—40 ng/dl, 500—1,500 pmol/l) may predict the onset of OHSS [15], a potentially life-threatening complication characterized by ovarian enlargement, high serum sex steroids and, secondary to increased vascular permeability, extravascular exudate accumulation primarily in the peritoneal cavity. However, it is unclear to what extent estradiol levels add to information generated by ultrasound alone.

**Gonadotropin preparations**

A recent meta-analysis comparing the effectiveness of daily urinary FSH to daily hMG for inducing ovulation in women with PCOS (polycystic ovary syndrome) who had not responded to clomiphene demonstrated no difference in pregnancy rate per treatment cycle [16]. However, the women given FSH were less likely to have moderately severe or severe OHSS.

With respect to rFSH, a recent multicenter prospective trial found that the cumulative ovulation rates were comparable with those achieved with purified urinary FSH (95% after three cycles) [17]. The total dose of rFSH needed was less and the duration of treatment was shorter, and the complication rates were similar. Two prospective randomized trials comparing rFSH and urinary purified FSH in women having in vitro fertilization were recently reported. One study of 123 women found that the two preparations were equally effective [18]. However, in two larger trials of 981 [19] and 235 [20] women, the dose of a different rFSH preparation and the duration of rFSH treatment needed to stimulate follicle development were less, and more oocytes were recovered, implying greater efficacy for rFSH. Whether or not rFSH improves the clinical outcome in these women is not known.

Purified urinary FSH has some LH activity, but rFSH does not. The experience with rFSH in hypogonadotropic hypogonadal women (WHO class 1) indicates that those women who have very low serum LH concentrations (< 0.5 IU/l) need exogenous hCG (or LH) to maintain adequate estradiol biosynthesis and follicle development [21].

**Outcomes**

With regard to the low-dose step-up regimen, the largest series published to date reported 225 women with PCOS treated over a 10-year period in one center and found rates of ovulation and pregnancy of 72 and 45%, respectively [22]. Multiple folliculogenesis and hyperstimulation are less common than seen with the standard protocol [23] and pregnancy rates appear similar [24]. However, the results of the low-dose step-up protocol are negatively influenced by age, obesity, and persistent raised serum LH concentrations [22].

Initial experience with the step-down protocol in a series of 82 women suggested that the duration of treatment and total gonadotropin dosage were reduced compared with the low-dose step-up protocol and that monofollicular growth was more frequently achieved [11]. These findings have recently been confirmed by a prospective randomized comparison of low-dose step-up and step-down regimens in 37 clomiphene-resistant women [25]. In comparison to the step-up regimen, the women treated with the step-down regimen were shown to have preovulatory estradiol levels within the normal range in 71% as opposed to 33%. The clinical benefits of a more physiological means of stimulating follicle development were reflected in an incidence of monofollicular cycles of 88% compared to 56% observed in women treated with the step-up regimen, presumably reducing the risk of multiple pregnancy and hyperstimulation. Potential health-economic benefits were suggested since those treated with the step-down regimen required a mean duration of treatment of just 9 days, as opposed to 18 days in women treated with the low-dose step-up regimen.

Other studies assessing outcomes with the step-down protocol have employed varied inclusion criteria and treatment protocols. Steinkampf et al. [26] reported in abstract form a randomized prospective multicenter study comparing a step-down regimen with an ascending-dose regimen. Ovulation and complication rates were equal, but pregnancy rates in the step-down group were significantly reduced. However, the starting dose employed was 3 ampules HMG/day, and may have been excessive [27]. Further, the dose was decreased according to fixed schedule which did not take account of individual differences in the FSH threshold [28]. Caution is required when interpreting the thus far published data in this area.

## Conclusion

Both the low-dose step-up and step-down regimens for gonadotropin ovulation induction provide safe and effective means of treating anovulatory infertility in appropriately selected women. However, studies of the endocrine physiology of normal follicular development carried out in our center and elsewhere have highlighted the essential unphysiological nature of step-up regimens. In an attempt to mimic in anovulatory women more closely the means by which monofollicular development is achieved in normally ovulatory women, the step-down regimen has been developed. Multicenter randomized trials should clarify the role of the step-down protocol in clinical practice.

## References

1. Imani B, Eijkemans MJC, Te Velde ER, Habbema JDF, Fauser BCJM. Predictors of patients remaining anovulatory during clomiphene citrate induction of ovulation in normogonadotropic

oligomenorrheic infertility. J Clin Endocrinol Metab (In press).

2. Dickey RP, Holtcamp DE. Development, pharmacology and clinical experience with clomiphene citrate. Hum Reprod 1996;2:483—506.

3. Fauser BCJM. Developments in human recombinant FSH technology: are we going in the right direction? Hum Reprod Suppl (In press).

4. Brown JB. Pituitary control of ovarian function- concepts derived from gonadotropin therapy. Austr NZ J Obstet Gynaecol 1978;18:47—54.

5. Hall JE, Schoen DA, Martin KA, Crowley WF. Hypothalamic gonadotropin-releasing hormone secretion and follicle-stimulating hormone dynamics during the luteal-follicular transition. J Clin Endocrinol Metab 1992;74:600—607.

6. Le Nestour E, Marraoui J, Lahlou N, Roger M, de Ziegler D, Bouchard P. Role of estradiol in the rise in follicle-stimulating hormone levels during the luteal-follicular transition. J Clin Endocrinol Metab 1993;77:439—442.

7. Fauser BCJM, Pache TD, Schoot DC. Dynamics of human follicle development. In: Hsueh AJ, Schomberg DW (eds) Ovarian Cell Interactions: Genes to Physiology. Serono Int. Symposia Series. New York: Springer-Verlag, 1993;134—147.

8. Groome NP, Illingworth PJ, O'Brien M, Pai R, Rodger FE, Mather JP, McNeilly AS. Measurement of dimeric inhibin B throughout the human menstrual cycle. J Clin Endocrinol Metab 1996;81:1401—1405.

9. Hsueh AJ, Adashi EY, Jones PB, Welsh TH Jr. Hormonal regulation of the differentiation of cultures ovarian granulosa cells. Endocrine Rev 1984;5:76—127.

10. Fauser BCJM, van Heusden AM. Manipulation of human ovarian function: physiological concepts and clinical consequences. Endocrine Rev 1997;18:71—106.

11. van Santbrink EJP, Donderwinkel PFJ, van Dessel TJHM et al. Gonadotrophin induction of ovulation using a step-down dose regimen: single center clinical experience in 82 patients. Hum Reprod 1995;10:1048—1053.

12. Schipper I, Hop WCJ, Fauser BCJM. The follicle-stimulating hormone (FSH) threshold/window concept examined by differential interventions with exogenous FSH during the follicular phase of the normal menstrual cycle: duration rather than magnitude of FSH increase affects follicle development. J Clin Endocrinol Metab 1998;83:1292—1298.

13. Pache TD, Wladimiroff JW, de Jong FH, Hop WC, Fauser BCJM. Growth patterns of non-dominant ovarian follicles during the normal menstrual cycle. Fertil Steril 1990;54:638—644.

14. van Santbrink EJP, Hop WC, van Dessel HJHM, Fauser BCJM. Decremental FSH and dominant follicle development during the normal menstrual cycle. Fertil Steril 1995;64:37—43.

15. Haning RV, Austin CW, Carlston IH et al. Plasma estradiol is superior to ultrasound and urinary estriol glucuronide as a predictor of ovarian hyperstimulation during induction of ovulation with menotropins. Fertil Steril 1983;40:31—36.

16. Hughes E, Collins J, Vanderkerkhove P. Ovulation induction with urinary follicle stimulating hormone vs. human menopausal gonadotropin for clomiphene-resistant polycystic ovary syndrome. Cochrane Libr 1996;3:1—8.

17. Coelingh Bennink HJ, Fauser BCJM, Out HJ. Recombinant FSH (puregon) is more efficient than urinary FSH (metrodin) in women with clomiphene-resistant normogonadotrophic chronic anovulatory women: a prospective, multi-center, assessor-blind, randomised clinical trial. Fertil Steril 1998;69:19—25.

18. Recombinant human FSH study group. Clinical assessment of recombinant human follicle-stimulating hormone in stimulating ovarian follicular development before in vitro fertilization. Fertil Steril 1995;63:77—86.

19. Out HJ, Mannaerts BMJL, Driessen SGAJ et al. A prospective, randomized, assessor-blind, multicenter study comparing recombinant and urinary follicle-stimulating hormone (puregon vs. metrodin) in in vitro fertilization. Hum Reprod 1995;10:2534—2540.

20. Bergh C, Howles CM, Borg K, Hamberger L, Josefsson B, Nilsson L, Wikland M. Recombinant human follicle stimulating hormone (r-FSH; gonal-F$^{®}$) versus highly purified urinary FSH

(metrodin HP®): results of a randomized comparative study in women undergoing assisted reproductive techniques. Hum Reprod 1997;12:2133—2139.

21. Kousta E, White DM, Piazzi A et al. Successful induction of ovulation and completed pregnancy using recombinant human luteinizing hormone and follicle stimulating hormone in a woman with Kallmann's syndrome. Hum Reprod 1996;11:70—71.

22. White DM, Polson DW, Kiddy D et al. Induction of ovulation with low-dose gonadotropins in polycystic ovary syndrome: an analysis of 109 pregnancies in 225 women. J Clin Endocrinol Metab 1996;81:3821—3824.

23. Buvat J, Buvat HM, Marcolin G et al. Purified follicle-stimulating hormone in polycystic ovary syndrome: slow administration is safer and more effective. Fertil Steril 1989;52:553—559.

24. Shoham Z, Patel A, Jacobs HS. Polycystic ovary syndrome; safety and effectiveness of a stepwise and low-dose administration of purified FSH. Fertil Steril 1991;55:1051—1056.

25. van Santbrink EJP, Fauser BCJM. Urinary follicle-stimulating hormone for normogonadotropic clomiphene-resistant infertility: prospective, randomized comparison between low-dose step-up and step-down dose regimens. J Clin Endocrinol Metab 1997;82:3597—3602.

26. Steinkampf MP, Banks KS. Step-down vs. conventional FSH treatment in patients with WHO group II amenorrhoea: results of a US multicenter clinical trial. Abstracts of the Annual meeting American Fertility Society, Montreal, Canada. 1993;S21—S22 (Abstract).

27. Schoot DC, Pache TD, Hop WC, de Jong FH, Fauser BCJM. Growth patterns of ovarian follicles during induction of ovulation with increasing doses of HMG following presumed selection in polycystic ovarian syndrome. Fertil Steril 1992;57:1117—1120.

28. Fauser BCJM, Donderwinkel P, Schoot DC. The step-down principle in gonadotrophin treatment and the role of GnRH analogues. Bailliére's Clin Obstet Gynaecol 1993;7:309—330.

# Ovarian drilling

Hisao Sumioki[1] and Takafumi Utsunomiya[2]

[1]*Division of Obstetrics and Gynecology, National Beppu Hospital, Beppu City; and* [2]*Saint Luke Clinic, Oita City, Japan*

**Abstract.** Ovarian drilling as a method of ovulation induction in PCO was reviewed with its various techniques. Clinically, ovulation rate and pregnancy outcome of this method are comparable to those of ovulation induction with gonadotropin and its various modifications. Low multiple pregnancy and ovarian hyperstimulation rates as well as a low abortion rate are beneficial points.

The hormonal changes before and after ovarian drilling were compared in the light of peripheral steroid levels and central gonadotropin secretory patterns. With the decline in testosterone and androstenedione levels, exaggerated LH pulsatile secretion and LH hypersensitivity to pituitary GnRH normalized, and resulted in successful ovulation. The mechanisms by which high intra-ovarian androgen environment and resultant monofollicular ovulation occur by this method raise the question on monofolliculogenesis and follicular recruitment and atresia.

**Keywords:** laparoscopic ovarian drilling, monofolliculogenesis, ovarian wedge resection, polycystic ovary syndrome, pulsatile LH secretion.

## Historical background of ovarian drilling

Although the distinct definition of ovarian drilling has not yet been determined, it obviously originated from the first report of Stein and Leventhal (1935) [1], who demonstrated that the wedge resection (WR) of the ovary in polycystic ovary syndrome (PCO) leads to effective ovulation. However, WR by laparotomy caused peritubal and periovarian adhesion very frequently (15—100% evaluated by the second-look procedure) [2,3]. It was thought to be the main reason for the low pregnancy rate (mean 58.8% in 1,079 WR cases) [4] despite the high ovulation rate (80%). With the discovery and purification of human menopausal gonadotropin (HMG) and with a widespread usage of HMG for ovulation induction in PCO, WR became unfavored and unpopular in 1972—1983. The development of operative laparoscopy has resulted in the introduction of minimally invasive methods, where laparoscopic multiple biopsies [5,6] were reported to have the same effect as WR, irrespective of a smaller volume of ovarian resection.

Since Gjönnaess first reported on laparoscopic electrocautery in 1984 [7], which had a lower postoperative adhesion rate, several modifications of the technique [8] have been introduced. With the acceptance of laser technology and development of laser delivery systems through laparoscope, laparoscopic laser

*Address for correspondence:* Dr Hisao Sumioki, Department of Obstetrics and Gynecology, National Beppu Hospital, 1473 Uchikamado, Beppu City 874, Japan. Tel.: +81-977-67-1111. Fax: +81-977-67-5766. E-mail: sumiokih@beppu.hosp.go.jp

techniques [9,10] were also introduced in 1989 as they possess sharper excision and cautery capability than electrocautery. These techniques include not only the wide and superficial vaporization of thick ovarian capsule but also the vaporization of deep ovarian hypertrophic theca and perforation of the ovarian stroma [11]. This tendency to perforate and destroy the thick ovarian cortex led to the description of "ovarian drilling" in the literature. As a whole, the definition of ovarian drilling is comprised of multiple ovarian biopsy and resection, multiple electrocautery, laser vaporization, and laser perforation techniques.

## Indications before surgical procedure of PCO

Clomiphene citrate (CC) remains the first line of treatment for the chronic anovulation which accompanies PCO. If the treatment of PCO with increased dosage of CC fails, further therapy with gonadotropin and its modified treatment should be initiated using pure FSH only, or the combination with GnRHa, various modes of which will be discussed later.

## Various methods of ovarian drilling technique

1) Classical WR;
2) slice incision of ovary;
3) multifollicular puncture and resection (MPR);
4) care of the procedure;
5) laser superficial vaporization;
6) laser deep perforation; and
7) vaginal method of mutifollicular puncture and aspiration.

1) Classically wedge shaped resection (WR) of ovarian tissue was conducted in almost one-half to three-quarters of the ovarian volume described in the original report by Stein and Leventhal [1].

2) In the past (1972) we reported on the method of slice incision of the ovary, which is the mere incision with a cold knife deep inside the ovary and cutting at the middle of the ovarian tissue [12]. In comparison with classical WR, this method did not induce marked reduction of testosterone or LH/FSH ratio postoperatively. Originally, slice incision of the ovary was intended to clarify whether or not the mechanical decompression of the ovarian capsule is a key factor in the etiology of PCO. However, it did not improve the ovulation and pregnancy rate, so we terminated further trials of this procedure.

3) According to the Gjönnaess's operation [7], we performed multifollicular puncture and resection (MPR) [13] which consists of a multiple biopsy targeted mainly toward the transparent subcapsular cysts (about six to 10 follicles per ovary) underneath the thick capsule and resection of the capsular tissue. We prefer to use punch biopsy forceps which mimic the forceps used at the colposcopic cervical biopsy.

4) Care must be taken to avoid the hilum of the ovary to prevent disruption of the ovarian blood supply. In order to minimize postoperative adhesion, the whole pelvis should be thoroughly irrigated with saline not only to remove follicular fluid and cauterized debris but also to cool the heated ovary by the diathermy.

5) Generally, $CO_2$, KTP and argon laser vaporize the superficial (2—4 mm depth) ovarian capsule with 25—40 craters (per ovary) until the subcapsular cysts were drained of their follicular fluid [9], while in the case of noncontact type Nd-YAG laser, wedge-shaped area of ovarian tissue with a depth of 4—10 mm is usually coagulated (nonvaporized) by the defocused beam.

5) On the other hand, KTP or argon laser can be used to perforate the ovarian capsule to a depth of 2—4 mm and destroy the underlying stroma which open the subcapsular cyst and intraovarian tissue vaporization can be obtained [14,15].

6) Recently, Mio et al. [16] reported a transvaginal method of ovarian multiple follicle aspiration with a high ovulation rate and pregnancy outcome. They punctured and aspirated the persistent follicles which failed in ovulation at least three cycles after HCG injection (at midluteal phase). They emphasized that transvaginal US-guided follicular aspiration is preferable and less invasive than laparoscopic drilling and the key factor is the drainage of follicular content and not the ovarian stroma.

## Results of ovarian drilling in comparison with medical ovulation induction

Overall ovulation rate after laparoscopic ovarian drilling (LOD) has been reported to be 80—90% (mean 84.2% in 729 patients reviewed by Donnesky 1995) [17] and conception rate 45—65% (mean 55.7% in the same review), as compared to 76—95% ovulation rate and 28—66% conception rate by conventional gonadotropin therapy (724 patients reviewed by Wang and Gemzell 1980) [18]. We have reported a 91% ovulation rate among 23 PCO patients and a pregnancy rate of 52% after MPR [13] which was very similar to Gjönnaess's report (92 and 69% in 62 PCO patients, respectively) [7].

Likewise, similar results were obtained by laser vaporization. Reported ovulation rates and pregnancy rates by $CO_2$/KTP laser were 70—100% and 56—75%, respectively [9], and by Nd-YAG laser 70—83% and 36—58%, respectively [19]. The rates of multiple pregnancy and ovarian hyperstimulation are elevated compared with those of non-PCO subjects.

Abdel Gadir et al. [20] compared the incidence of multiple pregnancy and spontaneous abortion in 85 PCO patients among three groups of laparoscopic electrocautery, HMG treatment, and pure FSH group (Table 1).

Apparently, low miscarriage rates were reported after surgical LOD [21] and it is favorable for the incidence of multiple gestation and ovarian hyperstimulation that monofollicular ovulation is usually achieved by this method.

*Table 1.*

| Method of ovulation induction | Ref. | No. of cases | Ovulation rate | Pregnancy rate | Abortion rate | Multiple pregnancy rate |
|---|---|---|---|---|---|---|
| HMG-HCG treatment | [18] | 724 | 76—95% | 28—66% | 24—39% | 28.7%[a] (14—36)[a] |
| Laparotomic wedge resection (WR) | [4] | 1079 | 80% | 62.5% | 6—16% | |
| Laparoscopic ovarian drilling (LOD) | [17] | 729 | 84.2% (61—100) | 55.7% (20—75) | 15%[a] (11—15) | 15.8%[a] |
| Laparoscopic electrocautery | [7] | 62 | 92% | 69% | | |
| Laparoscopic MPR | [22] | 23 | 91% | 52% | | |
| Laparoscopic CO$_2$ & KTP laser | [9] | 85 | 71% | 56% | | |
| Laparoscopic Nd-YAG laser | [19] | 40 | 70% | 50% | | |
| Electrocautery | [20] | 88 | 71% | 52% | 21% | 0% |
| HMG | [20] | 88 | 71% | 55% | 53% | 20% |
| Pure FSH | [20] | 88 | 67% | 38% | 40% | 20% |

[a]Including other reports.

## Hormonal changes following ovarian drilling

Among various methods of LOD, we performed MPR in 23 patients of PCO and evaluated hormonal changes after MPR.

*Daily hormonal changes* (Fig. 1)

As was reported by coauthor Utsunomiya [22], MPR caused marked reduction (40—50%) of testosterone shortly after operation (3—5 days), which is invariably consistent with other investigator's results [23,24]. It is generally accepted that LOD results in a marked decline of testosterone, androstenedione and, in some reports, it also caused a decrease in estrone, free testosterone and elevated SHBG levels. Mostly, estradiol and other steroid hormones do not change significantly.

*Changes of pulsatile gonadotropin secretion* (Fig. 2)

Exaggerated pulsatile secretion of LH was markedly reduced, in which LH amplitude (but not LH pulse frequency) [24] was decreased with the decrement of mean LH level accompanied by the decline of testosterone. The FSH pulsatile release did not change markedly; rather they showed slight elevation [24].

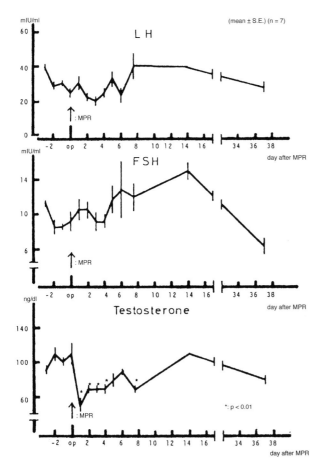

*Fig. 1.* The effects of laporoscopic multiple punch resection (MPR) on serum LH, FSH and testosterone levels.

### Changes in LH/FSH ratio

Imbalance between LH and FSH was generally corrected by the decrease in the LH/FSH ratio in accordance with reduced LH release without changes in FSH.

### Changes in normal control patients

In comparison, normal control patients at early follicular phase showed a rapid transient LH elevation after MPR without concomitant changes in testosterone levels [22], indicating that the mere destruction of ovarian capsule does not cause any specific hormonal change in a normal ovary. In contrast, in cases with hyperthesosis such as PCO, MPR causes a dramatic change in hormonal levels such as LH, testosterone and androstenedione.

542

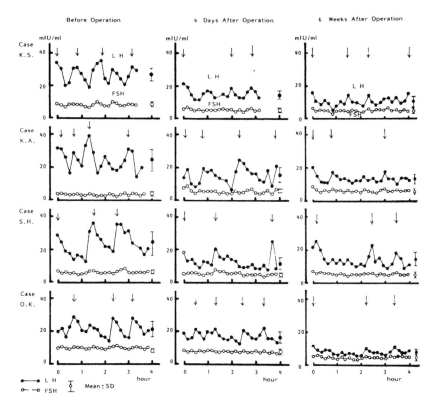

*Fig. 2.* The patterns of pulsatile gonadotropin secretion of PCO patients (four respresentative cases) who underwent laporoscopic multiple punch resection before the operation, 3–4 days after the operation. Arrows indicate the pulses. Closed circles indicate the changes in LH and open circles indicate FSH. The vertical line to the right of each figure expresses the mean ± SD of all LH and FSH values measured for 4 h.

*Comparison with the ovulatory and anovulatory patients after WR*

We have also investigated the difference between the patients who had their ovulatory cycle restored after WR and patients who did not. The testosterone change in patients who achieved ovulatory cycle was more prominent than those who failed in ovulation, indicating that the lower the testosterone level becomes after LOD, the higher the incidence of ovulatory cycle ensues after operation.

**Mechanism of monofolliculogenesis by wedge resection and ovarian drilling in PCO**

1) Vicious cycle of high androgen and high LH pulsation;
2) pituitary hyperresponse and positive feedback from high androgen;
3) high inhibin in atretic PCO follicle; and
4) high androgen and cytochrome P450 c17α enzyme activity.

1) The mechanism underlying the improvement in the vicious cycle of intraovarian hyperandrogenism and exaggerated pulsatile LH release with high LH/FSH ratio induced by the WR or LOD has not been clearly elucidated. Most of the investigators believe that the destruction of the androgen-producing ovarian stroma and drainage of follicles with high androgen and inhibin contents might be responsible for them. We [13,22] have demonstrated the similar hormonal changes by WR and MPR, and reported that the difference between WR and MPR depends on the extent of the impairment of the tissue deep inside the ovarian stroma and/or superficial ovarian capsule. However, these two impairments are not decernible even by the sharp laser destruction by limited focus area. It is not yet clarified which is the key factor for the improvement in the vicious cycle; the thick ovarian capsule or the hypertrophic ovarian stroma.

2) In our previous study, we and others [24] reported that the LH pulse frequency did not change significantly by LOD, which led us to speculate that the hypothalamic electrical activity needed to generate GnRH pulse was not influenced, but rather, the pituitary was influenced to release a less amount of LH.

Greenblatt and Casper [23] described that a decrease in androgen levels may result in lowered peripheral conversion of androgen to estrogen and decreased positive feedback on LH production centrally. Lowered LH levels might then decrease stromal androgen production and, along with increasing FSH levels, allow follicular development to proceed to ovulation.

3) The high inhibin contents in atretic follicle in PCO was observed [25,26], which might be related [27] with FSH suppression relative to high LH, and drainage of subcapsular follicle might result in elevated FSH levels.

4) Recently, it was reported [28,29] that abnormal regulation of cytochrome P450 c17 α causes the exaggerated secretion of ovarian androgen. On the other hand, enhanced LH secretion causes ovarian hyperandrogenism which might potentiate 17 α hydroxylase activity and 17, 20-lyase activity.

These intraovarian enzymes along with the local factors including inhibin- and insulin-like growth factor (IGF) system [30] might be related to the mechanism of monofolliculogenesis by LOD and WR in PCO.

## Complications and side effects of laparoscopic ovarian drilling (LOD)

Postoperative adhesion, which had been the main reason of WR to be unfavored in the 1970s, was found to be not an uncommon phenomena in LOD. Second-look laparoscopy following LOD revealed 19—86% adhesion rates by electrocautery, 0—43% by $CO_2$-KTP laser, and 0—80% by Nd-YAG laser as in Gürgan's review [31].

By second-look laparoscopy [8,11,32,33], most of these adhesions were detected as early as 3—4 weeks postoperatively and they were mostly filmy thin adhesion which was easily dissectable through laparoscope. Some investigators recommend its use, while other investigators [19] showed that the adhesiolysis during second-look laparoscopy did not improve short-term pregnancy outcome.

Direct complications of laparoscopy itself are the bowel injury and bleeding from the drilled hole of the ovary. Monopolar type of electrocautery is more prone to cause bowel injury by sparking and arcing, while bipolar type causes less frequent injury.

As a rare complication of WR, premature ovarian failure or ovarian atrophy [34] was reported, especially in cases where the damage occurred at the ovarian hilus. Therefore it is crucially important not to cauterize or apply laser to the ovarian hilus.

## Advantages and disadvantages of LOD

*Advantages of LOD*

1) Beneficial monofollicular growth (less possible multiple pregnancy and OHSS rate);
2) high ovulation and pregnancy rate comparable to those of gonadotropin therapy;
3) low spontaneous abortion rate;
4) ovulatory effect continues at least three to six cycles (easily with supplementation);
5) requires no intensive monitoring and expensive cost as gonadotropin therapy; and
6) useful for diagnostic laparoscopic examination of unexplained infertility.

*Disadvantages of LOD*

1) Surgery and anesthesia needed (although minimally invasive);
2) postoperative peritubal and periovarian adhesions (permanent if formed); and
3) anovulation might recur after 6 months or more (not permanent ovulatory effect).

As listed in the summary above [17,31,35], it is a controversial issue whether or not to choose the medical treatment (recently advanced modalities of gonadotropin treatment) or laparoscopic ovarian drilling.

## References

1. Stein IF, Leventhal ML. Amenorrhea associated with bilateral polycystic ovaries. Am J Obstet Gynecol 1935;29:181–191.
2. Kistner RW. Peri-tubal and peri-ovarian adhesions subsequent to wedge resection of the ovaries. Fertil Steril 1969;20:35–42.
3. Buttram VC, Vaquero C. Post-ovarian wedge resection adhesive disease. Fertil Steril 1975; 26:874–876.
4. Goldzieher JW, Axelrod LR. Clinical and biochemical features of polycystic ovarian disease. Fertil Steril 1963;14:631–653.

5. Neuwirth RS. A method of bilateral ovarian biopsy at laparoscopy in infertility and chronic anovulation. Fertil Steril 1972;23:361—366.

6. Campo S, Garcea N, Caruso A, Siccardi P. Effect of celioscopic ovarian resection in patients with polycystic ovaries. Gynecol Obstet Invest 1983;15:213—222.

7. Gjönnaess H. Polycystic ovarian syndrome treated by ovarian electrocautery through the laparoscope. Fertil Steril 1984;41:20—25.

8. Dabirashrafi H, Mohamad K, Behjatnia Y, Moghadami-Tabrizi N. Adhesion formation after ovarian electrocauterization on patients with polycystic ovarian syndrome. Fertil Steril 1991; 55:1200—1201.

9. Daniell JF, Miller W. Polycystic ovaries treated by laparoscopic laser vaporization. Fertil Steril 1989;51:232—236.

10. Huber J, Hosmann J, Spona J. Polycystic ovarian syndrome treated by laser through the laparoscope. Lancet 1988;2:215.

11. Keckstein J. Laparoscopic treatment of polycystic ovarian syndrome. Baillieres Clin Obstet Gynaecol 1989;3:563—581.

12. Kusuda M, Tsuda T. Research about the progress of ovulatory disorder. Acta Obstet Gynecol Jpn 1979;31:965—970.

13. Sumioki H, Utsunomiya T, Matsuoka K, Korenaga M, Kadota T. The effect of laparoscopic multiple punch resection of the ovary on hypothalamo-pituitary axis in polycystic ovary syndrome. Fertil Steril 1988;50:567—572.

14. Keckstein G, Rossmanith W, Spatzier K, Schneider V, Borchers K, Steiner R. The effect of laparoscopic treatment of polycystic ovarian disease by $CO_2$-laser or Nd:YAG laser. Surg Endosc 1990;4:103—107.

15. Heylen SM, Puttemans PJ, Brosens IA. Polycystic ovarian disease treated by laparoscopic argon laser capsule drilling: comparison of vaporization versus perforation technique. Hum Reprod 1994;9:1038—1042.

16. Mio Y, Toda T, Tanikawa M, Terado H, Harada T, Terakawa N. Transvaginal ultrasound-guided follicular aspiration in the management of anovulatory infertility associated with polycystic ovaries. Fertil Steril 1991;56:1060—1065.

17. Donesky BW, Adashi EY. Surgically induced ovulation in the polycystic ovary syndrome: wedge resection revisited in the age of laparoscopy. Fertil Steril 1995;63:439—463.

18. Wang CF, Gemzell C. The use of human gonadotropins for the induction of ovulation in women with polycystic ovarian disease. Fertil Steril 1980;33:479—486.

19. Gürgan T, Urman B, Aksu T, Yarali H, Develioglu O, Kisnisci HA. The effect of short-interval laparoscopic lysis of adhesions on pregnancy rates following Nd-YAG laser photocoagulation of polycystic ovaries. Obstet Gynecol 1992;80:45—47.

20. Abdel Gadir A, Mowafi RS, Alnaser HM, Alrashid AH, Alonezi OM, Shaw RW. Ovarian electrocautery versus human menopausal gonadotrophins and pure follicle stimulating hormone therapy in the treatment of patients with polycystic ovarian disease. Clin Endocrinol (Oxf) 1990;33:585—592.

21. Gjönnaess H. The course and outcome of pregnancy after ovarian electrocautery in women with polycystic ovarian syndrome: the influence of body-weight. Br J Obstet Gynaeol 1989; 96:714—719.

22. Utsunomiya T, Sumioki H, Taniguchi I. Hormonal and clinical effects of multifollicular puncture and resection on the ovaries of polycystic ovary syndrome. Horm Res 1990;33(Suppl 2):35—39.

23. Greenblatt E, Casper RF. Endocrine changes after laparoscopic ovarian cautery in polycystic ovarian syndrome. Am J Obstet Gynecol 1987;156:279—285.

24. Rossmanith WG, Keckstein J, Spazier K, Lauritzen C. The impact of ovarian laser surgery on the gonadotrophin secretion in women with polycystic ovarian disease. Clin Endocrinol (Oxf) 1991;34:223—230.

25. Tanabe K, Gagliano P, Channing CP, Nakamura Y, Yoshimura Y, Iizuka R, Fortuny A, Sulewski J, Rezai N. Levels of inhibin-F activity and steroids in human follicular fluid from normal

women and women with polycystic ovarian disease. J Clin Endocrinol Metab 1983;57:24.

26. Hurkadli KS, Jayaraman S, Gopalakrishnan K, Arbatti NJ, Sheth AR. Role of inhibin in polycystioc ovarian syndrome. Int J Fertil 1986;31:165—169.

27. Kovacs G, Buckler H et al. Treatment of anovulation due to polycystic ovarian syndrome by laparoscopic ovarian electrocautery. Br J Obstet Gynaecol 1991;98:30—35.

28. Sahin Y, Kelestimur F. 17-Hydroxyprogesterone responses to gonadotropin-releasing hormone agonist buserelin and adrenocortico-trophin in polycystic ovary syndrome: investigation of adrenal and ovarian cytochrome P450c17alpha dysregulation. Hum Reprod 1997;12:910—913.

29. Goudas VT, Dumesic DA. Polycystic ovary syndrome. Endocrinol Metab Clin North Am 1997;26:893—912.

30. Dunaif A. Insulin resistance and the polycystic ovary syndrome: mechanism and implications for pathogenesis. Endocr Rev 1997;18:774—800.

31. Gürgan T, Yarali H, Urman B. Laparoscopic treatment of polycystic ovarian disease. Hum Reprod 1994;9:573—577.

32. Gürgan T, Kisnisci H, Yarali H, Develioglu O, Zeyneloglu H, Aksu T. Evaluation of adhesion formation after laparoscopic treatment of polycystic ovarian disease. Fertil Steril 1991;56: 1176—1178.

33. Greenblatt EM, Casper RF. Adhesion formation after laparoscopic ovarian cautery for polycystic ovarian syndrome: lack of correlation with pregnancy rate. Fertil Steril 1993;60:766—770.

34. Dabirashrafi H. Complications of laparoscopic ovarian cauterization. Fertil Steril 1989;52: 878—879.

35. Greenblatt E. Surgical options in polycystic ovary syndrome patients who do not respond to medical ovulation induction. Bailliere Clin Obstet Gynaecol 1993;7:421—433.

# Menopause

Fertility and Reproductive Medicine.
R.D. Kempers, J. Cohen, A.F. Haney and J.B. Younger, editors.

549

# HRT forever

William Thompson
*Department of Obstetrics and Gynaecology, The Queen's University of Belfast, Belfast, UK*

**Abstract.** An increase in female life expectancy over the past century means that women now live more than one-third of their lives beyond the menopause. It has been estimated that by the year 2000 there will be 35 million women over the age of 65. Therefore, quality of life and psychological wellbeing related to ageing in women have assumed increasing importance to health professionals. Hormone replacement therapy provides an effective means of reducing two major diseases of old age, namely, arteriosclerosis and osteoporosis. In spite of this, less than 20% of women over 65 years of age receive hormonal therapy. A major obstacle to long-term therapy is poor compliance resulting from fear of breast cancer and vaginal bleeding problems. The recent introduction of selective oestrogen receptor modulators (SERMs) may prove to overcome many of the problems of conventional HRT.

**Keywords:** Alzheimer's disease, cardiovascular disease, osteoporosis, phyto-oestrogen, selective oestrogen receptor modulators (SERMs).

## Introduction

Few medical interventions have as great a potential of affecting morbidity and mortality as long-term hormone replacement therapy (HRT) in postmenopausal women. Furthermore, there is increasing evidence that HRT can be important in improving the quality of life and in particular psychological wellbeing [1]. With increasing life expectancy of the female population the problems of postmenopausal women is now a major public health concern. Women can now expect to live one-third of their life after the menopause.

For some women menopause is the beginning of an era of ageing with its connotations of diminishing abilities and competence. However, to others it is the beginning of a new and promising period of life, free from worries about contraception, pregnancy and menstruation. In this context, women in many cultures view the menopause as a natural process and thus consider that taking medication should be avoided. Health professionals, on the other hand, are much more likely to perceive the menopause as a "medical problem" or a deficiency disease requiring treatment. However, the wider use of HRT is not accepted by all; a recent survey reported that only 64% of gynaecologists and 56% of general practitioners thought that all women should be offered HRT [2].

One of the major limitations in the evaluation of long-term HRT is the identifi-

*Address for correspondence:* Prof William Thompson, Queen's University of Belfast, Institute of Clinical science, Grosvenor Road, Belfast, BT12 6BJ, UK. Tel.: +44-1232-894600. Fax: +44-1232-328247. E-mail: w.thompson@qub.ac.uk

cation of a control group. Women taking HRT often have healthier life styles and are more likely to seek medical advice than those women who decide against treatment [3]. In spite of this, the epidemiological evidence supporting the beneficial effects of HRT is overwhelming in its uniformity and consistency.

Against the background of increasing public awareness and expectations of HRT, tertiary referral menopause clinics are treating increasing numbers of patients with complicated medical histories. In our experience, these patients often have concerns which include protection against many of the diseases of ageing, especially osteoporosis and cardiac disease [4]. These findings suggest that menopausal women in both the UK and USA are well informed about the potential protective benefits of HRT, and now expect an improvement in the quality of their lives well beyond the relief of menopausal symptoms.

**The benefits of long-term HRT**

Protection against cardiovascular disease is a major benefit of long-term postmenopausal oestrogen treatment. This is particularly significant when we consider that diseases of the cardiovascular system are the leading cause of death in Western societies. Nearly one-third of heart disease mortality in women occurs before the age of 65 from atherosclerosis in major vessels [5]. Several case-control as well as cohort studies have shown that HRT reduces the risk of cardiovascular disease. Although it is accepted that there are limitations to such observational data the studies are large enough to control for a number of confounding factors. A meta-analysis of women using HRT shows that the relative risk of coronary artery disease is reduced to 0.5 [6]. The data on stroke is less clear and this is partly due to the fact that this condition occurs at a relatively more advanced age than myocardial infarction and few women at present use oestrogens beyond the age of 70 years of age [7]. Recent publications suggest a protective effect against Alzheimer's disease as HRT has been shown to increase cerebral blood flow and neuronal stimulation [8]. This is now supported by a meta-analysis which has demonstrated a 29% decrease in dementia in HRT users. This data on Alzheimer's disease suggests a positive effect but further study is required [9]. There is more convincing evidence that oestrogen helps to maintain verbal memory in ageing women [10].

Prevention of osteoporosis is one of the most important reasons for long-term or indeed forever HRT since its beneficial effect lessens with time off therapy. A 50-year-old woman has a 15% lifetime probability of suffering a hip fracture and a 1.5% probability of dying from this condition [11]. As the proportion of elderly women in the society increases so does the frequency of osteoporotic fractures which in turn place an additional burden on health resources. HRT offers protection from accelerated postmenopausal bone loss and an estimated reduction to 0.28 in the relative risk of death from femoral neck fracture as well as an ability to improve the quality of life.

## The problem of compliance

The two main reasons for poor compliance with HRT are fear of cancer and vaginal bleeding and both these factors are extremely important in the older woman requiring long-term therapy.

Breast cancer is the most common cancer in women. However, the leading cause of death in women is cardiac disease which accounts for 34% of deaths compared to 3—4% of deaths which result from breast cancer [12]. There have been many epidemiological studies of the relationship between HRT and breast cancer, however, a consistent pattern of risk has not been demonstrated.

The latest reports from the Nurses Health Study represent 16 years of follow up (1976—1992) [13,14]. The analysis revealed that women who had used oestrogen in the past were not at increased risk of breast cancer but there was an increased risk in current users. However, this finding of an increased relative risk in current users was not definitive and note free from confounding variables. In contrast, another recent case control study focused on long-term use and could not detect an adverse impact of HRT on the risk of breast cancer [15].

In an attempt to resolve these conflicting reports researchers formed a collaborative group and reanalysed 90% of the worldwide evidence on oestrogen and breast cancer. Among current and recent users of HRT there is a small increased risk of breast cancer, approximately 2.3% in RR for each year of use [16]. This report suggests that there will be an extra 12 cases of breast cancer by the age of 70 for every 1,000 women who start HRT at the age of 50 and continue for 15 years. The mortality rates of women who were taking estrogen at the time of breast cancer diagnosis have documented improved survival rates [16]. This probably reflects earlier diagnosis in users because the greater survival rate in current users is associated with a lower frequency of late stage disease. There is also evidence to suggest estrogen users develop better differentiated tumors and that detection bias is not the only explanation for better survival.

The data on breast cancer and estrogen therapy remains inconclusive and lacking in consistency. However, this lack of a definitive answer is actually very reassuring as this indicates that there is unlikely to be a major effect of estrogen therapy on breast cancer risk. This issue is being addressed in several new studies which include the National Institutes of Health-Funded Women's Health Initiative in the USA and a randomised trial of 18,000 women being coordinated by the Medical Research Council in the UK. Unfortunately, data from these studies will not be available until well into the next millennium.

With regard to other cancers, the Nurses Health Study has recently reported a reduced risk of colorectal cancer in past users of postmenopausal HRT [17].

In those with an intact uterus unopposed oestrogens should be avoided as there is a 20% incidence of endometrial hyperplasia after 1 year of use [18]. The endometrium can be protected by the addition of progestogen for a minimum of 10 days per month [19]. However, this will result in monthly withdrawal bleeding in 90% of women. Reluctance to accept menstrual bleeding is an important cause of poor continuance in women with an intact uterus [20]. Furthermore, there is evidence that the absence of withdrawal bleeding may improve long-term compliance [21].

The continuous-combined estrogen/progestin method of treatment was introduced as bleeding is avoided in 80% of patients after 6 months of treatment [22]. However, for those that continue to have bleeding problems, as yet, there is no effective method of drug alteration. However, a recent study demonstrated that 81% of women on continuous-combined preparations discontinued treatment at the end of the 3rd year compared with 76% on cyclical therapy [21]. We should not dismiss the importance of other nonlife-threatening side effects adversely affecting compliance especially in older women. There are now a wide variety of oestrogen preparations and routes of administration — e.g., patches and gels which avoid the first pass effect — and therefore reduce the dosage required and thus the side effects. Many women have an intolerance to progestogens. Intrauterine devices containing a progestogen offer an alternative to oral progestogens and appear to maintain an atrophic endometrium. Further studies are needed to confirm that such a treatment regimen would be acceptable to older women.

Women are concerned about the potential weight gain that may occur with hormonal therapy. This aspect was studied in a double-blinded prospective fashion by the PEPI Trial [28] in which patients had follow up on placebo and various HRT regimens. All groups in the study gained weight but the placebo group gained the most weight. In spite of this convincing evidence it is still difficult to convince women that weight gain is an effect of ageing and lowered basal metabolic rate and not a side effect associated with HRT.

**Other adverse effects of HRT**

Three studies published in a recent issue of the Lancet suggested that postmenopausal HRT was associated with a 2- to 3-fold risk of venous thromboembolism [23–25]. These studies tried to control for risk factors for venous thromboembolism (VTE) except a family history of VTE. In view of the recent knowledge regarding the Leiden mutation and its impact on VTE with OCPs this is a very important consideration and would inject bias into the case group.

The incidence of idiopathic VTE in this age group is approximately one per 10,000 women per year. If these studies are correct this would increase the incidence to about three cases per 10,000 per year which is a very small number. Even if we accept that this is a real risk it remains confined to short-term current users and would not diminish our emphasis on long-term use for preventative health benefits.

**Future prospects for HRT**

Recent studies have shown that the role of the estrogen receptor is not identical in all tissues. The antiestrogen tamoxifen may preserve bone mass in postmenopausal women with breast cancer [26]. Thus by targeting activities of the estrogen receptor it may be possible to develop agents for the modulation of specific tissues or processes. Such compounds will exert beneficial agonistic effects on bone, cardiovascular system and brain but have an antagonistic (antiostrogenic) effect on the uterus or breast. Preliminary data on a number of selective estrogen receptor modulators (SERMS) such as raloxifene, droloxifene and levormeloxifene are promising. Large multicentre studies, of these compounds, have been initiated and preliminary data is encouraging. They may prove to be the next generation of postmenopausal hormone therapy specifically targeted for the older patient.

Another promising development is phytoestrogens, which are compounds derived from plants that have a weak affinity for the estradiol receptors compared to estradiol. They appear to compete with estradiol for the oestrogen receptor. Foods containing phytoestrogens reduce cholesterol and human data shows benefit in treating osteoporosis. They also inhibit the growth of different cancer lines in cell culture. Human epidemiologic evidence supports the hypothesis that phytoestrogens inhibit cancer formation and growth in humans [27]. In all respects they appear to meet the health needs of the older woman.

### Conclusion

The benefits of long-term HRT outweigh the risks in the majority of women. The development of new formulations further enhance the risk/benefit profile of treatment. HRT forever is not an unrealistic prospect for the new millennium.

### References

1. Purdie DW, Empson JAC, Crichton CC, MacDonald L. Hormone replacement, sleep quality and psychological well-being. Br J Obstet Gynaecol 1996;102:735–739.
2. Norman SG , Studd JWW. A survey of views on hormone replacement therapy. Br J Obstet Gynaecol 1994;101:879–887.
3. Barrett-Connor E. Postmenopausal estrogen and prevention bias. Ann Int Med 1991;115; 455–456.
4. McKinney KA, Severino M, McFall P, Burry K, Thompson W. The treatment seeking women at menopause; a comparison between two university menopause clinics. Menopause (In press).
5. Wenger NK, Speroff L, Packard B. Cardiovascular health and disease in women. N Engl J Med 1993;329:247–256.
6. Stevenson JC, Crook D, Godland IF. Cardiovascular and skeletal effects of hormone replacement therapy. In: Seymour CA, Weetman AP (eds) Horizons in Medicine, No. 5. London: Blackwell Scientific Publications, 92–101.
7. Grodstein F, Stampfer MJ, Manson JE et al. Postmenopausal estrogen and progestin use and the risk of cardiovascular disease. N Engl J Med 1996;335:453–461.
8. Paganini-Hill A, Henderson VW. Estrogen deficiency and the risk of Alzheimer's disease in women. Am J Epidemiol 1994;140:256–261.
9. Yaffe K, Sawaya G, Lieberburg I, Grady D. Estrogen therapy in postmenopausal women. Effects on cognitive function and dementia. JAMA 1998;279:688–695.
10. Sherwin BB. Sex hormones and psychological functioning in postmenopausal women. Exp

Geront 1994;29:423—430.

11. Grady D, Rubin SM, Petitti DB, Fox CS, Black D, Ettinger B, Ernster VL, Cummings SR. Hormone therapy to prevent disease and prolong life in postmenopausal women. Ann Int Med 1992;117:1016—1037.

12. Cummings SR, Black DM, Rubin SM. Lifetime risks of hip, Colles or vertebral fracture and coronary heart disease among white postmenopausal women. Arch Intern Med 1989;149: 2445—2448.

13. Colditz GA, Stampfer MJ, Willett WC, Hunter DJ, Manson JE, Hennekens CH, Rosner BA, Speizer FE. Type of postmenopausal use and risk of breast cancer: 12-year follow-up from the Nurses Health Study, Cancer Causes Control 3, 1992;433—439.

14. Colditz GA, Hankinson SE, Hunter DJ, Willett WC, Manson J. Hennekens C, Rosner B, Speizer FE. The use of estrogens and progestins and the risk of breast cancer in postmenopausal women. N Engl J Med 1995;332:1589—1593.

15. Stanford JL, Weiss NS, Voight LF, Daling JR, Habel LA, Rossing MA. Combined estrogen and progestin hormone replacement therapy in relation to risk of breast cancer in middle-aged women. JAMA 1995;274:137—142.

16. Collaborative Group on Hormonal Factors in Breast Cancer. Breast cancer and hormone replacement therapy: collaborative re-analysis of data from 51 epidemiological studies of 52,705 women with breast cancer and 108,411 women without breast cancer. Lancet 1997;350: 1047—1059.

17. Chute CG, Willett WC, Colditz GA, Stampfer MJ, Rosner B, Speizer FE. A prospective study of reproductive history and exogenous estrogens on the risk of colorectal cancer in women. Epidemiology 1991;2:201—204.

18. Woodruff JD, Pickar JH. Incidence of endometrial hyperplasia in postmenopausal women taking conjugated estrogens (Premarin) with medroxyprogesterone acetate or conjugated estrogens alone. The Menopause Study Group. Am J Obstet Gynecol 1994;170:1213—1223.

19. Varma TR. Effect of long-term therapy with estrogen and progesterone on the endometrium of postmenopausal women. Acta Obstet Gynaecol Scand 1985;64:41—46.

20. Williams SR, Frenchek B, Speroff T, Speroff L. A study of combined continuous ethinyl estradiol and norethindrone acetate for postmenopausal hormone replacement. Am J Obstet Gynecol 1990;162:438—446.

21. Ettinger B, De-Kun I, Klein R. Continuation of postmenopausal hormone replacement therapy: comparisons of cyclic versus continuous combined schedules. Menopause 1996;3:185—189.

22. Archer DF, Pickar JH, Bottiglioni F. Bleeding patterns in postmenopausal women taking continuous combined or sequential regimens of conjugated estrogens with medroxyprogesterone acetate. The Menopause Study Group. Obstet Gynecol 1994;83:686—692.

23. Daly E, Vessey MP, Hawkins MM et al. Risk of venous thromboembolism in users of hormone replacement therapy. Lancet 1996;348:977—980.

24. Jick H, Derby LE, Myers MW et al. Risk of hospital admission for idiopathic venous thromboembolism among users of postmenopausal oestrogens. Lancet 1996;348:981—983.

25. Grodstein F, Stampfer MJ, Goldhaber SZ. Prospective study of exogenous hormones and risk of pulmonary embolism in women. Lancet 1996;348:983—987.

26. Love RR, Mazess RB, Barden HS, Epstein S. Neurcomb PA, Jordan VC et al. Effects of tamoxifen on bone mineral density in postmenopausal women with breast cancer. N Engl J Med 1992;326:852—856.

27. Knight DC, Eden JA. A review of the clinical effects of phyto-estrogens. Obstet Gynaecol 1996;87:897—904.

28. PEPI Trial — The Writing Group for the PEPI Trial. Effects on oestrogen or oestrogen/progestin on heart disease risk factor in postmenopausal women. JAMA 1995;273:199—208.

Fertility and Reproductive Medicine.
R.D. Kempers, J. Cohen, A.F. Haney and J.B. Younger, editors.

# Designer estrogens: clinical aspects

Rogerio A. Lobo

*Department of Obstetrics and Gynecology, College of Physicians and Surgeons of Columbia University, New York, New York, USA*

**Abstract.** Because estrogen affects many important physiological processes, the concept of designing an estrogen which would have selectivity for specific organ systems has become a popular notion. Theoretically, this may be accomplished by a selective delivery system or by selective receptor interactions. Our understanding of estrogen action has evolved recently with the realization that there are two receptors ERα and β, and that selectivity is determined by binding characteristics as well as the relative activities of domains within the receptor called transactivating factors. Selective estrogen receptor modulators (SERMs) are compounds which have mixed agonistic and antagonistic activities in various organs. SERMs may be utilized to target an organ (e.g., uterus) for antagonistic activity or to advance postmenopausal health by producing an optimum combination of agonistic and antagonistic activities. To date there is no ideal SERM, but second generation SERMs such as raloxifene have been developed for clinical use. The ideal SERM would be agonistic for the brain, cardiovascular system, bone and vagina but antagonistic to the breast and uterus. Several natural dietary products (phytoestrogens) function much like man-made SERMs.

**Keywords:** designer, estrogen, menopause, raloxifene, receptors, SERMs, tamoxifen.

## Introduction

Estrogen receptors are ubiquitous; thus, it is expected that estrogen exerts an influence throughout the body. Although in normal premenopausal women, all these effects are desirable, in disease states and after menopause some estrogenic effects should be avoided. Examples of these include estrogen-sensitive neoplasia and disorders such as leiomyomata and endometriosis in premenopausal women and estrogenic stimulation of the breast and uterus in postmenopausal women.

It would be ideal, therefore, to "design" an estrogen which would have selective agonistic or stimulatory effects on one organ system, and neutral or antagonistic effects on other organ systems. At least two approaches could be adapted to "design" such as estrogen. The first would involve targeted delivery of native estradiol using a vehicle or modified molecule such that estradiol could enter one organ and not another. The second approach would be to use an estrogen analog, which would selectively modulate receptors to express agonistic, neutral or antagonistic activities in different tissues.

*Address for correspondence:* Rogerio A. Lobo MD, Department of Obstetrics and Gynecology, Columbia University College of Physicians and Surgeons, 630 West 168th Street, New York, NY 10032, USA.

An example of the first approach is to couple estradiol to a quaternary salt, which would not have systemic effects, but which could pass through the blood-brain barrier. The molecule could be modified to release estradiol for direct action in the brain [1]. While this is an appealing approach, there are no clinical data to support its use at the present time.

The second approach involves a group of compounds called SERMs (selective estrogen receptor modulators). A list of SERMs may be found in Table 1. How SERMs "selectively" influence different tissues is not completely understood but will be reviewed briefly below.

## Estrogen action

It is now known that there are two estrogen receptors (ER) $\alpha$ and $\beta$ (Fig. 1). While the DNA-binding domains of ER$\alpha$ and $\beta$ are almost identical with about 97% homology, the ligand-binding domains are different and only have 60% homology [2]. Various estrogens have different affinities for ER$\alpha$ and $\beta$, which in turn are distributed differently throughout the body. For example, preliminary evidence suggests that in certain regions of the brain (e.g., frontal cortex) ER$\beta$ predominates over ER$\alpha$. In the cerebellum, only ER$\beta$ is expressed [3,4]. Phyto-estrogens as ligands appear to have a greater affinity for ER$\beta$ than ER$\alpha$.

Our understanding of ligand binding to the estrogen receptor has also changed over the last few years. SERMs may be classified according to their antagonistic and agonistic activities, which relate to how they bind to the receptor. This has been modeled after knowledge of the progesterone receptor [5,6]. Compounds which prevent receptor/DNA interactions are called type I antiestrogens. There are no known pure type I antiestrogens. A type II antiestrogen is one that induces conformation which is closest to that of an inactive receptor. An example of this is the antiestrogen, ICI 164, 384. A compound which exhibits partial agonistic effects is considered a type III antiestrogen and an example of this is raloxifene. A compound which stabilizes the estrogen receptor in a conformation allowing transcription on a certain number of estrogen receptor responsive genes is a type IV antiestrogen; this is exemplified by 4 OH-tamoxifen.

How does a type III antiestrogen, like raloxifene, exert agonistic vs. antagonistic

*Table 1.* Selective estrogen receptor modulators SERMs: a partial list.

Clomiphene
Tamoxifen, 4 OH tamoxifen
Nafoxidene
Droloxifene
Toremifene
Idoxifene
Raloxifene
Isoflavones (phytoestrogens)

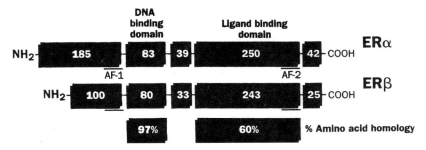

*Fig. 1.* Homology of ERα and ERβ.

activities? The estrogen receptor contains different transcription activating factors, TAF 1 and 2. TAF or AF1 is located near the N-terminus, and AF2 at the C-terminus (Fig. 1). Different tissues have different AF1 and AF2 activities. Thus far, tamoxifen is known to interact with AF2 exhibiting antagonistic activity and AF1 with agonistic activity. In the breast, a tissue exhibiting much AF2 activity, tamoxifen acts as an antagonist. In addition, as proposed by McDonnel, compounds like raloxifene induce a different and unique receptor conformation, which explains its activity.

**Clinical effects of SERMs**

In the future it is anticipated that many more SERMs will be identified which will have a more ideal profile of agonistic and antagonistic activities for various uses. However, there is considerable experience with two SERMs, which have been in use for some time. These are clomiphene and tamoxifen.

Clomiphene has mixed agonistic/antagonistic activity occurring as a racemic mixture of zu- or cis-, and en- or trans-clomiphene. Zu-clomiphene only constitutes 38% of a clomiphene tablet but exhibits higher concentrations and lasts longer in the circulation [7]. The en-clomiphene isomer, however, is the molecule which induces ovulation [8]. The estrogen antagonistic effects are responsible for ovulation induction by activating GnRH secretion in the hypothalamus. However, its antiestrogenic properties, which may be sustained, may cause problems with cervical mucus and endometrial maturation after its transient use in the early follicular phase.

Tamoxifen has been used almost exclusively for the treatment of estrogen receptor positive breast cancer. However, its use has been extended to chemoprotection for women at risk of breast cancer as well [9]. In addition, it has also been used as an alternate to clomiphene on occasion. While taxomifen is an antiestrogen for breast tissue, it exerts an agonistic (stimulatory) effect on the uterus and can lead to cases of endometrial disease (polyps and cancers) [10]. These effects are inconsistent, exhibit an unusual pattern of expression and are not predictable, possibly due to the activation of a spectrum of ligand-receptor interactions in tissues of different women. In addition, it is agonistic (to variable degrees) in bone and liver, but antagonistic in the vagina and certain brain regions, leading to hot flushes. Thus it is a protective to some degree against osteoporosis [11], induces some CV protection due to reduction in LDL and total cholesterol [12], but tends to increase vein thrombosis [13] and precipitate vaginal atrophy and hot flushes [14].

Ideally, the use of SERMs should fall into two categories. The first would be to relieve symptoms and improve the quality of life for postmenopausal women. The second, more selective use, would be to utilize the antiestrogenic effects for one purpose only, minimizing its effects on other organ systems.

For postmenopausal health, the following would be the ideal scenario: agonistic activity for the brain, bone, cardiovascular system (but not necessarily the liver), vagina and urinary system. Ideal antiestrogenic activity would be targeted at the breast and uterus in postmenopausal women.

Age increases the risk of breast cancer, independent of the effects of estrogen. Many lines of evidence suggest that a reduction in estrogen status, decreases the risk of breast cancer [15]. Thus, whether or not prolonged estrogen use increases the risk of breast cancer, any SERM ideally would lower this risk for postmenopausal women. Although not pathologic, uterine withdrawal bleeding is unacceptable to most postmenopausal women. Accordingly, a SERM which exerts agonistic effects on systems such as bone, but does not result in uterine/endometrial stimulation, would be ideal.

Estrogenic agonistic effects on the brain, CV system and bone improves morbidity and mortality. It improves cognitive function, reduces Alzheimer's risk, reduces cardiovascular risk and stroke mortality and reduces fractures from osteoporosis [16,17]. Ideally, these functions of estrogen could be substituted for with a SERM, resulting in a similar or greater effect than occurs with current doses of estrogen. The effect of estrogen or a SERM on the liver is viewed as being positive in that it induces increased HDL levels and reduces LDL and total cholesterol. However, this should be viewed as only a partial beneficial effect on CV function as at least 60–70% of the total effect of estrogen involves direct vascular effects. While these direct vascular effects are known to occur with estradiol, they are unlikely to occur with certain SERMs. Coronary vessels express both ERα and ERβ [18] ligands which interact differently with ERβ and ERα [19]. Moreover, hepatic effects of estrogen or SERMs, if excessive, increase the risk of venous thromboembolism, an effect known to occur with oral estrogen, tamoxifen and raloxifene.

What do we know of the effects of the currently available SERMs? Tamoxifen, a triphenyl ethylene, has been mentioned briefly above and has been shown in trials of "normal women" to exhibit a protective effect for osteoporosis and myocardial infarction, but increases the risk of uterine cancer and thrombosis [20]. In addition, tamoxifen induces and/or does not relieve hot flushes and induces vaginal atrophy.

Raloxifene, a benzothiophene, has recently been released for protection against osteoporosis. In head-to-head comparisons it prevents bone loss in a superior

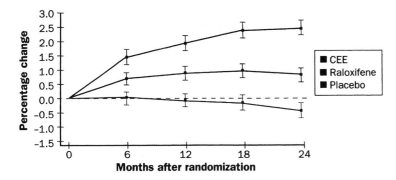

*Fig. 2.* Hip bone mass in women treated with placebo, raloxifene (middle line) and conjugated equine estrogen (CEE) – upper line. (Taken from [21].)

fashion to a placebo but not as well as conjugated equine estrogens (Fig. 2). The effects of raloxifene 60 mg are approximately 50–60% those of conjugated equine estrogens at a dose of 0.625 mg daily [21]. It has a beneficial effect on the liver in lowering total and LDL cholesterol, as well as triglycerides, but not in increasing HDL-C [22]. However, as stated earlier these lipid effects cannot be equated with significant CV protection or a reduction in atherosclerosis. In the cynamologous monkey model, raloxifene was shown not to decrease coronary atherosclerosis extent despite a lowering of total and LDL-cholesterol (Fig. 3) [23]. Of interest, however, again in the monkey model, tamoxifen was shown to lower coronary artery atherosclerosis extent, almost as much as conjugated equine estrogens [24], suggesting that not all SERMs are void of an arterial effect. In addition, raloxifene's antiestrogenic effects induces hot flushes and vaginal atrophy much like tamoxifen and is also associated with venous thrombosis.

Although human data are limited, certain isoflavones or phytoestrogens can

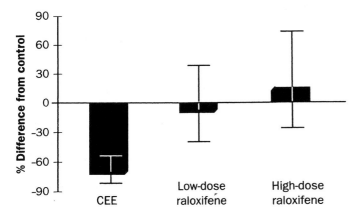

*Fig. 3.* Coronary plaque size in cynamologous monkeys treated with CEE (as percent difference from placebo) as compared to 2 doses of raloxifene. (Adapted from [23].)

*Table 2.* Effects of estradiol and SERMs on various organ systems as pertinent to postmenopausal use.

|  | Brain | Uterus | Vagina | Breast | Bone | CV |
|---|---|---|---|---|---|---|
| $E_2$ | ++ | ++ | ++ | ++ | ++ | ++ |
| Pure antiestrogen | – | – | – | – | – | – |
| "Ideal" | ++ | – | ++ | – | ++ | ++ |
| Tamoxifen | – | + | – | – | + | + |
| Raloxifene | – | – | – | – | + | + |
| Isoflavones | + | – | + | – | + | + |

also be considered to be SERMs. While having some positive effects on the brain, bone and coronary atherosclerosis, there may not be appreciable stimulatory effects on the breast or uterus [25]. Of interest, phytoestrogens appear to have a greater affinity for the β-estrogen receptor.

**Specific uses of SERMs**

In the future, it is reasonable to expect that these "designer" estrogens will be helpful in antagonizing certain organ systems. For example, there are in vitro data to suggest suppression of leiomyomata and endometriosis [26]. The suppression of endometrial hyperplasia, cancer and breast disease are also attractive goals. Thus, normal and specific therapies may be devised. The challenge, however, is that its use in premenopausal women in vitro is confounded by endogenous hormonal secretion. Adjunctive downregulation of ovarian steroid production by the use of a GnRH agonist may also lessen its effectiveness because of the potential downregulation of ERs. Preliminary short-term data are available for raloxifene in "normal", ovulating women. When given in doses up to 200 mg per day, a reduction in endometrial mitotic activity was witnessed, but the menstrual cycle was not adversely affected [27]. Although FSH levels increased slightly, as did estrogen, normal endogenous estrogen status appears to prevent much of the expected antiestrogenic effects.

**Conclusions**

Designer estrogens, specifically the SERMs, offer a range of opportunities for reproductive medicine and postmenopausal use. A scheme for the ideal profile as well as existing SERMs is provided in Table 2. Although there are some benefits to the use of the currently available SERMs, they have to be viewed as first generation products. In the future, novel modulatory design will lead to compounds with more ideal treatment profiles.

**References**

1.  Bodor N, Prokai L, Wu WM, Farag H, Jonalagadda S, Kawamura M, Simpkins J. A strategy for

delivering peptides into the central nervous system by sequential metabolism. Science 1992; 257:1698−1700.

2. McDonnell DP, Clemm DL, Hermann T, Goldman ME, Pike JW. Analysis of estrogen receptor function in vitro reveals three distinct classes of antiestrogens. Molec Endocrinol 1995;9: 659−669.

3. Kuiper GG, Carlsson B, Grandien K, Enmark E, Haggblad J, Nilsson S, Gustafsson JA. Comparison of the ligand binding specificity and transcript tissue distribution of estrogen receptors alpha and beta. Endocrinology 1997;138:863−870.

4. Shughrue PJ, Lane MV, Merchenthaler I. Comparative distribution of estrogen receptor-alpha and-beta mRNA in the rat central nervous system. J Comp Neurol 1997;388:507−525.

5. Klein-Hitpass L, Cato AC, Henderson D, Ryffel GU. Two types of antiprogestins identified by their differential action in transcriptionally active extracts from T47D cells. Nucl Acid Res 1991;19:1227−1234.

6. McDonnell DP, Wagner BL. The mechanism of action of estrogen and progesterone. In: Fraser I, Jansen R, Lobo RA, Whitehead M (eds) Estrogens and Progestrogens in Clinical Practice. London: Churchill-Livingstone, 1998;(In press).

7. Mikkelson TJ, Kroboth PD, Cameron WJ, Dittert LW, Chungi V, Manberg PJ. Single-dose pharmacokinetics of clomiphene citrate in normal volunteers. Fertil Steril 1986;46:392−396.

8. Glasier AF, Irvine DS, Wickings EJ, Hillier SG, Baird DT. A comparison of the effects on follicular development between clomiphene citrate, its two separate isomers and spontaneous cycles. Hum Reprod 1989;4:252−256.

9. Smigel K. Breast cancer prevention trial shows major benefit, some risk. J Natl Cancer Inst 1998;90:647−648.

10. Assikis VJ, Jordan VC. A realistic assessment of the association between tamoxifen and endometrial cancer. Endocrine Rel Cancer 1995;2:1−7.

11. Powles TJ, Hickish T, Kanis JA, Tidy A, Ashley S. Effect of tamoxifen on bone mineral density measured by dual-energy X-ray absorptiometry in healthy premenopausal and postmenopausal women. J Clin Oncol 1996;14:78−84.

12. Love RR, Wiebe DA, Feyzi JM, Newcomb PA, Chappell RJ. Effects of tamoxifen on cardiovascular risk factors in postmenopausal women after 5 years of treatment. J Natl Cancer Inst 1994;86:1534−1539.

13. Fisher B, Costantino JP, Redmond CK, Fisher ER, Wickerham DK, Cronin WM. Endometrial cancer in tamoxifen-treated breast cancer patients: findings from the National Surgical Adjunct Breast and Bowel Project (NSABP) B-14. J Natl Cancer Inst 1994;86:527−537.

14. Jennings TS, Creasman WT. Effects on the reproductive tract: Clinical aspects. In: Lindsay R, Dempster DW, Jordan VC (eds) Estrogens and Antiestrogens, chapter 15. Philadelphia: Lippincott-Raven Publishers, 1997;223−242.

15. Spicer DV, Pike MC. Epidemiology of breast cancer. In: Lob RA (ed) Treatment of the Postmenopausal Woman: Basic and Clinical Aspects, chapter 31. New York: Raven Press, 1993; 315−324.

16. Lobo RA. Benefits and risks of estrogen replacement therapy. Am J Obstet Gynecol 1995; 173:982−989.

17. Lobo RA. Therapeutic controversy: estrogen replacement in menopause. J Clin Endocrinol Metab 1996;81:3829−3838.

18. Register TC, Adams MR. Coronary artery and cultured aortic smooth muscle cells express mRNA for both the classical estrogen receptor and the newly described estrogen receptor beta. J Steroid Biochem Mol Biol 1998;64:187−191.

19. Paech K, Webb P, Kuiper GG, Nilsson S, Gustafsson J, Kushner PJ, Scanlan TS. Differential ligand activation of estrogen receptors ERalpha and ERbeta at AP1 sites. Science 1997;277: 1508−1510.

20. Thomas EJ, Walton PL, Thomas NM, Dowsett M. The effects of ICI 182,780, a pure antiestrogen, on the hypothalamic-pituitary-gonadal axis and on endometrial proliferation in premeno-

562

pausal women. Hum Reprod 1994;9:1191—1196.

21. Raloxifene [package insert]. International Multicenter Study. Indianapolis: Eli Lilly and Company, 1998.

22. Walsh BW, Kuller LH, Wild RA, Paul S, Farmer M, Lawrence JB, Shah AS, Anderson PW. Effects of raloxifene on serum lipids and coagulation factors in healthy postmenopausal women. J Am Med Assoc 1998;279:1445—1451.

23. Clarkson TB, Anthony MS, Jerome CP. Lack of effect of raloxifene on coronary artery atherosclerosis of postmenopausal monkeys. J Clin Endocrinol Metab 1998; 83:721—726.

24. Williams JK, Wagner JD, Li Z, Golden Dl, Adams MR. Tamoxifen inhibits arterial accumulation of LDL degradation products and progression of coronary artery atherosclerosis in monkeys. Arterioscl Thromb Vasc Biol 1997;17:403—408.

25. Anthony MS, Clarkson TB, Hughes CL Jr, Morgan TM, Burke GL. Soybean isoflavones improve cardiovascular risk factors without affecting the reproductive system of peripubertal rhesus monkey. J Nutr 1996;126:43—50.

26. Fuchs-Young R, Howe S, Hale L, Miles R, Walker C. Inhibition of estrogen-stimulated growth of uterine leiomyomas by selective estrogen receptor modulators. Molec Carcinogen 1996;17:151—159.

27. Baker VL, Draper M, Paul S, Allerheiligen, Glant M, Shifren J, Jaffe RB. Reproductive endocrine and endometrial effects of raloxifene hydrochloride, a selective estrogen receptor modulator, in women with regular menstrual cycles. J Clin Endocrinol Metab 1998;83:6—13.

# Beyond estrogen: DHEA and other androgens

John E. Buster and Peter R. Casson
*Baylor College of Medicine, Houston, Texas, USA*

**Abstract.** Age-related declines in dehydroepiandrosterone (DHEA) and dehydroepiandrosterone sulfate (DHEA-S) have been postulated to aggravate some diseases of aging. As a result, DHEA replacement, touted by some as youth restoring, is being used clinically without definitive evidence of efficacy or safety. The evidence is nonetheless compelling that DHEA, alone or in combination with estrogens, is insulin sensitizing, builds bone, provides cardioprotection, and enhances immunocompetance. This review addresses the current status of DHEA replacement with focus on issues of bioavailability, delivery systems, beneficial effects, and safety. At the present, DHEA replacement is not sufficiently proven for general clinical use, however, the potential for future DHEA alone or in combination with other replacement hormones is promising and deserves further investigation.

**Keywords:** aging, androgens, dehydroepiandrosterone (DHEA), dehydroepiandrosterone sulfate (DHEA-S), menapause.

DHEA-S levels decline markedly with age; in the elderly, they are about 10–20% of the reproductive age peak [1–4]. This decline is sometimes called "adreno-pause" and occurs concurrent with involution of the zona reticularis [5,6].

There is much lay speculation about DHEA; and it is now widely touted as a panacea for aging. Interest in DHEA replacement germinated with animal studies indicating it may have antioncogenic, cardioprotective, antiobesity, insulin-sensitizing, antiosteoporotic, and immune- and cognitive-enhancing properties. Unfortunately, extrapolation of these results to humans is limited, as the animal models used have negligible endogenous adrenal androgen levels, and the DHEA doses used were extremely supraphysiologic. It remains in the realm of clinical research to determine if the salutary effects of DHEA replacement exist. Epidemiologic studies addressing the relationship between endogenous serum DHEA-S levels and various disease outcomes are of limited utility. Single serum DHEA-S values may not accurately reflect adrenal androgen reserve or the rate of adrenal androgen decline with age in a particular individual. Finally, DHEA-S values are also subject to multiple confounding factors, including smoking, alcohol use, obesity, gender, and race.

Nonetheless, some 30 trials addressing DHEA replacement exist in the literature, with several more underway at the present time. This paper summarizes the clinical literature to date and provides an overview of the state-of-the-art of DHEA replacement.

*Address for correspondence:* Prof John E. Buster MD, Department of Obstetrics and Gynecology, Baylor College of Medicine, Division of Reproductive Endo, 6550 Fannin, Suite 801, Houston, TX 77030, USA. Tel.: +1-713-798-8399. Fax: +1-713-798-8431. E-mail: jbuster@bcm.tme.edu

## DHEA and cardioprotection

Animal evidence implies a cardioprotective effect from exogenously administered DHEA. In a rabbit model of accelerated atherogenesis (heterotopic heart transplantation or aortic balloon injury), DHEA retarded disease progression in a lipoprotein-independent fashion [7,8]. Despite these data, the epidemiologic literature on the cardioprotective effects of the adrenal androgens is more contentious. The initial evaluation of the Rancho Bernardo cohort indicated that an increase in serum DHEA-S of 100 µg/dl was associated with a 36% reduction in overall and a 48% reduction in cardiovascular mortality, even after adjustment for multiple risk factors [9]. This effect, however, was only seen in men, although another study of this cohort did demonstrate a significant association between high DHEA-S levels and elevated high-density lipoprotein (HDL) in women [10]. The most recent evaluation of this cohort, published in 1995, demonstrated a mild cardioprotective effect with elevated DHEA-S levels, in both men and women [11].

Other epidemiologic data is similarly equivocal. Some reports imply an inverse relationship between DHEA-S levels and premature myocardial infarction (MI) in young men [12,13]. DHEA-S is also lower in men with angiographically demonstrated coronary artery disease [14], and in heart transplant patients with accelerated posttransplant atherosclerosis [15]. However, other studies have not demonstrated a reproducible cardioprotective effect of DHEA [16—18]. Unrecognized confounding factors may impact DHEA levels and may explain these equivocal results. Factors that increase adrenal androgen levels include cigarette smoking [19], alcohol consumption [20], and obesity [21]. Conversely, DHEA-S levels are attenuated by estrogen replacement [20,22], chronic illness [23], and hyperinsulinemia [24]. There is also a strong heritable and racial component to individual DHEA-S levels [25].

Thus, it remains the venue of clinical trials of DHEA replacement to determine whether any cardioprotective effects exist. In a prospective double-blind, randomized trial of 10 healthy young men, Nestler and colleagues administered DHEA (1,600 mg/day) or placebo over 28 days, [26] and observed a decline in low-density lipoprotein (LDL) in the DHEA group. However, subsequent clinical trials of DHEA replacement in various populations have demonstrated either no effect on lipids [27], or overall androgenization [28]. We have shown 6 months of 25 mg of oral micronized DHEA given to postmenopausal women results in a 12% decline in HDL, with a concurrent decline in apolipoprotein $A_1$ (APO $A_1$), indicative of increased atherogenic risk [29]. In perimenopausal women, Barnhardt and colleagues observed that oral DHEA (50 mg/day) given over 3 months also induced a progressive decline in total cholesterol and HDL [30]. It may very well be, therefore, that oral administration of DHEA, even in low doses, may adversely effect the lipoprotein profile of women.

As with estrogen replacement, the cardioprotective effect of DHEA may not be entirely lipoprotein mediated. Other plausible cardioprotective mechanisms postulated on the basis of human trials include a fibroblast antiproliferative effect [31], glucose-6 phosphate dehydrogenase inhibition [32], decreased platelet aggregation [33], or increased fibrinolysis [34]. DHEA may also have an indirect inotropic effect on the aged heart by augmenting serum insulin-like growth hormone (IGF-1) levels [27,29,35]. It may also have secondary beneficial cardiac effects via its antiobesity and insulin-sensitizing actions.

## DHEA and obesity

In both rodents and dogs, DHEA supplementation appears to have antiobesity effects [36,37]. Again, the clinical trials are more equivocal. Nestler and colleagues, giving 1,600 mg/day of DHEA in young men over a month, demonstrated a decline in body weight and an increase in lean body mass [26]. However, two further investigations in the same population or in obese young men did not confirm these results [38,39]. In elderly men and women, Yen and colleagues performed a double-blind, parallel, randomized controlled trial of 100 mg/day of oral DHEA administration, showing increased lean body mass in both sexes, and decreased fat mass in men, but not in women [35]. We have done a 1-month study of 25 mg/day of oral micronized DHEA administered to older men and also noted decreased weight with increased lean body mass [40], but we have not seen any reproducible effects on body morphology in postmenopausal women. Thus, if there is an effect of DHEA replacement on obesity in humans, the effect appears mild, and may also be gender-limited.

## DHEA and insulin sensitivity

In rats, DHEA administration reduces the onset and ameliorates the severity of genetic and drug-induced diabetes [41]. A case report of DHEA treatment of severe type II diabetes with subsequent improvement has been described [42]. Seventeen-hour infusions of intravenous DHEA in women with polycystic ovarian disease has been noted to increase postreceptor pyruvate dehydrogenase (PDH) activity, thought a postreceptor marker of insulin effect [43].

These studies prompted us to examine whether DHEA replacement may augment insulin sensitivity in older men and women. In a placebo-controlled, double-blind crossover trial in postmenopausal women (with 3-week treatment periods, and a 2-week washout), we found that 50 mg/day of oral micronized DHEA augmented T-lymphocyte insulin binding and -degradation [44], a marker of clinical insulin sensitivity. This enhanced insulin effect was associated with a trend towards decreased areas under the curve (AUC) for glucose and insulin after an oral glucose load. Subsequently, we performed a parallel, blinded, randomized, controlled trial giving 50 mg/day of oral micronized DHEA to post-reproductive women [45]. We measured insulin sensitivity with an intravenous glucose tolerance test, with data analysis by the minimal modeling technique, and found DHEA replacement has an ameliorating effect on observed study-induced declines in insulin sensitivity.

Despite these data, other studies have not shown an insulin-sensitizing effect of DHEA [27]. However, Diamond and colleagues recently demonstrated that application of 10% DHEA cream for 12 months in older women resulted in significant declines in basal glucose and insulin levels [46]. In an early study of 1600 mg/day of DHEA replacement in obese young men, HgB A1c did decline [38]. In summary, it appears that if an insulin-sensitizing effect of DHEA exists, it may well not be dramatic and be gender-limited (to women).

**DHEA and bone turnover**

While data on DHEA and bone metabolism is limited, the observation that the pattern of bone gain and during loss in human life closely parallels adrenal androgen secretion, provides tantalizing evidence of an association between the two phenomena. Some epidemiologic investigations have correlated bone loss with DHEA-S levels, particularly in the very elderly [47]. Other rationale for a role of DHEA in bone turnover include the existence of frequent and disastrous bone loss with long-term corticosteroid administration, a situation where adrenal androgen secretion is greatly reduced, to negligible levels [48]. Interluken 6 (IL-6), a mediator of bone reabsorption in osteoporosis, decreases with DHEA supplementation [49].

In vitro studies in this area also show promise. In human osteoblast cell cultures, DHEA has a mitogenic effect, mediated through transforming growth factor-fβ (TGF-β) and the androgen receptor [50]. This effect is not blocked by 5α-reductase or 3β-hydroxysteroid dehydrogenase (3β-HSD) inhibition, indicating a direct DHEA/androgen receptor effect, or an effect mediated by $\Delta^5$-metabolites of DHEA.

Despite these hints that DHEA may play a role in bone turnover, the clinical data remain limited. In our 3-week and 6-month studies in postmenopausal women, we have measured urinary hydroxyproline, hydroxylysine, and collagen cross-links, and have not seen DHEA-induced effects [29,44]. In similar populations, others have not seen bone mineral density (BMD) changes with DEXA scans, albeit with short durations of treatment [35]. However, a recent study by Labrie and colleagues, using 12 months of DHEA 10% cream applied topically, demonstrated increases in BMD at the hip in conjunction with declines in plasma bone alkaline phosphatase and urinary hydroxyproline [51]. Serum osteocalcin, a marker of bone formation, was increased 2-fold over control values. Whether or not DHEA replacement has bone-sparing effects remains an area for further investigation.

## DHEA replacement and the growth hormone (GH)/IGF-1 axis

GH declines markedly with age and itself has been under scrutiny as a possible hormonal replacement therapy to prevent some of the sequelae of aging [52]. Studies with recombinant GH (rGH) demonstrate some promise in increasing muscle mass, strength, and also in elderly individuals [53,54]. However, this therapy is expensive and requires daily injection.

The effects of GH are in large part mediated by either hepatic or end-organ production of IGF-1, otherwise known as somatomedin [55]. In several clinical trials of DHEA replacement in aged individuals, serum IGF-1 levels, both total and free, were increased in concert with decreasing IGF-1 binding protein-3 (IGFBP-3) values. This was first demonstrated by Morales and colleagues in a placebo-controlled trial in men and women [27], and subsequently confirmed by Yen [35] and by the authors [29] in 6-month and 1-year long trials. Diamond and colleagues have also demonstrated an augmentation of serum IGF-1 levels and action with 12 months of 10% DHEA cream in 15 postmenopausal women [46]. Thus, it appears certain that in both men and women, physiologic DHEA replacement augments serum IGF-1 levels by about 50%, about the same magnitude of increases with rGH. This effect may be due to augmentation of hepatic and end-organ IGF-1 secretory response to circulating GH. That this augmentation of IGF-1 secretion may have clinical benefits is demonstrated by Yen and colleagues' finding of increased muscle strength in men with DHEA replacement [35].

## DHEA and immune function

In aging individuals, a decline in cellular mediated immune competence is thought to occur, a phenomenon termed "immunosenescence" [56]. This decline in immune function may be mediated by decreased interluken-2 (IL-2) or lymphocyte IL-2 receptor levels, and is also associated with increased IL-6. The concept that the age-related decline in DHEA levels may be linked to immunosenescence was first given credence by Schwartz and colleagues, who demonstrated that DHEA supplementation prevents spontaneous or mutagen-induced carcinogenesis in rats [57]. While the DHEA doses used were extremely high, subsequent studies in mice have demonstrated that both in vivo and in vitro DHEA augments lymphocyte IL-2 production [58]. In humans, an in vitro study indicates that DHEA augments lymphocyte IL-2 production [59].

There is now increasing clinical data demonstrating the immunoaugmentory effects of physiologic DHEA replacement in the elderly. A measurement of 50 mg of DHEA-S, given twice a day at the time of vaccination, increases influenza (but not tetanus) titer response over that seen with placebo [60]. In another randomized, blinded trial, 7.5 mg of subcutaneous DHEA-S given at the time of influenza vaccination increases hemagglutination inhibition (HI) antibody response, particularly in subjects with lower initial titers, and lower serum endogenous DHEA-S levels [61]. However, the effects seen in both studies are not large.

In 1993, we demonstrated that DHEA significantly augments natural killer cell (NK cell) cytotoxicity and number in postreproductive women, and decreases stimulated lymphocyte IL-2 response [49]. Yen's group subsequently confirmed these data in a 6-month study giving 100 mg of oral DHEA to elderly men and women [35], and also demonstrated increases in serum IL-2 levels and lymphocyte expression of surface IL-2 receptor.

It appears now that one of the more clearly delineated effects of DHEA replacement in humans is functional enhancement of the aging immune system. Whether this finding results in clinically significant beneficial effects is an issue that remains to be addressed.

## Cognitive effects

DHEA has demonstrated neurotropic action at the GABA receptor. This steroid enhances the maze performance of mice, and has a beneficial effect on memory in these animals [63,64]. It also promotes the growth of mouse brain explant in vitro [65].

Human studies are more limited. In a single-dose, double-blind, randomized, controlled trial, DHEA significantly augmented rapid eye movement (REM) sleep over placebo [66]. Given the benefits of REM sleep to overall sleep quality, this finding may contribute to the postulated enhancement in wellbeing seen in subjects given DHEA, as shown by Morales [27]. Morales and her colleagues demonstrated a libido-independent increase in a sense of wellbeing (as measured by objective scales) with DHEA (50 mg/day).

## Bioavailability of DHEA preparations

The bioavailability of orally administered adrenal androgens was first reported in 1982 in the form of a case report describing 1 year of administration of 25 mg/day of DHEA-S for 1 year to a 19-year old with hypogonadal hypogonadism [67].

Administration of this compound did not result in puberty, but serum DHEA-S rose to peripubertal levels (200–250 μg/dl), with development of high testosterone (T) levels (150 ng/dl). Thus, even at this early stage, significant bioconversion of orally administered adrenal androgen to more potent androgens was demonstrated. Later, Nestler and colleagues gave 1,600 mg/day of DHEA to five healthy young men for 28 days [26]. Surprisingly, at this dose they only increased serum DHEA-S levels 2.5- to 3.5-fold. Androstenedione increased 2-fold, and estrone, estradiol, SHBG, and total and free T remained unaltered. However, Mortola and colleagues later used the same doses given to postmenopausal women and demonstrated significant elevation in all downstream androgens to supraphysiologic levels, with androgenization of both glucose tolerance and lipid profiles [28].

The use of physiologic replacement doses were then considered by investigators working in the area, on the basis of the fact that the combined production rates of DHEA and DHEA-S are in the range of 50 mg/day. We performed an initial dose-ranging study to ascertain what levels of our oral micronized DHEA preparation (Belmar Pharmacy, Lakewood, CO) were needed to reproduce the premenopausal adrenal androgen milieu without adverse androgenization. On the basis of these single dose studies, we postulated that the optimal oral replacement dose of this preparation of DHEA was 50 mg/day. Concurrently, we addressed the issue of nonoral administration by performing a randomized, placebo-controlled, blinded, single-dose trial of oral, compared to vaginal micronized DHEA administration [68]. After DHEA administration, we sampled blood over a 12-h period and generated AUCs for DHEA, DHEA-S, and T. Comparison of the AUCs shows that with oral administration there is significant bioconversion to DHEA-S and T; but with vaginal administration, this bioconversion is dramatically attenuated, with most of the DHEA appearing in the circulation as the native steroid.

In our 3-week trial of 50 mg/day of oral micronized DHEA in postmenopausal women, we demonstrated supraphysiologic elevations of 23-h postdose DHEA-S and T, indicating that oral bioavailability of this preparation was more efficient than initially postulated, and that 25 mg/day may be a more appropriate dose [44]. However, in a subsequent study, 25 mg/day of oral micronized DHEA, administered to older women for over 6 months, was subject to significant dose attenuation [29]. At the end of the trial, serum DHEA and DHEA-S levels (again 23 h postdose) were not significantly different from placebo values. Thus we feel that any further trials of DHEA supplementation would require dose titration on the basis of serum DHEA-S and T values to overcome this dose-attenuation effect. Also, given the adverse lipid effects seen with oral administration, the possibility of nonoral (vaginal, sublingual, or transcutaneous) administration becomes germane to avoid putative hepatic first pass effect. Indeed, DHEA 10% cream has been effectively administered transcutaneously with physiologic elevations of downstream metabolites. Importantly, in these studies, there were also changes in the GH axis and in bone turnover, indicating that even with nonoral administration, beneficial salutary effects exist, and thus, may not be mediated by hepatic first pass effect [46,51].

Much more investigation needs to be done on doses of DHEA and routes of administration used in human trials. The future of DHEA replacement therapy may very well lie with nonoral administration.

## Side effects

While the possibility of adverse effects of this potent oral steroid exist, in the literature to date there is only one side effect noted [69]. This occurred in one of our single-dose studies, where a woman was given a 150-mg dose and developed transient jaundice and hepatic dysfunction a week later. Her baseline blood serum, assayed retrospectively, demonstrated false positive hepatitis C titers and positive antimitochondrial antibodies. Thus, whether or not her hepatic dysfunction was a direct result of DHEA administration is not known, but the previously documented effects of oral steroids, particularly androgens, give pause for concern [71].

While no other side effects have been noted, the lipid changes seen in women, both in our 6-month study and in Barnhardt and colleagues' investigation, raise some concern about chronic oral administration of this compound [29,30]. Additionally, the theoretic potential for side effects such as hirsutism are cogent because of the rapid biotransformation of this compound to the more potent androgens when administered orally. Finally, in animal models of oral DHEA administration, increases in liver size and induction in hepatic carcinoma are seen [71,72]. Finally, in men, the possible effects of chronic DHEA administration on subclinical prostate cancer or benign prostatic hyperplasia must also be considered carefully.

## Conclusion

It appears that physiologic DHEA administration to aging humans may have multiple beneficial effects. In men, but possibly not in women, it may have an antiobesity effect. Conversely, in women, but possibly not in men, DHEA may have an insulin sensitizing effect. DHEA may beneficially effect bone turnover, and clearly augments the GH/IGF-1 axis. Additionally, DHEA is quite likely an immunoaugmentory hormone, reducing some of the declines in immune competence seen with aging.

It is still puzzling how DHEA achieves these effects. Several investigators have noted either a membrane-bound or cytosolic DHEA receptor [73,74], but despite intensive effort, this work remains to be replicated. Alternately, Labrie and colleagues postulate that DHEA may act by virtue of end-organ bioconversion to a mix of estrogenic and androgenic metabolites, which in turn, would interact with androgen and estrogen receptors to create a set of tissue-unique physiologic effects [76]. This potential mechanism of action of DHEA is termed "intracrinology", and remains the most plausible theory of DHEA action at present.

DHEA may also act in humans to exert multiple beneficial effects by augmenting end-organ and hepatic production of IGF-1 in response to GH. It has now been well-demonstrated that IGF-1 is an immunoaugmentory substance in its own right [55], IGF-1 receptors and effects are noted in bone, muscle, and fat [55]. Such an augmentation of IGF-1 effect would also result in overall decline in serum GH levels by virtue of hypothalamic-pituitary negative feedback, and thus result in a beneficial effect on insulin sensitivity. Indeed, IGF-1 therapy is in clinical trials as a treatment for diabetes [76].

Clearly the issue DHEA replacement as an antiaging therapy is rapidly evolving. Future studies of DHEA replacement in humans are needed, with dose titration, possibly nonoral administration, and with and without concurrent estrogen replacement. Even more important are development of basic science investigations into this area, looking at the mechanism of adrenarche and adrenopause, and the secretory control of DHEA and DHEA-S. Finally, elucidating a mechanism of action explains the multiple beneficial effects of these compounds would lend credence to this field.

Unfortunately at this point, popularization of this compound has far outpaced credible scientific investigation. At present, we do not recommend using DHEA clinically because of its possible side effects. However, the future of DHEA replacement has great potential for attenuating some aspects of aging, and the subject is certainly worthy of further concentrated investigation.

## References

1. Casson PR, Buster JE. DHEA administration to humans: panacea or palaver? Sem Reprod Endocrinol 1995;13:247—256.
2. Endoh A, Kristiansen SB, Casson PR et al. The zona reticularis is the site of biosynthesis of dehydroepiandrosterone and dehydroepiandrosterone sulfate in the adult human adrenal cortex, resulting from its low expression of 3β-hydroxysteroid dehydrogenase. J Clin Endocrinal Metab 1996;81(10):3558—3365.
3. Dhom G. The prepuberal and puberal growth of the adrenal (adrenarche). Beitrage zur Pathologie 1973;150:357—377.
4. Orentreich M, Brind JL, Kizer RL et al. Age changes and sex differences in serum dehydroepiandrosterone sulfate concentrations throughout adulthood. J Clin Endocrinol Metab 1984; 59:551—555.
5. Kreiner E, Dohm G. Altersveranderungen de menschlichen Nebenniere. Zbl Allg Pathol Anat 1979;123:351—356.
6. Sapolsky RM, Vogelman JH, Orentreich N et al. Senescent decline in serum dehydroepiandrosterone sulfate concentrations in a population of wild baboons. J Gerontol 1993;48:B196—B200.
7. Eich DM, Nestler JE, Johnson DE et al. Inhibition of accelerated coronary atherosclerosis with dehydroepiandrosterone in heterotopic rabbit model of cardiac transplantation. Circulation 1993;87:261—269.
8. Gordon GB, Bush DE, Weisman HF. Reduction of atherosclerosis by administration of dehydroepiandrosterone. Adv Enzyme Regul 1987;26:355—382.
9. Barrett-Connor E, Goodman-Gruen D. Dehydroepiandrosterone sulfate does not predict cardiovascular death in postmenopausal women. Circulation 1995;91:1757—1760.
10. Barrett-Connor E, Khaw KT, Yen SSC. A prospective study of dehydroepiandrosterone sulfate, mortality, and cardiovascular disease. N Engl J Med 1986;315:1519—1524.
11. Barrett-Connor E, Goodman-Gruen D. The epidemiology of DHEA-S and cardiovascular disease. In: Bellino FL, Daynes RA, Hornsby PJ, Lavrin DH (eds) Dehydroeniandrosterone (DHEA) and Aging. New York: Ann NY Acad Sci 1995;774:259—270.
12. Mitchell LE, Sprecher DL, Borecki IB et al. Evidence for an association between dehydroepiatdrosterone sulfate and nonfatal premature myocardial infarction in males. Circulation 1995; 89:89—93.
13. Slowinska-Srzednicka J, Zgliczynski S, Ciswicka-Sznajderman M et al. Decreased plasma dehydroepiandrosterone sulfate and dihydrotestosterone concentrations in young men after myocardial infarction. Atherosclerosis 1989;79:197—203.
14. Herrington DM, Gordon GB, Achuff SC et al. Plasma dehydroepiandrosterone and dehydroepiandrosterone sulfate in patients undergoing diagnostic coronary angiography. J Am Coll Cardiol 1990;16:862—870.

15. Herrington DM. DHEA and coronary atherosclerosis. Ann NY Acad Sci 1995;774:271—280.
16. Contoreggi CS, Blackman MR, Andres R et al. Plasma levels of estradiol, testosterone, and DHEAS do not predict risk of coronary artery disease in men. J Androl 1990;11:460—470.
17. Rice T, Sprecher DL, Borecki IB et al. The Cincinnati myocardial infarction and hormone family study: family resemblance for dehydroepiandrosterone sulfate in control and myocardial infarction families. Metabolism 1993;42:1284—1290.
18. Newcomer LM, Manson JE, Barbieri RI et al. Dehydroepiandrosterone sulfate and the risk of myocardial infarction in US male physicians: a prospective study. Am J Epidemiol 1994; 140:870—877.
19. Khaw KT, Tazuke S, Barrett-Connor E. Cigarette smoking and levels of adrenal androgens in postmenopausal women. N Engl J Med 1987;318:1705—1709.
20. Tazuke S, Khaw KT, Barrett-Connor E. Exogenous estrogen and endogenous sex hormones. Medicine 1992;71:44—50.
21. Field AF, Colditz GA, Willett WC et al. The relation of smoking, age, relative weight, and dietary intake to serum adrenal steroids, sex hormones, and sex hormone-binding globulin in middle-aged men. J Clin Endocrinol Metab 1994;79:1310—1316.
22. Casson PR, Elkind-Hirsch KE, Carson SA et al. Effect of postmenopausal estrogen replacement on circulating androgens. Obstet Gynecol 1997;90(6):995—998.
23. Casson PR, Hornsby PJ, Buster JE. DHEA — adrenal androgens, insulin resistance and cardio-vascular disease. In: Speroff L, Wild B (eds) Seminars in Reproductive Endocrinology 1996;14(1):29—34.
24. Nestler JE, Clore JN, Strauss III JR , Blackard WG. The effects of hyperinsulinemia on serum testosterone, progesterone, dehydroepiandrosterone sulfate and cortisol levels in normal women and in a woman with hyperandrogenism, insulin resistance and acanthosis nigricans. Clin Endocrinol Metab 1987;64:180—184.
25. Rotter JI, Wong L, Lifrak ET et al. A genetic component to the variation of dehydroepiandrosterone sulfate. Metabolism 1985;34:731—736.
26. Nestler JE, Barlascini CO, Clore JN et al. Dehydroepiandrosterone reduces serum low density lipoprotein levels and body fat but does not alter insulin sensitivity in normal men. J Clin Endocrinol Metab 1987;64:180—184.
27. Morales AJ, Nolan JJ, Nelson JC et al. Effects of replacement dose of dehydroepiandrosterone in men and women of advancing age. J Clin Endocrinol Metab 1994;78:1360—1367.
28. Mortola J, Yen SSC. The effects of dehydroepiandrosterone on endocrine- metabolic parameters in postmenopausal women. J Clin Endocrinol Metab 1990;71:696—704.
29. Casson PR, Santoro N, Elkind-Hirsch KE et al. Postmenopausal dehydroepiandrosterone (DHEA) administration increases insulin-like growth factor-I (IGF-I) and decreases high density lipoprotein (HDL): a six month trial. Fertil Steril 1998;(In press).
30. Barnhart KT, Rader D, Freeman E et al. The Effect of DHEA Replacement on the Endocrine and Lipid Profiles of Perimenopausal Women. Fertil Steril 1997;0—081 (Abstract).
31. Saenger P, New M. Inhibitory action of dehydroepiandrosterone (DHEA) on fibroblast growth. Experientia 1976;33:966—967.
32. Lopez SA, Krehl WA. In vivo effect of dehydroepiandrosterone on red blood cells glucose-phosphate dehydrogenase. Proc Soc Exp Med 1967;126:776—778.
33. Lesse RL. The Effects of DHEA on Atherogenesis and Platelet Function. Dehydroepiandrosterone and Aging Conference. New York Academy of Sciences, Washington DC, June 1995 (Abstract).
34. Beer HA, Jakubowicz DJ, Matt DE et al. Oral Dehydroepiandrosterone (DHEA) Administration Produces Plasma Levels of Plasminogen Activator (t-PA) in Men. Dehydroepiandrosterone and Aging Conference. New York Academy of Sciences, Washington, D.C., June 1995 (Abstract).
35. Yen SCC, Morales AJ, Khorram O. Replacement of DHEA in aging men and women: potential remedial effects. In: Bellino FL, Daynes PA, Hornsby PJ, Lavrin DH, Nestler JE (eds) Dehydroeniandrosterone (DHEA) and aging. New York: Ann NY Acad Sci, 1995;775:128—142.

36. Yen TT, Allan JV, Pearson DV. Prevention of obesity in Avy/A mice by dehydroepiandrosterone. Lipids 1997;12:409–413.

37. MacEwen EG, Kurzman ID. Obesity in the dog: role of the adrenal steroid dehydroepiandrosterone (DHEA). J Nutr 1991;121:S51–S55.

38. Usiskin KS, Butterworth S, Clore JN et al. Lack of effect of dehydroepiandrosterone in obese men. Int J Obes 1990;14:457–463.

39. Welle NB, Jozefowics R, Statt M. Failure of DHEA to influence energy and protein metabolism in humans. J CIin Endocrinol Metab 1990;71:1259–1264.

40. Ghusn HF, Taffet G, Jaweed MM et al. DHEA improves lean body mass of older men. J Am Geriatr Soc 1998 (Submitted).

41. Coleman DL, Leiter EH, Schwizer RW. Therapeutic effects of dehydroepiandrosterone (DHEA) in diabetic mice. Diabetes 1982;31:830–833.

42. Buffington CK, Pourmotabbed G, Kitabchi AE. Case report: amelioration of insulin resistance in diabetes with dehydroepiandrosterone. Am J Med Sci 1993;306:3200.

43. Schriock ED, Buffington CK, Givens JR et al. Enhanced post-receptor insulin effects on women following dehydroepiandrosterone infusion. J Soc Gynecol Invest 1994;1:74–78.

44. Casson PR, Faquin LC, Stentz FB et al. Replacement of dehydroepiandrosterone (DHEA) enhances T-lymphocyte insulin binding in postmenopausal women. Fertil Steril 1995;3(5):1027–1031.

45. Bates GW, Egerman RS, Umstot ES et al. Dehydroepiandrosterone attenuates study-induced declines in insulin sensitivity in postmenopausal women. In: Bellino FL, Daynes RA, Hornsby PJ, Lavrin DH, Nestler JE (eds) Dehydroeniandrosterone (DHEA) and Aging. New York: NY Acad Sci, 1995;774:291–293.

46. Diamond P, Cusan L, Gomez JL et al. Metabolic effects of 12-month percutaneous dehydroepiandrosterone replacement therapy in postmenopausal women. J Endocrinol 1996;150:S43–S50.

47. Wild PA, Buchanan JR, Myers C et al. Declining adrenal androgens: an association with bone loss in aging women. Proc Soc Exp Biol Med 1987;186:355–360.

48. Abraham GE. Ovarian and adrenal contribution to peripheral androgens during the menstrual cycle. J Clin Endocrinol Metab 1974;39:340.

49. Casson PR, Anderson RN, Herrod HG et al. Oral dehydroepiandrosterone in physiologic doses modulates immune function in postmenopausal women. Am J Obstet Gynecol 1993;169:1536–1539.

50. Kasperk CH, Wakley GK, Hierl T et al. Gonadal and adrenal androgens are potent regulators of human bone cell metabolism in vitro. J Bone Min Res 1997;12(3):464–471.

51. Labrie T, Diamond P, Cusan L et al. Effect of 12-month dehydroepiandrosterone replacement therapy on bone, vagina, and endometrium in postmenopausal women. J Clin Endocrinol Metab 1997;82(10):3498–3505.

52. Lamberts SWJ, Vandenbeld AW, Vanderly AJ. The endocrinology of aging. Science 1997;278(5337):419–424.

53. Cuttica CM, Castoldi L, Ggorrini GP et al. Effects of six-month administration of recombinant human growth hormone to healthy elderly subjects. Aging 1997;9(3):193–197.

54. Sassolas G. Potential therapeutic applications of growth hormone in adults. Hormone Res 1994;42(1–2):72–78.

55. Clark R. The somatogenic hormones and insulin-like growth factor-1: stimulators of lymphopoiesis and immune function. Endocrine Rev 1197;18(2):157–179.

56. Thoman ML, Weigle WO. The cellular and subcellular bases of immunosenescence. Adv Immunol 1989;46:331–361.

57. Schwartz AG, Pashko LL. Cancer chemoprevention with the adrenocortical steroid dehydroepiandrosterone and structural analogs. J Cell Biochem 1993;17G:73–79.

58. Daynes RA, Dudley DJ, Araneo BA. Regulation of murine lymphokine production in vivo: dehydroepiandrosterone is a natural enhancer of interleukin 2 syntheses by helper T cells. Eur J

Immunol 1990;20:793—802.

59. Suzuki T, Suzuki N, Daynes RA et al. Dehyydroepiandrosterone enhances IL-2 production and cytotoxic effector function of human T cells. Clin Immunol Immunonpathol 1991;61:202—211.

60. Araneo BA, Dowell T, Woods MA et al. DHEAS as an effective vaccine adjuvant in elderly humans. In: Bellino FL, Daynes RA, Hornsby PJ, Lavrin DH, Nestler JE (eds) Dehydroeoiandrosterone (DHEA) and Aging. New York: Ann NY Acad Sci 1995;774:232—248.

61. Degelau J, Guay D, Hallgren H. The effect of DHEAS on influenza vaccination in aging adults. J Am Geriatr Soc 1997;45:747—751.

62. Robel P, Baulieu EE. Neurosteroids: biosynthesis and function. Trends Endocrinol Metab 1994;5:1—8.

63. Flood JF, Roberts E. Dehydroepiandrosterone sulfate improves memory in aging mice. Brain Res 1988;448:178—181.

64. Melchior CL, Ritzmann RF. Dehydroepiandrosterone enhances the hypnotic and hypothermic effects of ethanol and pentobarbital. Pharmacol Biochem Behav 1992;43:223—227.

65. Roberts E. Dehydroepiandrosterone (DHEA) and its sulfate (DHEAS) as neural facilitators: effects on brain tissue in culture and on memory in young and old mice. A cyclic GMP hypothesis of action of DHEA and DHEAS in nervous system and other tissues. In: Kalimi M, Regelson W (eds) The Biologic Role of Dehydroepiandrosterone (DHEA). Berlin: Walter de Gruyter, 1990:43—64.

66. Friess E, Trachsel L, Guldner J et al. DHEA administration increases rapid eye movement sleep and EEG power in the sigma frequency range. Am J Physiol 1995;268:E107—E113.

67. Cohen HN, Hay ID, Beastall GH et al. Failure of adrenal androgen to induce puberty in familial cytomegalic adrenocortical hypoplasia. Lancet 182;21:1471—1472.

68. Casson PR, Straughn AB, Milem CA et al. Delivery of dehydroepiandrosterone (DHEA) in premenopausal women: effects of micronization and non-oral administration. Am J Obstet Gynecol 1996;174:649—653.

69. Buster JE, Casson PR, Straughn AB et al. Postmenopausal steroid replacement with micronized dehydroepiandrosterone: preliminary oral bioavailability and dose proportionality studies. Am J Obstet Gynecol 1992;166:1163—1170.

70. Casson PR, Carson SA. Aildrogen replacement therapy in the menopause: myth and reality. Int J Fertil 1996;41(4):412—422.

71. Milewich L, Catalina F, Bennett M. Pleotropic effects of dietary DHEA. Ann NY Acad Sci 1995;774:149—170.

72. Rao MS, Subbarao V, Yelandi AV et al. Hepatocarcinogenicity of dehydroepiandrosterone in the rat. Cancer Res 1992;52:2977—2779.

73. Imai A, Ohno T, Tamaya T. Dehydroepiandrosterone sulfate-binding sites in plasma membrane from human uterine cervical fibroblasts. Experientia 1992;48:999—1002.

74. Miekle AW, Dorchuck RW, Araneo BA et al. The presence of dehydroepiandrosterone-specific receptor binding complex in murine t cells. J Steroid Biochem Molec Biol 1992;42:293—304.

75. Labrie F, Belanger A, Simard J et al. DHEA and peripheral androgen and estrogen formation: intracrinology. In: Bellino FL, Daynes RA, Hornsby PJ, Lavrin DH, Nestler JE (eds) Dehydroepiandrosterone (DHEA) and Aging, 774th edn. New York: Ann NY Acad Sci 1996;774:16—28.

76. Kolaczynski JW, Caro JF. Insulin-like growth factor-1 therapy in diabetes: physiologic basis, clinical benefits, and risks. Ann Intern Med 1994;120(1):47—55.

# In vitro maturation

# The practical aspects of in vitro maturation of human oocytes

Anthony J. Rutherford

*Clarendon Wing, The General Infirmary at Leeds, Leeds, UK*

**Abstract.** In vitro maturation (IVM) of human oocytes from antral-stage follicles, followed by in vitro fertilisation (IVF), has a number of potential practical advantages over conventional superovulation and IVF for the infertile patient. The most important are reduced cost, and a simpler, less invasive treatment. The ability of mammalian oocytes to undergo IVM has been known for some time, but it is only in the last decade that this technology has been applied to oocytes from small antral follicles. There are significant practical differences in the recovery and culture requirements of these immature oocytes, compared to standard IVF. In addition, embryo development seems to be generally retarded, and inatally the number of pregnancies was disappointingly low. However, recent reports would suggest that some of these preliminary difficulties have been overcome, with success rates akin to conventional IVF described. Nevertheless, further work on the general safety of the procedure should be considered before the widespread use of IVM in clinical practice.

**Keywords:** antral stage oocytes, serum-free culture.

## Introduction

At present, in vitro maturation (IVM) of human oocytes, in a clinical context, extends to immature oocytes from antral stage follicles, removed in the early to midfollicular phase [1], and to a lesser extent, to immature oocytes retrieved following conventional superovulation [2–5]. In theory, IVM from antral stage follicles is very attractive as it has a number of practical advantages over conventional superovulation. Most IVM protocols are relatively simple, both for the patient and clinician, with fewer consultations, a shorter period of treatment, and a significantly reduced drug bill. In addition, both short-term and any potential long-term sequelae of ovarian superovulation are completely avoided. As well as the obvious benefits to infertile patients, as the treatment is much less invasive more women may be prepared to donate oocytes, both for research and to help other infertile couples.

The initial discovery that mammalian oocytes would undergo in vitro maturation was in 1935, when Pincus and Enzmann [6] demonstrated that oocytes liberated from unstimulated rabbit Graafian follicles would undergo meiotic maturation spontaneously in vitro. This showed that the programme of cytoplasmic and nuclear events between the LH surge and subsequent ovulation could take place

*Address for correspondence:* Anthony J. Rutherford MD, Clarendon Wing, The General Infirmary at Leeds, Belmont Grove, Leeds LS2 9NS, UK. Tel.: +44-113-2926908. Fax: +44-113-2922971.
E-mail: anthonyR@ulth.northy.nhs.uk

in culture. In 1965 Edwards [7] confirmed and extended these results with a range of mammalian species including the human, and in 1969 [8] was able to demonstrate for the first time the fertilisation of in vitro matured human oocytes. The earliest recorded pregnancies following human IVM were in 1983 [2] arising from immature oocytes that had failed to respond appropriately to an ovulatory dose of human chorionic gonadotrophin (hCG) during a conventional IVF programme. There are only a handful of published clinical trials that have evaluated the exciting potential of IVM of immature oocytes from small antral follicles [1,9–11]. Each of these studies has addressed a different aspect of IVM, and all have recorded pregnancies. A review of these studies, and results of our own work, form the basis for the remainder of this chapter.

## Oocyte physiology

Before discussing the practical aspects of IVM, it is pertinent to briefly outline the principles of oocyte physiology that describe the changes that take place in the final days of oocyte development.

The oocyte has remained suspended at the dictyate-stage of the first meiotic prophase from fetal life, through to and beyond puberty, when, with the advent of ovulatory cycles, meiosis is resumed in response to the midcycle luteinising hormone (LH) surge. To be able to respond appropriately to the LH surge the oocyte needs to have acquired nuclear and cytoplasmic maturation.

### Nuclear maturation

During the prolonged period of follicular and oocyte growth, the oocyte acquires both the ability to resume meiosis, and the payload of RNA and proteins required to support complete meiotic maturation, a process known as meiotic competence. Oocytes from preantral follicles do not have the ability to resume meiosis. The final acquisition of meiotic competence in oocytes from antral follicles appears to take place in two sequential steps, firstly from the breakdown of the

*Table 1.* The effect of FSH pretreatment in vivo on human oocyte maturation in vitro.

|  | Control (n = 9) | FSH-treated (n = 17) |
| --- | --- | --- |
| Mean follicle diameter (mm) at collection ± SEM | 8.0 ± 0.5 | 8.9 ± 0.3 |
| Mean number of oocytes collected ± SEM | 5.2 ± 1.3 | 7.5 ± 1.2 |
| Total number of degenerate oocytes following 48 h culture | 8 (17.4%) | 6 (5.3%) |
| Number of germinal vesicle-stage oocytes after 48 h | 5 (10.9%) | 12 (10.5%) |
| Number of metaphase I oocytes after 48 h | 13 (28.3%) | 15 (13.2%) |
| Number of metaphase II oocytes after 48 h | 20 (43.5%) | 81 (71.1%) |
| Total number of oocytes cultured | 46 | 114 |

(Reproduced, with permission from [13].)

oocyte nucleus (germinal vesicle breakdown — GVBD) to the completion of metaphase I, and secondly, entry into anaphase, arresting again at metaphase II.

*Cytoplasmic maturation*

As the oocyte grows there are widespread changes in the infrastructure of the cytoplasm and its organelles. The pattern of protein production changes throughout this growth phase, right through to the second metaphase arrest. Cytoplasmic maturation is essential to prepare the oocyte for fertilisation, activation and then, early preimplantation development before the new embryonic genome is functional. Even though an oocyte may be capable of fertilisation, having attained meiotic competence, it may not have achieved the appropriate degree of cytoplasmic maturation necessary to sustain a viable embryo. It is therefore not surprising that a higher proportion of oocytes recovered from large antral follicles are competent to proceed to form blastocysts compared to those oocytes retrieved from small antral follicles [12].

*Patient selection*

The outcome of any assisted conception treatment cycle is dependant on the quality of the oocytes collected. Three main groups of patients have been used to investigate in vitro maturation of human oocytes. The first group consists of volunteers, some having oophorectomy for gynaecological pathology, such as adenomyosis, endometriosis, uterine fibroids and ectopic pregnancy [10], and another group of fertile women undergoing a sterilisation procedure [13]. The second group consists of those patients who have entered into clinical trials involving IVM as part of their infertility treatment. This includes patients with polycystic ovaries [9] (PCO) and, those with a wide range of diagnoses who had failed at least one cycle of IVF [1]. The third group consists of "rescue" IVM, where women who were undergoing routine superovulated IVF or ICSI, with or without hCG, and were found to have immature oocytes at collection [3–5].

The majority of these studies have used oocytes that are potentially suboptimal. All patients in the latter two groups suffered from infertility, and many had significant endocrine disturbance, such as raised serum androgens and LH which is commonly seen with PCOS and known to be detrimental to oocytes [14]. Others had unresolved infertility after failed conventional IVF [1], or had oocytes that had failed to respond to a normal ovulatory dose of hCG [2], despite being given at the appropriate time as judged by follicle size. In addition, in the volunteer group, 18 of the 23 of the oophorectomy specimens came from patients over the age of 36, with the majority from women aged over 40 years [10].

Barnes and colleagues [11] demonstrated that immature oocytes removed from regularly cycling women were found to have a greater developmental capacity, significantly better maturation and fertilisation rates and a trend to higher cleavage rates than women with anovular or irregular cycles. Therefore, in an attempt to gain a better understanding of the culture requirements and development capacity of immature human oocytes, we decided to study a group of healthy volunteer patients of proven fertility, age range 23–36 years, in a series of controlled studies [13].

*Oocyte cumulus priming*

One of the major theoretical advantages of IVM is the reduced requirement for ovarian stimulation. However, studies in rhesus monkeys [15] have indicated that mild ovarian stimulation prior to retrieval markedly improved the proportion of oocytes that were meiotically competent, and that after fertilisation would support normal embryonic development. Human evidence is limited, but, in a series of case reports immature oocytes have been collected after exposure to conventional follicle-stimulating hormone (FSH) stimulation with a follicular phase of relatively normal length. The subsequent maturation rates were generally high and pregnancies were recorded [2–5]. None of the major human trials investigating IVM of oocytes recovered from small antral follicle have utilised any type of ovarian pretreatment [1,9,10], and although it is not appropriate to make a direct comparison, the embryo cleavage rate, and the pregnancy rates in these studies have generally been disappointing.

To investigate the potential benefits of FSH priming on human oocyte in vitro maturation, Wynn et al. [13] randomly allocated a group of fertile volunteers to receive either mild FSH stimulation or no treatment, prior to egg retrieval on day 7 of the follicular phase. The stimulation group received a truncated course of recombinant FSH (Gonal F, Serono, Herts., UK): 300 IU on day 2, with additional doses of 150 IU FSH on days 4 and 6 of the menstrual cycle. The results of this study are summarised in Table 1. The mean diameter of the small antral follicles was similar in each group. However, there were significantly more follicles and hence immature oocytes recovered, in the stimulated group. Although the same proportion of immature oocytes initiated meiosis a significantly greater percentage of oocytes from pretreated patients progressed to reach metaphase II. Furthermore, within the FSH-treated group successful oocyte maturation was positively correlated with follicle size, which is in keeping with findings in other primates [15] and domestic animal species [12]. Interestingly no oocytes capable of maturation were found in follicles less than 5 mm in diameter. Although no attempt was made to fertilise these oocytes and assess embryo development, these findings suggest that FSH priming will be of value in the human setting.

It remains to be elucidated how FSH priming works. Humans and other primates have a much longer follicular phase than other species studied, and it has been postulated that this is to allow time for completion of cytoplasmic maturation [15]. The provision of additional FSH will promote follicular granulosa cell proliferation, steroid production and through intercellular signalling, additional oocyte RNA and protein synthesis.

*Oocyte collection*

As all experienced in oocyte retrieval will validate, recovering oocytes from "mature" follicles where hCG has been withheld can be extremely difficult. The classical microscopic appearance of the expanded cumulus oocyte complex is not found; instead oocytes are surrounded by tightly packed, corona and cumulus cells, which can be hard to differentiate from sheets of granulosa cells [4]. It is therefore surprising to find that with experience, immature oocytes can be recovered relatively easily from antral follicles between 5 and 12 mm [11,13].

Initial attempts at oocyte recovery using a conventional IVF ultrasound guided approach were generally unsuccessful [10]. Therefore, Trounson [9] introduced two major changes, firstly, a new more rigid aspiration needle with a shorter bevel at the tip (Cook, Australia Ltd.) and, secondly, a reduced aspiration pressure of 80 mmHg. These adaptations, combined with experience, led to much higher recovery rates, and a reduced need to resort to laparoscopic recovery. Our work indicated that decreasing the aspiration pressure was by far the most significant change. In our preliminary studies we utilised both the adapted Cook needle and a standard 16-gauge double lumen needle (DC1S/16G/Clarendon, Casmed, Surrey, UK) with no difference in recovery rates [13].

Most reports have described the use of a single lumen needle, under ultrasound guidance, with each small follicle aspirated in turn [1,9,11]. The needle and tubing were then flushed with a warm, pH buffered, heparinized culture medium to clear the contents. However, using a double lumen needle each follicle can be measured, then aspirated and flushed sequentially, using known volumes of culture medium, without having to remove the needle. This allows accurate identification of oocytes from follicles of known diameter and volume, which can be correlated with oocyte outcome.

The follicular aspirates are examined using a dissecting microscope to identify the immature cumulus-oocyte complex. To aid detection, embryo filters can be used to remove erythrocytes and other granulosa cell debris [1,9]. In time, and with practice, the recovery of immature oocytes from small follicles is no more complex than a routine IVF egg collection both for the clinician and laboratory.

*Culture media*

The mutual interdependence of oocytes and granulosa cells for survival and normal development has important practical implications for strategies aimed at successfully maturing oocytes in vitro. The granulosa-oocyte complex is a metabolically coupled unit. The granulosa cells represent the nutrient and regulatory conduits between the oocyte and its environment, both through their regulation of phosphorylation events within the oocyte, and through the glycolytic activity within the oocyte-cumulus complexes during the resumption of meiosis. Importantly, both the interassociation of granulosa cells and their differentiated status can be profoundly affected by components of the culture environment. Development of a culture medium which supports normal granulosa cell functions is therefore also likely to provide a suitable milieu for oocyte maturation. While the attainment of oocyte meiotic competence and developmental potential clearly requires inclusion of at least preovulatory levels of FSH and LH, by far the most critical component which can influence the success of IVM is supplementation of the culture medium with serum [1,9,10] or follicular fluid [10].

Historically, monolayers of granulosa cells cultured in the presence of serum have been used to investigate the effects of hormonal treatments on steroidogenesis [16,17]. While the inclusion of serum provides a complex mixture of hormones, nutrients, growth and attachment factors (including collagen and fibronectin), which are necessary to support cell proliferation, serum also exerts inhibitory effects on follicular-type functions of granulosa cells. Typically, rat and human granulosa cells cultured in the presence of serum or extracellular matrix proteins [18,19] rapidly proliferate to form flattened, epithelioid monolayers with a dramatically different morphology to that seen in vivo. Furthermore, in the presence of serum or attachment factors, cells spontaneously luteinize and lose the capacity to convert androgens to oestrogens. Aromatase activity and hence oestradiol production by granulosa cells, which are key biochemical markers of the maintenance of follicular phenotype in vitro, are also central to preovulatory follicle selection and oocyte development in vivo [20,21].

Optimisation of the novel serum-free culture system, developed for ovine [20], bovine [23] and porcine granulosa cells [24,25] to support IVM of human oocytes [13] offers major advantage over previously published cell culture systems. Using this approach it is possible to maintain oestradiol production in granulosa cells which are exquisitely sensitive to physiological concentrations of gonadotrophins. Furthermore, controlled luteinization of the cells can be induced by the addition of preovulatory surge levels of gonadotrophins (H.M. Picton, unpublished work). On the basis of this serum-free culture system, we have used a combination of insulin and the synthetic analogue Long-R3 IGF, for human IVM [13] with concentrations based on the follicular fluid levels of insulin and IGF-I measured in human antral follicles [26,27]. These additives enhance granulosa cell metabolism and induce, sustain and amplify the actions of FSH and LH on differentiated cell function.

Most importantly using this serum-free approach, cultured granulosa cells form distinct clumps of rounded cells [22–25] which closely resembles the morphology of granulosa cells in vivo [28]. In response to the FSH and insulin [29] in the culture medium, the extensive network of gap junctions between cumulus cells and between cumulus cells and the oocyte is maintained. Following exposure to high levels of FSH and LH in vitro the controlled luteinization of cumulus cells and paracrine signalling breaks these fragile connections and so aids the resumption of nuclear maturation in the oocyte. In contrast, cell proliferation and attachment to the culture surface, caused by inclusion of serum and follicular fluid in the incubation media, may lead to premature disruption of oocyte-cumulus communication and so compromise oocyte maturation potential. The morphological differences of cumulus cells cultured in the presence or absence of se-rum or follicular fluid and the associated changes in their actin-cytoskeleton [30] may therefore profoundly affect the success of in vitro maturation systems.

## In vitro maturation and fertilisation

In most circumstances, the cumulus oocyte complex is retrieved 3–7 days prior to natural ovulation and no attempt is made to mimic the physiological cycle by delaying resumption of meiosis in vitro. The basic assumption is made that the oocyte will have already achieved the necessary cytoplasmic maturation to allow nuclear maturation, fertilisation and subsequent normal embryonic development. However, data from human and animal work show that protein synthesis in the oocyte continues throughout the follicular phase until and beyond the time of germinal vesicle breakdown [31,32]. These late stages of cytoplasmic maturation may hold the key to explain the poor success in human IVM, but at present there has been no study to precisely define at what stage of follicular development the human oocyte achieves cytoplasmic competence.

Although the functional syncytium [33] found in the intact follicle is lost when the cumulus-oocyte complex is removed at egg collection, the speed at which the gap junctions between cumulus cells and the oocyte are degraded remains unknown. Evidence from human oocytes suggests that this close association con-tinues in culture, as denuded oocytes have reduced developmental potential [1,9]. In all of the human studies, oocytes were cultured "cumulus intact" [1,2,4,6,9–11,13] with the exception of those stripped for ICSI [3] or to study the time course of maturation [9,13].

The optimal length of culture for human oocytes to achieve nuclear maturation is impossible to determine from animal data, as there is such a wide species spe-cific variation, for example, mouse oocytes reach metaphase II by 12 to 16 h, and cow oocytes by 24 h [34]. Culture conditions and methology will also effect the rate of maturation [35]. In the first paper on human IVM in 1965 Edwards [7] demonstrated that maturation took place over a 40- to 48-h period. Conse-quently, many of the later studies adopted a 48-h culture period [4,5,13], although others have successfully used a slightly longer fixed culture period of 52 to 58 h prior to attempting fertilisation using ICSI [1].

Although acceptable fertilisation rates have been achieved with conventional insemination [9–11] ICSI minimises the potential detrimental effects of long-term culture on the zona pellucida [1]. Prolonged culture of the oocyte, in the absence of serum, may cause premature cortical granule release, which leads to hardening of the zona pellucida [36]. This would not only reduce the fertilisation potential using conventional insemination, but also could prevent embryo hatch-ing. Zona hardening has been shown to reduce the rate of blastocyst hatching in the rhesus monkey from 77% in serum-based medium to only 25% in serum-free culture [37]. Ultimately it may prove necessary to perform both ICSI and assisted hatching [1,38] for all IVM oocytes and embryos. Alternatively, with adaptations to the culture medium such as the addition of the serum-derived antioxidant fetuin we might be able to overcome the potential problem of zona hardening [39].

## Embryo development

Embryos derived from immature oocytes collected after a normal length follicular phase appear to cleave at a similar rate to oocytes matured in vivo, reaching four to six cells after 42 h [3]. In contrast embryos from immature oocytes collected from small antral follicles have a higher rate of arrest at the pronuclear stage, and a significantly lower average cleavage and development rate than in conventional IVF embryos [11]. Furthermore those embryos from anovulatory patients are even more retarded [11]. Cleavage rates are a good predictor of embryo health, and correlate well with the chance of pregnancy [40,41]. This appears to hold true for IVM-derived embryos, as pregnancy is more likely to occur with rapidly dividing embryos [9].

The failure of slowly dividing embryos may represent an intrinsic abnormality of the original oocyte, or indeed a failing of the culture system [9]. Theoretically both these factors could be implicated. The limited evidence available is reassuring, in that morphologically normal human oocytes matured in vitro have a similar incidence of gross meiotic aberrations (18%) [42] as those oocytes matured in vivo (20%), and apparently lower rates than those seen in oocytes recovered after gonadotrophin stimulation [43–45]. In addition, although morphology alone does not confer normality, the incidence of morphologically abnormal embryos is no greater following IVM than conventional IVF [10].

## Embryo transfer

Healthy viable embryos and a suitable intrauterine environment are both required for successful implantation. Therefore, the timing of embryo development in relation to the physiological stage and degree of development of the endometrium must be considered. Clearly, embryo/endometrial asynchrony does not arise if the developing embryos are either cryopreserved for replacement in a subsequent hormone replacement cycle [4] or used in oocyte donation [10]. In cases of "rescue IVM" the follicular phase is of normal length, and as patients have received stimulation with FSH, there is sufficient endogenous oestrogen, appropriately supplemented with progesterone after oocyte collection, to ensure a suitable endometrium [3]. However, when oocytes are collected in the midfollicular phase, with no prior ovarian stimulation, evidence suggests that the endometrium is unlikely to have developed sufficiently, despite adding progesterone supplements, to sustain a pregnancy [13,47]. Russell successfully overcame this hurdle by introducing midfollicular phase oestradiol supplementation, on cycle days 5 to 7, in combination with prolonged embryo culture, transferring the embryos on day 3 after fertilisation [1]. Interestingly, relatively high-dose oestradiol supplements, given early in the follicular phase, starting on day 2 or 3, were found to be detrimental, with poor oocyte maturation rates and a high rate of early cleavage arrest [1]. An alternative strategy is to prolong the period of oocyte and embryo culture, allowing time for endometrial development to occur. This could be achieved by maintaining meiotic arrest in immature oocytes through the addition of cyclic AMP analogues or phosphodiesterase inhibitors [48]. This approach may also provide a bonus through allowing time for the oocyte to undergo the final stages of cytoplasmic maturation in vitro before the resumption of meiosis.

*Pregnancy outcome*

There have been too few pregnancies to adequately access the safety of this new technique. So far, concerns about a high rate of aneuploidies in the children born from in vitro matured oocytes has not materialised. All 10 children, reported in the literature, are described as normal, and many have had their chromosomes analysed. The rate of pregnancy loss appears low with only one biochemical pregnancy [2]. As these studies are so diverse in their methodology, it would not be valid to collate the results together and calculate an overall pregnancy rate.

## References

1. Russell JB, Knezevich KM, Fabian KF, Dickson JA. Unstimulated immature oocyte retrieval: early versus midfollicular endometrial priming. Fertil Steril 1997;67:616—620.
2. Veeck LL, Wortham JWJ, Witmyer J et al. Maturation and fertilization of morphologically immature human oocytes in a program of in vitro fertilization. Fertil Steril 1983;39:594—602.
3. Nagy ZP, Cecile J, Liu J et al. Pregnancy and birth after intracytoplasmic sperm injection of in vitro matured germinal vesicle stage oocytes: case report. Fertil Steril 1996;65:1047—1050.
4. Liu J, Katz E, Garcia JE et al. Successful in vitro maturation of human oocytes not exposed to human chorionic gonadotropin during ovulation induction, resulting in pregnancy. Fertil Steril 1997;67:566—568.
5. Jaroudi KA, Hollanders JMG, Sieck UV et al. Pregnancy after transfer of embryos which were generated from in vitro matured oocytes. Hum Reprod 1997;12:857—859.
6. Pincus G, Enzmann EV. The comparative behaviour of mammalian eggs in vivo and in vitro. J Exp Med 1935;62:665—675.
7. Edwards RG. Maturation in vitro of human ovarian oocytes. Lancet 1965;2:926—929.
8. Edwards RG, Bavister BC, Steptoe PC. Early stages of fertilisation in vitro of human oocytes matured in vitro. Nature 1969;221:632—635.
9. Trounson AO, Wood C, Kausche A. In vitro maturation and fertilization and developmental competence of oocytes recovered from untreated polycystic ovarian patients. Fertil Steril 1994b;62:353—362.
10. Cha KY, Koo JJ, Choi DH et al. Pregnancy after in vitro fertilization of human follicular fluid oocytes collected from nonstimulated cycles, their culture in vitro and their transfer in a donor oocyte program. Fertil Steril 1991;55:109—118.
11. Barnes FL, Kausche A, Tiglias J et al. Production of embryos from in vitro matured primary human oocytes. Fertil Steril 1996;65:1151—1156.
12. Pavlok A, Lucas-Hahn A, Niemann H. Fertilisation and developmental competence of bovine

oocytes derived from different categories of antral follicles. Molec Reprod Devel 1992;31: 63—67.

13. Wynn P, Picton HM, Krapez JA et al. Hum Reprod 1998;(In press).

14. Homburg R, Armar NA, Eshel A et al. Influence of serum luteinising hormone concentrations on ovulation, conception and early pregnancy loss in polycystic ovary syndrome. Br Med J 1988;297:1024—1026.

15. Schramm, RD, Bavister BD. Follicle-stimulating hormone priming of rhesus monkeys enhances meiotic and developmental competence of oocytes matured in vitro. Biol Reprod 1994;51: 904—912.

16. Erickson GF, Wang C, Hsueh AJW. FSH induction of functional LH receptors in granulosa cells cultured in a chemically defined medium. Nature 1979;279:336—338.

17. Ham RG, McKeehan WL. Media and growth requirements. Meth Enzymol 1979;58:44—93.

18. Furman A, Rotmensch S, Dor J et al. Culture of human granulosa cells from an in vitro fertilization program: effects of extracellular matrix on morphology and cyclic adenosine 3',5' monopo-sphate production. Fertil Steril 1986;46:514—517.

19. Amsterdam A, Rotmensch S. Structure-function relationships during granulosa cell differentia-tion. Endocr Rev 1987;8:309—337.

20. Hsueh AJW, Adashi EY, Jones PBC, Welsh TH. Hormonal regulation of the differentiation of cultured ovarian granulosa cells Endocr Rev 1984;5:76—127.

21. Hutz RJ. Disparate effects of estrogens on in vitro steroidogenesis by mammalian and avian granulosa cells. Biol Reprod 1989;40:709—713.

22. Campbell BK, Scaramuzzi RJ, Webb R. Induction and maintenance of oestradiol and immuno-reactive inhibin production with FSH by ovine granulosa cells in serum-free media. J Reprod Fertil 1996;106:7—16.

23. Gutierrez CG, Campbell BK, Webb R. Development of a long term bovine granulosa cell culture system: induction and maintenance of estradiol production response to FSH and morphological characteristics. Biol Reprod 1997;56:608—616.

24. Picton HM, Campbell BK, Hunter MG. Maintenance of aromatase activity in porcine granulo-sa cells in serum free culture. J Reprod Fert Abst Series 1994;14:1.

25. Picton HM, Campbell BK, Hunter MG. Maintenance of oestradiol production and cytochrome P450 aromatase enzyme messenger ribonucleic acid expression in long-term serum-free cul-tures of porcine granulosa cells. J Reprod Fertil 1998;(Submitted).

26. Seifer DB, Giudice LC, Dsupin BA et al. Follicular fluid insulin-like growth factor-I and insulin-like growth factor-II concentrations vary as a function of day 3 serum follicle stimulating hor-mone. Hum Reprod 1995;10:804—806.

27. Homberg R, Orvieto R, Bar-Hara I et al. Serum levels of insulin-like growth factor-1, IGF bind-ing protein-1 and insulin and the response to human menopause gonadotrophins in women with polycystic ovary syndrome. Hum Reprod 1996;11:716—719.

28. Chang SCS, Anderson W, Lewis JC et al. The porcine ovarian follicle. II. Electron microscopic study of surface features of granulosa cells at different stages of development. Biol Reprod 1977;16:349—357.

29. Amsterdam A, May J, Schomberg DW. Synergistic effect of insulin and follicle stimulating hor-mone on biochemical and morphological differentiation of porcine granulosa cells in vitro. Biol Reprod 1988;39:379—390.

30. Ben-Ze'ev A, Amsterdam A. Regulation of cytoskeletal proteins involved in cell contact forma-tion during differentiation of granulosa cells on extracellular matrix. Proc Natl Acad Sci USA 1988;83:2894—2898.

31. Schultz GA, Gifford DJ, Mahadevan MM et al. Protein synthetic patterns in immature human oocytes. Ann NY Acad Sci 1988;541:237—247.

32. Wassarman P. Oogenesis: synthetic events in the developing mammalian egg. In: Hartmann J (ed) Mechanism and Control of Animal Fertilisation. New York: Academic Press, 1983;1—54.

33. Eppig JJ. The ovary: oogenesis. In: Hillier SG, Kitchener HC, Neilson JP (eds) Scientific Essen-

tials of Reproductive Medicine. London: WB Saunders, 1996;147—159.

34. Trounson AO, Pushett D, Maclellan LJ et al. Current status of IVM/IVF and embryo culture in humans and farm animals. Theriogenology 1994a;41:57—66.

35. Dekel N, Piontkewitz Y. Induction of maturation of rat oocytes by interruption of communication in the cumulus-oocyte complex. Bull Assoc Anat 1991;75:51—54.

36. Green DPL. Three-dimensional structure of the zona pellucida. Rev Reprod 1997;2:147—156.

37. Schramm RD, Bavister BD. Development of in-vitro-fertilized primate embryos into blastocysts in a chemically defined, protein-free culture medium. Hum Reprod 1996;11:1690—1697.

38. Barnes FL, Crombie A, Gardner DK et al. Blastocyst development and birth after in-vitro maturation of human primary oocytes, intracytoplasmic sperm injection and assisted hatching. Hum Reprod 1995;10:3243—3247.

39. Schroeder AC, Schultz RM, Kopf GS et al. Fetuin inhibits zona pellucida hardening and conversion of ZP2 to ZP2f during spontaneous mouse oocyte maturation in vitro in the absence of serum. Biol Reprod 1990;43:891—897.

40. Cummings JM, Breen TM, Harrison KL et al. A formula for scoring human embryo growth rates in in vitro fertilisation: its value in predicting pregnancy and in comparison with visual estimates of embryo quality. J In Vitro Fertil Embryo Transf 1986;3:284—295.

41. Bolton VN, Hawes SM, Taylor CT, Parsons JH. Development of spare human preimplantation embryos in vitro and analysis of the correlations among gross morphology, cleavage rates and development to the blastocyst. J In Vitro Fertil Embryo Transf 1989;6:30—35.

42 Racowsky C, Kaufman ML. Nuclear degeneration and meiotic aberrations observed in human oocytes matured in vitro: analysis by light microscopy. Fertil Steril 1992;58:750—755.

43. Gras L, McBain J, Trounson AO, Kola I. The incidence of chromosomal aneuploidy in stimulated and unstimulated (natural) uninseminated human oocytes. Hum Reprod 1992;7:1396—1401.

44. Munne S, Lee A, Rosenwaks Z et al. Diagnosis of major chromosomal aneuploidies in human preimplantation embryos. Hum Reprod 1993;8:2185—2191.

45. Delhanty JD, Harper JC, Handyside AH, Winston RM. Multicolour FISH detects frequent chromosomal mosaicisms and chaotic division in normal preimplantation embryos from fertile patients. Hum Genet 1997;99:755—760.

46. Gardiner DK, Vella P, Lane M et al. Culture and transfer of human blastocysts increases implantation rates and reduces the need for multiple embryo transfers (abstract O—002) American Society of Reproductive Medicine Annual Meeting 1997.

47. Navot D, Anderson TL, Droesch K et al. Hormonal manipulation of endometrial maturation. J Clin Endocrinol Metab 1989;68:801—807.

48. Downs SM, Daniel S, Bornslaeger EA et al. Maintenance of meiotic arrest in mouse oocytes by purines: modulation of cAMP levels and cAMP phosphodiesterase activity. Gamete Res 1989;23:323—334.

# Future directions of in vitro maturation

Kwang Y. Cha

*College of Medicine, Pochon CHA University and Infertility Medical Center of CHA General Hospital, Seoul, South Korea*

**Abstract.** Techniques for in vitro maturation (IVM) of human immature oocytes have recently been developed. This IVM technique is especially useful for establishing pregnancy in infertile patients with various ovarian disorders. By developing this technique, additional advantages are anticipated in the field of human reproductive medicine. In this article, therefore, we firstly described IVM of human immature oocytes retrieved from unstimulated polycystic ovarian syndrome (PCOS) patients. Newly concepted techniques in artificial reproductive technology, which are related to IVM, were further reviewed.

**Keywords:** cryopreservation, IVM, ovarian tissue preservation, PCOS.

## Introduction

Human reproductive medicine has been greatly developed by employing an assisted reproductive technology (ART), including techniques for in vitro fertilization (IVF), in vitro culture (IVC) of oocytes and embryo transfer (ET). However, the overall implantation and delivery rates still have much room for improvement (15—40%) and, for the patients having certain specific infertile disorders such as polycystic ovarian syndrome (PCOS) and premature ovarian failure (POF), it is extremely difficult to be pregnant. Recently, we developed the in vitro maturation (IVM) system for immature oocytes and could expect additional improvement of implantation and pregnancy rates. Further, this new technology becomes more efficient when combined with cryopreservation for oocytes and it greatly contributes to establishing an ovum donation program and an oocyte bank. In this article, we firstly review the details of our experimental results on the IVM of oocytes and the clinical application of these programs in POF or PCOS patients. Secondly, current research progress in cryopreservation of oocytes and ovarian tissues are briefly reviewed.

*Address for correspondence:* Dr Kwang Y. Cha, College of Medicine, Pochon CHA University and Infertility Medical Center of CHA General Hospital, 606-5 Yeoksam 1-Dong, Gangnam-gu, Seoul 135-081, South Korea. Tel.: +82-2-557-3937. Fax: +82-2-555-9007.

## IVM of immature oocytes and its clinical application

*IVM*

Meiotic maturation of mammalian oocytes, which commences during the embryonic period, is arrested at the diplotene stage after birth. Resumption of the meiosis, called oocyte maturation, does not occur until puberty, becoming a suitable in vivo environment for the final maturation of oocytes. Unlike oocyte development in vivo, however, the diplotene stage oocytes retrieved from ovaries can spontaneously undergo the final maturational process in vitro and reach the MII stage being ready for fertilization and further development. These biological aspects encouraged us to design a clinical use of immature (before the MII stage) oocytes obtained from infertile patients. In the previous study, we retrieved immature oocytes directly from ovarian follicles of 3–10 mm in diameter by an ultrasound-guided transvaginal oocyte aspiration technique. We used a specially designated aspiration needle for enhancing the efficiency of oocyte retrieval. After the retrieval, immature oocytes were cultured in a tissue culture medium (TCM)-199 supplemented with fetal bovine serum (FBS, 20%), human chorionic gonadotropin (hCG, 10 IU/ml) and pregnant mare serum gonadotropin (PMSG, 10 IU/ml) for their maturational process. In our IVM system, a different maturation protocol was employed for oocytes retrieved from either unstimulated or stimulated patients, since the major proportion of the oocytes reached the MII stage at 27 and 45 h after the culture in the stimulated and unstimulated patients, respectively (unpublished data). The final maturation rate (approximately 80%) obtained from our IVM system was comparable with the rates obtained from other IVM systems (58–100%; [1–5]).

There are few reports on the fertilization and cleavage of immature oocytes (Fig. 1). Veeck et al. [4] reported for the first time that a high rate of fertilization (formation of male and female pronuclei) was obtained after IVF of oocytes retrieved from the patients with stimulated cycle. Regardless of the IVF system (conventional in vitro insemination or intracytoplasmic sperm injection, ICSI), more than 50% of oocytes retrieved from stimulated patients were normally fertilized by spermatozoa and developed up to the two-cell stage following IVC [2,6–8]. Similar results after IVF and IVC were obtained in oocytes collected from unstimulated patients [8–10]. These results clearly indicated that, regardless of induction program, immature oocytes retrieved from infertile patients can normally develop up to the viable embryos following IVM, IVF and IVC procedures.

*Clinical application of IVM*

The results described above encouraged us to apply these ART techniques for obtaining a pregnancy with infertile patients. The clinical trials were conducted: 1) by an ovum donation program for the patients with POF and repeated IVF failure or menopausal women; and 2) by use of the IVM technique for unstimu-

In stimulated cycle

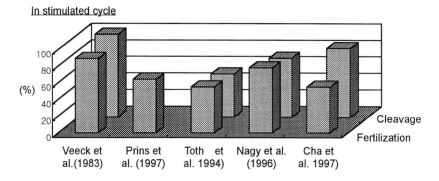

Unstimulated cycle

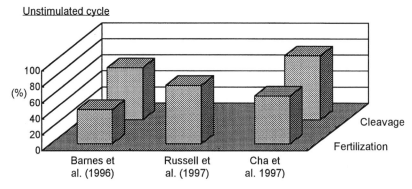

*Fig. 1.* Previous reports on fertilization and cleavage of immature oocytes retrieved from infertile patients with stimulated or unstimulated cycle following in vitro fertilization and in vitro culture.

lated PCOS patients. In the first case (Table 1), heterogeneous oocytes matured in culture were transferred to the patients. A total of seven pregnancies were achieved and we obtained four deliveries from these women. This was the first

*Table 1.* Pregnancy obtained from in vitro maturation and ovum donation program for patients with POF or repeated IVF failure and menopausal women in unstimulated cycle.

| No. | Media | Age (years) | Indication | No. ET | Results |
|---|---|---|---|---|---|
| 1 | Ham's F-10 + 50% hFF | 32 | POF | 5 | Triple/delivered |
| 2 | Ham's F-10 + 50% hFF | 43 | Repeated IVF failure | 1 | Single/delivered |
| 3 | Ham's F-10 + 50% hFF | 51 | Menopause | 3 | Clinical abortion (10 weeks) |
| 4 | Ham's F-10 + 50% hFF | 33 | POF | 5 | Clinical abortion (triploid) |
| 5 | TCM-199 + 50% hPF | 32 | POF | 10 | Clinical abortion (25 weeks) |
| 6 | TCM-199 + 50% hPF | 31 | POF | 5 | Twin/delivered |
| 7 | TCM-199 + 50% hPF | 29 | POF | 3 | Single/delivered |

hFF: human follicular fluid; hPF: human peritoneal fluid; POF: premature ovarian failure; IVF: in vitro fertilization.

report on the pregnancy and delivery of POF patients and demonstrated future prospectives of the clinical application of IVM.

In the second case for clinical application of IVM, a total of 76 PCOS patients (91 cycles) underwent IVM/IVF/ET programs from March 1995 through to February 1998. The mean age of the patients was 30.8 ± 3.2 years and the duration of their infertility was 6.3 ± 3.0 years. No hormonal treatment was performed before oocyte retrieval. An average of 12.3 ± 6.4 oocytes were retrieved from the patients by transvaginal oocyte aspiration and 61.8% of the retrieved oocytes developed to the MII stage. Among the matured oocytes, 68.7% were normally fertilized following IVF. Part of the normal pronucleus stage oocytes were transferred to the patients by ZIFT and the remaining were transferred by intrauterine transfer at 2 days after IVF. In the remaining cases, the cleavage rate was 91.6%. For the endometrial preparation, 4 mg E2 valerate was administered to the patients daily by PO from the day of oocyte aspiration through to 12 days after oocyte aspiration and 100 mg progesterone was administered daily by IM from 2 through to 12 days after oocyte aspiration. When the patients were hCG positive (pregnant), E2 valerate and progesterone were administered daily until 12 weeks of gestation. As shown in Table 2, a total of 82 cycles were conducted for ET and a mean of 4.2 ± 2.5 embryos were transferred to the patients. Among them, 22 (26.8%) patients were pregnant after ET and 10 patients delivered normal babies. A total of eight patients are presently in the stages of pregnancy. From the rest of the cases, four were aborted and one was an ectopic pregnancy.

**Cryopreservation**

*Cryopreservation of oocytes*

Particular interest has focused on developing an effective cryopreservation technique for immature oocytes in view of the many advantages of this program, e.g., attenuation of ethical concerns by avoiding the disposal of surplus oocytes and embryo freezing, and contribution to restoring fertility of women who suffer from various catastrophic diseases. We carried out some experiments in order to establish a cryopreservation technology for immature oocytes and a vitrification

*Table 2.* Pregnancy of unstimulated PCOS patients following IVM/IVF/ET program from March 1995 through to February 1998.

|  | Outcome |
| --- | --- |
| Total cycles for ET | 82 |
| No. of pregnant patients | 22 (26.8%) |
| No. of patients delivered | 10 |
| No. of patients with ongoing pregnancy | 8 |
| No. of patients with ectopic pregnancy | 1 |
| No. of aborted patients | 3 |

method using ethylene glycol (EG) and sucrose as a cryoprotectant and a copper electron microscope (EM) grid was selected. This method was designed by Martino et al. [11], but we have further modified it for human immature oocytes [12]. Use of the EM grid for this protocol may help rapid heat conduction from the outside to the oocyte and the relatively short protocol prevents oocytes from damage by the solution effect of the cryoprotectant. Also, we modified the equilibration and thawing method of our basic protocol to lessen osmotic damage and CPA toxicity, as shown in Table 2. GV stage oocytes retrieved from unstimulated PCOS patients were tested for this study and high rates of morphological normality (92%), maturation (91%), fertilization (60%) and blastocyst formation (17%) were obtained after vitrification.

*Clinical application using cryopreservation of immature oocytes*

Using our newly established vitrification method, we vitrified immature oocytes retrieved from unstimulated PCOS patients and transferred the embryos developed from the vitrified oocytes to the patients. A total of 301 oocytes were retrieved from 14 cycles and morphological normality of oocytes after vitrification was 83% (249/301). Among them, 68% of the oocytes matured in vitro and 68% of the matured oocytes (115/170) were normally developed to the pronuclear stage after IVF. The cleavage rate of those pronuclear stage oocytes was 90%. We transferred the embryos derived from vitrified oocytes to the uterus of the patients at 3 days after IVF. No implantation and pregnancy has yet been reported up to the present. However, we are continually attempting to use the cryopreserved oocytes for clinical treatment and we anticipate positive results (Table 3).

*Cryopreservation of ovarian tissue*

Ovarian cortex contains many primordial follicles that give rise to immature oocytes. The use of these primordial follicles provides infertile patients with more possibility of pregnancy, since more oocytes can be retrieved from it. An

*Table 3.* Renovated vitrification protocol for human immature oocytes retrieved from unstimulated PCOS patients.

| Procedures | Original[a] | Modified |
|---|---|---|
| Equilibration | 1) 5.5 M EG for 20 s | 1) 1.5 M EG for 5 min |
| | | 2) 5.5 M EG for 20 s |
| Thawing | 1) 0.5 M sucrose for 1 min | 1) 1M sucrose for 2.5 min |
| | 2) 0.25 M sucrose for 1 min | 2) 0.5 M sucrose for 2.5 min |
| | 3) 0.125 M sucrose for 1 min | 3) 0.25 M sucrose for 2.5 min |
| | | 4) 0.125 M sucrose for 2.5 min |

[a]Adapted from [11].

594

increase in efficiency of fertility treatment can be anticipated. Ovarian tissue banking can then become a new area contributing to the development of human reproductive medicine. There have been several reports concerning the preservation of ovarian tissue with improving results. In our preliminary study, ovarian tissue can be vitrified by our standard protocol that is slightly modified for tissue preservation, and survival of primordial follicles after vitrification and thawing was > 85%. We are carrying out extensive research on this project and we expect the growth of human primordial oocytes to viable oocytes.

## Conclusion

In our previous studies described above, IVM of human immature oocytes is a reliable technique for supporting oocyte development. The IVM technique combined with IVF and IVC programs is useful for the treatment of infertile patients. Vitrification has a potential to develop as an effective long-term preservation method for human oocytes in the near future. All of these research and clinical applications markedly contribute to developing human reproductive medicine, yielding a highly efficient program.

## References

1. Trounson A, Wood C, Kausche A. In vitro maturation and the fertilization and developmental competence of oocytes recovered from untreated polycystic ovarian patients. Fertil Steril 1994;62:353–362.
2. Nagy ZP, Cecile J, Liu J, Loccufier A, Devroey P, Van Steirteghem A. Pregnancy and birth after intracytoplasmic sperm injection of in vitro matured germinal-vesicle stage oocytes: case report. Fertil Steril 1996;65:1047–1050.
3. Liu J, Katz E, Garcia JE, Compton G, Baramki TA. Successful in vitro maturation of human oocytes not exposed to human chorionic gonadotropin during ovulation induction, resulting in pregnancy. Fertil Steril 1997;67:566–568.
4. Veeck LL, Wortham JW Jr, Witmyer J, Sandow BA, Acosta AA, Garcia JE, Jones GS, Jones HW Jr. Maturation and fertilization of morphologically immature human oocytes in a program of in vitro fertilization. Fertil Steril 1983;39:594–602.
5. Jaroudi KA, Hollanders JMG, Sieck UV, Roca GL, EL-Nour AM, Coskun S. Pregnancy after transfer of embryos which were generated from in vitro matured oocytes. Hum Reprod 1997;12:857–859.
6. Prins GS, Wagner C, Weidel L, Gianfortoni J, Marut EL, Scommegna A. Gonadotropins augment maturation and fertilization of human immature oocytes cultured in vitro. Fertil Steril 1987;47:1035–1037.
7. Toth TL, Baka SG, Veek LL, Jones HW Jr, Muasher S, Lanzendorf SE. Fertilization and in vitro development of cryopreserved human prophase I oocytes. Fertil Steril 1994;61:891–894.
8. Cha KY, Koo JJ, Ko JJ, Choi DH, Han SY, Yoon TK. Pregnancy after in vitro fertilization of human follicular oocytes collected from nonstimulated cycle, their culture in vitro and their transfer in a donor oocyte program. Fertil Steril 1991;55:109–113.
9. Russell JB, Knezevich KM, Fabian KF, Dickson JA. Unstimulated immature oocyte retrieval: early versus midfollicular endometrial priming. Fertil Steril 1997;67:616–620.
10. Barnes FL, Kausche A, Tiglias J, Wood C, Wilton L, Trounson A. Production of embryos from in vitro-matured primary human oocytes. Fertil Steril 1996;65:1151–1156.

11. Martino A, Songsasen N, Leibo SP. Development into blastocysts of bovine oocytes cryopreserved by ultra-rapid cooling. Biol Reprod 1996;54:1059—1069.
12. Hong SW, Chung HM, Yoon TK, Lee HK, Ko JJ, Cha KY. Morphological normality and development of vitrified human oocytes thawed by two dilution procedures. Abstracts, IFFS and American Society for Reproductive Medicine 2—8 October 1998 (Abstract).

# Gamete and tissue freezing

# Cryopreservation of human oocytes: state of the art

Eleonora Porcu, Raffaella Fabbri, Luca Savelli, Simone Petracchi and Carlo Flamigni
*Infertility and IVF Centre, Department of Gynecology and Obstetrics, University of Bologna, Bologna, Italy*

**Abstract.** The cryopreservation of female gametes might offer a solution to several religious, legal and ethical problems related to embryo freezing. Moreover, this technique would be able to insure the maintenance of fertility in women suffering from pathologies of the reproductive system which compromise the function of the ovaries, such as premature ovarian failure, endometriosis, cysts and pelvic infections. Finally, the use of frozen oocytes might be included in a program of oocyte donation. The cryopreservation of oocytes, however, has faced technical problems that ended in poor survival rates at thawing and in a low number of pregnancies. These difficulties are due to biological features of the oocytes and have raised various questions about the possibility of inducing aneuploidy after the exposition of the gametes to cryoprotectants and the process of freezing and thawing. However, recent basic research documented the absence of stray chromosomes and normal karyotypes in oocytes after thaw. In addition, our clinical results suggest that the association of oocytes cryopreservation and intracytoplasmic sperm injection produces good fertilization and implantation rates, and the birth of healthy children. These results are the first clinical proofs in favour of the efficiency and the safety of this technique.

**Keywords:** assisted reproductive techniques, cryoprotectant, freezing.

During recent decades the body of information concerning the cryopreservation of human embryos in liquid nitrogen has grown significantly. The utilization of this process was fostered by the problem of the excess number of human embryos which often occurs in the programs of IVF/ET. As it is not possible to transfer all the embryos developed, due to the risk of multiple pregnancies, their storage in liquid nitrogen provides the solution for the surplus embryos. However, the cryopreservation of human embryos presents legal, moral and religious problems to clinicians, patients, legislators and, above all, to the public. Some countries, such as Austria, Germany, Switzerland, Denmark and Sweden have forbidden or even strongly restricted the use of this technique [1]. The cryopreservation of female gametes may offer a solution to these problems. Analogously to the cryo-storage of sperms, the preservation of oocytes would avoid the condition of iatrogenic sterility after chemo/radiotherapy in neoplastic pathologies. Moreover, this technique would be able to insure a potential fertility, until now unimaginable even in women who suffer from pathologies of the reproductive system which

*Address for correspondence:* Eleonora Porcu, Infertility and IVF Centre, Department of Gynecology and Obstetrics, University of Bologna, via Massarenti, 13 40138, Bologna, Italy.

compromise the function of the ovaries: premature ovarian failure, endometriosis, cysts and pelvic infections. In order to face such pathologies, the use of frozen oocytes in a program of assisted fertilization would be able to guarantee the maintenance of fertility in such patients. The cryopreservation of oocytes could also function as an alternative in family planning for women who delay maternity due to career demands, the absence of a partner or because of pathologies which momentarily prevent the state of pregnancy. Finally, the utilization of frozen oocytes might be included in a program of oocyte donation. The cryopreservation of oocytes, however, has faced more problems than the storage of male gametes or human embryos. These difficulties are due to the biological features of the oocytes and have raised various questions about the possibility of inducing aneuploidy after the exposition of the gametes to cryoprotectants and the process of freezing and thawing. In fact, at ovulation the oocytes are blocked at metaphase of the second meiotic division with 23 dichromatidic chromosomes bound to the microtubules of the meiotic spindle. In this stage, the oocytes are extremely sensitive to temperature changes, the eventual depolymerization of microtubules of the spindle caused by the cryoprotectants or by the ice crystals formed during the process of freezing and thawing which could impair the normal separation of the chromatids at the moment of fertilization, thus inducing aneuploidy after the extrusion of the second polar body. The small number of pregnancies reported in the literature after the cryopreservation of oocytes [2–7] demonstrates the significant technical difficulties faced by this procedure.

The cryopreservation procedure follows five important stages: 1) initial exposition to cryoprotectants, substances which are able to reduce the cellular damage caused by the crystallization of water, 2) freezing until temperatures are below $0°C$, 3) storage, 4) thawing, and 5) dilution and removal of the cryoprotectants and the return to a physiological microenvironment permitting further development.

The two most potentially dangerous moments for cellular survival are constituted by the initial phase of freezing at a very low temperature and the final return to physiological conditions.

If the temperature reached is sufficiently low (normally $-196°C$, the temperature of liquid nitrogen) storage, even for a long period of time, has no effect on the successive survival rate.

In fact, at this temperature, insufficient energy is available for most physiological reactions and water molecules align themselves in a glassy, crystalline structure. The only known potential damage for gametes and embryos stored at this temperature is the breakdown of DNA caused by cosmic radiation.

When an oocyte is cooled at a temperature between $-5$ and $-15°C$ ice formation is first induced in the extracellular medium thanks to a process called seeding. As the temperature is decreased, the amount of ice is increased and the solutes concentrate in the extracellular medium. As a result, an osmotic gradient is created. Due to this gradient, water is attracted from the cytoplasm to the extracellular medium and the cell shrinks. If this process is sufficiently slow, the massive passage of the water out of the cell will be able to decrease the probable nucleation of ice within the cell, until approximately $-15°C$. A mathematical model has been created which represents the rate of volume modification of the cell as a function of its permeability, membrane area and temperature [8]. For those cells with a low surface/volume ratio, such as gametes, a low freezing rate is necessary to allow a sufficient amount of water to move out of the cell. In such a way, the intracellular ice crystals which form would be small enough to avoid any damage to the intracellular components. It is necessary to underline that, for any type of cell, an increase in the freezing rate reduces the survival rate.

The optimal freezing rate depends on various parameters: the cytosolic water content, the changing permeability constant of the membrane, the area of the membrane and the temperature. The intracellular water content, apart from causing mechanical damage at the moment of freezing, may also cause material damage at thawing, due to an increase in volume during this process. The survival rate in fact decreases if thawing occurs slowly, since, in this way, the crystals formed in the cytosol have a sufficient amount of time to grow, thus damaging intracellular structures.

Two phenomenon which occur during the thawing of frozen oocytes may effectively reduce the survival rate: 1) recrystallization, and 2) osmotic shock.

Recrystallization means the process by which water returns into the cell and assumes a solid state around small ice crystals previously formed in the cytosol. When the temperature is raised until $-40°C$ some water molecules may retrace the path followed during freezing, returning to the cytosol and reforming hydrogen bonds with ice crystals already present, thus significantly increasing the cellular dimension. The probability of recurrence of this phenomenon is influenced both by the thawing and the freezing rates. After rapid freezing, cellular dehydration is probably insufficient and would give way to the formation of large intracellular masses if the thawing process is carried out very slowly. The formation of intracellular ice is avoidable if rapid thawing takes place at the nucleation point of the ice. Osmotic shock may occur during rapid thawing. In fact, if the cryoprotectant which previously penetrated into the cell does not diffuse out rapidly enough to prevent an influx of water, the oocyte would swell and explode. During this period two opposing necessities must be faced: on one hand it is important to reduce to a minimum the contact time between the cell and the cryoprotectant at room temperature, as the cryoprotectant exercise a temperature-dependent cytotoxicity; on the other hand the process of dilution of the cryoprotectant in the cytosol must be very gradual in order to avoid the excessive reduction of the extracellular osmotic potential thus causing a massive influx of water into the cell with consequent cellular lysis.

As a result of an examination of the published literature, the studies performed until now concerning the cryopreservation of human oocytes have offered contrasting information regarding the ideal method which results in the least damage to cellular integrity. The principal factors which are most vitally involved in the success of cryopreservation regard the oocyte itself and the technique.

## Oocyte-related variables

The size influences the overall survival rate, as the probability of intracellular ice formation depends upon it. Human sperm offers a valid example of the influence of cytoplasmic volume on survival after cryopreservation: male gametes are 180 times smaller than female gametes, and their survival rate is much higher.

An optimal quality of the oocyte is essential in order to guarantee its survival upon freezing. Often low quality supernumerary oocytes are frozen, resulting in low survival rates. For this reason some authors, such as Chen [2], chose to freeze all the best oocytes available. Regarding this parameter, the four most important aspects involved in the evaluation of oocyte quality are: nuclear stage, cytoplasmic characteristics, aspect of the corona radiata, expansion of the cumulus cells.

Various authors argue both for and against the maintenance of cumulus oophorus to optimize the survival rate. Chen and Van Uem [2,4] affirmed that its absence facilitates the penetration of cryoprotectant into the cytoplasm; in effect the first pregnancies where achieved after thawing cryopreserved oocytes without cumulus. Even Gook et al. [9] reported an increased survival rate of frozen oocytes without the cumulus with respect to those maintaining cumulus (69 vs. 48%). On the other hand, several studies showed the importance of the presence of the cumulus which guarantees greater cellular survival at the end of the cryopreservation process [10,11]. Some authors hypothesized that the presence of cumulus cells is able to act as a protective barrier against sudden osmotic modifications and stress caused by the sudden concentration and dilution of cryoprotectants during the process of equilibrium and removal after thawing [12,13]. In our experience, the presence of the cumulus does not seem to significantly condition oocyte survival [7] in accordance with experience of Mandelbaum et al. [14].

All oocytes should be frozen shortly after being harvested, between 38 and 40 h after hCG [3]. The older oocytes cultured in vitro before freezing present a significantly reduced fertilization potential and an increase in anomalous fertilizations and polyploidy [15]. All the pregnancies achieved with frozen oocytes come from metaphase II oocytes. In fact, the mature oocytes at pick-up provide higher survival and fertilization rates [5]. The cryopreservation of oocytes in prophase I has been proposed as an alternative approach in the storage of female gametes. In fact, in these oocytes, meiosis is arrested and the chromosomes are inside the nucleus, not aligned along the spindle. Moreover, in this stage, the cells are small and undifferentiated, lacking a zona pellucida and relatively quiescent from a metabolic point of view. Given these theoretical data, various groups of researchers have examined the potentiality of cryopreserved oocytes in prophase I to mature, to become fertilized and to develop into embryos. Mandelbaum et al. [14] obtained discouraging results. In fact, given the low survival rate (37%) and the rate of in vitro maturation upon thawing (20%), these researchers deduced that prophase I, although theoretically not susceptible to the damages of "cold shock", is not the best stage in which to freeze oocytes. Toth et al. [15]

have studied fresh and cryopreserved immature oocytes again at prophase I in order to compare the maturation rate at metaphase (M) II, fertilization and maturation. The authors demonstrated that immature human oocytes are capable of surviving cryopreservation and maturing to M II. Moreover, frozen oocytes maintain the same possibilities of fertilizing and maturing in comparison to unfrozen control oocytes. In a subsequent study [16], two different methods for the cryopreservation of immature oocytes were compared. The two techniques differed in freezing and thawing rates, in the temperature chosen for the seeding, and in the utilization or not of sucrose as cryoprotectant. Method I consisted of the slow freezing/slow thawing rate, and a seeding at $-6°C$. On the contrary method II involved rapid freezing/rapid thawing, with the utilization of sucrose as cryoprotectant and seeding at $-7°C$. The results reported confirmed that oocytes at prophase I are capable of surviving cryoconservation and maturing to metaphase II after thawing. Both protocols result in the same amount of mature oocytes. Even if in the study the authors did not consider the fertilization capacity and the development of such treated oocytes, important clinical application may be observed.

In fact, those patients who desire to maintain their own reproductive potential despite chemo-/radiotherapy or ovariectomy, may benefit from this technique in combination with in vitro fertilization (IVF). A recent study by an Australian group [17] was conducted to evaluate the survival rate after freezing and thawing immature oocytes utilizing PROH as a cryoprotectant, where dosages and exposure time to cryoprotectant were the same used for storing mature oocytes. Encouraging results were obtained, demonstrating the efficacy of this method and proposing the strategy of freezing immature oocytes as a feasible therapeutic method for the future. Innovative strategies have recently been suggested to preserve fertility in those patients undergoing antineoplastic treatments or removal of the ovaries. Hovatta et al. [18] have investigated a new freezing technique, in order to store thin slices of ovarian parenchyma. The ovarian cortex is rich in follicles at different stages of maturation, in particular primordial follicles. Utilizing two different freezing protocols (DMSO 1.5 M o PROH 1.5 M + sucrose 0.1 M) it has been possible to store slices of ovarian cortex for a variable period from 24 h to 5 weeks. In both cases, the thawing procedure was carried out quickly in a water bath at $37°C$. The authors did not find any difference on histological examination before and after freezing in either protocol. The authors affirm that, due to the normal state of follicles after freezing and thawing, the oocyte should be capable of in vitro maturation and fertilization, under adequate stimuli. Newton et al. [19] and Gosden et al. [20], demonstrated that thin slices of ovarian parenchyma frozen and successively thawed could be grafted in the abdomen in order to permit the maturation of primitive and primordial follicles. The authors showed that cryoprotectants ethylenglicol and DMSO effectively reduce the damage done to the parenchyma caused by ice crystals and obtained quite high survival rates of the follicles. The authors concluded that, despite the necessary improvement of the technique of cryopreservation and transplantation, the results are sufficiently encouraging and suggest ovarian tissue banking as a valid method in preserving fertility in selected cases. If orthotopic autograft is capable of re-establishing ovulatory menstrual cycles, the necessity of ovulation induction and in vitro fertilization is eliminated. Even pediatric patients may benefit from this technique. In fact, most primordial follicles and the prepubertal quiescent state of the ovary may improve the possibility of success, and in certain cases ovarian tissue banking is the only available option to maintain fertility.

## Technical variables

Cryoprotectants are substances which present different chemical compositions and share a high water solubility associated with toxicity directly proportional to their concentration and temperature. Their role is to protect cells from damage which may occur during the entire procedure of freezing, storing and thawing. This damage is called "cold shock".

The cryoprotectants are divided into two categories according to their capacity to penetrate inside the cells: intracellular and extracellular agents. From a biochemical point of view it is possible to distinguish three classes of cryoprotectant compounds: alcohols (methanol, ethanol, propanol, 1,2-propanediol, glycerol), sugars (glucose, lactose, sucrose, starch), and dimethylsulfoxide (DMSO).

### DMSO and glycerol
DMSO and glycerol have a low molecular weight and for the past 30 years have been recognised as a cryoprotectant against freezing damage. They have both been used in different protocols. In 1988 Friedler [21] demonstrated that DMSO was more effective than glycerol.

### 1,2-Propanediol (PROH)
PROH has been largely used in blastocysts and pre-embryo cryopreservation both in humans and other species. In combination with other agents that reduce its toxicity and osmotic power, PROH seems to obtain a better oocytes survival rate after thawing [22]; this characteristic may be due to the fact that PROH penetrates the oolemma more rapidly; it is also more water soluble [21] and less toxic [12].

### Sucrose
Sucrose is often used in association with other cryoprotectants. It is not able to penetrate through the cellular membrane and its presence in extracellular media can exert a significant osmotic effect. Sucrose is protective during the dilution phase or after rapid thawing, when cells begin to rehydrate and swell. This risk may be reduced by removing the intracellular cryoprotectants (e.g., PROH) in a stepwise dilution (1.5; 1.0; 0.25 M) so as to reduce the amount of cellular swelling. An alternative and more rapid method of removing permeating cryoprotectants involves the addition of nonpermeating molecules such as sucrose to the

thawing solution. The elevated extracellular concentration of these molecules balances the high concentration of intracellular cryoprotectant, reducing the osmolarity differences in the two sides of the plasmatic membrane. Up till now sucrose was the only nonpenetrating cryoprotectant routinely utilized in human oocyte cryopreservation. The mechanism of action of cryoprotectants is quite complex and is attributable to a series of properties. First of all, cryoprotectant presence in the solution determines a slight lowering of the cryoscopic point of the solution, approximately $-2$ or $-3°C$. The protective effects are mainly due to the capacity of these molecules to form hydrogen bonds which alter the normal crystal structure of water, thus reducing its dimension. Through their $-OH$ groups glycerol and PROH, for example, may form hydrogen bonds with water as does DMSO through its oxygen atoms. Cryoprotectant agents reduce the damaging effects of the high concentration of electrolytes in the portion of liquid water. In systems which are constituted by two phases such as ice and water, at a constant pressure, the total concentration of solutes in a liquid phase is constant for each concentration. Since the total concentration of the solutes must be constant, the addition of cryoprotectants reduces the amount of water which crystallizes [21].

Their efficacy is directly related to the temperature at which these compounds are added to the culture medium. In 1991 Pickering [23] demonstrated that human oocytes exposed to DMSO at $37°C$ temperature lose the capacity to be fertilized, while at $4°C$ this capacity is maintained. Even though the author did not freeze the oocytes, the results of this study suggest that the addition of cryoprotectant to the medium must take place at a temperature below $10°C$ in order to avoid fertilization failure. The optimal cryoprotectant concentration varies according to the type of cell and to the type of species under examination [24].

In 1988 Sathananthan [25] demonstrated that exposure time to DMSO is able to influence the amount of damage to the meiotic spindle: only 60 min of exposure at a concentration of 1.5 M is enough to determine important modifications of its structure, not reversible in the majority of the oocytes, while after $10-20$ min the spindle still presented structural integrity. Van der Elst et al. [26] found that the exposition of the oocytes to PROH 1.5 M for a brief period was harmless.

The removal of the permeating cryoprotectant from the cytoplasm is an important step in the process of cryopreservation [23]. The procedure consists of a series of passages of the oocyte in solutions of gradually diminishing concentrations. In fact if the cells were placed in a medium without cryoprotectant immediately upon thawing, they would swell until explosion, due to the effect of osmotic pressure.

The freezing and thawing rates condition the water diffusion through the cellular membrane. Furthermore, the choice of the optimal thawing rate depends upon the rate at which freezing has taken place as described above. Several protocols for oocyte cryopreservation have been used, based on different rates of freezing and thawing.

Oocyte storage is often performed with a slow freeze-rapid thaw procedure.

Chen [2] achieved the first worldwide pregnancy with this protocol. The same strategy was adopted by Siebzehnruebl et al. in [27].

Although uncommon and rarely reported in literature, slow freezing/slow thawing resulted in the second pregnancy with a frozen oocyte [4]. The authors used DMSO 1.5 M as cryoprotectant and oocyte thawing was performed at room temperature.

Ultrarapid freezing/rapid thawing avoids the formation of ice crystals and induces a glassy, amorphous medium using high concentrations of cryoprotectants.

Trounson [28] first applied this strategy to human oocyte cryopreservation by direct immersion of ova in liquid nitrogen (ultrarapid freezing). Rapid thawing was performed at 37°C, in water bath. Nine of 18 mature human ova thus treated survived to thawing, but all of them degenerated in culture.

In another process called vitrification, a high concentrated solution of cryoprotectants solidifies during freezing without the formation of ice crystals, in a supercooled, highly viscose fluid. It shows some clear advantages as compared to simple freezing because it avoids the damage caused by intracellular ice crystal formation. A high cooling rate (nearly 1,500°C/min) and high concentrations of cryoprotectants as DMSO, acetamide, propylene-glycol and polyethylene-glycol are requested for vitrification. The theoretic basis of vitrification was clearly expressed by Rall and Fahy [29] as a technique to preserve the embryos. However, results are discordant and the toxicity of the cryoprotectants is confirmed by experimental studies [21]. Trounson [28] reported acceptable survival and fertilization rates but low cleavage rates. The cleavage block may be related to the irreversible damage induced in the cytoskeleton by the association of cooling and vitrification solution. Recently, Hunter et al. [30] investigated human oocyte vitrification in order to demonstrate the feasibility of this procedure. Their data suggest that mature human oocytes are able to tolerate vitrification at room temperature but survival rates decrease if vitrification is performed at −196°C. The researchers obtained good survival and fertilization rates but the oocytes thus treated showed a strongly impaired cleavage rate. This phenomenon may be due to irreversible cytoskeletal damages when freezing is associated to vitrification.

*Effect of freezing on oocytes structure*

Several cell structures can be damaged during the entire process of freezing/thawing and by the cryoprotectants.

*Chromosome and meiotic spindle*

The meiotic spindle is constituted by fragile fibers which originate from the opposing poles of the cell, from a structure called the centriole and extending to the chromosomes. Any loss of the microtubules during freezing could separate the chromosomes and cause a condition of aneuploidy [11,21,25,26,31].

Gook et al. demonstrated in 1994 [13] that normal fertilization can be achieved in cryopreserved oocytes, suggesting that reasonable integrity is preserved after cryopreservation. In addition, karyotyping and DNA staining showed that chromosomes have not been lost from the spindle during fertilization of frozen oocytes. Thus the suggestion that oocytes cryopreservation would result in a high rate of aneuploid embryos due to loss of chromosomes from the spindle since unfounded for human oocytes. Probably the chromosomes are anchored via the associated kynetochores and are not free to move in the cytoplasm. It is likely that the spindle in human oocytes is less sensitive to freezing, compared to the mouse. Chromosomal loss from the spindle is minimal in human oocytes after freezing/thawing and fertilization, suggesting that the cryodamages documented in animals is not so common in human oocytes.

*Cytoskeleton*

The cytoskeleton is a complex fibrillary cytoplasmic structure. Its function is to maintain and modify the form, thus permitting the movement of cytoplasmic organelles, exocitosis and even the movement of intrinsic membrane proteins. The major components of the cytoskeleton are microtubules, microfilaments of actin and intermediate filaments. All of these components are rather sensitive to the various stimuli and are capable of rapid depolymerization of the subunits. Vincent et al. [32] demonstrated that the cryoprotectant DMSO produces important damage in the microfilaments of murine oocytes, in a manner directly proportional to its concentration. When DMSO is utilized at a temperature close to 0°C, this effect seems to be reduced. Alterations in the components of the cytoskeleton, produced in frozen/thawed oocytes by ice crystals or by cryoprotectants have also been postulated by Hunter et al. [33] and Van Blerkom and Davis [34]. Younis et al. [35] obtained identical results and even if it was not possible to affirm whether or not the damage of the cryoprotectant to the cytoskeleton is mediated directly by the components used or subsequently by osmotic modifications, it is clear that the alterations are directly proportional to the concentration of the cryoprotectants, their exposure time and the temperature at which they are added to the culture medium.

*Cortical granules*

According to some investigations, the oocytes which survive thawing demonstrate a high aneuploidy rate when fertilized in vitro [36]. Normally cortical granules in mature oocytes are aligned just under the oolemma. The zona reaction takes place after the movement of these granules to the periphery of the cytoplasm. This reaction is responsible for the block of polyspermy. A study performed on human and murine oocytes with the use of electron microscope [37] revealed a significant reduction in the number and morphological alterations of cortical granules after thawing. This observation might explain the high incidence of aneuploidy in frozen/thawed oocytes. Van Blerkom and Davis [34] noticed that the premature exocytosis of cortical granules may lead to a sudden zona hardening and, as a consequence, to a reduction of the fertilization rate (IVF). The premature release of cortical granules might be due to the damage caused by ice crystals or by cryoprotectants on the microfilaments of actin present just below the oolemma [24,34]. In a study, Gook et al. [9] showed a high number of cortical granules in frozen thawed oocytes suggesting that neither the cryoprotectants nor the low temperature reduce the release of these organelles.

*Zona pellucida*

A common characteristic of all mammalian oocytes is the presence of a glycoprotein layer, the zona pellucida, just external to the oolemma. The functions of the zona pellucida are multiple and only partially understood. The best known ones include: the presentation of receptors to sperms, the induction of the zona reaction, the block of polyspermy and the physical protection of the embryo. Various researchers have warned of the risk of damaging the zona pellucida during cryopreservation [1,38]. In particular, lesions have been observed in 20–29% of the oocytes. The damage to the zona pellucida is attributed to the formation of cleavage planes in the ice or to the growth of large crystals during the process of freezing and thawing, which may trap and perforate the cell.

*Parthenogenetic activation*

Since 1940 it has been shown that parthenogenetic activation can be induced by physical conditions such as freezing. Successively it was found that the thermal shock in the form of heat and cold could either effective as parthenogenetic activator in some animal species. Gook et al. [39] observed that fresh and aged cryopreserved human oocytes underwent parthenogenesis in 27 and 29% of oocytes, respectively.

**Survival and fertilization rates of frozen/thawed oocytes**

The survival rate of human oocytes at thawing reported in literature varies considerably (Table 1). The results of Chen [3], who reported a 76% survival rate, are classified among the highest ones. It must be emphasized that this author has frozen only oocytes of optimum quality in metaphase II. Mean survival rates inferior to those of Chen were reported by Al-Hasani et al. [5] (25%) who froze only supernumerary oocytes and not always of good quality. Substantially low percentages were obtained by Kazem et al. [1] (34.4%) and Tucker et al. [6] (24.7%). Gook et al. [40] documented a variable survival rate between 48 and 95%. This author utilized 1,2-propanediol and observed a greater survival rate freezing oocytes without the cumulus (69%) with respect to those with the cumulus oophorus (48%). The number of thawed oocytes is substantially low in all the studies and this partially accounts for the variability of the results. Our centre has presented the largest case study of thawed oocytes until now reported in the literature, and our mean survival rate varies from 57 to 58% [7].

The in vitro fertilization rate of frozen/thawed oocytes is quite variable and ranges from little more than 13% [1] to 71% [3]. In most of the studies the varia-

Table 1. Survival and fertilization rates of cryopreserved mature human oocytes.

| Author | No. oocytes | Cumulus | Cryo-protectant | Freeze thaw | Survival | IVF Total | IVF Normal | IVF Abnormal | ICSI Total | ICSI Normal | ICSI Abnormal | Cleavage |
|---|---|---|---|---|---|---|---|---|---|---|---|---|
| Trounson, 1986 | 3 | yes | DMSO | Slow Rapid | 0% | | | | | | | |
| | 6 | yes | PROH | Slow Rapid | 67% (4/6) | 100% (4/4) | | | | | | |
| Chen, 1986, 1987 | 50 | partial | DMSO | Slow Rapid | 76% | 71% | | | | | | 85% (23/27) 100% (2/2) |
| Van Uem, 1987 | 4 | no | DMSO | Slow Rapid | 100% (4/4) | 50% (2/4) | | | | | | |
| Al-Hasani, 1987 | 205 | partial | DMSO PROH | Slow Rapid | 25% | 56% 50% 75% | 40.3% 40% 41.6% | 15.3% 10% 33.3% | | | | 42% (3/7) |
| Mandel-baum, 1988 | 25 35 38 30 | yes no | DMSO PROH | Slow Rapid Slow Rapid | 36% (9/25) 43% (15/43) 26% (10/38) 37% (11/30) | 32% (7/22) | 18% (4/22) | 14% (3/22) | | | | |
| Siebzehn-ruebl, 1989 | 38 | yes | DMSO | Slow Rapid | 37% (14/38) | | | | | | | 50% (2/4) |
| Hunter, 1991 | 13 15 | | GLYCER. DMSO | Slow Rapid | 61.5% (8/13) 73.3% (11/15) | 37.5% 45.4% | | | | | | |
| Imoedehme E. Sigue, 1992 | 33 30 | yes no | PROH | Slow Rapid | 54.5% 26.6% | 44.4% 25% | | | | | | 85% (6/8) 50% (1/2) |
| Van Bler-kom, 1994 | 183 | | | | 55% (101/183) | 38% | 29% | 9% | | | | 32% (12/38) |
| Kazem, 1995 | 220 | no | PROH | Slow Rapid | 34.4% (74/220) | 13.5% (5/37) | 2.7% (1/37) | 10.8% (4/37) | 45.9% (17/37) | 43.2% (16/37) | 2.7% (1/37) | |
| Gook, 1995 | 32 | no | PROH | Slow Rapid | 48−95% (80.4%) | 55% (10/18) | 50% (9/18) | 5% (1/18) | 71% (10/14) | 50% (7/14) | 21% (3/14) | |
| Tucker, 1996 | 81 | no | PROH | Slow Rapid | 24.7% (20/81) | | | | | 65% (13/20) | | 100% (13/13) |
| Porcu, 1997 | 522 | no | PROH | Slow Rapid | 57.5% (300/522) | | | | 71.3% (162/227) | 64.3% (146/227) | 7% (16/227) | 88.3% (129/146) |

bility is between 30 and 55%, which is inferior to the fertilization rate of "fresh" oocytes. Anomalous fertilizations, generally polyploids, calculated on the number of inseminated oocytes, range from 5 [40] to 15.3% [5]. The often reduced percentage of fertilization and the rather high incidence of anomalous fertilizations in cryopreserved oocytes have been related to the possible damage to zona pellucida and cortical granules which impede the correct interaction with the spermatozoa. The intracytoplasmic sperm injection (ICSI) has recently been proposed as a solution to these problems. Gook's group in 1995 [40] obtained in 50% of cases normal fertilization with this technique, associated, however, with a 21% abnormal fertilizations. It is important to note that with respect to those embryos obtained with traditional IVF, those embryos derived from the ICSI technique demonstrated a greater capacity of cell division for many days.

Analogous experiences were conducted by Kazem et al. [1], who documented 43.2% of normal fertilizations with ICSI and by Tucker et al. [6], who obtained 65% of normal fertilizations and three pregnancies, all of which resulted in abortions.

After the preliminary experience with IVF which involved frozen oocytes and resulted in a fertilization rate of 46% we undertook a study associating the ICSI technique with the freezing of female gametes. Superovulation was induced through a combination of a GnRH analogue and gonadotropins [40]. The oocytes were cryopreserved using a slow freeze/rapid thaw protocol and PROH plus sucrose as cryoprotectants. During ICSI, technical damages occurred in 7% of the oocytes [42], a lower rate than those reported by Kazem et al. in 1995 [1] (32%) and by Gook et al. [40] in the same year (26%). The percentage of normal fertilizations obtained in our study was 64.3% [43—45], similar to those reported by Tucker et al. (1996) [6]. The percentage of abnormal fertilizations was 7.2%, the same as that found by our group using IVF and in the ICSI of "fresh" oocytes. Most of the embryos were found to be of good quality and demonstrated a good tendency to subsequent division.

*Pregnancies and births*

In 1986 Chen [2] reported the first pregnancy from frozen thawed oocytes (Table 2). One year later two additional pregnancies and births were reported [3,4]. Ten years later our group reported the first birth of a healthy female conceived associating the techniques of freezing oocytes and ICSI [7]. At the moment we have obtained nine pregnancies and the birth of six normal and healthy babies [46]. The best results were obtained with the transfer of the embryos in a delayed, hormonal replacement cycle.

Until recently the cryopreservation of oocytes was considered an inefficient technique, with poor survival, fertilization and cleavage rates. With the introduction of the ICSI technique, the results in terms of fertilization, embryo development and implantation have become similar to those obtained with fresh oocytes. The only limiting step of the process at the moment appears to be the survival

*Table 2.* Births from frozen oocytes reported in the literature.

| Author | Year | Births |
|---|---|---|
| Chen (Adelaide, Australia) | 1986 | 2 (IVF) |
| | 1987 | 1 (IVF) |
| Van Uem (Erlangen, Germany) | 1987 | 1 (IVF) |
| Porcu (Bologna, Italia) | 1997 | 1 (ICSF) |

rate of the oocytes after thawing, which should be improved upon.

The safety of this technique has been widely debated. One of the most important concerns regards the possible damage to the meiotic spindle and the consequent induction of aneuploidy.

Nevertheless, the studies of Gook et al. [9,13,39] have reassuringly demonstrated a normal genetic patrimony and the absence of stray chromosomes in cryoconserved oocytes. It is therefore most probable that the process of freezing selects only the best and most resistant oocytes, able to survive different stresses.

## References

1. Kazem R, Thompson LA, Srikantharajah A, Laing MA, Hamilton MPR, Templeton A. Cryopreservation of human oocytes and fertilization by two techniques: in-vitro fertilization and intracytoplasmic sperm injection. Hum Reprod 1995;10:2650–2654.
2. Chen C. Pregnancy after human oocyte cryopreservation. Lancet 1986;i:884–886.
3. Chen C. Pregnancies after human oocyte cryopreservation. Ann NY Acad Sci 1987;541:541–549.
4. Van Uem JFHM, Siebzehnrubl ER, Schun B, Koch R, Trotnow S, Lang N. Birth after cryopreservation of unfertilized oocytes. Lancet 1987;i:752–753.
5. Al-Hasani S, Diedrich K, Van der Ven H, Reinecke A, Hartje M, Krebs D. Cryopreservation of human oocytes. Hum Reprod 1987;2:695–700.
6. Tucker M, Wright G, Morton P, Shanguo L, Massey J, Kort H. Preliminary experience with human oocyte cryopreservation using 1,2-propanediol and sucrose. Hum Reprod 1996;11:1513–1515.
7. Porcu E, Fabbri R, Seracchioli R, Ciotti PM, Magrini O, Flamigni C. Birth of a healthy female after intracytoplasmic sperm injection of cryopreserved human oocytes. Fertil Steril 1997;4:724–726.
8. Mazur P. Limits to life at low temperatures and at reduced water activities. Orig Life 1980;10:137.
9. Gook D, Osborn S, Johnston W. Cryopreservation of mouse and human oocytes using 1,2-propanediol and the configuration of the meiotic spindle. Hum Reprod 1993;8:1101–1109.
10. Pellicer A, Lightman A, Parmer TG, Behrman HR, De Cherney AH. Morphologic and functional studies of immature rat oocyte-cumulus complexes after cryopreservation. Fertil Steril 1988;50:805–810.
11. Sathananthan AH, Kirby C, Trounson A, Philipatos D, Shaw J. The effects of cooling mouse oocytes. J Assist Reprod Genet 1992;9:139–148.
12. Imoedmhe DG, Sigue AB. Survival of human oocytes cryopreserved with or without the cumulus in 1,2-propanediol. J Assist Reprod Genet 1992;9:323-327.
13. Gook D, Osborn S, Bourne H, Johnston W. Fertilization of human oocytes following cryopreservation; normal karyotipes and absence of stray chromosomes. Hum Reprod 1994;9:684–691.

612

14. Mandelbaum J, Junca AM, Tibi C, Plachot M, Alnot MO, Rim H, Salat-Baruox J, Cohen J. Cryopreservation of immature and mature hamster and human oocytes. In Vitro Fertil Assist Reprod 1988;541:550—561.
15. Toth T, Baka S, Veeck L, Jones H, Muasher S, Lanzendorf S. Fertilization and in vitro development of cryopreserved human prophase I oocytes. Fertil Steril 1994;61:891—894.
16. Toth TL, Lazendorf SE, Sandow BA, Veeck L, Hassen W, Hassen K, Hodgen GD. Cryopreservation of human prophase I oocytes collected from unstimulated follicles. Fertil Steril 1994; 61:1077—1082.
17. Gook D, Osborn SM, Bourne H, Johnston WIH, Speirs AL. Mature and immature human oocyte cryopreservation. In: Porcu E, Flamigni C (eds) Human Oocytes: From Physiology to IVF. Bologna: Monduzzi Editore, 1998;279—284.
18. Hovatta O, Silye R, Krausz T, Abir R, Margara R, Trew G, Lass A, Winston RML. Cryopreservation of human ovarian tissue using dimethylsulphoxide and propanediol-sucrose as cryoprotectants. Hum Reprod 1996;11:1268—1272.
19. Newton H, Aubard Y, Rutherford A, Sharma V, Gosden R. Low temperature storage and grafting of human ovarian tissue. Hum Reprod 1996;11:1487—1491.
20. Gosden R. Ovarian tissue banking. In: Porcu E, Flamigni C (eds) Human Oocytes: From Physiology to IVF. Bologna: Monduzzi Editore, 1998;265—269.
21. Friedler S, Giudice L, Lamb E. Cryopreservation of embryos and ova. Fertil Steril 1988;49: 743—764.
22. Baka SG, Toth TL, Veeck LL, Jones HW, Muasher SJ, Lanzendorf SE. Evaluation of the spindle apparatus of in-vitro matured human oocytes following cryopreservation. Hum Reprod 1995; 10:1816—1820.
23. Pickering S, Braude P, Johnson M. Cryoprotection of human oocyte: inappropriate exposure to DMSO reduces fertilization rates. Hum Reprod 1991;6:142—143.
24. Vincent C, Pruliere G, Pajot-Augy E, Campion E, Garnier V, Renard JP. Effects of cryoprotectants on actin filaments during cryopreservation of one-cell rabbit embryos. Cryobiology 1990;127:9—23.
25. Sathananthan AH, Trounson A, Freeman L, Brady T. The effects of cooling human oocytes. Hum Reprod 1988;8:968—977.
26. Van Der Elst J, Van Den Abbeel E, Nerinckx S, Van Steirteghem A. Parthenogenetic activation pattern and microtubular organization of the mouse oocyte after exposure to 1,2-propanediol. Cryobiology 1992;29:549—562.
27. Siebzehnruebl ER, Todorow S, Van Uem J, Koch R, Wildt L, Lang N. Cryopreservation of human and rabbit oocytes and one-cell embryos: a comparison of DMSO and propanediol. Hum Reprod 1989;4:312—317.
28. Trounson A. Freezing human eggs and embryos. Fertil Steril 1986;46:1—12.
29. Rall WF, Fahy GM. Ice free cryopreservation of mouse embryos at −196°C by vitrification. Nature 1985;313:573.
30. Hunter JE, Fuller B, Bernard A, Jackson A, Shaw RW. Vitrification of human oocytes following minimal exposure to cryoprotectants; initial studies on fertilization and embryonic development. Hum Reprod 1995;10:1184—1188.
31. Pickering S, Braude P, Johnson M, Cant A, Currie J. Transient cooling to room temperature can cause irreversible disruption of the meiotic spindle in the human oocyte. Fertil Steril 1990;54: 102.
32. Vincent C, Pickering SJ, Johnson MH, Quick SJ. Dimethylsulfoxide affects the organization of microfilaments in the mouse oocyte. Development 1990;26:227—235.
33. Hunter JE, Bernard A, Fuller B, Amso N, Shaw RW. Fertilization and development of the human oocyte following exposure to cryoprotectants, low temperatures and cryopreservation: a comparison of two techniques. Hum Reprod 1991;6:1460—1465.
34. Van Blerkom J, Davis P. Cytogenetic, cellular and developmental consequences of cryopreservation of immature and human oocytes. Microsc Res Tec 1994;27:165—193.

35. Younis AI, Toner M, Albertini DF, Biggers JD. Cryobiology of non-human primate oocytes. Hum Reprod 1996;11:156—165.
36. Al-Hasani S, Kirsch J, Diedrich K, Blanke S, Van Der Ven H, Krebs D. Successful embryo transfer of cryopreserved and in-vitro fertilized rabbit oocytes. Hum Reprod 1989;4:77—79.
37. Al-Hasani S, Diedrich K. Oocyte storage. In: Grudzinskas JG, Yovich JL (eds) Gametes — The Oocyte. Cambridge: Cambridge University Press, 1995.
38. Dumoulin JCM, Marij Bergers Janssen J, Pieters HEC, Enginsu ME, Geraedts JPM, Evers JLH. The protective effects of polymers in the cryopreservation of human and mouse zonae pellucidae and embryos. Fertil Steril 1994;62:793—798.
39. Gook D, Schiewe MC, Osborn S, Asch RH, Jansen RPS, Johnston WIH. Intracytoplasmic sperm injection and embryo development of human oocytes cryopreserved using 1,2-propanediol. Hum Reprod 1995;10:2637—2641.
40. Gook D, Osborn S, Johnston W. Partenogenetic activation of human oocytes following cryopreservation using 1,2-propanediol. Hum Reprod 1995;10:654—658.
41. Porcu E, Dal Prato L, Seracchioli R, Fabbri R, Longhi M, Flamigni C. Comparison between depot and standard release triptoreline in in vitro fertilization: pituitary sensitivity, luteal function, pregnancy outcome and perinatal results. Fertil Steril 1994;62:126—132.
42. Porcu E, Fabbri R, Petracchi S, Ciotti PM, Magrini O, Savelli L, Flamigni C. Microinjection of cryopreserved oocytes. In: Porcu E, Flamigni C (eds) Human oocytes: From Physiology to IVF. Bologna: Monduzzi, 1998,285—290.
43. Porcu E, Fabbri R, Seracchioli R, Ciotti PM, Magrini O, Savelli L, Ghi T, Flamigni C. Intracytoplasmic sperm injection of cryopreserved human oocytes. In: Gomel V, Leung PCK (eds) In Vitro Fertilization and Assisted Reproduction, Vancouver. Bologna: Monduzzi, 1997;1150—1157.
44. Porcu E, Fabbri R, Petracchi S, Ciotti PM, Seracchioli R, Savelli L, Marsella T, De Cesare R, Giunchi S, Flamigni C. Fertilization of cryopreserved human oocytes with ICSI. In: Ambrosini A, Melis GB, Dalla Pria S, Dessole S (eds) Infertility and Assisted Reproductive Technologies. Bologna: Monduzzi, 1997;173—177.
45. Porcu E, Fabbri R, Seracchioli R, Ciotti PM, Savelli L, Ghi T, Flamigni C. Birth and pregnancy after microinjection of human oocytes. Abstracts, 53rd annual Meeting of The American Society for Reproductive Medicine, Cincinnati, 1997:75.
46. Porcu E, Fabbri R, Seracchioli R, Ciotti PM, Petracchi S, Savelli L, Ghi T, Flamigni C. Birth of six healthy children after intracytoplasmic sperm-injection of cryopreserved human oocytes. Hum Reprod 1998;13:124.

# The cryopreservation of human ovarian tissue

Roger Gosden, Helen Newton and S. Samuel Kim
*Centre for Reproduction, Growth and Development, School of Medicine, University of Leeds, Leeds, UK*

**Abstract.** Ovarian tissue cryopreservation is being developed as a method for conserving the fertility of young women at risk of early ovarian failure. Experimental animal studies have demonstrated that, following freezing and thawing to liquid nitrogen temperatures and autografting, ovarian cortical slices restore ovulatory cycles and even fertility. Likewise, high rates of primordial follicle survival have been obtained using human tissue xenografted into immunodeficient animals. Progress towards the goal of growing follicles from frozen-thawed tissue to maturity for IVF is slower. Cryopreservation of immature oocytes appears to present fewer problems than at the metaphase II stage and, when grafting and culture methods become fully effective, ovarian tissue storage will be an attractive and routine option in reproductive medicine.

**Keywords:** cryopreservation, fertility, follicle, oocyte, ovary.

## History and Background

The first attempts to cryopreserve ovarian tissue were made in the 1950s in London. Ovarian tissue from rats and mice was frozen to $-79°C$ in glycerol-saline, thawed and grafted into oophorectomised host animals. Some follicular tissue survived and produced enough estrogen to cornify the vaginal epithelium, but fertility was not tested [1−4]. In a later series of experiments, inbred mice were restored to fertility which, although producing small litters, was proof of the principle of conserving female fertility [5]. These developments followed the breakthrough in sperm freezing in the late 1940s, but this potentially effective technology had been pioneered without any specific applications in mind.

Over the next 30 years there was little interest or further research, even though cryotechnology was progressing with other cell types as better cryoprotectants were developed and automated freezers were introduced. Application of these methods to mouse ovarian tissue was found to produce good results with restoration of fertility [6], and subsequently it was found that primordial follicles can be isolated for cryostorage and returned as grafts, which provide another strategy for conserving female fertility [7]. The success with immature follicles seemed to be at variance with results in secondary oocytes, although careful comparisons have never been made. Nevertheless, it is evident that human oocytes are particularly difficult to cryopreserve and, until more progress was reported recently [8] only five successful pregnancies from many attempts worldwide had been

---

*Address for correspondence:* Roger Gosden, Division of Obstetrics and Gynaecology, D floor, Clarendon Wing, Leeds General Infirmary, Leeds LS2 9NS, UK.

reported in the literature [9,10]. Greater success is now being achieved with oocyte freezing, but metaphase II is not always the most appropriate stage for storage. Therefore further efforts are being made to develop ovarian banking.

Whilst it was clear that the delicate ovaries of small laboratory animals can be stored, it was unclear whether the protocols would be effective with the bulkier and more fibrous organs in humans. With this in mind, experiments were conducted to test the feasibility of storing sheep ovaries, which are more comparable to humans in size, composition and follicle density. Ovaries were removed at laparotomy and autografted either immediately as fresh tissue slices onto the ovarian pedicle or after freezing and thawing 3 weeks later [11]. The animals were bled weekly and slaughtered 9 months later. All grafts, whether fresh or cryopreserved, were recovered and all except one still contained follicles and most follicles ranged up to the Graafian stage. Two animals out of six had become pregnant and delivered normal lambs, and sufficient follicles remained at autopsy to suggest that a second breeding cycle was a possibility in some animals. A lag of about 3 months occurred between grafting and the onset of cyclical activity. This was presumably the time required for primordial follicles to grow to the Graafian stage, since virtually all of the growing follicles are lost by ischemia during and after the grafting procedure, and only primordial follicles survive.

Subsequently, the cycles of animals bearing cryopreserved ovarian autografts have been investigated. The cycles were of normal length and endocrinologically similar to control animals except in respect of their elevated serum gonadotropin (especially FSH) and depressed $\alpha$ inhibin levels [12]. Serum estradiol and progesterone levels were normal. The animals had cycled for two breeding seasons after grafting only a small fraction of the original ovaries. There were endocrine indications of imminent graft failure but, were longer function required, the spare cortical strips in the freezer bank could probably have reinitiated cycles for some years to come. It is now important to test the fertility of grafted animals more rigorously.

These results provide the best evidence so far that autografting can restore function to frozen-thawed ovarian tissue. Other studies have demonstrated that primate tissue can be effectively cryopreserved. Ovarian tissue from marmoset monkeys, which has been frozen and grafted into immunodeficient mice, has shown that the total number of follicles were similar in fresh and frozen grafts, and also that estrogenic activity was restored in 16 days after transplantation of the frozen grafts [13]. What is more, thin biopsies of human ovarian cortex have been transplanted after freezing and thawing under the kidney capsules of SCID mice (see below).

## Applications

To understand the applications it is important to appreciate the relevant ovarian biology and toxicology.

The ovary is endowed with a nonrenewable store of $1-2$ million primordial follicles at birth which declines steadily with age. By the time of the first ovulation at puberty, the number has fallen to 250,000 and by age 35 to about 25,000 [15,16]. At the average age of the natural menopause, only 1,000 remain and these are evidently incapable of completing maturation and disappear within a few months or years. Once the store of follicles has disappeared, there is no further chance of conception (although egg donation remains a possibility). Additionally the quality of the eggs has also deteriorated by the fourth decade of life. The current tendency of American women to defer child-bearing is therefore on a collision course with the loss of functional ovarian reserve and desire of reproduction during aging. Perhaps some women anticipating to have a child after the optimal years of fertility will wish to store oocytes while they are still young. A more pressing reason is to conserve fertility in young women who are at risk of premature ovarian failure ($< 40$ years).

There are many causes of ovarian failure: genetic, infectious, autoimmune, or iatrogenic. Although the mean age of menopause has remained fairly stable, the numbers of young women and children who are being sterilized by high-dose chemotherapy and total body irradiation has been increasing. Because of long-term survival and cure with therapeutic advances, infertility is often a concern to these individuals [17].

The ovaries are susceptible to cytotoxic treatment, even though the majority of follicles are nongrowing primordial stages. Yet, animal studies demonstrate that these are paradoxically more sensitive to ionizing radiation and probably to alkylating agents than growing follicles [18]. Attempts have been made to protect the ovaries from radiation or chemotherapy induced damage using GnRH agonists to suppress gonadotropin levels, but the evidence for clinical benefit is inconclusive [19] and some experimental studies revealed no protective effect of hypogonadotrophism on radiation sensitivity [20]. Oophoropexy is only suitable in certain cases, and never for chemotherapy. Embryo cryopreservation, while a proven technique, has limited application because IVF requires a lengthy protocol and is unsuitable for preadolescent children. Oocyte cryopreservation is an attractive option, but it is not practical until further development of this technology. Ovarian tissue banking could therefore meet these needs. At present it is clinically unproven and there are concerns whether malignant cells might be stored in the tissue [21−23].

The risk of transferring the cancer cells back to the patient depends on the disease type and stage, and some cancers appear unsuitable for tissue transplatation. High-dose chemotherapy is now being used for an increasing number of nonmalignant conditions, such as autoimmune diseases and thalassemias, for which tissue storage is also potentially attractive.

Additionally, fertility conservation will be desirable for the women whose family history anticipates early ovarian failure.

## Technology

Cryopreservation of ovarian tissue is deceptively simple and effective but a better understanding of the physiology and biophysics will no doubt improve the results. In principle, three strategies are available. First, storage of the whole organ followed by autografting with vascular reanastomosis is the ultimate technique since this holds the promise of restoring normal ovarian function. So far, no adult organ of any kind has been successfully restored to function after freeze-storage, although the ovary is probably a better candidate than other organs.

Second, storage of isolated follicles is also possible, and has been effectively carried out in mice [7]. Primordial follicles can be isolated from human ovaries using a two-step enzymatic-dissection procedure [24]. Successful freeze storage is possible but the follicles are very delicate and the prospects of long-term culture are poor at present. Also it is less practical grafting them back as isolated follicles than leaving them in situ.

However, the most promising method at present is to collect thin slices of cortical tissue using a customized biopsy instrument. Since only the primordial follicles are required and they are superficial, a slice < 1 mm thick is adequate. A thin slice is more suitable for rapid equilibration of cryoprotectants, and NMR spectroscopy has been used to investigate the rate of penetration of the familiar ones [25]. After 30 min in a rotating bottle at 4°C, the tissue is 80% equilibrated and ready for freezing. The freezing protocols for ovarian tissue have not yet been optimized but a slow cooling — rapid thawing method has been found effective (Table 1).

## Cryoprotectant

The efficiency of several cryoprotectants has been compared by freeze-thawing and xenografting human ovarian tissue into immunodeficient mice [14]. The results indicated that dimethylsulphoxide, ethylene glycol and 1,2 propanediol were much more effective than glycerol. Glycerol, although relatively less toxic, was poor, probably because it penetrated slowly and caused osmotic stress. The study was carried out quantitatively so that the percentage of follicles surviving 3 weeks after grafting could be assessed in histological sections. By this time, necrotic tissue had cleared and follicles remaining were long-term survivors. With the best cryoprotectants 70—80% or more of the estimated original popula-

*Table 1.* The freeze-thawing protocol for human ovarian tissue

Cool samples from room temperature to − 9°C at 2°C/min
Seed manually
Cool samples to − 40°C at 0.3°C/min
Cool to − 140°C at the faster rate of 10°C/min
Plung into liquid nitrogen to store
Thaw rapidly by agitating vials in a water bath at 20°C

tion of follicles survived. These results bode well for ovarian storage and have practical implications. The methods should minimise long-term exposure to the cryoprotectant since it is at high concentration and potentially toxic. After thawing rapidly, the tissue is washed through several steps in fresh saline solution. Whether it is beneficial to cryopreservation to add protein or sucrose, as in single cell freezing, has not been established, although it is a sensible precaution until more information is available.

## The future

Ovarian tissue has been stored already at a number of centers in several countries, even though it is not yet clinically proven. The procedures for collection and storage of the tissue are straightforward and the experimental evidence is encouraging. A careful trial to evaluate the method is warranted before it is launched as a clinical service and casual use of the technique should be discouraged until further progress has been made. There are important questions about safety, efficacy and optimization to be settled, not to speak of the importance of careful registration of details and a mechanism to keep in touch with patients for what may turn out to be a lengthy period of storage.

At present, there are uncertainties about the optimum use of the tissue when it is required. Simple autografts, like those carried out in sheep, seem most promising, but the length of function will depend on the numbers of follicles present. Where few follicles remain and early graft exhaustion is expected, it may be better to use a heterotopic site and recover oocytes for an IVF procedure. In the long term, however, it is hoped that oocytes can be matured in vitro from frozen-thawed tissue. The potential success of in vitro follicle growth has been demonstrated with primordial follicles from the ovaries of infant mice [26].

The challenge of growing human follicles should not be underestimated, because the length of the growing phase may extend to 6 months, and it may be impractical to grow a human follicle to full size. Nevertheless, innovation will no doubt overcome or bypass the problems in due course. For the present the fact that there is more than one option for using frozen-thawed tissue gives confidence in this new technology.

## Acknowledgements

We thank the Leukaemia Research Fund and Well-Being (Royal College of Obstetricians and Gynaecologists) for grants supporting our research.

## References

1. Parkes AS, Smith AU. Regeneration of rat ovarian tissue grafted after exposure to low temperatures. Proc Roy Soc 1953;140:455—467.
2. Deanesly R. Immature rat ovaries grafted after freezing and thawing. J Endocrinol 1954;

11:197—200.

3. Parkes AS. Grafting of mouse ovarian tissue after freezing and thawing. J Endocrinol 1956; 14:30—31.

4. Parkes AS. Viability of ovarian tissue after freezing. Proc Roy Soc 1957;147:520—528.

5. Parrot DMV. The fertility of mice with orthotopic grafts derived from frozen tissue. J Reprod Fertil 1996;1:230—241.

6. Harp R, Leibach J, Black J, Keldahl C, Karow A. Cryopreservation of murine ovarian tissue. Cryobiology 1994;31:336—343.

7. Carroll J, Gosden RG. Transplantation of frozen-thawed mouse primordial follicles. Hum Reprod 1993;8:1163—1167.

8. Porcu E, Fabbri R, Seracchioli R, Ciotti PM, Magrini O, Flamigni C. Birth of a healthy female after intracytoplasmic sperm injection of cryopreserved human oocytes. Fertil Steril 1997;68: 724—726.

9. Chen C. Pregnancy after human oocyte cryopreservation. Lancet 1986;i;884—886.

10. Van Uem JFHM, Siebzehnrubl ER, Schuh B, Koch R, Trotnow S, Lang N. Birth after cryopreservation of unfertilised oocytes. Lancet 1987;ii;752—753.

11. Gosden RG, Baird DT, Wade JC, Webb R. Restoration of fertility to oophorectomised sheep by ovarian autografts stored at −196°C. Hum Reprod 1994;9:597—603.

12. Baird DT, Webb R, Campbell B, Harkness L, Gosden RG. Autotransplantation of frozen ovarian strips in sheep results in normal oestrus cycles for at least 22 months. Hum Reprod 1996; 11(Abstract book 1):58.

13. Candy CJ, Wood MT, Whittingham DG. Follicular development in cryopreserved marmoset ovarian tissue after transplantation. Hum Reprod 1995;10:2334—2338.

14. Newton H, Aubard Y, Rutherford A, Sharma V, Gosden RG. Low temperature storage and grafting of human ovarian tissue. Hum Reprod 1996;11:1487—1491.

15. Block E. Quantitative morphological investigation of the follicular system in women. Acta Anat 1952;14:108—123.

16. Faddy MJ, Gosden RG, Gougeon A, Richardson SJ, Nelson JF. Accelerated disappearance of ovarian follicles in midlife-implication for forecasting menopause. Hum Reprod 1992;7: 1342—1346.

17. Nicholson HS, Byrne J. Fertility and pregnancy treated for cancer during childhood or adolescence. Cancer supplement 1993;71(10):3392—3399.

18. Baker TG. Radiosensitivity of mammalian oocytes with particular reference to the human female. Am J Obstet Gynecol 1971;110:746—761.

19. Blumenfeld Z, Avivi I, Linn S et al. Prevention of irreversible chemotherapy induced ovarian damage in young women with lymphoma by gonadotrophin releasing hormone agonist in parallel to chemotherapy. Hum Reprod 1996;11:1620—1626.

20. Gosden RG, Wade JC, Fraser HM et al. Impact of congenital or experimental hypogonadotrophism on the radiation sensitivity of the mouse ovary. Hum Reprod 1997;12:2483—2488.

21. Shaw JM, Bowles J, Koopman P, Wood EC, Trounson AO. Fresh and cryopreserved ovarian tissue samples from donors with lymphoma transmit the cancer to graft recipients. Hum Reprod 1996;11:1668—1673.

22. Shaw J, Trounson A. Oncological implications in the replacement of ovarian tissue. Hum Reprod 1997;12:403—405.

23. Gosden RG, Rutherford AJ, Norfolk DR. Transmission of malignant cells in ovarian grafts. Hum Reprod 1997;12:403.

24. Oktay K, Nugent D, Newton H, Salha O, Chatterjee P, Gosden RG. Isolation and characterization of primordial follicles. Fertil Steril 1997;67:481—486.

25. Newton H, Fisher J, Arnold JR, Faddy M, Gosden RG. Permeation of human ovarian tissue with cryoprotective agents in preparation for cryopreservation. Hum Reprod 1998;13:376—380.

26. Eppig JJ, O'Brien MJ. Development in mouse oocyte from primordial follicles. Biol Reprod 1996;8:1163—1167.

Fertility and Reproductive Medicine.
R.D. Kempers, J. Cohen, A.F. Haney and J.B. Younger, editors.

621

# Cryopreservation of testicular tissue: a highly effective method to provide sperm for successful TESE/ICSI procedures

W. Schulze[1], H. Hohenberg[2] and U.A. Knuth[3]

[1]Department of Andrology, University of Hamburg (UKE), Hamburg; [2]Heinrich-Pette-Institut, University of Hamburg, Hamburg; [3]Gemeinschaftspraxis BKS, Hamburg, Germany

**Abstract.** *Background.* This article presents an optimal treatment procedure to extract spermatozoa from cryopreserved testicular biopsies, "cryo-TESE", from infertile men.

*Methods.* A total of 770 men underwent unilateral or bilateral testicular biopsies according to the cryo-TESE concept. This concept involves the subdivision of a testicular biopsy into at least four fragments. Of these, one fragment is used for a histological examination. Two fragments are exponentially frozen using HEPES-buffered human serum albumin with glycerol as cryoprotectant. A fourth fragment is immediately subjected to a sperm extraction attempt by enzymatic digestion to assess the likelihood of the presence of spermatozoa in the cryopreserved samples.

*Results.* Spermatozoa could be isolated from the testicular tissue of 629 men (81.7%) in total. In azoospermic patients with normal FSH concentrations ($< 8$ IU/l) 94.9% (187 of 197 patients) had a positive TESE result. But even when the FSH concentrations were elevated there was a 65.1% chance to isolate sperms. In only 13 (0.9%) of all biopsy samples (n = 1,426) was complete maturation arrest at the stage of the "round" spermatids recorded. In seven biopsies (from four patients) histological analysis revealed the presence of a carcinoma in situ. The yield of viable spermatozoa from cryopreserved samples did not differ from that using fresh material. The fertilization and pregnancy rates are similar to those obtained by microinjection (ICSI) of ejaculated spermatozoa.

*Conclusions.* The cryo-TESE concept combines the diagnostic evaluation of male infertility with the option of repeated TESE/ICSI attempts. It allows a comprehensive andrological investigation previous to an IVF procedure and improves the chance for a successful sterility treatment of the couple.

**Keywords:** andrology, assisted reproduction, male infertility, testis.

It has been demonstrated that sperm extracted from testicular tissue taken by biopsies (TESE) can be used for intracytoplasmic sperm injection (ICSI) to induce a pregnancy [1]. For the first time this procedure offers an effective treatment, even for those couples in whom the male suffers from azoospermia due to a defect of the spermatogenetic tissue. Past experience has shown that even in testes of apparently azoospermic men there are areas with sufficient spermatogenetic activity to form the basis for our recently developed "cryo-TESE concept". This concept combines the removal of testicular tissue via biopsies for the diagnostic evaluation of the infertility with the possibility of a TESE/ICSI option [2—4]. It involves the subdivision of a biopsy sample into at least four portions

---

*Address for correspondence:* Prof Dr W. Schulze, Department of Andrology, University of Hamburg (UKE), Martinistr. 52, 20246 Hamburg, Germany.

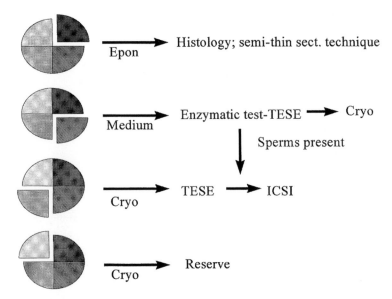

Epon → Histology; semi-thin sect. technique

Medium → Enzymatic test-TESE → Cryo

Sperms present

Cryo → TESE → ICSI

Cryo → Reserve

*Fig. 1.* The cryo-TESE/ICSI concept. The testicular biopsy is divided into four portions. One part is analysed histologically using the semi-thin sectioning technique. A second part is transferred to IVF medium containing collagenase (type Ia) and subjected to a preliminary enzymatic sperm extraction (test-TESE). The remaining portions are cryopreserved. When the preliminary diagnosis indicates the presence of sperm, then the definitive TESE/ICSI treatment can be carried out at a later time-point using the cryopreserved fragments.

(Fig. 1). One portion, in which fragments of three testicular lobules are included, is subjected to a histological examination by means of the semi-thin sectioning technique. A second portion, which spatially overlaps the first, is immediately used for a mild enzymatic sperm extraction procedure (test-TESE) using collagenase type Ia. The remaining two biopsy portions are cryopreserved. This tissue can be used even many months later for the definitive TESE/ICSI treatment, when sperm were detected by the test-TESE or during histological examination. Testicular samples taken for the diagnostic procedure (histology, test-TESE) and storage overlap and cover several layers of tissue, "sandwich pattern". This guarantees a high predictive value as to the suitability of the cryopreserved portions for TESE [3,5] (Fig. 2).

The protocols for freezing/thawing and subsequent preparation of the testicular

*Table 1.* Freezing of human testicular biopsies.

SpermFreeze (MediCult, Denmark) as ready-to-use medium: Earle's balanced salt solution + 15% glycerol as cryoprotectant, HEPES-buffered (18 mM)

Submerge biopsies into 0.5 ml SpermFreeze within Nunc Vials, equilibrate for a maximum of 15 min

In Nicoolbag 10 System (Air Liquide, Germany): cool to $-60°$ C within 5 min

Start exponential cooling to $-120°$ C over 55 min

Submerge samples into liquid nitrogen until use

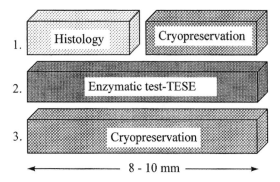

*Fig. 2.* The "sandwich pattern" for portioning a testicular biopsy. Following an incision in the tunica albuginea, testicular tissue is extruded and cut into three layers. The upper layer is divided into two portions. One portion is analysed histologically, the adjacent piece of tissue is cryopreserved. The test-TESE is performed on the central layer of the biopsy. The lower layer is cryopreserved in toto. Because of the overlapping manner in which the biopsy is apportioned, the diagnostic steps (histology, test-TESE) acquire a high predictive value as to the suitability of the cryopreserved portions for TESE.

tissue are listed in Tables 1 and 2.

The application of cryoprotectant can lead — presumably as a consequence of local hyperosmolarity — to a shrinkage of cell nuclei and cytoplasm in some immature germ cells. Primary spermatocytes are the most likely cells to be affected. Spermatids, on the other hand, hardly ever exhibit such changes. Occasionally the acrosome appears swollen, although both the acrosome membrane and the outer cell membrane remain intact (Fig. 3). These changes show that the cryoprotectant itself causes impairment of cell function, although it prevents even greater damage from the freezing process. The best preservation of germ cell structures is observed when testicular tissue is incubated in the cryoprotectant for 3 to 15 min. During this short time period no equilibrium is reached and a gradient of cryoprotectant with lower concentrations towards the center of the tissue sample is formed. Accordingly cells at the outside shrink to a higher

*Table 2.* Enzymatic sperm extraction from frozen testicular tissue.

1. Thaw sample in $37°C$ water bath for approximately 3 min
2. Transfer to 1 ml culture medium (MediCult) and dissect gently
3. Incubate sample for 30 min ($37°C$; 5% $CO_2$)
4. Add collagenase (Sigma type Ia) at a final concentration of 400 U/ml
5. Incubate for 30 min, dissect further without squeezing the tubules
6. Incubate for another 60 min with collagenase (total incubation time can be modified according to the previous finding in the test-TESE, in severe cases overnight)
7. Squeeze remaining tubules, remove debris mechanically
8. Suspend the sediment, transfer to test tube and centrifuge ($500-800$ g, 10 min)
9. Remove collagenase supernatant, resuspend pellet in small volume of culture medium
10. Transfer suspension into medium droplets under oil and incubate for at least 30 min
11. Collect sperm from the edges of the droplets and transfer into PVP
12. Perform ICSI as usual

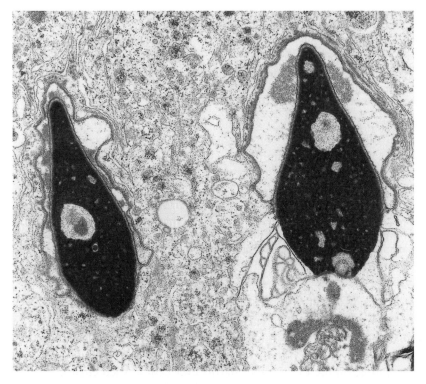

*Fig. 3.* Electron micrograph showing mature spermatids in the seminiferous epithelium following the freezing/thawing procedure. Occasionally a swelling of the acrosome can be noticed. However, all cytomembranes remain intact. Magnification × 17,000.

degree than in the middle of the sample. Upon freezing this protects peripheral tissue from cell damage, since the outer layers are dehydrated and vitrify without formation of ice crystals. Consequently, no heat is generated. Towards the centre cells are less protected by the cryoprotectant, but this is compensated for by two mechanisms: less osmotic damage by the lower concentrations of cryoprotectant and an almost optimal cooling rate. The adaption of the cooling rate is caused by the poor heat conductivity of the amorphously solidified outer tissue layer, which slows the cooling process towards the centre of the biopsy sample. Thus the cells of the whole tissue sample are frozen in an ideal way.

Upon thawing the sample, no heat of recrystalisation is set free in the outer regions of the biopsy (because little water is present). Therefore, only little heat is transferred to the inner part of the sample, and the cells there, which are probably less cryoprotected, can thaw without formation of larger ice crystals.

Until December 1997 complete data sets were available from 770 patients who underwent testicular biopsies according to the cryo-TESE concept. This group comprised men in whom previous semen analyses had shown azoospermia or such low numbers of viable sperm, that there was a high risk of a futile ICSI treatment if relying on ejaculated sperm only. The indications for the application of the cyo-TESE concept are listed in Table 3.

The postsurgical testicular sperm extraction (test-TESE) was successful in 629 (81.7%) cases in total. In the remaining 141 (18.3%) cases neither the histological evaluation nor the analysis of the test material revealed the presence of sperm.

Merely 0.9% (n = 13) of all biopsy samples (n = 1,426) showed a spermatogenetic arrest at the early ("round") spermatid stage (step 1–3 according to Holstein and Roosen-Runge [6]). These data clearly indicate that a complete maturation arrest at the stage of the "round" spermatids is a rare phenomenon.

A total of 538 patients suffered from complete azoospermia. A positive TESE result was obtained in 409 (76.0%) cases. If the analysis is limited to azoospermic men with FSH serum concentrations below 8 IU/l, which represent the majority of obstructive azoospermia, 187 of 197 patients (94.9%) had a positive TESE result. However, even when the FSH concentrations were elevated (> 8 IU/l) in azoospermia (341 patients), there was still a 65.1% chance of isolating sperm from the test material. A subgroup of these hypergonadotropic men with azoospermia had a history of testicular cancer and other malignant tumours with subsequent irradiation and/or chemotherapy. Surprisingly, in 67.9% of these patients spermatogenetic activity sufficient for a TESE/ICSI treatment could still be noticed in at least one of the testes.

During the evaluation of the histological analyses and TESE it became evident that the predictive value of the histological examination in regard to the TESE outcome is highly dependent on the pattern and extent of the pathological features in the testis tissue. It decreases significantly with increased incidence of pathological features. These observations were corroborated in 552 biopsies. Although no mature spermatids were detectable in the histological examination, enough sperm suitable for ICSI could be extracted in 37.9% of the cases (209 biopsies). Nevertheless, the importance of a careful histological analysis is overwhelmingly supported by the fact that in seven of the biopsies an early stage, treatable testicular tumour (carcinoma in situ; CIS) could be diagnosed.

The experience to date has shown that microinjection of frozen/thawed testicular sperm yields very similar fertilization and pregnancy rates to those obtained with spermatozoa from the ejaculate. The actual results (state: December 1997) of our group (Fischer, Naether, Baukloh, Schulze, Hamburg, Germany) are pre-

*Table 3.* Indications for testicular biopsy with cryo-TESE option.

During surgery for posttesticular obstruction
Inoperable posttesticular obstruction
Bilateral aplasia of the vasa deferentia
Idiopathic normogonadotropic azoospermia
Hypergonadotropic azoospermia
Anejaculation (resistant to treatment)
Cryptozoospermia
Necrozoospermia

626

*Table 4.* Overview over cryo-TESE/ICSI treatments between 1995 and 1997.

| | | |
|---|---|---|
| Patients treated | 246 | |
| No. of oocyte retrievals | 406 | 1.65 per patient |
| Embryo transfers | 367 | 90.4% of cycles |
| Pregnancies | 75 | 18.5% per puncture |
| | | 20.4% per transfer |
| | | 30.5% per patient |
| Abortions | 9 | 12% per pregnancy |
| Intact pregnancies | 37 | 24.5% of patients |
| Deliveries: | | |
|    Singletons | 26 | |
|    Twins | 7 | |
|    Triplets | 1 | |

sented in Table 4.

In conclusion, the cryo-TESE/ICSI concept offers optimal conditions for a successful clinical treatment of severe male fertility disturbances. Based upon an extensive andrological diagnostic approach in the initial stage (histology; test-TESE) it is possible to reasonably predict the chance of a successful TESE/ICSI treatment and minimize the risk of costly and futile preparations of the female partner for an IVF procedure. Moreover, if the preliminary diagnosis indicates the presence of sperm, the cryopreserved samples can be used for repeated TESE/ICSI cycles without the need for further surgery of the male. Also in terms of preventive medicine, e.g., potential CIS, the concept described here is superior to other methods which are directed solely towards retrieval of sperm.

## References

1. Devroey P, Liu J, Nagy Z, Tournaye H, Silber SJ, Van Steirteghem AC. Normal fertilization of human oocytes after testicular sperm extraction and intracytoplasmic sperm injection. Fertil Steril 1994;62:639—641.
2. Fischer R, Baukloh V, Naether OGJ, Schulze W, Salzbrunn A, Benson DM. Pregnancy after intracytoplasmic sperm injection of spermatozoa extracted from frozen-thawed testicular biopsy. Hum Reprod 1996;11:2197—2199.
3. Jezek D, Knuth UA, Schulze W. Successful testicular sperm extraction (TESE) in spite of high serum follicle stimulating hormone and azoospermia: correlation between testicular morphology, TESE results, semen analysis and serum hormone values in 103 infertile men. Hum Reprod 1998;13:1230—1234.
4. Salzbrunn A, Benson DM, Holstein AF, Schulze W. A new concept for the extraction of testicular spermatozoa as a tool for assisted fertilization (ICSI). Hum Reprod 1996;11:752—755.
5. Schulze W, Knuth UA, Jezek D, Benson DM, Fischer R, Naether OGJ, Baukloh V, Ivell R. Intratesticular sperm extraction. Basis for a successful treatment of infertility in men with ejaculatory azoospermia. In: Ivell R, Holstein AF (eds) The Fate of The Male Germ Cell. New York: Plenum Press, 1997;81—88.
6. Holstein AF, Roosen-Runge EC. Atlas of Human Spermatogenesis. Berlin: Grosse Verlag, 1981.

# Oocyte and embryo micromanipulation

# In vitro maturation (IVM) of human preovulatory oocytes reconstructed by germinal vesicle (GV) transfer

John Zhang[1], Chia-Woei Wang[1], Lewis Krey[1], Hui Liu[1], Li Meng[2], Anna Blaszczyk[1], Alexis Adler[1] and Jamie Grifo[1]

[1]*New York University Medical Center — Program for In Vitro Fertilization, New York, New York; and* [2]*Oregon Regional Primate Research Center, Beaverton, Oregon, USA*

**Abstract.** A micromanipulation-electrofusion procedure is described to transfer germinal vesicles (GVs) between immature human oocytes. This procedure consists of the removal of a GV-containing karyoplast and its subzonal insertion and subsequent electrofusion into an enucleated host oocyte at the same developmental stage. The reconstructed GV oocyte is then subjected to in vitro maturation. Initially, GV removal and transfer was performed on the same oocyte; these "self-reconstructed" oocytes were then cultured in vitro for up to 50 h and examined periodically for maturation as judged by the extrusion of the first polar body. In a second study GVs from "old" oocytes (patient age > 38 years) were successfully transferred into enucleated immature "young" oocytes (patient age < 31 years) and similarly matured and examined.

"Reconstructed" oocytes matured to meiosis stage II and displayed a normal second meiotic metaphase complement. In view of these findings, GV transfer may have several important applications. It may be a potentially attractive alternative to whole oocyte donation. It may also be a valuable research tool to generate the cell models needed to characterize the cytoplasmic-nuclear interplay regulating cell cycle, maturation and fertilization in the human oocyte.

**Keywords:** aneuploidy, electrofusion, germinal vesicle transfer, immature oocytes, karyoplast, micromanipulation.

## Introduction

In vitro fertilization clinics throughout the USA have reported that the clinical pregnancy and embryo implantation rates drop precipitously when the age of the female partner is greater than 40 years [1]. These declines in clinical pregnancy and implantation rates are associated with an increase in the incidence of chromosomal aneuploidies in the oocytes and embryos of older women [2–7]. These anomalies in chromosome segregation arise during a dysfunctional first or second meiotic division [8].

In the oocytes of laboratory animals and humans, interactions between the nuclear genome and numerous factors in the cytoplasm influence meiosis — the reduction in chromosome number from 4n (germinal vesicle or GV stage) to 2n (metaphase II stage) to n (fertilization stage) that is necessary if fertilization is

*Address for correspondence:* John Zhang MD, PhD, NYU Medical Center, Program for In Vitro Fertilization, 660 First Avenue, Fifth Floor, New York, NY 10016, USA. Tel.: +1-212-2638990. Fax: +1-212-2638827.

630

to proceed normally [9—15]. These cytoplasmic factors initiate and organize the construction of meiotic spindles from microtubules during LH- or hCG-stimulated final maturation and following sperm penetration [13—15]. Moreover, structurally abnormal spindles identified by tubulin immunocytochemical staining are thought to result in aneuploidy [15,16].

Presently, we do not understand the nuclear-cytoplasmic interactions necessary for normal meiosis in oocytes because we cannot assess the relative contribution(s) of each compartment. In this report, we describe a cell model to study nuclear-cytoplasmic interrelationships and meiosis in human oocytes. In this model germinal vesicles (GVs) are transferred by a micromanipulation-electrofusion procedure to transfer GV between immature oocytes retrieved from patients of different ages. Such "reconstructed" oocytes mature in vitro through the first stage of meiosis.

**Materials and Methods**

*Source of oocytes*

GV stage oocytes were obtained from patients (25—42 years old) who were undergoing ICSI following controlled ovarian stimulation. These oocytes were considered to be unsuitable for fertilization and were, therefore, routinely discarded for use in research upon patient consent (NYUMC-IBRA Protocol H 6902). Oocytes were divided into two groups according to patient age: oocytes from "young" patients (< 31 years old); and oocytes from "old" patients (> 38 years old). Oocyte manipulation, GV transfer, and in vitro maturation were usually initiated within 6 h after transvaginal oocyte retrieval.

*Germinal vesicle removal and transfer*

Initially, the oocytes were stripped of cumulus cells by repeated pipetting in HTF medium (Irvine Scientific, Santa Ana, California) containing 80 IU/ml hyaluronidase (Sigma Chemical, St. Louis, Missouri). Immature oocytes (GV stage) were collected in HTF supplemented with 10% fetal bovine (v/v, HyClone, Road Logan, Utah).

GV removal was modified from that previously described by Meng and coworkers [17]. The oocytes were preincubated in HTF containing 7.5 µg/ml cytochalasin B (Sigma Chemical, St. Louis, Missouri) for approximately 1 h. A slit made in the zona pellucida with a sharp needle as developed by Tsunoda et al. [18] and the GV was removed directly with a small amount of local cytoplasm (karyoplast) with an enucleation pipette (ID: approximately 20 µm) inserted through a slit. We have found that this procedure is more efficient than increasing the pressure inside the holding pipette to expel the GV-karyoplast through the slit.

The GV-karyoplast was then inserted subzonally into an enucleated oocyte which was then washed in HTF medium. Membrane fusion between oocyte and karyoplast was achieved by electrofusion in a microfusion chamber (BTX, San Diego, California) containing a solution of 0.3 M mannitol, 0.01 mM magnesium sulfate, 0.1 M calcium chloride and 0.05 mg/ml bovine serum albumin — Fraction V (BSA, Sigma Chemical, St. Louis, Missouri). The oocyte was aligned by an alternating current pulse (8 V; 6 s); fusion was accomplished by a direct current pulse (1.36 kV/cm; 30—40 µs) using an ElectroCell Fusion instrument (BTX 2001, BTX, San Diego, California). Routinely, oocytes and karyoplasts was fused within 15 min after which time the "reconstructed" oocytes were cultured in vitro.

*In vitro maturation*

Granulosa cells routinely discarded during oocyte donation retrievals were harvested upon consent and dispersed by repeated pipetting in HTF medium containing 0.3% trypsin (w/v, Sigma Chemical, St. Louis, Missouri) and 10% fetal calf serum (v/v, HyClone, Road Logan, Utah). After washing twice in HTF, the cells were plated at a concentration of $0.5 \times 10^6$ cells/ml Medium 199 (Sigma Chemical, St. Louis, Missouri) in a central well dish.

Oocytes were cocultured with the granulosa cells (36—50 h; 37°C in 5% $CO_2$) in medium supplemented with 10% fetal bovine serum, 0.075 IU/ml FSH (Metrodin, Serono, Oakville, Ontario), 35 ng/ml insulin (Sigma Chemical, St. Louis, Missouri), and 20% pooled human follicular fluid (v/v) obtained from oocyte donation cycles with consent. Oocytes were examined microscopically for maturation at 24, 36, 42 and 50 h. Oocytes were considered to be mature when the first polar body was observed (MII stage).

*Analysis of chromosome number in MII oocytes*

Some in vitro maturated, "reconstructed" oocytes were analyzed to assess chromosome number. The oocytes were incubated in a hypotonic solution of 0.8% sodium citrate (w/v) solution supplemented with 0.3 mg/ml BSA (Sigma Chemical, St. Louis, Missouri) for 10 min and fixed sequentially in methanol: acetic acid: water (5:1:4) and methanol: acetic acid (3:1) for 5 min each [19]. Following gradual air-drying, the fixed chromosomes were stained with Giemsa and their distribution in the metaphase spread was analyzed using a Cytovision 2.21 Imaging System (Applied Imaging).

*Experiment design*

Initially oocyte "self-reconstruction" was performed by GV removal and transfer itself compromised oocyte maturation. Additional oocytes were manipulated without microsurgery and were matured in vitro to serve as controls.

In a second study, the GV was removed from oocytes of older patients (> 38 years) and transferred into enucleated oocytes of young patients (< 31 years). Following electrofusion, these "reconstructed" oocytes were cultured in vitro and nuclear maturation was monitored. Additional "old" oocytes (group II) were not manipulated but matured in vitro to serve as controls.

**Results**

*Experiment 1*

A total of 32 immature oocytes were manipulated. A GV-karyoplast was successfully removed without lysis in 21 oocytes and transferred subzonally in 16. Karyoplast fusion was accomplished in 14 oocytes. Following coculture, nine "self-reconstructed" oocytes extruded the first polar body within 50 h. Similar results were noted for the manipulated-only control oocytes: eight of 14 reached metaphase.

*Experiment 2*

GV removal was accomplished in 28 of 47 ooplasm hosts and 33 of 60 GV donor oocytes. Intact GV-karyoplasts were successfully inserted subzonally in 19 of 28 host oocytes and 12 fused to form a "reconstructed " oocyte. Seven of these "reconstructed" oocytes extruded a polar body. By comparison, nine of the 13 control group oocytes similarly matured. We were able to analyse the karyotype of five "reconstructed" MII oocytes; four displayed a normal second meiotic chromosome complement. We also analyzed the karyotype of seven control oocytes from the older patients; only two had a normal second meiotic complement, the remainder displaying various abnormalities in the metaphase plate, including no segregation with predivision and hyperploidy with monodyads or dyads [4].

**Discussion**

In this study we demonstrate that germinal vesicles can be transferred between preovulatory human oocytes in the same developmental stage using micromanipulation and electrofusion techniques. Furthermore, these "reconstructed" oocytes mature in vitro to experience a morphologically normal first meiotic division to the second stage. These observations support our view that such "reconstructed" oocytes may be an appropriate cell model to investigate the relative contributions of cytoplasmic and nuclear factors for meiosis.

These cell models may also identify what intracellular factors and/or mechanisms underlie the increase in aneuploidy reported in older women's oocytes. Tarin [13] has suggested that in oocytes from older women, compromised mitochondrial function and a resultant increase in oxidative stress results in an incompetent regulation of meiosis. Battaglia and co-workers [15] and Plachot and Crozet [16] have noted meiotic spindle abnormalities in aged oocytes. Such observations suggest that aneuploidy frequency might decrease when the nuclei of oocytes of older women are transferred at the germinal vesicle stage to enucleated oocytes of young women. Significantly, we did note a normal second meiotic chromosome complement in 80% of such "reconstructed" oocytes. However, our data is still limited and current studies are directed to increase our numbers of observations. In addition, we plan to analyze the structure of the meiotic spindle in reconstructed oocytes using immunocytochemical probes for tubulin.

In this report each step in GV transfer was accomplished at a success rate of 40–60%. We have improved these rates to > 80% in the past 6 months. Clearly there is a "learning curve" for this micromanipulation technique as there was for others such as intracytoplasmic sperm injection [20].

Electrofusion is still a relatively new procedure in human reproduction and different pretreatments and electrical parameters may result in higher rates of fusion with fewer potential side effects. In vitro maturation of human oocytes is currently under study in many research and clinical laboratories [21].

Clearly, the maturation rate of "reconstructed" oocytes will only increase when the optimal conditions have been identified to mature the human oocyte in vitro. In this regard, it is important to note that, in both our studies, the maturation rates of reconstructed GV oocytes were similar to those of control oocytes that were simply handled. These observations suggest that the experimental source of oocytes may actually determine the maturation rate for any experimental group. As a result, one may conclude that, following GV transfer, virtually 100% of the "reconstructed" oocytes retain the ability to undergo meiosis at least to the metaphase II stage.

Although devised for research, GV transfer also offers the potential for a unique form of oocyte donation, the donation of ooplasm only. Oocyte donation has been widely used to treat female infertility, but as currently practiced, it has the drawback that the oocyte recipient is the biologic, but not the genetic, mother of her child. She could be both, however, if a GV from her oocyte normally and reliably matures in vitro within an enucleated oocyte from a young donor. Recently, cryopreservation banking of ovarian tissue has been performed as a future treatment option for patients about to undergo chemotherapy or irradiation [22]. Considering that primordial follicles are in the GV stage, they can be used for transfer as has been successfully done in mice [23]. Clearly, such an approach would bypass the long period required to grow primordial follicles to the antral stage. However, before GV transfer can even be considered for donation purposes additional research must be conducted in three areas. First, we must establish that "reconstructed" oocytes mature normally through both stages of meiosis. Assessments of meiotic spindle morphology and chromosomal anomalies must be performed after the first and second meiotic division. Secondly, we must optimize in vitro maturation of human oocytes; currently the pregnancy rates with in vitro matured eggs is significantly lower than that of conventional IVF with controlled ovarian stimulation [21,25]. Thirdly, we need to obtain information about the interplay of cytoplasmic and nuclear factors that

634

determine cell cycle regulation, maturation and fertilization of the human oocyte. The "reconstructed" cell models that can be generated by GV transfer will be valuable in our attempts to obtain this information.

## References

1. Society for Assisted Reproductive Technology, American Society for Reproductive Medicine, American Society for Reproductive Medicine. Assisted reproductive technology in the United States and Canada: 1992 results generated from the American Society for Reproductive Medicine/Society for Assisted Reproductive Technology registry. Fertil Steril 1995;64:13–21.
2. Hook E. Rates of chromosomal abnormalities at different maternal ages. Obstet Gynecol 1981;58:282–285.
3. Hollander D, Breen JL. Pregnancy in the older gravida: how old is old? Obstet Gynecol Surv 1991;45:106–112.
4. Angell RR, Xian J, Keith J, Ledger W, Baird DT. First meiotic division abnormalities in human oocytes:mechanism of trisomy formation. Cytogenet Cell Genet 1994;65:194–202.
5. Munne S, Alikani M, Tomkin G, Grifo J, Cohen J. Embryo morphology, developmental rates and maternal age are correlated with chromosome abnormalities. Fertil Steril 1995;64: 382–391.
6. Benadiva CA, Kligman I, Munne S. Aneuploidy 16 in human embryos increases significantly with maternal age. Fertil Steril 1996;66:248–255.
7. Verlinsky Y, Kuliev A. Preimplantation diagnosis of common aneuploidies in fertile couples of advanced maternal age. Hum Reprod 1996;11:2076–2077.
8. Moore DP, Orr-Weaver TL. Chromosome segregation during meiosis: building an unambivalent bivalent. Curr Topic Devel Biol 1998;37:263–299.
9. Masui Y, Markert CL. Cytoplasmic control of nuclear behavior during meiotic maturation of frog oocytes. J Exp Zool 1971;177:129–146.
10. Hashimoto N, Kishimoto T. Regulation of meiotic metaphase by a cytoplasmic maturation-promoting factor during mouse oocyte maturation. Devel Biol 1988;126:242–252.
11. Flood JT, Chillik CF, van Uem JFHM, Iritani A, Hodgen G. Ooplasmic transfusion: prophase germinal vesicle oocytes made developmentally competent by microinjection of metaphase II egg cytoplasm. Fertil Steril 1990;53:1049–1054.
12. Plancha CE, Albertini DF. Hormonal regulation of meiotic maturation in the hamster oocyte involves a cytoskeleton-mediated process. Biol Reprod 1994;51:852–864.
13. Tarin JJ. Etiology of age-associated aneuploidy: a mechanism based on the 'free radical theory of ageing'. Molec Hum Reprod 1995;10:1563–1565.
14. Van Blerkom J, Davis PW, Lee J. ATP content of human oocytes and developmental potential and outcome after in vitro fertilization and embryo transfer. Hum Reprod 1995;10:415–424.
15. Battaglia DE, Goodwin P, Klein NA, Soules MR. Influence of maternal age on meiotic spindle in oocytes from naturally cycling women. Hum Reprod 1996;11:2217–2222.
16. Plachot M, Crozet N. Fertilization abnormalities in human in vitro fertilization. Hum Reprod 1992;7:89–94.
17. Meng L, Rutledge J, Kidder G, Khamsi F, Armstrong DT. Influence of germinal vesicle on the variance of patterns of protein synthesis of rat oocytes during maturation in vitro. Molec Reprod Devel 1996;43:228–235.
18. Tsunoda Y, Tokunaga T, Imai H, Uchida T. Nuclear transplantation of male primordial germ cells in the mouse. Development 1989;107:407–411.
19. Kamiguchi Y, Rosenbusch B, Sterzik K, Mikamo K. Chromosomal analysis of unfertilized human oocytes prepared by a gradual fixation-air drying method. Hum Genet 1993;90: 533–541.
20. Grimbizis G, Vandervorst M, Camus M, Tournaye H, Van Steirteghem A, Devroey P. Intracyto-

plasmic sperm injection, results in women older than 39, according to age and the number of embryos replaced in selective or non-selective transfers. Hum Reprod 1998;13:884–889.

21. Cha KY, Chung HM, Han SY, Yoon TK, Oum KB, Chung MK. Successful in vitro maturation, fertilization and pregnancy by using immature follicular oocytes collected from unstimulated polycystic ovarian syndrome patients. 1996 ASRM annual meeting, Abstract O-044.

22. Gosden RG, Rutherford AJ, Norfolk DR. Ovarian banking for cancer patients: Transmission of malignant cells in ovarian grafts. Hum Reprod 1997;12:403.

23. Czolowska R, Tarkowski AK. First meiosis of early dictyate nuclei from primordial oocytes in mature and activated mouse oocytes. Zygote 1996;4:73–80.

24. Gougeon A. Dynamics of follicular growth in the human: a model from preliminary results. Hum Reprod 1997;1:81.

25. Barnes FL, Crombie A, Gardner DK, Kausche A, Lacham-Kaplan O, Suikkari A, Tiglias J, Wood C, Trounson A., Blastocyst development and birth after in vitro maturation of human primary oocytes, intracytoplasmic sperm injection and assisted hatching. Hum Reprod 1995; 10:3243–3247.

# Biochemical-assisted hatching

Sung Il Roh

*Infertility Research Center, Jeil Women's Hospital, Seoul, Korea*

**Abstract.** Human-assisted reproductive technology (ART) programs have been developed remarkably during this decade. However, implantation rates following embryo replacement remain low, regardless of increased fertilization rates by ICSI (intracytoplasmic sperm injection). One proposed possibility limiting successful implantation is impaired hatching caused by suboptimal culture conditions. As to improving the hatching potential of blastocysts, assisted hatching by an artificial alteration of zona pellucida (ZP) has been carried out in many laboratories using the various methods. We have tried to investigate whether the supplementation of proteases into the culture media has any effect on development, zona structure, and/or hatching of mouse embryos. Supplementation of either pronase E (PE) or proteinase K (PK) in culture media did not affect development up to blastocyst but significantly increased the hatching rate. Furthermore, we observed the alteration of ultrastructure and casein binding properties of ZP in mouse embryos. We also investigated the effects of protease on the development of human embryos and pregnancy rates in the human ART program. From July 1994 to December 1996, 792 cycles (for study I) and 1,095 cycles (for study II) undergoing the IVF-ET program in Jeil Women's Hospital were randomly selected for biochemical-assisted hatching (BAH). The concentrations of proteases used in this study were 1 μg/ml PE, 0.1 μg/ml PK and 1 μg/ml PE + 0.1 μg/ml PK in human tubal fluid (HTF) with 0.5% human serum albumin (HSA), and in vitro fertilized embryos were cultured for 24 h. We analyzed the efficiency and stability of BAH according to the clinical profiles of patients and fertilization methods. After being cultured in HTF with proteases for 24 h of human embryos, the thinning in ZP of embryos was observed but its development was not disturbed. Also, clinical pregnancy rates were higher in the PE, PK and PE+PK groups than the control group without proteases (36.0% (32/89), 35.3% (36/102), 35.1% (39/111) vs. 25.5% (125/490), $p < 0.05$). The live birth rate in the PE, PK and PE+PK groups was increased compared to the control, and the abortion rates were not different. They showed the effect and safety of proteases treatment in human embryos. We selected PE as BAH for study II because of the slightly better embryonic morphology and pregnancy rate. In patients over 35 years of age, clinical pregnancy rates of the BAH group were higher than that of the control group (31.4% (58/185) vs. 22.2% (51/230); $p < 0.05$). In the cases with low oocyte retrieval, or with less than three cycles of IVF-ET, clinical pregnancy rates of the BAH group were significantly higher than that of the control group (36.8% (86/234) vs. 27.2% (93/342), $p < 0.05$; 36.8% (148/402) vs. 29.9% (168/562), $p < 0.05$). In BAH groups, the clinical pregnancy rate was similar between conventional IVF and ICSI groups. From the above results, it is suggested that improved hatching by protease treatment is due to physiological alteration of ZP structure, giving rise to the similar hatching process as that in vivo. We suggest that BAH using protease is a simple, safe and economic technique compared to the other known assisted hatching techniques in the human ART program.

**Keywords:** assisted hatching, IVF-ET program, proteases.

---

*Address for correspondence:* Sung Il Roh MD, Clinical Associate Professor of Obstetrics and Gynecology, Infertility Research Center, Jeil Women's Hospital, 1021-4, Daschi-Dong, Kangnam-Gu, Seoul 135-280, South Korea. Tel.: +82-2-3467-3700. Fax: +82-2-501-3472.

## Introduction

Human-assisted reproductive technology (ART) programs have developed remarkably during this decade. One of the recently developed techniques, the intracytoplasmic sperm injection method, markedly increased the fertilization rate overcoming the unexplained and male factor- induced failure of fertilization in IVF. However, implantation rates following embryo replacement remain low, regardless of the increased fertilization rates by this method. One proposed possibility limiting the successful implantation is an impaired hatching caused by suboptimal culture conditions [1]. In mice, in vitro culture of embryos causes hardening of the zona pellucida and impairs embryonic ability to implant. It is possible that enzymes and other molecules in the reproductive tract might assist embryos to grow normally by maintaining the zona in a soft state and/or by helping the blastocyst escape from the zona. The proportion of blastocysts failing to hatch in vivo is unknown, and empty zonas have never been observed in or recovered from the human reproductive tract. Therefore, it would be meaningful to investigate whether the culture environment causing thinning or softening to the zona may influence the embryonic ability to hatch and/or implant following embryo transfer.

The zona pellucida (ZP) is an extracellular matrix that surrounds the oocyte and is known to have a variety of functions. Prior to fertilization, the ZP presents a species-specific sperm barrier or receptor. Immediately following fertilization, the ZP acts as a major block to polyspermy [2]. The ZP may act to protect against the infiltration of leukocytes and infection by bacterial or fungal agents and to protect the fragile oocytes and embryos from physical damage from the environment. Also, the ZP functions to prevent the separation of blastomeres from cleaving embryos and to maintain the blastomeric arrangement to ensure successful subsequent development [3].

In mammals, embryonic development up to the blastocyst and hatching from ZP are prerequisites for implantation and successful pregnancy. Before implantation, the ZP must be shed to ensure contact between the implanting embryo and the endometrium. In vitro experiments have shown that hatching, oozing out of the blastocyst from the surrounding ZP is achieved through a hole formed in the zona. The mechanisms of hatching are not well characterized but may involve two physicochemical events: one is lysis of the ZP by substances elaborated either from the embryos or the female reproductive tract, the other is hydrostatic pressure exerted on the ZP, which is developed by expansion of the blastocyst [4]. Perona and Wassarman observed that a trypsin-like protease activity appeared in mural trophectoderm of mouse blastocyst immediately before hatching [5]. It was also reported that a trypsin-like protease could be identified in culture medium in which mouse embryos had been allowed to hatch [6] and that the addition of protease inhibitors to the culture medium could inhibit hatching of mouse embryos [7].

Gordon and Dapunt suggested that the main mediator of hatching was lysis of the ZP, but not pressure against it, based on their experimental results using a blastomere destruction and mineral oil droplet insertion model in mice [8]. Recently, Gonzales and Bavister have suggested a different mechanism whereby blastocysts hatch through uniform lysis of the entire ZP, not by a focal lysis of the ZP [9]. They observed that hamster embryos in vivo exhibited total zona lysis which occurred progressively but uniformly around the entire ZP and suggested that the lytic event might be due to extrinsic factor(s) present in the uterine environment rather than intrinsic factor(s) of embryos themselves (Table 1). However, a similar observation has not been made in other species.

## Development of biochemical-assisted hatching using protease supplementation into culture media in mouse model

Whether or not the hatching takes place with the aid of hydrostatic pressure exerted on the ZP by expansion of the blastocyst, it is rather obvious that enzymatic lysis is involved in the event. While the embryonic enzyme activity has been suggested to be responsible for the zona lysis [5,10], several investigators reported that the hatching time and behavior in vivo were somewhat different from those in vitro, suggesting the presence of uterine factor(s) which are unidentified. We have tried to investigate whether the supplementation of proteases in culture media has any effect on embryonic development, zona structure, and/or hatching of mouse in vitro, and thus can be used as a new assisted hatching technique.

*Effects of protease on the development and hatching of mouse embryos*

Firstly, we evaluated the effects of proteases on embryonic development and hatching. Two-cell mouse embryos were cultured for 72 h in 0.5% bovine serum albumin (BSA, Gibco BRL, Grand Island, New York, USA) supplemented human tubal fluid medium (HTF) with or without proteases. Supplementation of 1.0 µg/ml pronase E (PE; from *Streptomyces griseus*, type XIV, 4 units/mg,

*Table 1.* The characteristics of zona escape during hatching in vivo vs. in vitro of hamster embryo.

| In vivo | In vitro |
| --- | --- |
| Zona escape window 68.5–74 h | Delayed zona escape ≥ 29 h |
| (escape t-50, 70.9 h) | (escape t-50, 101 h) |
| Global lysis thinning of zona | Focal lysis intact zona |
| Small blastocoele cavity | Expanded blastocoele |
| Retarded embryos (e.g., eight-cell) | Retarded embryos are entrapped in zona |
|    Global lysis with successful escape | |
| All embryos escape | Only   63% : one-cell stage culture |
| |        92% : blastocyst culture |

Reproduced from [9].

P-5147; Sigma Chemical Co., St. Louis, Missouri, USA) and/or 0.1 µg/ml proteinase K (PK; from *Tritirachium album*, 10—20 units/mg, P-6556; Sigma) did not affect embryonic development up to blastocyst but significantly increased the hatching rate (Table 2). In contrast, supplementation of α-chymotrypsin (Chymo; from bovine pancreas, type II, 40—60 units/mg, C-4129; Sigma) was a little detrimental to mouse embryos and thus they showed retarded development.

The effects of combined treatment with proteases on the embryonic development and hatching are shown in Table 3. When two-cell mouse embryos were cultured in 0.5% BSA-HTF with combined proteases, either supplementation of 0.1 µg/ml PE and 0.01 µg/ml PK, or 1 µg/ml PE and 0.1 µg/ml PK increased the hatching rate. In contrast, the developmental rate to blastocyst was significantly reduced in the medium supplemented with 1.0 µg/ml PE, 0.1 µg/ml PK and 1.0 µg/ml Chymo, although all of the blastocysts that developed have hatched.

In short, supplementation of either PE or PK in culture media did not affect the development up to blastocyst but significantly increased the hatching rate, while supplementation of Chymo was detrimental to embryonic development and hatching. Similarly, combined supplementation of both PE and PK increased the hatching rate. However, the presence of chymotrypsin in the culture medium retarded the development of mouse embryos.

*Structural changes of zona pellucida of mouse embryos during protease treatment*

To evaluate whether the functional structure of ZP was affected by protease treatment during in vitro culture, ZP of mouse embryos was examined using a scanning electron microscope and a fluorescence microscope. For in vivo grown blastocysts (in vivo blastocyst), mouse embryos obtained from the uterus at 100 h after hCG (human chorionic gonadotropin) injection were used. For in vitro

*Table 2.* Developmental and hatching rates of two-cell mouse embryos cultured in HTF media containing 5% BSA according to proteases and concentrations for 72 h.

| Proteases | Concentration (µg/ml) | No. of exp. embryos | No. of embryos (%) | | |
|---|---|---|---|---|---|
| | | | Morula | Blastocyst | Hatched |
| PE[b] | Control | 102 | 12 | 90 (88.2) | 40 (39.2) |
| | 1.0 | 101 | 6 | 95 (94.1) | 61 (60.4)[a] |
| | 0.1 | 102 | 18 | 84 (82.4) | 21 (20.6) |
| PK[c] | Control | 102 | 10 | 92 (90.2) | 36 (35.3) |
| | 0.1 | 103 | 8 | 95 (92.2) | 74 (71.8)[a] |
| | 0.01 | 103 | 7 | 96 (93.2) | 40 (38.8) |
| Chymo[d] | Control | 103 | 14 | 89 (86.4) | 25 (24.3) |
| | 1.0 | 103 | 8 | 71 (68.9) | 7 (6.8)[a] |
| | 0.1 | 101 | 7 | 94 (93.1) | 29 (28.7) |

[a] p < 0.01; [b] pronase E; [c] proteinase K; [d] α-chymotrypsin.

*Table 3.* Developmental and hatching rates of two-cell mouse embryos cultured in HTF media containing 0.5% BSA with or without combined protease for 72 h.

| Experimental groups | Total no. of embryos | No. of embryos (%) | | |
|---|---|---|---|---|
| | | Morula | Blastocyst | Hatched |
| Control | 103 | 8 | 95 (92.2) | 38 (36.9) |
| 1.0 PE[b] + 0.1 PK[c] | 103 | 19 | 84 (81.6) | 62 (60.2)[a] |
| 0.1 PE + 0.01 PK | 103 | 9 | 94 (91.3) | 64 (62.1)[a] |
| 1.0 PE + 0.1 PK + 1.0 Chymo[d] | 102 | 19 | 65 (63.7)[a] | 65 (63.7)[a] |

[a]$p < 0.01$; [b]pronase E; [c]proteinase K; [d]$\alpha$-chymotrypsin. The unit of protease concentration is $\mu$g/ml.

grown blastocysts, two-cell mouse embryos obtained from the oviduct at 48–50 h after hCG injection were cultured in 0.5% BSA-HTF with or without 1 $\mu$g/ml PE (PE-treated blastocysts; in vitro blastocyst) for 72 h. After culture, only those developed to blastocysts were collected and examined. Each group of embryos (in vivo, in vitro, PE-treated) was observed with a scanning electron microscope. The ZP of in vivo grown blastocysts exhibited uniform, compact fiber-mass structures, whereas that of in vitro cultured blastocysts showed a fenestrated structure. Interestingly, the ZP of PE-treated blastocysts showed a structure similar to that of in vivo ones. Since the ZP structures of in vitro grown blastocysts were similar to that of two- or four-cell embryos, compact, fiber-mass structures of ZP observed in both in vivo grown and PE-treated blastocysts are believed to differentiate during development in the presence of specific environmental factors.

In the mouse, the biochemical properties of perivitelline space (PVS) of oocytes and embryos undergo changes by the influence of the oviductal environment. These changes are believed to be due to proteinaceous material(s) secreted by the oviduct and are distinguished by the distinct staining of PVS with fluorescein-isothiocyanate-conjugated (FITC)-casein. The staining pattern of PVS by FITC-casein continued to the morula stage and gradually disappears around the blastocyst stage both in vivo and in vitro, and did not disappear by washing [11]. Thus the changes of staining patterns were examined in embryos treated with proteases in the present study. The mouse embryos treated with 1 $\mu$g/ml PE and 0.1 $\mu$g/ml PK for 24 h were stained with FITC-casein. The PVS of in vitro-matured MII oocytes was not stained with FITC-casein. However, when they were introduced into the oviduct, a distinct fluorescence staining within PVS was shown and these staining patterns did not change by PBS-washing. The two-cell embryos were cultured in 0.5% BSA-HTF for 24 h and then stained with FITC-casein. Their PVS was stained and a fluorescence staining within PVS was not removed by PBS-washing. In contrast, PVS of the eight-cell embryos cultured in media containing PE and PK were not stained with FITC-casein. When these embryos were introduced into the oviduct and cultured together, their PVS were strongly stained with FITC-casein and these stains were removed by PBS-washing [12].

In this study, we observed good development and a higher hatching rate in mouse embryos, and protease supplementation in culture medium, which is accompanied by the induction of alteration of the zona structure was revealed by the disappearance of fluorescence PVS staining. Therefore, we suggest that the uterine factor(s), assumed to be proteolytic enzyme(s), play an important role in the hatching process in vivo, though not eliminating the possible involvement of intrinsic factors of the embryo itself and hydrostatic pressure against ZP.

**Application of biochemical-assisted hatching in human IVF-ET program**

Generally, the hatching rate of domestic animal embryos is lower in vitro compared to in vivo. The differences may be caused by zona hardening or reduction of zona lysin activity [8,13,14]. Therefore, induction of in vitro hatching seems to be a major hurdle for human embryos grown in vitro in an IVF program as only about one-quarter of those becoming blastocyst hatch successfully. As in the human, the ZP is known to become hardened when human oocytes are obtained by controlled ovarian hyperstimulation and with an increasing duration of culture in vitro. Adverse ultrastructural changes often occur in early embryonic cells during prolonged culture of 48–72 h. The oocytes of women with over 38 years of age or elevated basal FSH levels exhibited abnormally thick ZP and low hatching rates when they were fertilized, and resulted in low pregnancy rates.

As to improving the hatching potential of blastocysts, assisted hatching by an artificial alteration of the ZP have been carried out in many laboratories using the following methods: partial zona dissection (PZD) using mechanical force [15] and zona drilling (ZD) using acidic Tyrode's solution [16]. Many studies have reported that assisted hatching techniques can improve the hatching rate and successful pregnancy in many human IVF-ET cases [1,17]. It is possible that these techniques may enhance the implantation not only by facilitating the embryonic hatching process but also by allowing the earlier embryo-endometrium contact [18].

However, Cohen et al. reported that assisted hatching was effective mostly in patients aged $\geq 38$ years and in those with elevated basal FSH levels, whereas patients whose embryos have thin ZP might be jeopardized by assisted hatching [16]. In contrast, Bider et al. have not observed increased implantation rates in women of advanced age, despite differences in the number of embryos transferred [19]. Also, Malter and Cohen suggested that PZD could inhibit the embryonic development [20]. Besides, a possibility remains that partial loss of embryonic blastomeres or the whole embryo would happen due to the contractions of the female reproductive tract following transfer of the embryos. To avoid these drawbacks, several methodologies were adopted. Khalifa et al. attempted cruciate thinning of the mouse ZP, obtaining a significant enhancement of blastocyst hatching [21]. Also, zona thinning using an Er: YAG laser on embryos at 48 h after oocyte retrieval significantly increased the implantation and pregnancy rates [22]. However, these techniques using micromanipulator and/or acid Tyrode may be harmful to embryonic development and thus requires skillful techniques, since the use of a micromanipulator could expose the embryo to the external environment for a long time and the acid Tyrode solution is toxic to embryos.

Although human and other mammalian embryos exhibited delayed development and a lower hatching rate in vitro than in vivo, the reason for this is not yet clarified. The difference may lie in deficiency of paracrine factors and enzymes in reproductive tracts, which affects the development of embryos. It has long been suggested that proteolytic activity is present in uterine fluid. Some investigators have proposed that the embryonic hatching enzyme "strypsin" and/ or a uterine proteolytic component may contribute to the hatching process [5,9,23]. We observed that the supplementation of PE and/or PK in culture media did not affect the development of two-cell mouse embryos to blastocysts but increased the hatching rate significantly and the morphology of ZP of the blastocyst, cultured with protease, was similar to the morphology of ZP of blastocyst grown in vivo [12]. Recently, Fong et al. reported that day-5 or -6 blastocysts whose ZP was removed enzymatically, or day-5 or -6 blastocysts that hatched naturally on their own in vitro, attached tightly, spread out and grew on a variety of feeder layers irrespective of the source of supporting cells in their ongoing ES cell studies. Therefore, it is suggested that protease treatment may be very safe and is a convenient technique for the improvement of hatching and implantation in the human IVF-ET program.

In this study, we investigated the effects of protease, which is thought to be found in female reproductive tracts, on the development of human embryos and pregnancy rates following embryo transfer. We analyzed the efficiency and stability of biochemically assisted hatching (BAH) by the supplementation of protease into the culture medium according to the clinical profiles of patients and fertilization methods. The project was approved by the Institutional Review Board on the Human Subjects in Research at the Infertility Research Center, Jeil Women's Hospital.

*Study I*

In order to titrate an optimal concentration of proteases, a preliminary study was done using an abnormally fertilized (3PN) human zygote. The dissolution time of the human ZP upon protease treatment was shorter than that of the mouse ZP, although there was no difference in embryonic development of both of the species (data are not shown). Therefore, treatment of human embryos with proteases was done for only 24 h in this study.

From July 1994 to December 1995, 792 cycles undergoing the IVF-ET program in Jeil Women's Hospital were randomly selected for protease treatment. The concentrations of proteases used in this study were 1 µg/ml PE, 0.1 µg/ml PK and 1 µg/ml PE + 0.1 µg/ml PK in HTF with 0.5% human serum albumin (HSA). Media containing protease(s) were quality controlled by using 3PN zygotes, and aliquoted and stored in $-20°C$ until use. We thawed and warmed it in a 5% $CO_2$ incubator for 6 h, and also used it for embryonic culture. In vitro fertilized embryos were cultured for 24 h in HTF with 10% human serum (HS) or synthetic serum substitute (SSS, Irvine Scientific, Santa Ana, California, USA). Then the embryos were transferred to HTF with proteases and cultured for 24 h. After protease treatment, their development and clinical pregnancy were investigated after embryo transfer to the uterus of the patient. The results were compared with those of the control group.

Patient age, the number of retrieved oocytes, and fertilization rates among control, PE, PK and PE+PK groups are not different. After being cultured in HTF with proteases for 24 h, the thinning in zona pellucida of embryos was observed but its development was not disturbed (Table 4). Also, clinical pregnancy rates were higher in the PE, PK and PE+PK groups than the control group without proteases (36.0% (32/89), 35.3% (36/102), 35.1% (39/111) vs. 25.5% (125/490), $p < 0.05$, Table 5). The live birth rate in the PE, PK and PE+PK groups were higher than in the control, and the abortion rates were not different. They showed the effect and safety of protease treatment in human embryos. We selected PE as BAH for later study because of slightly better embryonic morphology and pregnancy rate.

*Study II*

From July 1994 to December 1996, 1,095 cycles undergoing the IVF-ET program in Jeil Women's Hospital were randomly selected for BAH (using proteases). The concentration of PE used in this study was 1 μg/ml in HTF with 0.5% HSA. In vitro fertilized embryos were cultured for 24 h in HTF with 10% HS or SSS. In the BAH group, embryos were transferred to HTF with PE and

*Table 4.* Development of human embryos cultured in HTF media containing 0.5% HSA with or without proteases.

| Exp. groups | No. of total fertilized embryos | No. of frozen embryos | Quality of embryonic development | | |
|---|---|---|---|---|---|
| | | | Good (%)[c] | Poor (%)[d] | Bad (%)[e] |
| Control | 2500 | 342 | 1330 (61.6) | 591 (27.4) | 237 (11.0) |
| PE[a] | 616 | 36 | 390 (67.2) | 121 (20.9) | 69 (11.9) |
| PK[b] | 814 | 129 | 425 (62.0) | 187 (27.3) | 73 (10.7) |
| PE[a] + PK[b] | 849 | 238 | 364 (59.6) | 179 (29.3) | 68 (11.1) |

[a]The concentration of pronase E was 1.0 μg/ml; [b]the concentration of proteinase K was 0.1 μg/m; [c]embyos with blastomere of equal size and < 20% cytoplasmic fragmentation; [d]embryos with blastomere of unequal size and 20−50% cytoplasmic fragmentation; [e]embryos with blastomere of distinctly unequal size and > 50% cytoplasmic fragmentation.

*Table 5.* Effects of biochemical assisted hatching by proteases on pregnancy rate and live baby birth rate in human IVF-ET program.

| | Control | Biochemical-assisted hatching | | |
| --- | --- | --- | --- | --- |
| | | PE[a] | PK[b] | PE[a] + PK[b] |
| No. of cycles | 490 | 89 | 111 | 102 |
| Age (years)[c] | 32.3 ± 4.0 | 33.6 ± 4.0 | 33.9 ± 4.3 | 32.2 ± 3.9 |
| No. of oocytes[c] | 10.7 ± 7.1 | 12.6 ± 6.8 | 13.2 ± 8.4 | 13.4 ± 8.5 |
| No. of fertilized oocytes[c] | 5.4 ± 3.9 | 6.9 ± 3.5 | 7.4 ± 4.0 | 8.3 ± 5.9 |
| No. of ET | 490 | 89 | 111 | 102 |
| No. of transferred embryos[c] | 3.1 ± 1.5 | 3.8 ± 1.3 | 3.6 ± 1.4 | 3.3 ± 1.4 |
| No. of clinical pregnancies (%) | 125 (25.5) | 32 (36.0)[d] | 39 (35.1)[d] | 35 (34.3)[d] |
| No. of live baby births (%) | 84 (17.1) | 24 (27.0)[d] | 28 (25.2)[d] | 26 (25.5)[d] |

[a]The concentration of pronase E was 1.0 µg/ml in HTF-0.5% HSA; [b]the concentration of proteinase K was 0.1 µg/ml in HTF-0.5% HSA; [c]values are means ± SD; [d]$p < 0.05$.

cultured for 24 h. The development of embryos was observed and they were transferred to the uterus of the patients. After embryo transfer to the uterus of the patient, clinical pregnancy rates were compared with those of the control group. The pregnancy rate according to patient age, the number of stimulation cycles, the number of retrieved oocytes and the fertilization method were analyzed, comparing between the BAH and control groups.

In patients under 34 years of age, clinical pregnancy rates increased in the BAH group but not significantly (36.7% (102/278) vs. 33.3% (134/402)). In patients over 35 years of age, clinical pregnancy rates of the BAH group were higher than that of the control group (31.4% (58/185) vs. 22.2% (51/230); $p < 0.05$). In the cases with few oocytes ($4 \leqslant n \leqslant 12$), or less than three cycles of IVF-ET, clinical pregnancy rates of the BAH group were significantly higher than that of the control group (36.8% (86/234) vs. 27.2% (93/342), $p < 0.05$; 36.8% (148/402) vs. 29.9% (168/562), $p < 0.05$). However, in the case of many oocytes ($\geqslant 13$) or more than four cycles of IVF-ET, clinical pregnancy rates were no different in either group. In the BAH groups, the clinical pregnancy rate was similar between the conventional IVF and ICSI (intracytoplasmic sperm injection) group (Table 6).

Assisted hatching of human embryos has proven to be beneficial in IVF-ET treated patients [13,16,18]. In this study using several proteases, we observed improved pregnancy rates in women $\geqslant 35$ years of age and the outcome was comparable to the other assisted hatching programs [24–26].

BAH of human embryos increased clinical pregnancy rates in few oocytes or less than three cycles of IVF-ET. But, in the case of many oocytes or more than four cycles of IVF-ET, clinical pregnancy rates did not differ. It was suggested that BAH in culture improved hatching and pregnancy rates in the former group, and that similar results were observed in other assisted hatching techniques. However, we acquired different results in patients with many retrieved oocytes

*Table 6.* Comparison of pregnancy rate between biochemical assisted hatching and control group according to patients characteristics

| Patient characteristics | No. of pregnancies/No. of stimulations (%) | |
| --- | --- | --- |
| | BAH[b] | Control |
| No. of stimulation cycles | | |
| $\geqslant 4$ | 12/61 (20.0) | 17/70 (24.3) |
| $\leqslant 3$ | 148/402 (36.8)[a] | 168/562 (29.9) |
| Patients age (years) | | |
| $\leqslant 34$ | 102/278 (36.7) | 134/402 (33.3) |
| $\geqslant 35$ | 58/185 (31.4)[a] | 51/230 (22.2) |
| Fertilization method | | |
| ICSI | 78/227 (34.4) | 49/148 (33.1) |
| conventional IVF | 82/236 (34.7) | 136/483 (28.3) |
| No. of retrieved oocytes | | |
| $\leqslant 3$ | 4/40 (10.0) | 15/89 (16.9) |
| $4\leqslant$ and $\leqslant 12$ | 86/234 (36.8)[a] | 93/342 (27.2) |
| $\geqslant 13$ | 70/189 (37.0) | 77/201 (38.3) |

[a]$p < 0.05$; [b]biochemical assisted hatching by 1.0 µg/ml pronase E.

($\geqslant 13$) and many repetitive ($\geqslant 4$) failed IVF. If we can retrieve many oocytes, it is believed that we will increase the incidence of pregnancy because a large number of good embryos are acquired in the non-BAH group. We also think that the low pregnancy rate in many repetitively ($\geqslant 4$) failed patients may indicate that implantation failures in these patients were caused by other components, not zonal factors [27].

Using the BAH method in the human IVF-ET program gave a similar benefit as other assisted hatching techniques. Moreover, when the medium containing protease(s) was used after freezing at $-20°C$ and thawing, there were no differences in the hatching rate compared to the freshly prepared medium. Therefore, BAH using proteases, specifically pronase E, may be simple and convenient in clinical applications. Additionally, it has the advantage of not needing expensive tools or skillful technique, and avoids prolonged exposure to the external environment.

## Conclusions

In the present study, we obtained a better development and higher hatching rate of mouse and human embryos after culture in media with protease(s). Using a scanning electron and fluorescence microscope, the structure of the ZP of blastocysts that were cultured with protease was shown to be similar to that of blastocysts grown in vivo. Therefore, it is suggested that improved hatching by protease treatment is due to an alteration of ZP structure, giving rise to the similar hatching process to that in vivo.

In human IVF-ET programs, the oocytes of women with higher ages or elevated basal FSH levels exhibited abnormally thick ZP and low hatching, which resulted in the low pregnancy rate. To overcome these difficulties and to increase implantation rates, investigators have adopted various techniques to assist hatching during culture in vitro. Although these methods were proved to give better IVF-ET results, several limitations must be considered — exposure of eggs against the external environment including toxic acid Tyroid for a long time, requirements of expensive tools and skillful experts, etc. In contrast, the BAH method, as reported here, provides rather a convenient and economic achievement. By using this method in the human IVF-ET program, we obtained good pregnancy rates and normal deliveries particularly in patients over 35 years of age or patients with a low oocyte retrieval rate. However, the precise mechanism whereby protease supplementation could increase hatching and implantation of mammalian embryos remains to be elucidated. We suggest that BAH using proteases(s) is a simple, safe and economic technique compared to the other known assisted hatching techniques in the human ART program.

## References

1. Cohen J, Elsner C, Kort H et al. Impairment of the hatching process following IVF in the human and improvement of implantation by assisting hatching using micromanipulation. Hum Reprod 1990;5:7—13.
2. Wassarman PM. Mouse gamete adhesion molecules. Biol Reprod 1992;46:186—191.
3. Suzuki H, Togashi M, Adachi J et al. Developmental ability of zona-free embryos is influenced by cell association at the 4-cell stage. Biol Reprod 1995;53:78—83.
4. Massip A, Mulnard J. Time lapse cinematographic analysis of hatching of normal and frozen-thawed cow blastocysts. J Reprod Fertil 1980;58:475—478.
5. Perona RM, Wassarman PM. Mouse blastocysts hatch in vitro by using a trypsin-like proteinase associated with cells of mural trophoectoderm. Devel Biol 1986;114:42—52.
6. Sawada H, Yamasaki K, Hoshi M. Trypsin-like protease from mouse embryos: evidence for the presence in culture medium and its enzymatic properties. J Exp Zool 1990;254:83—87.
7. Yamazaki K, Kato Y, Hoshi M. Protease inhibitors block the zona shedding of mouse embryos in vitro. Devel Growth Differ 1985;27:491.
8. Gordon JW, Dapunt U. A new mouse model for embryos with a hatching deficiency and its use to elucidate the mechanism of blastocyst hatching. Fertil Steril 1993;59:1296—1301.
9. Gonzales DS, Bavister BD. Zona pellucida escape by hamster blastocysts in vitro is delayed and morphologically different compared with zona escape in vivo. Biol Reprod 1995;52:470—480.
10. Confino E, Rawlin R, Binor Z, Radwanska E. The effect of the oviduct, uterine, and in vitro environments on zona thinning in the mouse embryo. Fertil Steril 1997;68:164—167.
11. Kim H, Kim H, Kim SR et al. Oviductal protein produces fluorescence staining of the perivitel-line space in mouse oocytes. J Exp Zool 1996;274:351—357.
12. Lee DR, Lee JE, Yoon HS et al. The supplementation of protease in culture medium improves the hatching rate of mouse embryos. Hum Reprod 1997;12:2493—2498.
13. Cohen J. Assisted hatching of human embryos. J In Vitro Fertil Embryo Transfer 1991;8:179—190.
14. Schiewe MC, Hazeleger NL, Sclimenti C et al. Physiological characterization of blastocyst hatching mechanisms by use of a mouse antihatching model. Fertil Steril 1995;63:288—294.
15. Malter HE, Cohen J. Partial zona dissection of the human oocyte: a nontraumatic method using micromanipulation to assist zona pellucida penetration. Fertil Steril 1989a;51:139—148.
16. Cohen J, Alikani M, Trowbridge J et al. Implantation enhancement by selective assisted hatching

using zona drilling of human embryos with poor prognosis. Hum Reprod 1992;7:685–691.

17. Tucker MJ, Cohen J, Massey JB et al. Partial dissection of the zona pellucida of frozen thawed human embryos may enhance blastocyst hatching, implantation and pregnancies. Am J Obstet Gynecol 1991;165:341–345.
18. Liu HC, Cohen J, Alikani M et al. Assisted hatching facilitates earlier implantation. Fertil Steril 1993;60:871–875.
19. Bider D, Livshits A, Yonish M et al. Assisted hatching by zona drilling of human embryos in women of advanced age. Hum Reprod 1997;12:317–320.
20. Malter HE, Cohen J. Blastocyst formation and hatching in vitro following zona drilling of mouse and human embryos. Gamete Res 1989b;24:67–80.
21. Khalifa E-AM, Tucker MJ, Hunt P. Cruciate thinning of the zona pellucida for more successful enhancement of blastocyst hatching in the mouse. Hum Reprod 1992;7:532–536.
22. Antinori S, Panci C, Selman HA et al. Zona thinning with the use of laser: a new approach to assisted hatching in humans. Hum Reprod 1996;11:590–594.
23. Bavister BD. Culture of preimplantation embryos: facts and artifacts. Hum Reprod Update 1995;1:91–148.
24. Schoolcraft WB, Schlenker T, Johns GS et al. In vitro fertilization in women age 40 and older: the impact of assisted hatching. J Assist Reprod Genet 1995;12:581–584.
25. Stein A, Rufas O, Amit S et al. Assisted hatching by partial zona dissection of human pre-embryos in patients with recurrent implantation failure after in vitro fertilization. Fertil Steril 1995;63:838–841.
26. Tucker MJ, Morton PC, Wright G et al. Enhancement of outcome from intracytoplasmic sperm injection: does co-culture or assisted hatching improve implantation rates? Hum Reprod 1996;11:2434–2437.
27. Munne S, Alikani M, Tomkin G et al. Embryo morphology, developmental rates, and maternal age are correlated with chromosome abnormalities. Fertil Steril 1995;64:382–391.

# Implantation and placentation

# Metalloproteinases, cell adhesion and invasion molecules in human implantation and placentation

P. Bischof, A. Meisser and A. Campana

*Department of Obstetrics and Gynecology, University of Geneva, Geneva, Switzerland*

**Abstract.** The metastatic potential of tumour cells largely depends on their capacity to secrete proteolytic enzymes capable of degrading the constituents of the basement membrane and the extracellular matrix (ECM) of the host tissue. Several enzymes are implicated in the invasive process but only matrix metalloproteinases (MMP) have the capacity to digest the different collagens which constitute the immediate cell environment. MMPs form a family of 12 structurally homologous enzymes having all an atom of zinc in their active domain. They are secreted as inactive enzymes (zymogens) and activation occurs upon proteolysis. The local activity of MMPs is under the control of inhibitors: Tissue Inhibitor of Metalloproteinases (TIMP-1 and TIMP-2).

Like tumour cells, human cytotrophoblastic cells (CTB) are constitutively invasive. CTB obtained from legal abortions secrete MMPs such as the 72- and 92-kDa gelatinases. These gelatinases are responsible for the invasive behaviour of CTB since inhibitors of MMP abolish their invasiveness. Trophoblast invasion is also controlled by endometrial signals. Medium conditioned by decidual cells inhibits invasion of trophoblast cells. These effects are due to cytokines and other decidual proteins but also to constituents of the ECM. Thus, depending on their integrin (ECM protein receptors) repertoire, CTB differentiate along an invasive phenotype or fuse to form secretory syncytia. A normal pregnancy can thus be viewed as a state of equilibrium between invasive and antiinvasive regulatory mechanisms. Excessive trophoblastic invasion leads to pathologies such as hydatidiform moles and choriocarcinoma whereas a shallow invasion induces preeclampsia.

**Keywords:** adhesion molecules, gelatinases, implantation, integrins, metalloproteinases, placentation, trophoblast.

## Introduction

Although human blastocysts resulting from IVF programs have been examined by conventional and electron microscopy, neither the stage of adhesion to the uterine surface nor penetration into the endometrium have been observed in the human. Consequently the nature of these crucial events are deduced from information gathered in other primates or from in vitro observations. The implantation process can be divided in two phases: 1) an attachment phase, and 2) a penetration phase.

Attachment consists of two steps: apposition and adhesion. During apposition, no visible connections are established between the blastocyst and the endometrium, and the blastocyst can be dislodged by simple washing of the uterine cav-

*Address for correspondence:* Dr Paul Bischof MD, Department of Obstetrics and Gynecology, Laboratoire d'Hormonologie, 1211 Geneva 14, Switzerland. Tel.: +41-22-382-4336. Fax: +41-22-382-4310, E-mail: pail.bischof@hcuge.ch

ity. Adhesion is the step during which functional connections are established although the nature of these connections is still very speculative.

Penetration of the blastocyst is said to be intrusive. In vitro, trophoblast cells penetrate an endometrial epithelial cell monolayer by forming long slender ecto-plasmic protrusions which insinuate between endometrial cells and disrupt their desmosomes [1]. This not only occurs at implantation, but also later during pla-centation when cytotrophoblastic cells (CTB) leave the villous tree to invade the endometrium.

Studying attachment implies the identification of molecules which allow two different epithelial cells (the trophectodermal cells of the blastocyst and the endo-metrial epithelial cells) to make contact through their apical membranes. Study-ing penetration implies understanding the mechanisms which allow a cell (or a group of cells) to invade a neighboring tissue. Thus, in the first case one will have to study cell-cell adhesion molecules, whereas in the second case one will study the expression of proteolytic enzymes which allow a cell to digest the extra-cellular matrix in which it is embedded.

## Mediators of attachment

Attachment of two epithelial cells through their apical membrane domains is a biological paradox [2]. The trophectoderm of the blastocyst and the uterine lining are epithelia formed by polarized cells. Polarized cells have two membrane domains: a baso-lateral domain which anchors the cells to each other (through desmosomes and other specialized areas) and to the basement membrane (through integrins), and an apical domain which exhibits microvilli but which is usually devoid of adhesion molecules.

Lectin-binding studies indicate that modulation of cell-surface glycoconjugates on both uterine epithelium and trophectoderm occurs at implantation in rodents [3]. The appearance of new glycoproteins on the apical surface of the uterine luminal epithelium during the period of endometrial receptivity has been demon-strated biochemically in the rabbit [4]. Lindenberg and co-workers [5] tested seven oligosaccharides for their effects in an in vitro model of mouse blastocyst attachment and trophoblast outgrowth on endometrial epithelial monolayers. Only one compound, lacto-N-fucopentaose 1 (LNF-1) significantly inhibited attachment and outgrowth. It was later shown that mouse blastocysts carry LNF-1 receptors [6,7]. LNF-1 is specifically expressed on the mouse uterine epithelial lining during the first 4 days of pregnancy and expression can be induced in castrated animals by estrogen treatment [8]. LNF-1 is a pentasaccha-ride which contains the H-type-1 epitope. This epitope is a fucosylated blood group antigen in humans but a tissue antigen in rodents. $\alpha$-(1-2)-Fucosyltransfer-ase is the enzyme that catalyses the final step in the formation of H-type-1 epi-tope. Since estrogen stimulate and progesterone inhibit this enzyme in the uterine luminal epithelium, it is believed that this fucosyltransferase is the rate-limiting factor of the hormonal control of blastocyst attachment in mice [9]. There is probably more than only one glycoprotein involved in blastocyst attachment in mice [10] but clearly estrogen-induced carbohydrates play a crucial role in this important step. In rodents, implantation is notoriously dependent on estrogen. This is, however, not the case in primates [11]. Nevertheless, oligosaccharides and particularly glycosaminoglycans have been implicated in the attachment of the human blastocyst to the endometrium [12]. Perlecan is such a gycosaminogly-can, appearing on the surface of mouse blastocyst at the time of attachment [13]. Since perlecan can bind to the integrin $\alpha v \beta 3$ [14] and since this integrin is specifically expressed on human uterine epithelium only at the time of implanta-tion [15], it is tempting to speculate that these molecules are implicated in the attachment of the human blastocyst [16]. Recently, more direct evidence has implicated E-cadherin (an epithelial cell adhesion molecule) and integrin $\alpha 6 \beta 1$ in human trophoblast-epithelial cell adhesiveness [17].

## Mediators of penetration

Penetration (or invasion) of trophoblastic cells into the endometrium is not due to passive growth pressure, but to an active biochemical process. A cell is invasive by virtue of its ability to secrete proteases and trophectodermal cells and CTB are no exception [18,19]. Serine proteases, cathepsins and metalloproteinases (MMP) have been implicated in the invasive process [20].

MMP form a family of homologous enzymes (Table 1) which have all a $Zn^{++}$

*Table 1.* Biochemical properties of metalloproteinases.

|  | Other names | M.W. | Substrates | Location of the gene |
|---|---|---|---|---|
| MMP-1 | Interstitial collagenase fibroblast collagenase | 54007 | Col I, II, III, VII, X, MMP-5, entactin | 11q22-q23 |
| MMP-2 | Gelatinase A 72 kD gelatinase | 73882 | Col IV, V, VII, X, gelatin fibronectin, elastin | 16q13 |
| MMP-3 | Stromelysin-1 Transin-1 | 53977 | Col III, IV, IX, X, gelatin, laminin fibronectin, elastin, casein | 11q23 |
| MMP-7 | PUMP-I matrilysin | 29677 | Casein, fibronectin, gelatin | 11q21-q22 |
| MMP-8 | Neutophil collagenase PMNL collagenase | 53412 | Col I, III | 11q21-q22 |
| MMP-9 | Gelatinase B 92 kD gelatinase | 78427 | Col IV, V, gelatin | 20q11.2-q13.1 |
| MMP-10 | Stromelysin-2 Transin-2 | 54151 | Col II, IV, V, fibronectin, gelatin | 11q22.3-q23 |
| MMP-11 | Stromelysin-3 | 54595 | Col IV | 22q11.2 |
| MMP-13 | Collagenase-3 | 53819 | Col I | 11q22.3 |
| MMP-14 | MT1-MMP, MMP-X1 | 65883 | MMP-2 | 14 q11-q12 |
| MMP-15 | MT2-MMP | 75807 | MMP-2 |  |
| MMP-16 | MT3-MMP, MMP-X2 | 69158 | MMP-2 |  |

atom in their active site. They are secreted as inactive proenzymes (zymogens) which become activated upon partial hydrolysis whereby they lose their propeptide. Activation of the proMMPs into active MMPs can be reproduced in vitro by the addition of different agents such as mercurial salts. Although the physiological activators of the different MMPs are unknown, it has been shown that plasmin [21], MMP-3 [22] and membrane bound MMPs (MT-MMPs, [23–25]) are potent activators of several MMPs. This means that MMPs act in cascade similar to the enzymes involved in blood coagulation.

MMPs are classified in four subfamilies according to their substrate specificity (Table 1):

1. Gelatinases are represented by two enzymes, gelatinase A and B (72- and 92-kDa gelatinases or MMP-2 and MMP-9, respectively). These proteases digest collagen type IV (the major constituent of basement membranes) and denatured collagen (gelatin).

2. Collagenases include three proteases: the interstitial collagenase (MMP-1 or collagenase-1), the neutrophil collagenase (MMP-8) and collagenase-3 (MMP-13). These enzymes digest collagen type I, II, III, VII and X. They are thus appropriately designed for digesting the collagen of the extracellular matrix of the interstitium.

3. Stromelysins is a subfamily of four enzymes: MMP-3, -7, -10 and -11 (also called stromelysin-1, matrilysin, stromelysin 2 and 3, respectively). These proteases have a relatively broad substrate specificity and digest collagen type IV, V, VII as well as laminin, fibronectin, proteoglycans and gelatin.

4. Membrane metalloproteinases (MT-MMP) include three membrane-bound enzymes (MMP-14, -15, -16). The substrate of these MMPs is essentially proMMP-2, and these enzymes allow activation of MMP-2 at the cell surface of the invasive front.

Direct evidence links the expression of MMPs, and particularly MMP-9 [26] to the metastatic phenotype, and the tissue inhibitor of metalloproteinases (TIMP) to the inhibition of metastatisation [27]. In vitro CTB invade an acellular amniotic membrane or a reconstituted basement membrane (Matrigel [28]), they thus behave like metastatic cells. This invasive behavior is due to the ability of CTB to secrete MMPs since TIMP inhibits their invasiveness [29]. Several studies have localized MMP proteins and mRNA [30] in human trophoblast. Furthermore, cultured CTB secrete MMPs [18,19,31] but CTB from early pregnancy are more invasive and secrete more MMPs than CTB isolated from term placenta. All MMPs are not equally important for trophoblast invasion. Gelatinase B has been shown to mediate CTB invasion into matrigel [19,29] but one must ask if this is also true in vivo, particularly since the nature of the matrix in which the cells are embedded plays such a crucial role in the regulation of MMP secretion [31]. Whatever the exact mechanism in vivo, one must admit that CTB behave like metastatic cells and that they secrete MMPs from very early on in their development since human blastocysts [32] or even triploid eight-cell human embryos [19] produce MMPs.

## The role of adhesion molecules

Cell adhesion molecules (CAM) are represented by four subfamilies of molecules: cadherins, immunoglobulins, selectins, and integrins. Cadherins and selectins are membrane glycoproteins involved in Ca-dependent cell-cell binding, immunoglobulins allow cell-cell binding in a Ca-independent way, whereas integrins regulate mainly (but not exclusively) Ca-dependent cell-substrate interactions. We purposely limit our discussion to integrins since very few studies have investigated the role of other CAMs in implantation and placentation.

Integrins are widely expressed cell-surface adhesion receptors. They are $\alpha$ $\beta$ heterodimers. Depending on the type of $\alpha$-$\beta$ combination, the integrin will bind to one or another matrix-glycoprotein, i.e., $\alpha 5 \beta 1$ to fibronectin, $\alpha 2 \beta 1$ to laminin, etc. Both integrin subunits are transmembrane glycoproteins with a short cytoplasmic domain, a single transmembrane segment and a large extracellular domain. Integrins are transducers signaling the nature of the extracellular environment to the interior of the cell. This signal is then translated into events which allow the cell to change shape, migrate, adhere to other matrices and release proteases. This will in turn modify the microenvironment of the cell to which it will readapt by changing its integrin repertoire. How the transduction mechanism works precisely is unclear to date but it involves the clustering of integrins at focal contacts on the cell membrane, the phosphorylation of the kinase FAK 125 (focal adhesion kinase) and possibly the induction of gene transcription [33]. Integrins are causally related to invasion as demonstrated by transfection of Chinese hamster ovary cells with cDNA for the integrin $\alpha 5 \beta 1$ [34]. Increased expression of $\alpha 5 \beta 1$ (a fibronectin receptor) on these cells inhibited their capacity to form tumors and to migrate. This suggests that enhancing adhesion of a cell reduces its invasive potential.

Trophoblast and particularly CTB also express integrins (Fig. 1). Immunohistochemical studies [35,36] and functional studies [37] have shown a fascinating new property of CTB: they modulate their integrin repertoire during invasion of the endometrium. The villous CTB are immotile stem cells resting on the villous basement membrane, they express the integrin a6β4 (a laminin receptor) in a clustered manner towards the basement membrane. When these cells leave the villous tree to form CTB cell columns they still express the integrin $\alpha 6 \beta 4$ but in an unclustered way. Delocalisation of $\alpha 6 \beta 4$ probably allows the CTB to become motile and to start invasion of the endometrium. CTB located deeper in the decidualised endometrium have lost their capacity to express the integrin $\alpha 6 \beta 4$ but express instead the integrin $\alpha 5 \beta 1$, the major fibronectin receptor. CTB that have invaded the endometrial blood vessels express yet another integrin: the integrin $\alpha 1 \beta 1$, a known collagen receptor. These observations show that during invasion CTB adapt to their successive environments, the placental basement membrane, the cell columns, the placental bed and the endometrial blood vessels. This adaptation not only changes the integrin repertoire of the CTB but also their metabolism. We observed recently [38,39] that CTB isolated from first

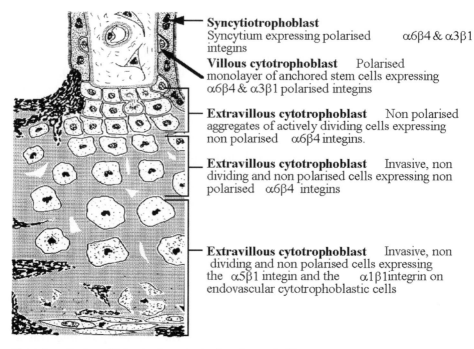

**Syncytiotrophoblast**
Syncytium expressing polarised          α6β4 & α3β1
integins

**Villous cytotrophoblast**     Polarised
monolayer of anchored stem cells expressing
α6β4 & α3β1 polarised integins

**Extravillous cytotrophoblast**     Non polarised
aggregates of actively dividing cells expressing
non polarised    α6β4 integins.

**Extravillous cytotrophoblast**     Invasive, non
dividing and non polarised cells expressing non
polarised    α6β4  integins

**Extravillous cytotrophoblast**     Invasive, non
dividing and non polarised cells expressing
the   α5β1 integin and the       α1β1integrin on
endovascular cytotrophoblastic cells

*Fig. 1.* Localization of integrins in an anchoring placental villous.

trimester trophoblast and expressing the α6 integrin subunit secrete significantly higher concentrations of gelatinases and significantly lower concentrations of fibronectin than the CTB expressing the α5 integrin subunit. In contrast, both CTB subsets secreted similar amounts of hCG. We conclude from these in vitro studies that during trophoblast invasion, extravillous CTB expressing the α6β4 integrin (in an unclustered way) represent the invasive population of CTB. Once the cells express the α5β1 integrin, their invasive behavior and their gelatinase (MMP-9) secretion has almost stopped, and the cells become immotile and secrete more fibronectin. This fibronectin is deposited in the extracellular matrix and contributes to anchoring the CTB into the endometrium. It is tempting to speculate that delocalisation of the α5β1 integrin (possibly induced by insulin-like growth factor binding protein-1, IGFBP-1, [40]) and acquisition of the α1β1 integrin will secondarily allow the CTB to invade the endometrial spiral arteries.

### Conclusions

Although CTB behave like metastatic cells, in vivo they are only transiently invasive (first trimester) and their invasion is limited only to the endometrium and to the proximal third of the myometrium. This temporal and spatial regulation of trophoblast invasion is believed to be essentially mediated by uterine factors including the glycoproteins of the extracellular matrix (fibronectin, laminin) and secretory products of the different endometrial cells (IGFBP-1 and different cytokines). It is not the aim of this review to deal with these matters and the reader is referred to several recent reviews [41–44].

# References

1. Lindenberg S, Pedersen B, Hamberger L, Kimber SJ. Models for human implantation derived from implantation in vitro. Reprod Fertil Devel 1992;4:653–670.
2. Denker HW. Implantation: a cell biological paradox. J Exp Zool 1993;266:541–558.
3. Chavez DJ. Cell surface of the mouse blastocysts at the trophectoderm-uterine interface during the adhesive stage of implantation. Am J Anat 1996;176:153–158.
4. Anderson TL, Olsen GE, Hoffman LH. Stage specific alterations in the apical membrane glycoproteins of endometrial epithelial cells related to implantation in the rabbit. Biol Reprod 1986;34:701–720.
5. Lindenberg S, Sundberg K, Kimber SJ, Lundblad A. The milk oligosaccharide, lacto-N-fucopentaose I, inhibits attachment of mouse blastocysts on endometrial monolayers. J Reprod Fertil 1988;83:149–158.
6. Lindenberg S, Kimber SJ, Kallin E. Carbohydrate binding properties of mouse embryos. J Reprod Fertil 1990;89:431–439.
7. Yamagata T, Yamazaki K. Implanting mouse embryo stain with a LNF-I bearing fluorescent probe at their mural trophectodermal side. Biochem Biophys Res Commun 1991;181:1004–1009.
8. Kimber SJ, Lindenberg S. Hormonal control of a carbohydrate epitope involved in implantation in mice. J Reprod Fertil 1990;89:13–21.
9. White S, Kimber SJ. Changes in a (1-2)-fucosyltransferase activity in the murine endometrial epithelium during the oestrous cycle, early pregnancy, and after ovariectomy and hormone replacement. Biol Reprod 1994;50:73–81.
10. Fenderson BA, Eddy EM, Hakomori SI. Glycoconjugate expression during embryogenesis and its biological significance. Bioessays 1990;12:173–180.
11. Ghosh D, De P, Sengupta, J. Luteal phase ovarian oestrogen is not essential for implantation and maintenance of pregnancy from surrogate embryo transfer in rhesus monkey. Hum Reprod 1994;9:629–637.
12. Rohde LH, Carson DD. Heparin like glycosaminoglycans participate in binding of human trophoblastic cell line (Jar) to human uterine epithelial cell line (RL 95). J Cell Physiol 1993;155:185–196.
13. Carson DD, Tang JP, Julian J. Heparan sulphate proteoglycan (perlecan) expression by mouse embryo during acquisition of attachment competence. Devel Biol 1993;155:97–106.
14. Hayashi K, Madri J, Yurchenco P. Endothelial cells interact with the core protein of basement membrane perlecan through alpha 1 and beta 3 integrins: an adhesion modulated by glycosaminoglycan. J Cell Biol 1992;119:945–955.
15. Lessey BA, Damjanovich L, Coutifaris C, Castelbaum, Albelda SM, Buck CA. Integrin adhesion molecules in human endometrium. J. Clin Invest 1992;90:188–195.
16. Damsky C, Sutherland A, Fisher S. Extracellular matrix 5: Adhesive interactions in early mammalian embryogenesis, implantation and placentation. FASEB J 1993;7:1320–1329.
17. Thie M, Harrach-Ruprecht, B Sauer H, Fuchs P, Albers A, Denker HW. Cell adhesion to the apical pole of epithelium: a function of cell polarity. Eur J Cell Biol 1995;66:180–191.
18. Fisher SJ, Cui T, Zhang L, Hartmann L, Grahl K, Guo-Yang Z, Tarpey J, Damsky. CH Adhesive and degradative properties of human placental cytotrophoblast cells in vitro. J Cell Biol 1989;109:891–902.
19. Bischof P, Martelli M, Campana A, Itoh Y, Ogata Y, Nagase H. Importance of metalloprotein-

ases (MMP) in human trophoblast invasion. Early Pregn Biol Med 1995;1:263—269.

20. Cawston TE. Proteinases and inhibitors. Br Med Bull 1995;51:385—401.

21. Murphy G, Atkinson S, Ward R, Gavrilovic J, Reynolds JJ. The role of plasminogen activators in the regulation of connective tissue metalloproteinases. Ann NY Acad Sci 1992;667:1—12.

22. Ogata Y, Enghild JJ, Nagase H. Matrix metalloproteinase 3 (stromelysin) activates the precursor for human matrix metalloproteinase 9. J Biol Chem 1992;267:3581—3584.

23. Sato H, Takino T, Okada Y, Cao J, Shinagecuna A, Yamamoto E, Seiki M. A matrix metallopro-teinase expressed on the surface of invasive tumour cells. Nature 1994;370:61—65.

24. Takino T, Sato H, Shinigawa A, Seiki M. Identification of the second membrane type matrix metalloproteinase (MT-MMP-2) gene from a human placenta cDNA library. J Biol Chem 1995;270:23013—23020.

25. Will H, Heinzmann B. cDNA sequence and mRNA tissue distribution of a novel human matrix metalloproteinase with a potential transmembrane segment. Eur J Biochem 1995;231:602—608.

26. Bernhard EJ, Gruber SB, Muschel RJ. Direct evidence linking expression of matrix metallopro-teinase 9 (92-kDa gelatinase/collagenase) to the metastatic phenotype in transformed rat embryo cells. Proc Natl Acad Sci 1994;91:4293—4297.

27. DeClerck YA, Perez N, Shimada H, Boone TC, Langley KE, Taylor SM. Inhibition of invasion and metastasis in cells transfected with an inhibitor of metalloproteinases. Cancer Res 1992; 52:701—708.

28. Graham CH, Connelly I, MacDougall JR, Kerbel RS, Stetler-Stevenson WG, Lala PK. Resis-tance of malignant trophoblast cells to both the anti-proliferative and anti-invasive effects of transforming growth factor beta. Exp Cell Res 1994;214:93—99.

29. Librach CL, Werb Z, Fitzgerald ML, Chiu K, Corwin NM, Esteves RA, Grobelny D, Galardy R, Damsky CH. 92 kDa type IV collagenase mediates invasion of human cytotrophoblasts. J Cell Biol 1991;113:437—449.

30. Polette M, Nawrocki B, Pintiaux A, Massenat C, Maquoi E, Volders L, Schaaps JP, Birembaut P, Foidart JM. Expression of gelatinases A and B and their tissue inhibitors by cells of early and term human placenta and gestational endometrium. Lab Invest 1994;71:838—846.

31. Bischof P, Friedli E, Martelli M, Campana A. Expression of extracellular matrix-degrading metalloproteases by cultured human cytotrophoblast cells: effect of cell adhesion and immuno-purification. Am J Obstet Gynecol 1991;65:1791—1801.

32. Puistola U, Ronnberg L, Martikainen H, Turpéenniemi-Hujanen T. The human embryo pro-duces basement membrane collagen (type IV collagen)-degrading protease activity. Hum Reprod 1989;4:309—311.

33. Kornberg L, Juliano RL. Signal transduction from the extracellular matrix: the integrin-tyro-sine kinase connection. TIPS 1992;13:93—95.

34. Giancotti FG, Ruoslahti E. Elevated levels of the alpha5 beta1 fibronectin receptor suppress the transformed phenotype of Chinese hamster ovary cells. Cell 1990;60:849—859.

35. Damsky CH, Fitzgerald M, Fisher SJ. Distribution patterns of extracellular matrix components and adhesion receptors are intricately modulated during first trimester cytotrophoblast differen-tiation along the invasive pathway in vivo. J Clin Invest 1992;89:210—222.

36. Bischof P, Redard M, Gindre P, Vassilakos P, Campana A. Localisation of alpha 2, alpha 5 and alpha 6 integrin subunits in human endometrium, decidua and trophoblast. Eur J Obstet Gyne-col Reprod Biol 1993;51:217—226.

37. Burrows TD, King A, Loke YW. Expression of integrins by human trophoblast and differential adhesion to laminin and fibronectin. Hum Reprod 1993;8:475—484.

38. Bischof P, Martelli M, Campana A, Itoh Y, Ogata Y, Nagase H. Importance of metalloprotein-ases (MMP) in human trophoblast invasion. Early Pregn Biol Med 1995;1:263—269.

39. Bischof P, Haenggeli L, Campana A. Gelatinase and oncofetal fibronectin secretion are depend-ent upon integrin expression on human cytotrophoblasts. Hum Reprod 1995;10:734—742.

40. Bischof P, Meisser A, Campana A, Tseng L. Effects of decidua-conditioned medium and insulin-like growth factor binding protein-1 on trophoblastic metalloproteinases and their inhibitors.

Placenta 1998;(In press).

41. Cross JC, Werb Z, Fisher SJ. Implantation and the placenta: key pieces of the development puzzle. Science 1994;266:1508–1518.

42. Tabibzadeh S, Babaknia A. The signals and molecular pathways involved in implantation, a symbiotic interaction between blastocyst and endometrium involving adhesion and tissue invasion. Mol Hum Reprod 1995;10:1579–1602.

43. Loke YW, King A. Human implantation. Cell biology and immunology. Cambridge, New York, Melbourne: Cambridge University Press, 1995;1–ff.

44. Bischof P, Campana A. A model for implantation of the human blastocyst and early placentation. Hum Reprod Update 1996;50:73–81.

# The fetal transplant: is HLA-G important?

Michael T. McMaster[1] and Susan J. Fisher[1-4]

*Departments of [1]Stomatology, [2]Anatomy, [3]Pharmaceutical Chemistry, and [4]Obstetrics, Gynecology, and Reproductive Sciences, University of California, San Francisco, California, USA*

**Abstract.** *Background.* The location of human placental trophoblasts at the maternal-fetal interface suggests they could play an important role in maternal immunologic tolerance of the fetal semiallograft. Central to this hypothesis is the fact that they suppress class Ia production while expressing HLA-G, a class Ib molecule.

*Methods.* Using monoclonal antibodies that recognize HLA-G, we immunostained tissue sections of the maternal-fetal interface containing cytotrophoblasts in all stages of differentiation and used immunoblotting to study the HLA-G isoforms produced by cytotrophoblasts in vitro and by the amnion-chorion in vivo.

*Results.* Immunolocalization studies showed that HLA-G is expressed by cytotrophoblasts that invade the uterus, and by both amniocytes and cytotrophoblasts in the amnion-chorion. Cytotrophoblasts, their conditioned medium and amniotic fluid contained heterodisperse immunoreactive bands ($M_r$ 35,000–50,000). *N*-deglycosylation by PNGase F digestion resolved these isoforms into two distinct bands. Cell samples contained primarily a $M_r$ 37,000–42,000 protein, most likely encoded by the full-length mRNA. Conditioned medium and amniotic fluid contained a slightly smaller protein, most likely the secreted form lacking the transmembrane and cytoplasmic regions. Removal of polylactosamine chains by *endo*-β-galactosidase digestion significantly reduced the electrophoretic mobility of the immunoreactive bands, suggesting that HLA-G, unlike class Ib molecules studied to date, carries *N*-acetyllactosamine units.

*Conclusion.* HLA-G production is upregulated as an integral part of cytotrophoblast differentiation along the invasive pathway and in the amnion-chorion. Cytotrophoblasts that are in direct contact with maternal tissues express this class Ib molecule. In addition, the fetus is also surrounded by cells (amniocytes) that express, and fluid that contains, HLA-G. The molecular weight heterogeneity of the HLA-G protein is due to an unusual type of glycosylation rather than to the translation of alternatively spliced mRNAs.

**Keywords:** amnion-chorion, amniotic fluid, class I MHC, placenta, pregnancy, trophoblast.

## Introduction

A central question in pregnancy immunology is how the fetal-placental unit, a semiallograft, avoids maternal immune rejection during pregnancy. Trophoblasts, the specialized epithelial cells of the placenta, are presumed to be essential to this unique phenomenon because they lie at the maternal-fetal interface. Here they come into direct contact with cells of the fully competent maternal immune system (for a recent review see [1,2]). Exactly how this occurs depends on their

*Address for correspondence:* Dr Michael McMaster, HSW 604, University of California San Francisco, San Francisco, CA 94143-0512, USA. Tel.: +1-415-476-6037. E-mail: mcmaster@cgl.ucsf.edu

location within the placenta, i.e., whether they are components of floating or anchoring villi. In floating villi, cytotrophoblast stem cells detach from the underlying basement membrane and fuse to form a syncytium that covers the villus and is in direct contact with maternal blood. In anchoring villi, cytotrophoblast stem cells differentiate by detaching from their basement membrane and aggregating to form columns of mononuclear cells that attach to and invade the uterine decidua (interstitial invasion) and its arterial system (endovascular invasion). Interstitial invasion puts cytotrophoblasts in direct contact with the highly specialized subset of leukocytes that home to the uterus during pregnancy. Endovascular invasion puts cytotrophoblasts (like syncytiotrophoblasts) in direct contact with maternal blood. Another subpopulation of extravillous cytotrophoblasts lies adjacent to the amniotic epithelium. Collectively, these chorionic cytotrophoblasts, the amniocytes, and the connective tissue with which they are associated are termed the amnion-chorion. Cytotrophoblasts in the amnion-chorion are also directly juxtaposed to maternal cells (decidua capsularis). Thus, antigen presentation by trophoblasts in several locations at the maternal-fetal interface is likely to be an important component of maternal immunological responses during pregnancy.

MHC class I molecules and the peptides they present are critical to alloreactivity (reviewed in [3,4]). Thus, one key to understanding maternal tolerance of the fetal semiallograft lies in studying trophoblast expression of class I molecules. None of the trophoblast populations express HLA-A, HLA-B, or class II (HLA-D) MHC molecules. Whether these cells express HLA-C is controversial [6,7]. But it is well established that cytotrophoblasts which invade the uterus express the full-length nonclassical (class Ib) HLA protein, HLA-G [8—13] and secrete a truncated form of this molecule (sHLA-G; [9,13]). Although HLA-G mRNA has been detected in other adult and fetal tissues by RT-PCR analyses (for a review see [14]), a subpopulation of thymic epithelia are the only other normal cells known to express the protein [15]. Interestingly, Paul et al. recently reported HLA-G mRNA and protein production by melanoma cells [16].

The HLA-G gene has an intron/exon organization identical to that of the class Ia genes (HLA-A, -B and -C), and the HLA-G protein product has 86% sequence identity to the class I consensus sequence [17]. With regard to the 5' flanking region of the gene, the HLA-G promoter has elements (e.g., AP-1, NFκB) that are similar to sequences found in class Ia genes but lacks an interferon response element [18], suggesting potentially novel transcriptional regulatory mechanisms. HLA-G has a lower molecular mass (37—39 kDa) than class Ia molecules due to a premature stop codon in exon 6 that results in deletion of all but six amino acids in the cytoplasmic tail [19]. The single $N$-linked glycosylation site (Asn 86) present in all class I molecules is conserved, as are the structurally important cysteines in the α2 and α3 domains [18].

Studies of HLA-G expression at the mRNA level suggest a high degree of complexity. To date, six different alternatively spliced mRNAs have been reported. In addition to the full-length (G1) form, transcripts lacking exon 3 (G2), exons 3 and 4 (G3), or exon 4 (G4) have been described [20,21]. These mRNAs encode proteins that lack either the α2, α2 and α3, or α3 domains. Additionally, cDNAs that potentially encode soluble molecules have been reported [22,23]. Thus, protein products of the HLA-G gene could vary widely in both molecular weight and function.

We have a long-standing interest in understanding the role of trophoblast HLA-G expression in maternal tolerance of the fetal semiallograft [9,12,13,24,25]. Toward this end we produced monoclonal antibodies (mAbs) that specifically recognize HLA-G. We used these antibodies to study trophoblast HLA-G protein expression in vivo and in vitro. The data presented here show that HLA-G production is upregulated as an integral part of cytotrophoblast differentiation along the invasive pathway and in the amnion-chorion. Taken together, our studies of HLA-G expression in various locations within the placenta and the amnion-chorion suggest that cytotrophoblasts that are in direct contact with maternal tissues express this class Ib molecule. In addition, we now know that the fetus is also surrounded by cells (amniocytes) that express, and fluid that contains, HLA-G. Immunoblotting studies of HLA-G produced by these tissues in vivo and in vitro showed that the molecular weight heterogeneity of HLA-G observed at the protein level is due to an unusual type of glycosylation, rather than to the translation of alternatively spliced mRNAs.

## Materials and

## ethods

### Monoclonal antibody production

The 1B8, 3F6 and 4H84 anti-HLA-G mAbs were produced as described [12,13]. Briefly, BALB/c mice (Charles River, Wilmington, MA) were immunized with a peptide corresponding to amino acids 61–83 of the α1 domain of HLA-G (EEETRNTKAHAQTDRMNLQTLRG) coupled to keyhole limpet hemocyanin. Hybridomas that secreted antibodies reactive with the peptide immunogen were initially screened by ELISA. Monoclonal Ab 16G1 was produced by using a synthetic peptide immunogen corresponding to the amino acid sequence encoded by intron 4 in an HLA-G mRNA interrupted by this intron [22]. Details of the methodology were published [26].

### Tissue and amniotic fluid collection

Informed consent was obtained from all patients from whom tissue, fluid, and blood samples were collected. Placentas and amnion-chorion were obtained from elective pregnancy terminations. Leukocytes were isolated from blood by centrifugation through Ficoll-Hypaque 1027 (Sigma, St. Louis, MO). Amniotic fluid samples collected during weeks 16 to 18 of pregnancy were obtained from the UCSF Cytogenetics Laboratory. Amniotic fluid samples collected during the third trimester of pregnancy were obtained after amniocentesis for fetal lung maturity assessment. Fluids were stored at 4°C before centrifugation to remove cells, then stored at − 20°C until analyzed.

## Immunofluorescence

Immunofluorescence was performed as previously described on frozen sections of either first trimester placental bed samples or second trimester amnion-chorion [12]. Hybridoma conditioned medium was diluted 1:100. All sections were double stained with anti-HLA-G mAbs and anticytokeratin (7D3).

## Preparation of cell lysate and conditioned medium samples

Highly purified cytotrophoblasts were isolated from first, second and third trimester chorionic villi as previously described. Cells ($1 \times 10^6$) were plated in 35-mm culture wells coated with the extracellular matrix preparation Matrigel (Collaborative Research, Bedford, MA) in 2 ml MEM (UCSF Cell Culture Facility) containing 2% Nutridoma (Boehringer Mannheim Biochemicals, Indianapolis, IN). After 36 to 48 h, the conditioned medium was centrifuged to remove any cellular debris, aliquotted, and frozen at − 80°C until analysis. The cells were collected in cold lysis buffer containing 150 mM NaCl, 10 mM Tris (pH 8.0), 0.5% Nonidet P-40 (Sigma), and protease inhibitors (1 mM PMSF, 5 mM EDTA, 5 μg/ml aprotinin). Lysates were clarified by centrifugation at $16,000 \times g$ for 15 min at 4°C. Anchoring chorionic villi were dissected from placentas and cultured for 12 to 36 h, as previously described [29], before the cells and conditioned medium were processed as described for cytotrophoblasts. JEG-3 cells were cultured in MEM (UCSF Cell Culture Facility) supplemented with 10% fetal bovine serum (Hyclone Laboratories, Logan, UT) and processed as for the cytotrophoblasts and their conditioned medium. PBL lysates were also prepared as described above for the cytotrophoblasts.

## Immunoblotting

Samples were resolved in 10% SDS-PAGE gels and electroblotted to nitrocellulose membranes (Schleicher and Schuell, Keene, NH) according to published methods. Immunoblotting was performed using standard methods as described [13].

## Glycosidase treatments

Peptide-$N$-glycosidase F (peptide $N^4$-[$N$-acetyl-β-glycosaminyl]asparagine amidase F; PNGase F) was obtained from Boehringer Mannheim. Prior to $N$-deglycosylation, cell lysates, conditioned media, amniotic fluid, and cervical swab samples were boiled for 5 min in 20 mM $NaPO_4$, pH 7.2, 50 mM EDTA, 10 mM Na azide, and 0.05% SDS. PNGase was then added (8 U/ml) and the samples were incubated overnight at 37°C. Endo-β-D-galactosidase was obtained from V-Labs Inc. (Covington, LA). Digestions with this enzyme (overnight at 37°C) were carried out in 50 mM sodium acetate, pH 5.5. Following glycosidase treatment, samples were boiled in SDS-PAGE sample buffer and either electrophoresed immediately or stored at − 80°C for later analyses.

## Results

*HLA-G is expressed by invasive cytotrophoblasts and by both amniocytes and cytotrophoblasts in the amnion-chorion*

Immunohistochemical analysis using fluorescent detection was carried out on frozen sections of placenta and placental bed prepared from tissues obtained during the first, second and third trimesters of pregnancy. Sections contained floating chorionic villi and anchoring villi (including cytotrophoblast cell columns) as well as decidualized endometrium and myometrium. Thus, cytotrophoblast stem cells, as well as differentiated trophoblasts (syncytiotrophoblasts and invasive cytotrophoblasts), were evident. Sections were double stained with an anticytokeratin antibody (7D3), which in the placental bed is specific for trophoblast cells [27], and with anti-HLA-G mAbs (1B8, 3F6 or 4H84).

Figure 1 shows the staining pattern when the anticytokeratin (panels A, C and E) and 1B8 (panels B, D and F) mAbs were reacted with sections of second-trimester (18-week) placenta and placental bed. None of the components of floating villi, including undifferentiated cytotrophoblasts anchored to the villus basement membrane and fetal elements within the villus core, reacted with the anti-HLA-G antibodies. In contrast, invasive cytotrophoblasts within the cell columns of anchoring villi stained brightly (Fig. 1, panel B). Antibody reactivity was first detected in the distal part of the cell columns as the cytotrophoblasts made contact with the uterine wall. Cytotrophoblasts participating in interstitial invasion also stained brightly (Fig. 1, panel D). During this stage of pregnancy, when endovascular invasion peaks, cytotrophoblasts within blood vessels also showed intense reactivity with the anti-HLA-G antibodies (Fig. 1, panel F). Incubation of tissues with primary or secondary antibodies alone, or with nonimmune mouse serum or normal mouse IgG, showed no reactivity (data not shown).

Cytotrophoblast staining in first trimester samples was nearly identical to that in second trimester tissue. None of the floating villi components reacted with either antibody. The only exception was occasional syncytial brush border staining. Third trimester tissue exhibited the same pattern; floating villi (including the syncytial brush border) did not stain whereas interstitial and endovascular cytotrophoblasts reacted with the antibodies. However, by the third trimester, cytotrophoblasts within the uterine wall appeared to stain less brightly than cells in a comparable location earlier in gestation.

We also stained frozen sections of second trimester (18-week) amnion-chorion

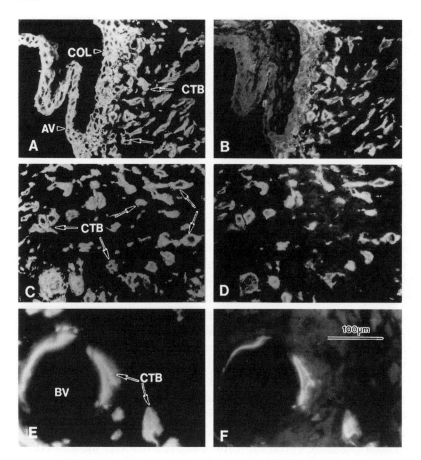

*Fig. 1.* HLA-G protein is produced by invasive cytotrophoblasts in-vivo. Frozen sections of 18-week placenta and placental bed were double-labeled with rat mAb 7D3 (anticytokeratin) and mouse mAb 1B8 (anti-HLA-G). Panels **A, C** and **E** show cytokeratin staining detected with rhodamine-conjugated antirat secondary antibodies. Panels **B, D** and **F** show HLA-G staining detected with fluorescein-conjugated antimouse secondary antibodies. Panels **A** and **B** show a section containing an anchoring villus (AV) with associated cytotrophoblast cell column (COL) and decidua. Panels **C** and **D** show interstitial trophoblasts within the decidua. Panels **E** and **F** show a blood vessel (BV) within the deep decidua that has been infiltrated with trophoblasts. Individual cytotrophoblast cells (CTB) are indicated by arrows. (Reprinted from McMaster et al. with permission.)

with anticytokeratin (7D3), to distinguish amniocytes and cytotrophoblasts (Fig. 2C,E), and with anti-HLA-G (4H84). All cells of the amnion layer reacted with the mAb that specifically recognized HLA-G (Fig. 2D). Many of the multilayered cytotrophoblasts within the chorion also reacted with the antibody, but not all cells stained with equal intensity, and some cells failed to demonstrate any immunoreactivity (Fig. 2F). In addition, a few cells that did not express cytokeratin reacted weakly with 4H84.

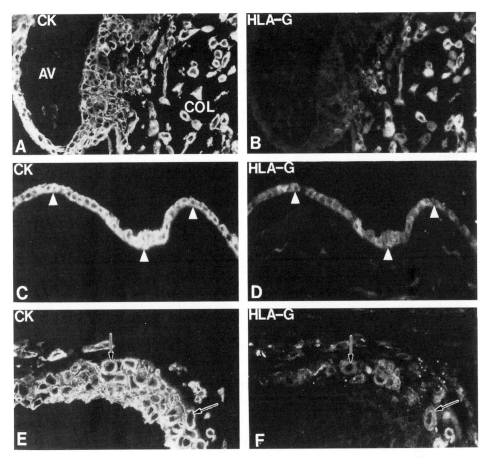

*Fig. 2.* Invasive cytotrophoblasts, as well as cytotrophoblasts and amniocytes in the amnion-chorion (extraembryonic membranes), express HLA-G protein in vivo. Frozen sections of 18-week placental bed and amnion-chorion tissue samples were double stained with mAb 7D3 (rat anticytokeratin) and mAb 4H84 (mouse anti-HLA-G). Panels **A**, **C** and **E** show cytokeratin (CK) staining detected with rhodamine-conjugated secondary antibodies. Panels **B**, **D** and **F** show HLA-G staining detected with fluorescein-conjugated secondary antibodies. Panels **A** and **B** show a section of placental bed containing an anchoring villus (AV) with an associated cell column (COL) of invasive cytotrophoblasts. Panels **C** and **D** demonstrate staining of the amnion layer of the fetal membranes (arrowheads). Panels **E** and **F** show staining of cytotrophoblasts within the chorion (individual cytotrophoblasts indicated by arrows). (Reprinted from McMaster et al. with permission.)

*Immunoblot characterization of the HLA-G heavy chain protein produced by placental villi, invasive cytotrophoblasts and JEG choriocarcinoma cells*

SDS-PAGE and immunoblotting of detergent extracts of early gestation (12-week) chorionic villi showed the HLA-G heavy chains as heterodisperse immunoreactive bands smeared across a molecular weight range of approximately $M_r$ 39,000—48,000 (Fig. 3). Conditioned medium from first trimester (12-week) pla-

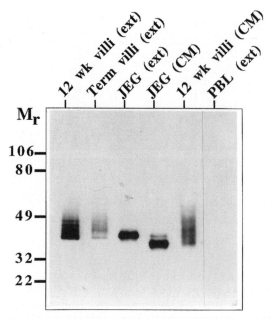

*Fig. 3.* Placental HLA-G heavy chains migrate as heterodisperse bands. In immunoblot analyses the 4H84 mAb reacted with a broad array of HLA-G isoforms present in extracts (ext) of placental chorionic villi, and in conditioned medium (CM) collected from villus explant cultures. In contrast, JEG cell extracts and conditioned medium samples contained much more discrete bands of $M_r$ 40,000-43,000 and 37,000—40,000, respectively. The anti-HLA-G mAb did not react with any proteins in extracts of peripheral blood leukocytes (PBL). (Reprinted from McMaster et al. with permission.)

cental villi cultured for 48 h contained bands that spanned a similar molecular weight range and also included isoforms of slightly lower molecular weight. These results were typical of those we obtained from early gestation samples, although some contained isoforms of even higher molecular weight. Analysis of extracts prepared from term placental villi showed that they contained less HLA-G per mg protein and that the bands detected were less heterodisperse. We then investigated whether a cytotrophoblast cell line (JEG-3) that produces HLA-G makes a similar array of heavy chain proteins. 4H84 reacted with a $M_r$ 40,000 − 43,000 protein in extracts prepared from JEG cells (Fig. 3). In contrast, the major band identified in conditioned medium from these cells was a $M_r$ 37,000—40,000 protein. Both these bands displayed much less molecular weight heterogeneity than those detected in placenta-derived samples. We also investigated the nature of the HLA-G heavy chains produced by primary cultures of purified first trimester cytotrophoblasts that were allowed to differentiate along the invasive pathway in vitro. Both cell extracts (Fig. 4) and conditioned medium samples contained heterodisperse immunoreactive bands that resembled those detected in samples of placental villi rather than the HLA-G produced by JEG cells.

It was also important to know whether 4H84 cross-reacted with classical MHC class I molecules expressed by other cells. A sample of a detergent lysate of pe-

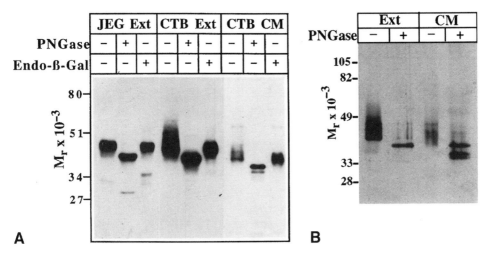

*Fig. 4.* Placental HLA-G molecular weight heterogeneity is due primarily to glycosylation. **A:** JEG and cytotrophoblast cell extracts and cytotrophoblast-conditioned medium (CM) were analyzed by immunoblotting without treatment ( − ) or after digestion (+) with either PNGase F, which *N*-degly-cosylates the molecule, or endo-β-D-galactosidase (Endo-β-Gal), which removes polylactosamine chains, leaving the oligosaccharide core intact. In comparison to HLA-G in JEG cell extracts, re-moval of oligosaccharide units from placental HLA-G significantly reduced the molecular weight heterogeneity of the molecule. **B:** Enzymatic *N*-deglycosylation of HLA-G in extracts of early gesta-tion chorionic villi similarly resulted in a single major band of $M_r$ 37,000−39,000. PNGase F treat-ment of conditioned medium from villus explant cultures revealed a prominent band that comigrated with cell-associated HLA-G. A slightly lower molecular weight band, migrating as a doublet in some samples, was consistently detected and presumably represents the soluble form of the molecule. (Re-printed from McMaster et al. with permission.)

ripheral blood leukocytes (PBLs) obtained from a single individual contained no 4H84-immunoreactive proteins (Fig. 3). PBLs from at least 20 other individuals were analyzed with identical results (data not shown). In addition, we have used this mAb for immunolocalization on tissue sections prepared from at least 30 dif-ferent placental samples and have never seen cross-reactivity with other class I (Ia) molecules on maternal and nontrophoblast fetal cells within these speci-mens. Thus, although it is not technically feasible to test this mAb for cross-reac-tivity against all alleles, 4H84 does not appear to cross-react with the commonly expressed classical class I molecules.

*Placental HLA-G does not contain epitopes encoded by intron 4*

Previous reports suggested that soluble HLA-G is the product of an alternatively spliced mRNA that contains intron 4 [22]. This mRNA has a stop codon 21 ami-no acids after the α3 domain, thus excluding the transmembrane region. LCL.221 cells transfected with a construct that expresses this mRNA released the corresponding protein, $G_{sol}$. To determine if the $G_{sol}$ molecule contributed to the molecular weight heterogeneity of the placental HLA-G heavy chains, we

670

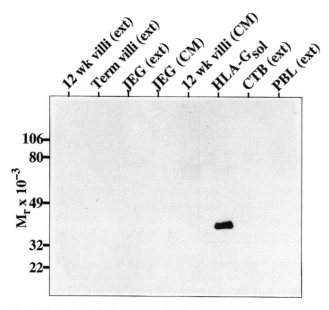

*Fig. 5.* Placental cells do not translate into protein an alternatively spliced HLA-G mRNA that contains intron 4. Placental cell extracts and conditioned medium were analyzed by immunoblotting with mAb 16G1, raised against a synthetic peptide corresponding to a portion of the intron 4 sequence. A recombinant $G_{sol}$ sample served as a positive and PBL extracts as a negative control. Among these samples the mAb 16G1 reacted only with the recombinant protein. (Reprinted from McMaster et al. with permission.)

analyzed placental cell extracts and conditioned medium by immunoblotting with mAb 16G1 (Fig. 5). This mAb was raised against a synthetic peptide corresponding to a portion of the intron 4 sequence [22]. As a positive control we included a recombinant $G_{sol}$ sample and as a negative control we analyzed PBL extracts. The mAb 16G1 reacted strongly with the recombinant protein but failed to react with the cell extracts or conditioned medium from placental villi, purified cytotrophoblasts, or JEG-3 cells.

*The array of placental HLA-G isoforms is primarily due to glycosylation*

The broad molecular weight range of the HLA-G immunoreactive bands in placental villi and cytotrophoblast samples could be due to the presence of other splice variants of the molecule or to heterogeneous glycosylation. To assess the role of glycosylation, we treated cytotrophoblast and JEG-3 cell lysates with PNGase F, an asparagine amidase that releases $N$-linked oligosaccharide chains, and then analyzed the products by immunoblotting with 4H84. The results are shown in Fig. 4A. After N-deglycosylation, the antibody primarily reacted with a more discrete band ($M_r$ 37,000–42,000) in cytotrophoblast extracts; a great deal of the smearing previously observed was eliminated. This band had an electrophoretic mobility similar to that of HLA-G in JEG cell extracts that had also been treated with peptide-$N$-glycosidase F. Likewise, enzymatic $N$-deglycosylation of HLA-G in extracts of early gestation chorionic villi resulted in a single major band of $M_r$ 37,000—39,000 band (Fig. 4B). PNGase F treatment of conditioned medium from villus explant cultures revealed a prominent band that comigrated with cell-associated HLA-G. One slightly lower molecular weight band, presumably the soluble form of the molecule, was consistently detected. In some samples this band migrated as a doublet (Fig. 4B). Thus, $N$-deglycosylation resolved the HLA-G isoforms into more discrete bands, indicating that the molecular weight heterogeneity observed before treatment was primarily due to $N$-linked glycosylation, which could add $\sim M_r$ 10,000 to the estimated molecular weight of the molecule.

Our previous work shows that trophoblasts add polylactosamine carbohydrate chains (repeating units of either Galβ1,3GlcNAc (type 1) or Galβ1,4GlcNAc (type 2) to fibronectin and certain integrin receptors — molecules that carry simple bi- and triantennary chains when they are isolated from other cellular sources [31,32]. The 4H84-immunoreactive bands observed in the chorionic villus and cytotrophoblast samples had a ladder-like appearance that was reminiscent of the polylactosaminylated placental glycoproteins we described previously [33]. This suggested that HLA-G from placental sources might carry this unusual modification. To test this hypothesis we treated cytotrophoblast samples with endo-β-D-galactosidase (V-Labs, Inc., Covington, LA), an enzyme that hydrolyzes polylactosamine oligosaccharide units but leaves the rest of the saccharide core intact. This treatment increased the mobility of placental HLA-G and decreased the molecular mass heterogeneity and ladder-like appearance of the bands (Fig. 4A). As expected since this enzyme only partially deglycosylates the molecule, the endo-β-D-galactosidase-treated HLA-G was intermediate in mobility between untreated and PNGase-treated samples. The mobility of JEG-3 HLA-G was unaffected by treatment with this enzyme, indicating that this cell line does not add polylactosamine units to the oligosaccharides it carries.

*Polylactosaminylated HLA-G isoforms are detected in amniotic fluid*

We have been very interested in the possibility that biological fluids of either maternal or fetal origin contain HLA-G. Given the pattern of HLA-G protein expression in the amnion-chorion, it seemed likely that this molecule might be detected in amniotic fluid. To test this hypothesis, 30 samples were collected from women undergoing amniocentesis for prenatal genetic testing at 16 to 18 weeks of pregnancy; 10 samples were obtained from women undergoing amniocentesis for fetal maturity assessment in the third trimester of pregnancy. By immunoblot analysis, we detected HLA-G in every sample. Representative results are shown in Fig. 6. 4H84 reacted with bands of varying intensity that had different degrees of molecular weight heterogeneity in all of these samples. These differences did not correlate with gestational age. Treatment of the samples with

672

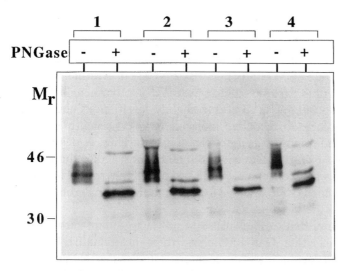

*Fig. 6.* Highly glycosylated HLA-G isoforms are detected in amniotic fluid by immunoblotting. Lanes 1 and 2 contained early gestation samples (5 µl); lanes 3 and 4 contained third trimester samples (5 µl). Treatment of the samples with PNGase F collapsed the broad bands detected in the untreated samples into a prominent $M_r$ 35,000−36,000 band. Most samples also contained a much less intense band corresponding to the mobility of the cell-associated form of the molecule ($\sim M_r$ 38,000). The faint $M_r$ 47,000 band in the enzyme-treated samples was due to nonspecific reactivity with the secondary antibody. (Reprinted from McMaster et al. with permission.)

PNGase F collapsed the broad bands detected in the untreated samples into a prominent $M_r$ 35,000−36,000 band corresponding to the estimated molecular weight of the secreted form of HLA-G detected in placental villus conditioned medium. A much less intense band, corresponding to the mobility of the cell-associated form of the molecule ($\sim M_r$ 38,000), was also detected in most of these samples. The faint $M_r$ 47,000 band in the enzyme-treated samples was due to nonspecific reactivity of the secondary antibody used in this experiment. As with the placental samples, endo-β-D-galactosidase treatment of amniotic fluid resulted in a significant reduction in molecular weight heterogeneity of the immunoreactive bands (data not shown).

## Discussion

The discovery that HLA-G is expressed by the human placenta represents a major advance in our understanding of factors that govern interactions between maternal and fetal cells during pregnancy. This finding resolves the long-standing controversy regarding trophoblast class I molecule expression and provides a framework for developing testable hypotheses concerning the role of specific molecules. In this regard, knowing the exact location of the placental cells that express this Ib molecule is important for formulating hypotheses about how HLA-G functions. As to which of the organ's component cells express HLA-G, most published studies suggest that only its specialized epithelial cells, termed cytotrophoblasts, synthesize HLA-G mRNA and protein [12—14,34].

Another layer of complexity is added to the interpretation of the immunolocalization data by the fact that whereas cytotrophoblasts are found in three different locations, in only two of these sites do they express HLA-G. With regard to the first location, our early immunolocalization study with anti-HLA-G antibodies [12] showed that cytotrophoblast stem cells anchored to the basement membranes of chorionic villi do not express this class Ib molecule. But extravillous cytotrophoblasts that detach from this basement membrane and migrate through the columns that connect the placenta to the uterus upregulate HLA-G expression. Expression in this second location is maintained once the cells have reached their final destination — either the interstitium of the uterine wall or the maternal vessels that traverse this region [12]. Our findings have since been confirmed by a different group using yet another anti-HLA-G antibody [34]. The fact that our second-generation antibodies (e.g., 4H84; [13]) failed to react with cytotrophoblast stem cells but stained the extravillous population confirmed these results.

Much less is known about cytotrophoblast expression of HLA-G in the third location — the amnion-chorion. The possibility that this subpopulation of cells expresses HLA-G was first suggested by the work of Ellis et al. [8] who found, by using Northern hybridization, that cytotrophoblasts isolated from the amnion-chorion expressed HLA-G mRNA. Subsequently, other studies confirmed this finding [35] and showed that amniotic epithelia also express this mRNA [10]. To our knowledge, the present study is the first report of the results of immunolocalization experiments using an HLA-G-specific antibody to study expression of this antigen in the amnion-chorion. In accordance with the mRNA data, we found that both cytotrophoblasts and amniocytes stained brightly with mAb 4H84. This prompted us to consider whether HLA-G produced by either cell type may also be a component of amniotic fluid. Immunoblot analyses, performed with the same antibody, confirmed this hypothesis. Taken together, our studies of HLA-G expression in various locations within the placenta and the amnion-chorion suggest that cytotrophoblasts that are in direct contact with maternal tissues express this class Ib molecule. In addition, we now know that the fetus is also surrounded by fluid that contains HLA-G.

We are interested in using the 4H84 mAb and the results of the studies reported here to design experiments to understand how HLA-G affects the maternal, and possibly the fetal, immune response during pregnancy. In this regard our immunoblotting data suggest that the biological activity of this molecule resides in either the full-length protein or a previously described truncated form [9], the exact origin of which remains elusive. We found no evidence that placental cells produce a soluble protein encoded by an HLA-G mRNA species that contains intron 4. Likewise, we failed to detect any immunoreactive bands corresponding to the predicted molecular weights of the proteins that would be encoded by the other alternatively spliced mRNAs that have been described (G2, $M_r$ 26,000; G3, $M_r$ 15,000; G4, $M_r$ 25,000; "intron 4" HLA-G, $M_r$ 31,000). In support of this conclusion, extensive Northern hybridization experiments carried out in our laboratory and by other investigators failed to detect transcripts that correspond to the predicted size of these splice variants [9,11,12,36,37]. Thus, it seems likely that the alternatively spliced mRNAs that are frequently detected using RT-PCR (reviewed in [4]) are not translated into protein.

A number of recent studies have focused on the role that HLA-G plays in regulating the maternal immune response to the fetus. In vivo, cytotrophoblasts in two locations could be involved in this phenomenon. Whereas little is known about maternal leukocyte interactions with fetal cells in the amnion-chorion, a great deal of evidence suggests that the HLA-G-positive cytotrophoblasts within the uterine wall are in direct contact with the unusual maternal natural-killer (NK) cells that reside in this location. Cell−cell interactions within the uterine wall have been simulated in vitro by coculturing LCL.221 cells that overexpress HLA-G with peripheral or decidual NK clones. Using this approach, several groups have reported HLA-G-specific inhibitory receptors on NK cells [38−41].

These observations led several groups to conclude that HLA-G, like class Ia molecules, downregulates NK cell activity by interacting with an inhibitory receptor complex − CD94/NKG2A. Data in support of this theory [38,40,42,43], have recently been shown to be an artifact of the LCL.221 targets in which HLA-G was expressed. Initially, McMichael and colleagues made the surprising discovery that HLA-E preferably binds peptides that are derived from the signal sequences of other MHC class I molecules, but cannot bind its own leader peptide [44]. This unexpected result caused them to investigate the consequences of transfecting MHC class I genes into LCL.221 cells, which normally express free HLA-E heavy chains that are retained intracellularly. They found that the transfectants showed cell surface expression of both HLA-E and the newly introduced class I molecule. This finding has a great many implications with regard to class I studies that have utilized LCL.221 cells. With specific regard to inhibitory receptor ligands, the McMichael group proved that the CD94/NKG2A complex interacts with HLA-E, but not with HLA-G or other class Ia molecules [45,46]. Thus, the mechanisms by which HLA-G inhibits immune activity are once again open to question.

While the identification of HLA-G-specific receptors on maternal effector cells remains elusive, it is suggestive that some inhibitory receptors are lectin-type molecules. This raises the possibility that the types of carbohydrate chains HLA-G carries might be relevant to its biological activity. Thus, it is interesting to note that HLA-G carries an unusual type of glycosylation. Like all other human class I molecules, it contains a single $N$-linked glycosylation site (Asn 86). But here the similarities end. Whereas the MHC class Ia molecules carry simple biantennary structures [47], HLA-G oligosaccharides are modified by the addition of numerous polylactosamine units. We hypothesize that such a modification could increase the stability of the molecule in the proteinase-rich environment of the uterus. This appears to be one function of the polylactosaminylated saccharides carried by placental fibronectins [33]. Additionally, we are intrigued by the possibility that the unusual glycosylation HLA-G carries might enhance its ability to interact with receptors on NK or other maternal effector cells.

The finding that HLA-G produced by chorionic cytotrophoblasts and amniocytes is easily detected in amniotic fluid raises the additional possibility that this class Ib molecule could function during development of the fetal immune system. In this regard it is interesting to note that, beginning in early pregnancy, the fetus swallows amniotic fluid. Oral exposure is known to have efficacy in re-establishing tolerance to antigens that are implicated in autoimmune diseases such as multiple sclerosis [48] and diabetes [49]. Whether this route of exposure could explain how tolerance to HLA-G is established remains to be determined.

Together, these observations probably reflect the fact that the placenta performs many unique functions, some of which change dramatically during pregnancy. Enhanced metalloproteinase expression [28] and integrin switching [50] are characteristics of the early gestation cytotrophoblasts that mediate uterine invasion. Downregulating the expression of these genes is probably one mechanism that controls cytotrophoblast invasiveness. In contrast, extravillous cytotrophoblasts of all gestational ages express HLA-G in vivo and retain the ability to upregulate its production in vitro. These observations are consistent with the fact that the cells need only transiently express invasive characteristics, but must consistently avoid maternal immune surveillance.

# References

1. Fisher SJ, Damsky CH. Human cytotrophoblast invasion. Semin Cell Biol 1993;4:183—188.
2. Cross JC, Werb Z, Fisher SJ. Implantation and the placenta: key pieces of the development puzzle. Science 1994;266:1508—1518.
3. Sherman LA, Chattopadhyay S. The molecular basis of allorecognition. Ann Rev Immunol 1993;11:385—402.
4. Maffei A, Harris PE. Peptides bound to major histocompatibility complex molecules. Peptides 1998;19:179—198.
5. Bulmer JN, Johnson PM. Antigen expression by trophoblast populations in the human placenta and their possible immunobiological relevance. Placenta 1985;6:127—140.
6. Redman CW, McMichael AJ, Stirrat GM, Sunderland CA, Ting A. Class 1 major histocompatibility complex antigens on human extravillous trophoblast. Immunology 1984;52:457—468.
7. King A, Boocock C, Sharkey AM, Gardner L, Beretta A, Siccardi AG, Loke YW. Evidence for the expression of HLAA-C class I mRNA and protein by human first trimester trophoblast. J Immunol 1996;156:2068—2076.
8. Ellis SA, Palmer MS, McMichael AJ. Human trophoblast and the choriocarcinoma cell line BeWo express a truncated HLA Class I molecule. J Immunol 1990;144:731—735.
9. Kovats S, Main EK, Librach C, Stubblebine M, Fisher SJ, DeMars R. A class I antigen, HLA-G, expressed in human trophoblasts. Science 1990;248:220—223.
10. Yelavarthi KK, Fishback JL, Hunt JS. Analysis of HLA-G mRNA in human placental and extraplacental membrane cells by in situ hybridization. J Immunol 1991;146:2847—2854.
11. Chumbley G, King A, Holmes N, Loke YW. In situ hybridization and northern blot demonstration of HLA-G mRNA in human trophoblast populations by locus-specific oligonucleotide. Hum Immunol 1993;37:17—22.
12. McMaster MT, Librach CL, Zhou Y, Lim KH, Janatpour MJ, DeMars R, Kovats S, Damsky C, Fisher SJ. Human placental HLA-G expression is restricted to differentiated cytotrophoblasts.

J Immunol 1995;154:3771−3778.

13. McMaster MT, Zhou Y, Shorter S, Kapasi K, Geraghty D, Lim KH, Fisher SJ. HLA-G isoforms produced by placental cytotrophoblasts and found in amniotic fluid are due to unusual glycosylation. J Immunol 1998;160:5922−5928.

14. Le Bouteiller P, Lenfant F. Antigen-presenting function(s) of the nonclassical HLA-E, -F and -G class I molecules: the beginning of a story. Res Immunol 1996;147:301−313.

15. Crisa L, McMaster MT, Ishii JK, Fisher SJ, Salomon DR. Identification of a thymic epithelial cell subset sharing expression of the class Ib HLA-G molecule with fetal trophoblasts. J Exp Med 1997;186:289−298.

16. Paul P, Rouas-Freiss N, Khalil-Daher I, Moreau P, Riteau B, Le Gal FA, Avril MF, Dausset J, Guillet JG, Carosella ED. HLA-G expression in melanoma: a way for tumor cells to escape from immunosurveillance. Proc Natl Acad Sci USA 1998;95:4510−4515.

17. Parham P, Lomen CE, Lawlor DA, Ways JP, Holmes N, Coppin HL, Salter RD, Wan AM, Ennis PD. Nature of polymorphism in HLA-A, -B, and -C molecules. Proc Natl Acad Sci USA 1988; 85:4005−4009.

18. Geraghty DE, Koller BH, Orr HT. A human major histocompatibility complex class I gene that encodes a protein with a shortened cytoplasmic segment. Proc Natl Acad Sci USA 1987;84: 9145−9149.

19. Shimizu Y, Geraghty DE, Koller BH, Orr HT, DeMars R. Transfer and expression of three cloned human non-HLA-A,B,C class I major histocompatibility complex genes in mutant lymphoblastoid cells. Proc Natl Acad Sci USA 1988;85:227−231.

20. Ishitani A, Geraghty DE. Alternative splicing of HLA-G transcripts yields proteins with primary structures resembling both class I and class II antigens. Proc Natl Acad Sci USA 1992; 89:3947−3951.

21. Kirszenbaum M, Moreau P, Gluckman E, Dausset J, Carosella E. An alternatively spliced form of HLA-G mRNA in human trophoblasts and evidence for the presence of HLA-G transcript in adult lymphocytes. Proc Natl Acad Sci USA 1994;91:4209−4213.

22. Fujii T, Ishitani A, Geraghty DE. A soluble form of the HLA-G antigen is encoded by a messenger ribonucleic acid containing intron 4. J Immunol 1994;153:5516−5524.

23. Moreau P, Carosella E, Teyssier M, Prost S, Gluckman E, Dausset J, Kirszenbaum M. Soluble HLA-G molecule. An alternatively spliced HLA-G mRNA form candidate to encode it in peripheral blood mononuclear cells and human trophoblasts. Hum Immunol 1995;43:231−236.

24. Kovats S, Librach C, Fisch P, Main EK, Sondel PM, Fisher SF, DeMars R. Expression and possible functions of the HLA-G alpha chain in human cytotrophoblasts. In: Chaouat G, Mowbray J (eds) Cellular and Molecular Biology of the Materno-Fetal Relationship, vol 212. London: John Libbey Eurotext Ltd., 1991;21−29.

25. Roth I, Corry DB, Locksley RM, Abrams JS, Litton MJ, Fisher SJ. Human placental cytotrophoblasts produce the immunosuppressive cytokine interleukin 10. J Exp Med 1996;184: 539−548.

26. Lee N, Malacko AR, Ishitani A, Chen MC, Bajorath J, Marquardt H, Geraghty DE. The membrane-bound and soluble forms of HLA-G bind identical sets of endogenous peptides but differ with respect to TAP association. Immunity 1995;3:591−600.

27. Fisher SJ, Cui TY, Zhang L, Hartman L, Grahl K, Zhang GY, Tarpey J, Damsky CH. Adhesive and degradative properties of human placental cytotrophoblast cells in vitro. J Cell Biol 1989;109:891−902.

28. Librach CL, Werb Z, Fitzgerald ML, Chiu K, Corwin NM, Esteves RA, Grobelny D, Galardy R, Damsky CH, Fisher SJ. 92-kD type IV collagenase mediates invasion of human cytotrophoblasts. J Cell Biol 1991;113:437−449.

29. Genbacev O, Powlin SS, Miller RK. Regulation of human extravillus trophoblast (EVT) cell differentiation and proliferation in vitro − role of epidermal growth factor (EGF). Troph Res 1994;8:427−442.

30. Towbin H, Staehelin T, Gordon J. Electrophoretic transfer of proteins from polyacrylamide gels

to nitrocellulose sheets: procedure and some applications. Proc Natl Acad Sci USA 1979;76: 4350—4354.

31. Zhu BC, Laine RA. Polylactosamine glycosylation on human fetal placental fibronectin weakens the binding affinity of fibronectin to gelatin. J Biol Chem 1985;260:4041—4045.

32. Moss L, Prakobphol A,Wiedmann TW, Fisher SJ, Damsky CH. Glycosylation of human trophoblast integrins is stage- and cell-type specific. Glycobiology 1994;4:567—575.

33. Zhu BC, Fisher SF, Pande H, Calaycay J, Shively JE, Laine RA. Human placental (fetal) fibronectin: increased glycosylation and higher protease resistance than plasma fibronectin. Presence of polylactosamine glycopeptides and properties of a 44-kilodalton chymotryptic collagen-binding domain: difference from human plasma fibronectin. J Biol Chem 1984;259:3962—3970.

34. Loke YW, King A, Burrows T, Gardner L, Bowen M, Hiby S, Howlett S, Holmes N, Jacobs D. Evaluation of trophoblast HLA-G antigen with a specific monoclonal antibody. Tissue Antigens 1997;50:135—146.

35. Houlihan JM, Biro PA, Harper HM, Jenkinson HJ, Holmes CH. The human amnion is a site of MHC class Ib expression: evidence for the expression of HLA-E and HLA-G. J Immunol 1995;154:5665—5674.

36. Risk JM, Johnson PM. Northern blot analysis of HLA-G expression by BeWo human choriocarcinoma cells. J Reprod Immunol 1990;18:199—203.

37. Yang Y, Geraghty DE, Hunt JS. Cytokine regulation of HLA-G expression in human trophoblast cell lines. J Reprod Immunol 1995;29:179—195.

38. Pazmany L, Mandelboim O,Vales-Gomez M, Davis DM, Reyburn HT, Strominger JL. Protection from natural killer cell-mediated lysis by HLA-G expression on target cells. Science 1996;274:792—795.

39. Soderstrom K, Corliss B, Lanier LL, Phillips JH. CD94/NKG2 is the predominant inhibitory receptor involved in recognition of HLA-G by decidual and peripheral blood NK cells. J Immunol 1997;159:1072—1075.

40. Rouas-Freiss N, Marchal RE, Kirszenbaum M, Dausset J, Carosella ED. The alpha1 domain of HLA-G1 and HLA-G2 inhibits cytotoxicity induced by natural killer cells: is HLA-G the public ligand for natural killer cell inhibitory receptors? Proc Natl Acad Sci USA 1997;94:5249—5254.

41. Rouas-Freiss N, Goncalves RM, Menier C, Dausset J, Carosella ED. Direct evidence to support the role of HLA-G in protecting the fetus from maternal uterine natural killer cytolysis. Proc Natl Acad Sci USA 1997;94:11520—11525.

42. Pende D, Sivori S, Accame L, Pareti L, Falco M, Geraghty D, Le Bouteiller P, Moretta L, Moretta A. HLA-G recognition by human natural killer cells. Involvement of CD94 both as inhibitory and as activating receptor complex. Eur J Immunol 1997;27:1875—1880.

43. Münz C, Holmes N, King A, Loke YW, Colonna M, Schild H, Rammensee HG. Human histocompatibility leukocyte antigen (HLA)-G molecules inhibit NKAT3 expressing natural killer cells. J Exp Med 1997;185:385—391.

44. Braud V, Jones EY, McMichael A. The human major histocompatibility complex class Ib molecule HLA-E binds signal sequence-derived peptides with primary anchor residues at positions 2 and 9. Eur J Immunol 1997;27:1164—1169.

45. Braud VM, Allan DS, O'Callaghan CA, Söderström K, D'Andrea A, Ogg GS, Lazetic S,Young NT, Bell JI, Phillips JH, Lanier LL, McMichael AJ. HLA-E binds to natural killer cell receptors CD94/NKG2A, B and C. Nature 1998;391:795—799.

46. Lanier LL. Follow the leader: NK cell receptors for classical and nonclassical MHC class I. Cell 1998;92:705—707.

47. Barber LD, Patel TP, Percival L, Gumperz JE, Lanier LL, Phillips JH, Bigge JC, Wormwald MR, Parekh RB, Parham P. Unusual uniformity of the N-linked oligosaccharides of HLA-A, -B, and -C glycoproteins. J Immunol 1996;156:3275—3284.

48. Weiner HL, Mackin GA, Matsui M, Orav EJ, Khoury SJ, Dawson DM, Hafler DA. Double-blind pilot trial of oral tolerization with myelin antigens in multiple sclerosis. Science 1993;259:1321—1324.

678

49. Weiner HL. Oral tolerance for the treatment of autoimmune diseases. Ann Rev Med 1997; 48:341−351.
50. Damsky CH, Librach C, Lim K-H, Fitzgerald ML, McMaster MT, Chun S-H, Zhao Y, Logan S, Fisher SJ. Integrin switching regulates normal cytotrophoblast invasion. Development 1994;120:3657−3666.

# Implantation and placentation: glycodelins

M. Seppälä[1], H. Koistinen[1], R. Koistinen[1] and T. Timonen[2]

*Departments of [1]Obstetrics and Gynecology, and [2]Pathology, Helsinki University Central Hospital, Helsinki, Finland*

**Abstract.** Glycodelin-A is a glycoprotein with immunosuppressive properties. This property is probably related to a specific glycosylation pattern, which appears at the fetomaternal interphase and varies according to the tissue synthesizing glycodelins. Increased activity of the NK (natural killer) cells in peripheral blood has been related to an increased risk of recurrent miscarriage. Here, the role of endometrial/decidual GdA (glycodelin-A) may be to locally inhibit NK cell activity. This mechanism is of interest because retarded endometrial maturation is related to infertility, to an increased risk of miscarriage, and to decreased concentration of GdA in the endometrium and peripheral blood.

**Keywords:** immunosuppression, implantation, NK cells, PP14.

## Introduction

Natural implantation of the human blastocyst usually takes place during the period from LH +5 to LH +9 days. While quality of the blastocyst is the major determinant, maternal factors involved in the transport of the fertilized ovum and uterine receptivity must play a significant role [1]. There is a minimum endometrial thickness for a good outcome following assisted reproductive technologies [2]. All different components of endometrial tissue are likely to be involved in the implantation process, and our knowledge on the interplay between various bioactive substances produced by the epithelium, stroma, vessels and the transiently resident cells is still fragmentary. Such factors include growth factors and their binding proteins, components of the complement system, cytokines, integrins, mucins, receptors for steroids, prostaglandins and cytokines, proteases and carbohydrates [3—12].

Immunomodulatory cells are present in varying numbers in the female genital tract. They are usually migratory in nature and some appear in a temporal fashion. In the endometrium they include macrophages, T cells, endometrial granulated lymphocytes, B cells and polymorphonuclear lymphocytes, intraepithelial lymphocytes and natural killer (NK) cells [13]. The human decidua of early pregnancy contains considerable numbers of NK cells [14]. Yet these decidual lymphocytes do not destroy the antigenically foreign fetus, and they exhibit greatly

*Address for correspondence:* Prof Markku Seppälä MD, PhD, Department of Obstetrics and Gynecology, Helsinki University Central Hospital, FIN-00290 HYKS, Helsinki, Finland. Fax: +358-9-479-102. E-mail: marseppa@cc.helsinki.fi

decreased cytotoxic activity [15].

There are many hypotheses to explain why the embryo is protected from maternal immune rejection. There are probably many overlapping mechanisms to safeguard effective protection. Since women are not generally immunocompromised during pregnancy, the protection must be localized at the fetomaternal interface.

## Glycodelins

The mechanism considered in this article is based on secretion of a 28-kDa glycoprotein designated glycodelin-A (GdA). In the female, the most abundant tissue that synthesizes GdA is decidua, and it can be purified from either this source or from amniotic fluid [16,17]. In the past, this protein was called by many names and abbreviations, e.g., CAG-2, PAMG-2, PAEP and PP14. Some of them were quite misleading. For instance, PP14 is an abbreviation of placental protein 14, but in fact PP14 is not produced by the placenta at all, and its molecular weight is not 14 kDa [16—18]. Moreover, this protein is not solely an endometrial protein, as it is also found in the bone marrow [19], seminal plasma and seminal vesicles [20—22] and various glands in the body [23,24]. Therefore the authors who first introduced these names and distributed the protein to many laboratories worldwide have agreed to replace these abbreviations by the name "glycodelin" [25].

## Decidua produces immunosuppressive glycodelin

Amniotic fluid glycodelin-A probably represents decidua-derived glycodelin. This is based on the likely pathway through the membranes and the very similar structure of the glycodelins purified from either source. In the endometrium, GdA is absent during the periovulatory period, and it usually appears in the glands on the 5th postovulatory day [26]. After ovarian stimulation and oocyte retrieval it may appear earlier [27]. This protein has been shown to inhibit the synthesis of interleukin-2 and the release of soluble interleukin-2 receptors from phytohaemagglutinin-stimulated lymphocytes [28], and the production of interleukin-1 from mitogenically stimulated mononuclear cell cultures [29]. Moreover, GdA inhibits the activity of NK cells [30]. Inhibition is seen at concentrations which have been reported to occur in uterine fluid during the peri-implantation period [30,31]. One of the characteristics of the NK cells is that they can destroy foreign cells even when there has been no prior exposure. Therefore, an antigenically foreign embryo should be a target for maternal NK cells, but usually it is not.

## Glycosylation dictates function

Based on the different glycosylation patterns of the glycodelins produced by various tissues it became necessary to relate these structural differences to biological actions [32]. Thus, GdA has been found to inhibit binding of spermatozoa to zona pellucida, the specialized membrane around the oocyte [33]. This inhibition is dose-dependent and it takes place at concentrations which normally occur in uterine fluid during the latter part of the luteal phase [31]. The contraceptive activity of GdA is probably due to its unique carbohydrate structure, as no similar effect was found in differentially glycosylated GdS from seminal plasma [32,34]. We have previously suggested that there is convergence in the types of carbohydrate sequences recognized during the initial human gamete binding and immune cell interactions [11]. Therefore we have studied the effects of purified GdA [17] and purified GdS [21] in NK cell activity.

We used NK cells from peripheral blood. Their activity was measured by chromium-51 release assay using K562 cells as target cells. Prior exposure of peripheral NK cells to purified GdA rendered them incapable of acting on the target cells, whereas GdS had no inhibitory activity. Because GdA is abundant at the fetomaternal interphase it is possible that reduced activity of decidual NK cells is due to the presence of GdA. The role of NK cells in reproductive failure is suggested by a study showing that women with high NK cell activity in peripheral blood have a significantly higher miscarriage rate than do women with normal NK cell activity [35]. In this respect, the NK cell inhibitory activity of GdA becomes of interest because women with retarded endometrial maturation have less GdA in endometrial tissue compared to those women with normal endometrial maturation [36].

As in sperm-egg interaction [33], the inhibitory effect of GdA on the NK cells is likely to be glycosylation-dependent, because differentially glycosylated GdS from seminal plasma had no similar effect. The major protein backbone of GdA and GdS is the same and, therefore, the immunosuppressive effect of GdA is likely to depend on its unique carbohydrate structure, which consists of sialylated and fucosylated lacdiNAc sequences that are potent inhibitors of selectin-mediated cell adhesions. Of all GdA oligosaccharides, 60% contain at least one antenna terminated with sialic acid $\alpha$2-6 linked to either Gal or GalNAc [34]. These oligosaccharides have been reported to bind to CD22, the human B-cell receptor [37]. The high concentration of GdA at the fetomaternal interphase is not reflected in peripheral blood where the glycodelin concentration is 1,000-fold lower [38]. We have found no detectable immunosuppressive effect of GdA at the low concentrations present in pregnancy serum, perhaps explaining why high local immunosuppression is not associated with significant systemic immunocompromise during pregnancy.

## Acknowledgements

The original papers referred to in this article were supported by grants from the Academy of Finland, Federation of the Finnish Life Insurance Companies, and the Helsinki University Central Hospital Research Fund.

682

## References

1. Cooke ID. Implantation and the endometrium. Curr Opin Obstet Gynecol 1995;7:233–238.
2. Abdalla HI, Brooks AA, Johnson MR, Kirkland A, Thomas A, Studd JWW. Endometrial thickness: a predictor of implantation in ovum recipients? Hum Reprod 1994;9:363–365.
3. Lessey BA, Killam AP, Metzger DA, Haney AF, Greene GL, McCarty KS Jr. Immunohistochemical analysis of human uterine estrogen and progesterone receptors throughout the menstrual cycle. J Clin Endocrinol Metab 1988;67:334–340.
4. Lessey BA. The use of integrins for the assessment of uterine receptivity. Fertil Steril 1994;61:812–814.
5. Mellor SJ, Thomas EJ. The actions of estradiol and epidermal growth factors in endometrial and endometriotic stroma in vitro. Fertil Steril 1994;62:507–513.
6. Simon C, Piquette GN, Frances A, el-Danasouri I, Irvin JC, Plan ML. The effect of interleukin-1β (IL-1β) on the regulation of IL1 receptor type I messenger ribonucleic acid and protein levels in cultured human endometrial stromal and glandular cells. J Clin Endocrinol Metab 1994;78:675–682.
7. Seppälä M, Koistinen R, Rutanen E-M. Uterine endocrinology and paracrinology: insulin-like growth factor binding proteins-1 and placental protein 14 revisited. Hum Reprod 1994;9:917–925.
8. Rutanen E-M, Nyman T, Pekonen F. The role of the insulin-like growth factor system in uterine cell proliferation and differentiation. In: Genazzani AR, Petraglia F, Genazzani AD (eds) Frontiers in Gynecologic Investigation. Cranforth, UK: The Parthenon Publishing Group, 1993;231–239.
9. Hasty LA, Lambris JD, Lessey BA, Pruksananonda K, Little CR. Hormonal regulation of complement components and receptors throughout the menstrual cycle. Am J Obstet Gynecol 1994;170:168–175.
10. Hey NA, Graham RA, Seif MW, Aplin JD. The polymorphic epithelial MUC1 in human endometrium is regulated with maximal expression in the implantation phase. J Clin Endocrinol Metab 1994;78:337–342.
11. Clark GF, Oehninger S, Patankar MS, Koistinen R, Dell A, Morris HR, Koistinen H, Seppälä M. A role for glycoconjugates in human development: the human feto-embryonic defense system hypothesis. Hum Reprod 1996;11:467–473.
12. Aplin JD. Adhesion molecules in implantation. Rev Reprod 1997;2:84–93.
13. Lea RG, Clark DA. Macrophages and migratory cells in endometrium relevant to implantation. Balliere's Clin Obstet Gynecol 1991;5:25–59.
14. Sato S, Kanzaki H, Yoshida M, Tokushige M, Wang HS et al. Studies on T-lineage cells in human decidua of the first trimester pregnancies. Am J Reprod Immunol 1990;24:67–72.
15. Deniz G, Christmas SE, Brew R, Johnson PM. Phenotypic and functional differences between human CD3-decidual and peripheral blood leukocytes. J Immunol 1994;152:4255–4261.
16. Julkunen M, Seppälä M, Jänne OA. Complete amino acid sequence of human placental protein 14: a progestogerone-regulated uterine protein homologous to β-lactoglobulins. Proc Natl Acad Sci USA 1988;85:8845–8849.
17. Riittinen L, Julkunen M, Seppälä M, Koistinen R, Huhtala ML. Purification and characterization of endometrial protein PP14 from mid-trimester amniotic fluid. Clin Chim Acta 1989;184:19–30.
18. Julkunen M, Koistinen R, Sjöberg J, Rutanen EM, Wahlström T, Seppälä M. Secretory endometrium synthesizes placental protein 14. Endocrinology 1986;118:1782–1786.
19. Kämäräinen M, Riittinen L, Seppälä M, Palotie A, Andersson LC. Progesterone-associated endometrial protein (PAEP) — a constitutive marker of human erythroid precursors. Blood 1994;84:467–473.
20. Julkunen M, Wahlström T, Seppälä M, Koistinen R, Koskimies AI, Stenman UH, Bohn H. Detection and localization of placental protein 14-like protein in human seminal plasma and

in the male genital tract. Arch Androl 1984;12(Suppl):59—67.

21. Koistinen H, Koistinen R, Dell A, Morris HR, Easton RL, Patankar MS, Oehninger S, Clark GF, Seppälä M. Glycodelin from seminal plasma is a differentially glycosylated form of contraceptive glycodelin-A. Molec Hum Reprod 1996;2:759—765.

22. Koistinen H, Koistinen R, Kämäräinen M, Salo J, Seppälä M. Multiple forms of messenger ribonucleic acid encoding glycodelin in male genital tract. Lab Invest 1997;76:683—690.

23. Kämäräinen M, Seppälä M, Virtanen I, Andersson LC. Expression of glycodelin in MCF-7 breast cancer cells induces differentiation into organized acinar epithelium. Lab Invest 1997; 77;565—573.

24. Kämäräinen M, Miettinen M, Seppälä M, von Boguslawsky K, Benassi MS, Böhling T, Andersson LC. Epithelial expression of glycodelin in synovial sarcomas. Int J Cancer 1998; 78:487—490.

25. Seppälä M, Tatarinov Y, Bohn H. Glycodelins. Tumor Biol 1998;19:213—220.

26. Seppälä M, Wahlström T, Julkunen M, Vartiainen E, Huhtala M-L. Endometrial protein as indicators of endometrial function. In: Tomoda Y, Mizutani S, Narita O, Klopper A (eds) Placental and Endometrial Proteins: Basic and Clinical Aspects. Utrecht: VNU Science Press, 1988; 35—42.

27. Wahlström T, Koskimies AI, Tenhunen A, Rutanen EM, Yki-Järvinen H, Julkunen M, Sjöberg J, Seppälä M. Pregnancy proteins in the endometrium after follicle aspiration for in vitro fertilization. Ann NY Acad Sci 1985;442:402—407.

28. Pockley AG, Bolton, AE. Placental protein 14 (PP14) inhibits the synthesis of interleukin-2 and release of soluble interleukin-2 receptors from phytohaemagglutinin-stimulated lymphocytes. Clin Exp Immunol 1989;77:252—256.

29. Pockley AG, Bolton, AE. The effect of human placental protein 14 (PP14) on the production of interleukin-1 from mitogenically stimulated mononuclear cell cultures. Immunology 1990;69: 277—281.

30. Okamoto N, Uchida A, Takakura K, Kariya Y, Kanzaki H, Riittinen L, Koistinen R, Seppälä M, Mori T. Suppression by human placental protein 14 of natural killer cell activity. Am J Reprod Immunol 1991;26:137—142.

31. Li TC, Dalton C, Hunjan KS, Warren MA, Bolton AE. The correlation of placental protein 14 concentrations in uterine flushing and endometrial morphology in the peri-implantation period. Hum Reprod 1993;8:1923—1927.

32. Morris HR, Dell A, Easton RL, Panico M, Koistinen H, Koistinen R, Oehninger S, Patankar MS, Seppälä M, Clark GF. Gender specific glycosylation of human glycodelin affects contraceptive activity. J Biol Chem 1996;271:32159—32167.

33. Oehninger S, Coddington CC, Hodgen GD, Seppälä M. Factors affecting fertilization: endometrial placental protein 14 reduces the capacity of human spermatozoa to bind to the human zona pellucida. Fertil Steril 1995;63:377—383.

34. Dell A, Morris HR, Easton R, Panico M, Patankar M, Oehninger S, Koistinen R, Koistinen H, Seppälä M, Clark GF. Structural analysis of the oligosaccharides derived from glycodelin, a human glycoprotein with potent immunosuppressive and contraceptive activities. J Biol Chem 1995;270:24116—24126.

35. Aoki K, Kajiura S, Matsumoto Y, Ogasawara M, Okada S, Yagami Y, Gleicher N. Preconceptional natural-killer activity as a predictor of miscarriage. Lancet 1995;345:1340—1342.

36. Klentzeris LD, Bulmer JN, Seppälä M, Li TC, Warren MA, Cooke ID. Placental protein 14 in cycles with normal and retarded endometrial differentiation. Hum Reprod 1994;9:394—398.

37. Powell LD, Varki A. The oligosaccharide binding specificities of CD22, a sialic acid-specific lectin of B cell. J Biol Chem 1994;269:10628—10636.

38. Julkunen M, Rutanen EM, Koskimies AI, Ranta T, Bohn H, Seppälä M. Distribution of placental protein 14 in tissues and body fluids during pregnancy. Br J Obstet Gynaecol 1985;92:1145—1151.

# Diagnostic accuracy in preimplantation diagnosis

# Diagnostic accuracy in preimplantation diagnosis single-cell PCR for mendelian disorders

K. Sermon

*University Hospital and Medical School of the Dutch-speaking Brussels Free University, Brussels, Belgium*

**Abstract.** Preimplantation genetic diagnosis (PGD) has become possible since the development of the polymerase chain reaction (PCR) which has become the method of choice for PGD of monogenic disorders. However, a number of pitfalls have to be taken into account when carrying out single-cell PCE. Contamination of the reaction mixture with genomic DNA (e.g., from sperm or corona cells surrounding the embryo) or by carry-over with PCR products as well as allele-dropout are two phenomena specific to single-cell PCR which can lead to misdiagnosis. Examples of misdiagnoses and how to avoid them are discussed in this chapter.

**Keywords:** preimplantation diagnosis, PCE, contamination, allele-dropout.

## Introduction

The idea of preimplantation genetics is not new: already in 1967 Bob Edwards succeeded in sexing rabbit embryos at the blastocyst stage after which they were successfully transferred [1]. In this article, the author predicted the use of similar technology in the human to prevent genetic disease. However, we had to wait until the beginning of the 1990s for a useful technology allowing us to detect mutations in single cells to emerge: the polymerase chain reaction (PCR) [2]. PCR allows us to amplify exponentially a well-defined DNA sequence and to end up with a workable amount of DNA, even when starting from only one single cell. Shortly, the principle of PCR is as follows: two short single-stranded DNA-stretches (oligonucleotides) of between 20 and 30 bp are designed so that they are complementary to a stretch of the DNA of interest, one on each side and complementary to the opposite strand. The genomic DNA is first denatured, after which these short oligonucleotides, called primers, are allowed to bind to the complementary sequences. A thermostable DNA polymerase, taq polymerase, synthetises the complementary strand starting from the primer sequences. This synthesis is repeated several cycles, so that an exponential amplification of the DNA in between the two primers results.

The first clinical application of this technique for PGD was described in 1991 [3]: Y-chromosome-specific sequences were amplified using the PCR reaction to

*Address for correspondence:* Dr K. Sermon, Department of Medical Genetics, AZ — Vrije Universiteit Brussels, Laarbeeklaan 101, B-1090 Brussels, Belgium. Tel.: +32-2-477-60-73. Fax: +32-2-477-60-72. E-mail: Igensnk@az.vub.ac.be

determine the sex of embryos obtained from couples at risk for X-linked diseases. Only female embryos were transferred and several healthy girls were born following this procedure. However, due to the risk of misdiagnosis (one male pregnancy had to be terminated [4]), sexing using PCR has now largely been abandoned in favor of the fluorescent in situ hybridization (FISH) technique [5]. Shortly after, other applications for PCR were developed, such as for cystic fibrosis (CF), a monogenetic disease inherited in an autosomal recessive manner [6,7]. The problem of contamination was easily solved, but a new problem soon emerged: allelic dropout (ADO), i.e., the nonamplification of one of both alleles in a heterozygous single cell. This phenomenon even probably led to two misdiagnoses in PGD for CF [8,9]: in both cases, both parents were carriers of different mutations, complicating accurate diagnosis even more. ADO has since been well studied and a number of improvements have been proposed. One of these improvements is the fluorescent PCR, where PCR fragments are not detected on ethidiumbromide-stained gels, which is done routinely, but are labelled with a fluorophore so that they can be detected when excited by the correct laser [10]. This fairly new technology will also be discussed.

**The difference between PCR on purified DNA and on single cells**

It would be a mistake to assume that, if a routine PCR can be done on 500 ng of purified DNA, PCR on a single cell, containing 6-pg DNA, is just a matter of doing more cycles. Three important hurdles, more or less specific to single-cell PCR, had to be taken before single-cell PCR could be called efficient and accurate enough to use it for diagnostic purposes: the specificity of the PCR, the problem of contamination, and the problem of ADO.

**Specificity of the PCR**

A well-designed PCR, using primers chosen with care and using the optimal conditions of reaction mix composition, should give one, clear band. However, the taq polymerase makes mistakes when incorporating deoxynucleotides, and when more and more cycles are used in the PCR, these mistakes accumulate and cause the result to be nonspecific: aspecific bands appear which do not have the correct expected length, and sometimes even a smear of PCR product appears. To amplify the small amount of DNA present in a single cell, something like 50–60 PCR cycles would be necessary. This explains why the first PGDs for sexing were possible: here, repetitive sequences on the Y-chromosome were amplified, so that 30 cycles were enough to obtain a visible signal on a plain agarose gel. However, when attempts were made to amplify a single-copy gene (CF), the results were less successful. A new method for increasing the specificity of single-cell PCR was then introduced: nested PCR [11]. The principle is the following: a relatively small number of cycles is carried out (usually 20 or less), after which the PCR product obtained is used as a template for a second round of

PCR (usually 20 cycles or more), using primers within the boundaries of the first PCR. Any mistake incorporated into the products obtained after the first PCR at the sites of the primers is thus eliminated by the second PCR. Until recently, this was the method of choice for single-cell PCR in our laboratory, and is still used in most laboratories performing PGD for monogenic disease.

Most of our assays are now performed using fluorescent PCR: one of the primers is fluorescently labeled, so that the resulting PCR product is also fluorescent. This product can be detected on a denaturing acrylamide gel: when the PCR product passes a laser beam, the fluorescent tag is excited to emit light at a certain wavelength. This light is measured by a photocell (one cell for each lane) and the signal transmitted to a computer with adapted software. Other systems, using columns to separate the DNA, are also available and work on the same principle. Fluorescent PCR is much more sensitive than conventional PCR with ethidiumbromide staining: less cycles are necessary to obtain a signal. As an example: for myotonic dystrophy (DM) we carry out 55 PCR cycles when using conventional PCR, while for fluorescent PCR, 43 cycles are sufficient. Moreover, fluorescent PCR is more accurate, which also has repercussions on the rate of ADO as we will see later.

*Contamination control*

When we amplify DNA from a single cell, containing two copies of the DNA of interest, the presence of a third DNA molecule originating from outside the cell can lead to a wrong genotyping of this cell. This is what is called contamination. Two types of contamination can be distinguished: contamination with cellular or genomic DNA, such as DNA from sperms sticking to the zona which can be coamplified with the biopsied blastomere, and carry-over contamination, i.e., contamination with PCR products from a former PCR reaction. In practice, the source of contamination cannot always be traced and the measures taken against contamination are the same for both types.

Contamination is not restricted to single-cell PCR: in the first days of PCR, investigators were not aware of the problem, and soon massive contamination occurred in many laboratories. Simple measures, like using different pipette sets to set up the PCR reactions and to process the samples after the PCR reaction, had not been taken, leading to carry-over contamination of pipettes, reaction components, bench tops, etc. There is one anecdote of Cetus Corporation, which developed many PCR applications, moving to another building because the old one was full of contaminated PCR products.

The measures taken at our laboratory are aimed specifically at contamination control for single-cell PCR:
1. PCR mixes are prepared in a vertical flow in a separate room. A freezer and a fridge in this room contain products only used for preparation of PCR mixes. No DNA (except single cells) is ever brought into this laboratory, and certainly not amplified products. Fresh green surgical coats and latex gloves are

worn during work in the flow. When the flow is not in use, a UV light is on to destroy DNA strands in the flow. This flow is thoroughly cleaned weekly.

2. Special, dedicated plasticware is used in this flow: PCR and other tubes are autoclaved and kept in a cupboard separate from other material. Gamma-sterilized filtered tips are used, which are also kept separately. A pipette set is used exclusively for the preparation of the PCR mixes and never leaves the room.

3. Water and solutions are autoclaved whenever possible and aliquoted. These aliquots are used a restricted number of times. Primers are ordered and custom made especially for single-cell PCR; to borrow primers from a routine genetic laboratory is a certain way to introduce contamination.

4. Cell preparation is also carried out in a flow where no PCR products are ever brought in. In our case, cells are prepared in the laboratory for reproductive biology, where primarily embryo culture takes place.

5. To eliminate DNA contamination that could possibly be present in reaction components, the PCR reaction mix is treated with an appropriate restriction enzyme before it is used in a PCR reaction. This restriction enzyme should cut within the target DNA sequence, should be active in a low-salt environment (such as PCR mixes) and should be heat inactivated. Usually, we prepare our reaction mixes the evening before the PCR and incubate the reaction mix overnight with the restriction enzyme. In the morning, the restriction enzyme is heat inactivated (incubation at $65°C$ for 20 min), after which the reaction mix is ready for the PCR.

6. Every sample containing a cell should have a blank counterpart for detection of possible contamination.

From this, it is clear that single-cell PCR demands an important infrastructure. Despite all our combined efforts at eliminating contamination, we still routinely have about 5% contamination when working with lymphoblasts, which are used for routine development of single-cell assays. This figure falls below 2% when we consider contamination encountered during clinical preimplantation genetic diagnoses (PGDs). Unfortunately, as is explained below, contamination led to a misdiagnosis during a PGD for DM. More and more laboratories are now developing methods to not only prevent contamination, but also to detect it. Multiplex PCRs, coamplifying the sequence of interest together with linked polymorphic markers, allow the detection of contaminating cellular or genomic DNA [12].

*ADO*

Navidi and Arnheim [13] calculated what the effects of contamination and (partial) failure of amplification would have on the diagnosis of autosomal-recessive and -dominant, and on X-linked genetic diseases. Failure of amplification of one allele was later dubbed ADO. They concluded that ADO would pose a particular problem for the correct diagnosis of autosomal dominant diseases, when the affected allele would fail to amplify, and recessive diseases involving two different mutations, when only one mutation would be analyzed and would fail to amplify. Ray et al. [14] recognized for the first time the phenomenon when they found that 25% of the blastomeres heterozygous for the $\Delta$F508 mutation in the CF gene analyzed during clinical PGD showed.ADO. Two misdiagnosis were reported, concerning PGD in compound heterozygotes for CF, as predicted by Navidi and Arnheim: the first misdiagnosis concerned a couple where one parent was carrier of the $\Delta$F508 mutation and the other of the W1282X mutation; only the $\Delta$F508 mutation was analyzed and ADO led to the transfer of an embryo carrying both mutations [8]. The second misdiagnosis also occurred in CF with compound heterozygosity [9]. ADO was also already present in a number of publications, although not under that name. Levinson et al. [15] described a multiplex PCR for the sexing of embryos in which they amplified the amelogenin gene on the X- and Y-chromosomes as well as the repetitive DYZ1 sequence on the Y-chromosome. Their table shows that they had an amplification efficiency of 92% and an ADO rate of 21%. We [16] have also encountered ADO in a blastomere heterozygous for the $\Delta$F508 mutation in the CF gene although at that time the interpretation was that the cell in question was monosomic or haploid. Since then, ADO has been described in different PCR assays and different DNA sequences. Strom et al. [17] can sport the lowest ADO rates: in a series of 203 heterozygous cells only one cell showed ADO (0.005%).

ADO can have a number of causes. Firstly, chromosomal mosaicism, which is now a well-documented feature of many embryos, could lead to misdiagnosis especially in autosomal-dominant diseases. This type of misdiagnosis can be avoided by the biopsy of two cells from the embryo after which a diagnosis is accorded only to embryos in which the two cells show the same genotype.

Secondly, it was shown that the method used for cell lysis before PCR has a tremendous effect not only on the efficiency of the PCR, but also on the ADO rate. Wu et al. [18] and Gitlin et al. [19] showed a dramatic difference in ADO rate between different lysis methods: a decrease from 19% (DTT and proteinase K) to 10% (alkaline lysis) for CF/$\Delta$F508 as shown by Wu et al., and a decrease from 89% (freeze-thawing) to 9% (alkaline lysis) for Tay-Sachs disease as shown by Gitlin et al.

Thirdly, Ray et al. [20] showed in a series of experiments on blastomeres and lymphocytes that the denaturation temperature at the start of the first PCR is of great importance. It was demonstrated for the CF/$\Delta$F508 mutation that at a denaturation temperature of $90°C$, 21% of heterozygous lymphocytes showed ADO, at $93°C$ the ADO rate decreased to 13%, to finally reach 5% when a denaturation temperature of $96°C$ was used. We found the same effect of the denaturation on the ADO rate: for the 1278ins4 mutation causing Tay-Sachs disease, we were able to decrease the ADO rate from 53% (16 out of 30 cells) when using $94°C$, to 30% (9 out of 30 cells) when using $96°C$ (unpublished data). Ray et al. [20] hypothesized that the effect of the higher denaturation temperature could be explained by the need for efficient separation of the native double-stranded DNA. As other causes of ADO, they proposed a strand break or other

DNA damage by, e.g., endogenous endonucleases.

Apart from raising the denaturation temperature, a number of strategies have been proposed to decrease the ADO rate, or at least to avoid misdiagnoses as a result of ADO. Findlay et al. [21] have presented a large body of evidence that fluorescence PCR, which is much more sensitive than conventional PCR, further decreases the ADO rate, because a number of ADO cases are in fact preferential amplifications which are classified as ADO by conventional PCR. The ADO rate is decreased dramatically by fluorescent PCR: they found an ADO rate for CF/ΔF508 of 4.3% using a denaturing temperature of 94°C. Another possibility would be that, since less PCR cycles are applied in fluorescent PCR and PCR is exponential, a difference in amplification efficiency between two alleles would be less obvious in the first cycles of PCR. Since we found a high rate of ADO for our single-cell PCR for DM (21% in blastomeres, [22]), we adapted this assay for fluorescent PCR. A substantial decrease in ADO was noted: 24% (9/38) heterozygous lymphoblasts showed ADO when assayed with conventional PCR, whereas only 6.5% (3/46) lymphoblasts showed ADO with fluorescent PCR (Sermon et al., in press). Similar results were obtained with blastomeres: 1/22 (4.5%) of the heterozygous cells showed ADO. Another application of fluorescent PCR would be multiplex PCR, which is notoriously difficult with conventional PCR. Findlay et al. [21] described a simultaneous fingerprinting, diagnosis of sex and mutation analysis for CF in single cells. Successful amplification (i.e., amplification of all microsatellites and both sexing alleles) was obtained in 71% of the samples, whereas partial amplification (i.e., amplification of some but not all microsatellite fragments) occurred in 25% of the samples. Although these results are not different from the ones obtained by Wu et al. [18] for a conventional multiplex amplifying CF/ΔF508 and HLA DQA1 (72% of the samples showed successful amplification as defined above), it must be taken into account that the microsatellite chosen by Findlay et al. is far more complex (six different loci per genome) and thus much more subject to ADO.

Another possibility to decrease ADO is to develop a PCR strategy in which ADO is detected, or alternatively, where ADO does not lead to misdiagnosis. An example of the first strategy is the simultaneous amplification of two different mutations in a compound heterozygous embryo using only one primer pair in the first PCR (remember these are the cases where misdiagnoses were reported), as described by Ray et al. [23] and Van de Velde et al. [24] for β-thalassemia major and Sermon et al. [25] for Tay-Sachs disease. As a result of ADO, the embryo would appear to be homozygous affected for either of both mutations, which is an impossible result. Another example is the multiplex PCR described above by Rechitsky et al. [12], where the ΔF508 mutation and a nearby polymorphism in intron 6 of the CF gene are amplified in multiplex and definite diagnosis is only ascribed to cells showing concordant results for both loci. We developed a single-cell PCR-assay for Steinert's disease, where only the healthy alleles of both parents, and not the expanded allele of the affected parent are amplified [22]. Thus, only the presence of the healthy allele of the affected parent would lead to a diagnosis of healthy embryo, whereas dropout of this allele would lead to the diagnosis of affected embryo and to nontransfer of this embryo.

### Diagnostic accuracy in preimplantation diagnosis using single-cell PCR for Mendelian disorders: the Brussels experience

*Overview of PGD cycles up to biopsy* (Table 1)

The first Mendelian disease which we performed on was CF, incidently in this case the husband suffered from CBAVD. We have diagnosed different CF mutations such as ΔF508, N1303K, 1414-1G→A and M/V476 polymorphism. We treated 10 patients in 17 cycles who carried CF without CBAVD, resulting in five pregnancies. Two of these were delivered and the babies are doing well, three are ongoing, of which two were shown to be unaffected after CVS. Five couples were treated where the husband suffered from CBAVD and the mother carried a CF mutation. Twelve treatment cycles resulted in three pregnancies (two delivered and one ongoing).

The second large group of patients for which we developed a PGD, was for patients suffering from DM. Fifteen patients underwent 42 treatment cycles, resulting in seven pregnancies. Two of these delivered and are doing well, one was a biochemical pregnancy, one was a blighted ovum, two are ongoing (one had a CVS showing the pregnancy was unaffected) and one was a misdiagnosis and was terminated. This misdiagnosis was most probably due to contamination,

*Table 1.* Summary of PGD cycles for PCR going up to analysis.

| Indication | No. of patients | No. of cycles | 2PN embryos | Embryos biopsied | Embryos without diagnosis | Unaffected embryos | Affected embryos | Carrier embryos | Embryos transferred | Pregnancy |
|---|---|---|---|---|---|---|---|---|---|---|
| CF | 6 | 11 | 87 | 51 | 2 | 20 | 11 | 18 | 17 | 2 |
| CF with CBAVD | 4 | 9 | 56 | 44 | 1 | 15 | 4 | 22 | 18 | 2 |
| DM | 15 | 42 | 348 | 262 | 44 | 94 | 115 | 9ᵃ | 70 | 7 |
| Duchenne's and Becker's muscular dystrophy | 4 | 6 | 72 | 50 | 2 | 34 | 15 | 0 | 13 | 2 |
| Huntington's disease | 4 | 6 | 64 | 36 | 9 | 9 | 18 | — | 9 | 0 |
| β-thalassemia | 1 | 2 | 14 | 8 | 3 | 1 | 2 | 2 | 3 | 0 |
| Charcot-Marie-Tooth disease type 1A | 1 | 2 | 18 | 15 | 3 | 2 | 10 | — | 2 | 1 |
| Marfan's disease | 1 | 3 | 22 | 15 | 0 | 9 | 6 | — | 6 | 0 |
| Adrenogenital syndrome | 1 | 2 | 13 | 12 | 1 | 4 | 3 | 5 | 6 | 1 |

ᵃThese embryos are "uninformative" embryos in couples who were only 50% informative.

since the embryo was diagnosed as healthy on the day of PGD because it showed the presence of the healthy allele of the mother. During prenatal diagnosis, however, the presence of this healthy allele could not be confirmed, and on the contrary, the presence of the mutated allele (a 2,000-bp expansion) was shown to be present on southern blotting. We concluded that maternal DNA, possibly coming from granulosa cells or from a polar body, was transferred into the PCR tube together with the embryo's blastomere.

Our third largest group of patients concerns the patients carriers for Duchenne's and Becker's muscular dystrophy. Two different assays were used: one amplifying exon 17 and one amplifying intron 45. With these two assays, we could treat four patients in six cycles. This resulted in two pregnancies: one is already delivered, the other pregnancy is ongoing.

Recently we have started to carry out PGDs for Huntington's disease. Four couples at risk underwent six cycles. Although a transfer took place in all of these cycles, no pregnancies ensued.

Two cycles were performed for a couple of carriers for $\beta$-thalassemia. The assay was based on the amplification of both mutations in the first PCR, followed by separate second PCRs for both mutations. Unfortunately, this patient did not conceive. One patient was treated in two cycles for Charcot-Marie-Tooth disease type 1A. The ensuing pregnancy is ongoing and was shown after CVS to be unaffected. One patient underwent three cycles for Martan syndrome, but unfortunately did not conceive.

Two cycles were carried out in a couple carrying the same mutation for adrenogenital syndrome. The second cycle ended successfully in a pregnancy. A CVS at 12-weeks pregnancy showed both fetuses to be heathy carriers. Not described in this list are two cycles (one for DM and one for HD) in which the diagnosis failed. In the first case, the patient accepted to receive the three morphologically best embryos, but did not conceive. In the second case, the patient declined to have a rebiopsy of the embryos at day 4 followed by transfer at day 4. The embryos were donated for research.

## References

1. Edwards RD, Gardner RL. Sexing of live rabbit blastocysts. Nature 1967;214:576—577.
2. Saiki RK, Scharf ST Faloona F et al. Enzymatic amplification of P-globin genomic sequences and restriction site analysis for diagnosis of sickle cell anemia. Science 1985;230:1350—1354.
3. Handyside AH, Kontogianni IEH, Hardy K, Winston RML. Pregnancies from biopsied human preimplantation embryos sexed by Y-specific DNA amplification. Nature 1990;344:768—770.
4. Hardy K, Handyside AH. Biopsy of cleavage stage human embryos and diagnosis of single-gene defects by DNA amplification. Arch Pathol Lab Med 1992;116:388—392.
5. Munné S, Grifo J, Cohen J, Weier HUG. Chromosome abnormalities in human arrested preimplantation embryos: a multiple-probe FISH study. Am J Hum Genet 1994;55:150—159.
6. Handyside AH, Lesko JG, Tarin JJ, Winston RM, Hughes MR. Birth of a normal girl after in vitro fertilization and preimplantation diagnostic testing for cystic fibrosis. N Engl J Med 1992;327:905—909.
7. Liu J, Lissens W, Silber SJ, Devroey P, Liebaers I, Van Steirteghem AC. Birth after preimplanta-

tion diagnosis of the cystic fibrosis AF508 mutation by polymerase chain reaction in human embryos resulting from intracytoplasmic sperm injection with epididymal sperm. JAMA 1994;272:1858−1860.

8. Grifo JA, Tang YX, Munné S, Alikani M, Cohen J, Rosenwaks Z. Healthy deliveries from biopsied human embryos. Hum Reprod 1994;9,912−916.

9. Harper JC, Handyside AH. The current status of preimplantation diagnosis. Curr Obstet Gynecol 1994;4:143−149.

10. Hattori M, Yoshioka K, Sakaki Y. Highly-sensitive fluorescent DNA sequencing and its application for detection and mass-screening of point mutations. J Electrophoresis 1992;13:560−565.

11. Holding C, Monk M. Diagnosis of beta-thalassemia by DNA amplification in single blastomeres from mouse preimplantation embryos. Lancet 1989;532−535.

12. Rechitsky S, Strom C, Verlinsky O, Amet T, Ivakhnenko V, Kukharenko V, Kuliev A, Verlinsky Y. Allele dropout in polar bodies and blastomeres. J Assist Reprod Genet 1998;5:253−257.

13. Navidi W, Arnheim N. Using PCR in preimplantation genetic diagnosis. Hum Reprod 1991;6:836−849.

14. Ray P, Winston RML, Handyside AH. Single cell analysis for diagnosis of cystic fibrosis and Lesch-Nyhan syndrome in human embryos before implantation. Miami Bio/Technology Short Reports: Proceedings of the 1994 Miami Bio/Technology European Symposium, Advances in Gene Technology: Molecular Biology and Human Genetic Disease 1994;5:46.

15. Levinson G, Fields RA, Harton GL, Palmer FT, Maddalena A, Fugger EF, Schulman JD. Reliable gender screening for human preimplantation embryo using multiple DNA target-sequences. Hum Reprod 1992;7:1304−1313.

16. Liu J, Lissens W, Devroey P, Van Steirteghem A, Liebaers I. Polymerase chain reaction analysis of the cystic fibrosis ΔF508 mutation in human blastomeres following oocyte injection of a single sperm from a carrier. Prenatal Diagn 1993;13:873−880.

17. Strom CM, Rechitsky S, Wolf G, Verlinsky Y. Reliability of polymerase chain reaction (PCR) analysis of single cells for preimplantation genetic diagnosis. J Assist Reprod Genet 1994;11:55−62.

18. Wu R, Cuppens H, Buyse I, Decorte R, Marynen P, Gordts S, Cassiman JJ. Co-amplification of the cystic fibrosis ΔF508 mutation with the HLA DQA1 sequence in single-cell PCR: implications for improved assessment of polar bodies and blastomeres in preimplantation diagnosis. Prenatal Diagn 1993;13:1111−1122.

19. Gitlin SA, Lazendorf SE, Gibbons WE. Polymerase chain reaction amplification specifity: incidence of allele dropout using different DNA preparation methods for heterozygous single cells. J Assist Reprod Genet 1996;13:107−111.

20. Ray PF, Handyside AH. Increasing the denaturation temperature during the first cycles of amplification reduces allele dropout from single cells for preimplantaiton diagnosis. Molec Hum Reprod 1996;2:213−218.

21. Findlay I, Quirke P, Hall J, Rutherford A. Fluorescent PCR: a new technique for PGD of sex and single-gene defects. J Assist Reprod Genet 1996;13:96−103.

22. Sermon K, Lissens W, Joris H, Seneca S, Desmyttere S, Devroey P, Van Steirteghem A, Liebaers I. Clinical application of preimplantation diagnosis for myotonic dystrophy. Prenatal Diagn 1997;17:925−932

23. Ray PF, Kaeda JS, Bingham J, Roberts I, Handyside AH. Preimplantation diagnosis of β-thalassemia major. Lancet 1996;1696.

24. Van de Velde H, Sermon K, Lissens W, De Vos A, Van Steirteghem A, Liebaers I. Development of a single-cell PCR for simultaneous detection of two β-thalassaemia mutations and its application for preimplantation genetic diagnosis. J Assist Reprod Genet 1997;14:474−475.

25. Sermon K, Lissens W, Nagy ZP, Van Steirteghem A, Liebaers I. Simultaneous amplification of the two most frequent mutations of infantile Tay-Sachs disease in single blastomeres. Molec Hum Reprod 1995;1:2214−2217.

# Preimplantation genetic diagnosis of aneuploidy and translocations

Santiago Munné[1], Carmen Márquez[1], Jingly Fung[2,3], Muhterem Bahçe[1], Larry Morrison[4], Ulli Weier[3] and Jacques Cohen[1]

[1]*The Institute for Reproductive Medicine and Science, Saint Barnabas Medical Center, Livingston, New Jersey;* [2]*Reproductive Genetics Unit, Department of Obstetrics, Gynecology and Reproductive Sciences, University of California, San Francisco, California;* [3]*Resources for Molecular Cytogenetics, Life Sciences Division, University of California, E.O. Lawrence Berkeley National Laboratory, Berkeley, California; and* [4]*Vysis, Downersgrove, Illinois, USA*

## Introduction

Ploidy assessment of single blastomeres by FISH using a combination of autosomal and gonosomal probes has been achieved in a time-frame compatible with IVF [1]. It has the potential of reducing the chances of delivering a trisomic baby, increasing pregnancy rates in women of advanced maternal age, and of reducing embryo loss during pregnancy.

Numerical chromosome abnormalities are the major cause of inherited diseases, with an incidence of 21% in spontaneous abortions [2]. Of these, trisomies for gonosomes and chromosomes 21, 18, 16 and 13 account for 50% of chromosomally abnormal abortions. In contrast to single gene defects, numerical chromosome abnormalities occur de novo, and the only risk factor known is maternal age, with trisomies increasing from 2% in recognized pregnancies of women 25 years old, up to 19% in women 40 years or over [2]. The screening of chromosome aneuploidies in human embryos by FISH using X, Y, 18, 13 and 21 probes should significantly reduce the risk in older IVF patients of delivering trisomic offspring.

On the other hand, PGD of aneuploidy may increase the pregnancy rate in women of advanced maternal age undergoing IVF. The causes of the decline in implantation observed with increasing maternal age are still under debate. Nevertheless, the high implantation rates obtained using oocyte donation strongly indicate that the major factor is maternal age [3]. Ooplasmic components may be a factor involved [4–6], but the only clear link between maternal age and embryo competence is aneuploidy. The increase in aneuploidy with maternal age in spontaneous abortuses and live offspring was also found in both cleavage-stage embryos [7] and unfertilized oocytes [8]. The rate of chromosomal abnormalities

*Address for correspondence:* Santiago Munné, The Institute for Reproductive Medicine and Science, Saint Barnabas Medical Center, Livingston, NJ 07052, USA.

in embryos was higher than the one reported in spontaneous abortions, suggesting that a sizable part of chromosomally abnormal embryos are eliminated before prenatal diagnosis can be performed. Such loss of embryos could account for the decline in implantation with maternal age. For instance, the rate of embryonic monosomy is similar to the one for trisomy [7], while with the exception of monosomy 21 (1/1,000 karyotyped abortions), the other autosomal monosomies are normally undetected in clinically recognized pregnancies. Furthermore, monosomies in mice die before implantation [9]. Other evidence comes from the observation that blastocyst formation declines with maternal age in women over 30, and more embryos arrest at the morula stage, which are supposed to be monosomic or grossly abnormal embryos [10]. Furthermore, although it is not known whether trisomies that arrive to term (13, 18, 21) have a lower implantation rate than normal embryos, even recognized pregnancies with trisomy 21, which have the greater survival rate of all trisomies, spontaneously abort in 84—93% of cases depending on the age of the mother [2]. This screening could be further advantageous if we consider that 52% of IVF stimulation cycles in the USA are performed in women 35 years or older (ASRM-SART 1998).

Because of the correlation between aneuploidy and declining implantation rates with maternal age, it was hypothesized that negative selection of chromosomally abnormal embryos could reverse this trend [1]. Currently, negative selection of aneuploid embryos can only be done through preimplantation genetic diagnosis (PGD), either by polar body or blastomere analysis. Low metaphase yield and less than 30% of karyotypable metaphases, together with the requirement of overnight culture in antimitotics [11—13], make karyotype analysis unsuitable for PGD. Fluorescence in situ hybridization (FISH) allows chromosome enumeration to be performed on interphase cell nuclei, i.e., without the need for culturing cells or preparing metaphase spreads. FISH has been applied to PGD of common aneuploidies using either human blastomeres (cells from 2- to 16-cell stage embryos) or oocyte polar bodies [1,7,14—18]. Currently, probes for X, Y, 13, 14, 15, 16, 18, 21 and 22 chromosomes are being used simultaneously (Munné et al., unpublished), with the potential of detecting 70% of the aneuploidies detected in spontaneous abortions.

## PGD of aneuploidy

### Fish technique for PGD of aneuploidy

FISH protocols for simultaneous detection of multiple chromosomes with specific probes for each chromosome are being used for PGD. These protocols are based on the use of ratios of fluorochromes labeling five or more chromosomes with only three fluorochromes [19,20]. For blastomere studies, the protocols include X, Y, 13, 18 and 21 chromosomes with or without chromosome 16 [1,16,21]. For polar body studies probes for X, 13, 18 and 21 chromosomes have been used [7,14,15,17,18]. The most complex protocol [21], uses probes for chromosome 13 (RB-1 locus, 13q14, expanding 440 Kb, Vysis,‹Inc. Downers Grove, IL), 21 (region 21q22.13-q22.2, Vysis), 16 (α satellite, Vysis), 18 (α satellite, D18Z1, Vysis), X (α satellite, DXZ1, Vysis) and Y (satellite III, DYZ1, Vysis). These probes are labeled with Spectrum-Orange[TM], Spectrum-Green[TM], and/or Spectrum-Aqua[TM] fluorochromes (Vysis). Chromosome X is labeled with Spectrum-Aqua, 16 with Spectrum-Green, and 21 with Spectrum-Orange. The other chromosomes are labeled with mixtures of fluorochromes, with 13 in Spectrum-Orange and Green, 18 with Spectrum-Orange and Aqua and chromosome Y with a combination of the three fluorochromes. When they are observed with a triple band pass filter, chromosome 13 appears as yellow, 18 as pink and Y as white. New fluorochromes are being developed, such gold (yellow) and blue (light blue), which will render the mixture of fluorochromes unnecessary for analysis of up to five chromosomes.

Once the cells are analyzed for a set of chromosomes, they can be reanalyzed with a different set of probes as demonstrated by Benadiva et al. [22]. This, coupled with fast protocols either with conventional denaturation and hybridization protocols (2 h [23]) or with microwave devices (6 min with α-satellite probes [24,25]), allows the analysis of 10 or more chromosomes simultaneously in a single interphase nucleus in a time frame compatible with regular IVF. For instance, we are currently reanalyzing blastomeres with probes for chromosomes 14 (binding to the 14q11.2 region), labeled with Spectrum-Aqua, 15 (binding to the α-satellite region) labeled with Spectrum-Orange, and 22 (binding to the 22q13.3) labeled with Spectrum-Green (Munné et al. unpublished). Therefore, by analyzing chromosomes X, Y, 13, 14, 15, 16, 18, 21 and 22 we can detect 70% of the aneuploidies found in spontaneous abortions.

*Scoring criteria and error rate of PGD of aneuploidy*

A scoring criterion for differentiating false-positives and false-negatives from mosaicism has been previously described [26–28]. Obviously this criteria only applies when all the cells of an embryo are analyzed, so it is necessary to determine the rate of misdiagnosis in PGD of numerical chromosome abnormalities. The specific FISH signals detected in a given blastomere were considered to reflect a true chromosome constitution in the following instances:

1) Blastomeres with two specific signals for gonosomes and two signals for each autosome analyzed; these were considered diploid blastomeres.
2) Embryos in which all the blastomeres had the same abnormality, such aneuploid, haploid or polyploid embryos.
3) Individual blastomeres that had only one signal per chromosome pair. These were considered haploid cells.
4) Individual blastomeres that had three or more signals per chromosome pair. These were considered polyploid cells.
5) Individual blastomeres that had extra or missing signals that were compensated by extra or missing signals in sibling blastomeres. We considered that

these blastomeres belonged to an embryo with mosaicism generated by mitotic nondisjunction.

6) Blastomeres showing less signals than their sibling blastomeres and belonging to mosaic embryos resulting from the uneven cleavage of a blastomere without previous DNA synthesis. An example would be an embryo with mostly XX 1313 1818 2121 cells, plus XO 13O 1818 OO and XO 13O OO 2121 cells.

7) The same criteria (1 to 6) were also used for multinucleated blastomeres.

8) Blastomeres with more or less than two gonosomes or chromosome-13, 18 or 21 specific signals were considered, respectively, FISH false-negative or false-positive errors unless one of the prior criteria (1 to 7) applied.

The method of differentiation between a split target producing two hybridization signals, and two targets close together was as follows: when their distance apart was at least 2 domain diameters this was taken to be two separate signals. Any others were considered split signals. A domain is the diameter of one signal, and domain areas for each chromosome type have different sizes. This criterion was applied to PGD using probes for chromosomes X, Y, 13, 18 and 21 with or without chromosome 16. After PGD, 198 embryos that were not replaced were fully biopsied and all cells analyzed. The PGD results were confirmed in 91% of these embryos, with 1.1% (1/88) of the embryos classified as normal embryos being abnormal and 17% (19/110) of the embryos classified as abnormal being normal [16,21]. Compared to previous protocols [1], the above criterion minimizes the risk of transferring abnormal embryos after PGD analysis, but a fraction of normal embryos are not being transferred after erroneous abnormal classification.

From these studies it is also evident that some probes produce more misdiagnosis than others. For instance, use of the 13/21 α-satellite probe has been discontinued because it produced more misdiagnosis than the individual- and locus-specific probes for chromosomes 13 and 21 [16]. Other probes, such as the one for chromosome Y and 18, produce more errors than those for chromosomes X, 13, 16 and 21, probably because they are bigger and tend to split more often [21]. These probes could be substituted for smaller ones and would presumably produce fewer errors.

**Limitations of PGD of numerical chromosome abnormalities**

*Mosaics*

Mosaicism cannot be detected efficiently by PGD unless all cells lines are abnormal. Misdiagnosis from mosaicism probably depends on the mosaic type and three major groups can be differentiated:

1) Mosaics produced by mitotic nondisjunction or anaphase lag of one of the chromosome pairs being analyzed. This is the most common source of misdiagnosis. They account for 11% of all mosaics.

2) The second group consists of mosaics involving two cell lines with different

numbers of haploid chromosome complements. They account for 25% of the mosaics. If the biopsied cell is 4N, this type of mosaicism can be readily detected with a few probes. These types of mosaicism are not considered seriously detrimental for the embryo because tetraploid cells usually end up forming the trophectoderm [29]; thus, if the 4N cell passes undetected, no serious misdiagnosis occurs. In addition, 12% of mosaics have different polyploid and/or haploid cell lines (i.e., one cell line 3N and another 4N), which will not produce misdiagnosis because the embryo will be classified as abnormal regardless of the cell biopsied.

3) Chaotic mosaics account for 17% of mosaics, half of them having all cells abnormal (but different cell lines) and the others have a few normal cells. Again, with a few probes most of these mosaics can be detected.

Therefore, only normal/aneuploid mosaics (11%) and normal/chaotic mosaics (9%) can produce misdiagnosis (20%). In morphologically normal embryos we found 40% mosaicism, therefore the error rate produced by mosaicism could be about 8%.

Recent results have shown that in normally developing embryos mosaicism occurs at the second or later divisions, with at least half or more mosaics being generated at the third or later divisions [28]. Consequently, even the analysis of three cells per eight-cell embryo would not be enough to find all mosaic embryos. However, the importance of mosaicism decreases when the percentage of abnormal blastomeres per mosaic embryo is considered, instead of the total number of embryos with mosaicism. Results in our center suggests that up to 40% of normally developing embryos are mosaics, but only 13% show more than 3/8 abnormal cells when all the cells are analyzed. Based on 17% frequency of extensive mosaicism found in nonarrested embryos [14], and 20% of mosaics producing misdiagnosis, mosaicism is estimated to produce about 5% misdiagnosis.

*Fish false negative errors and overlaps*

The occurrence of missing signals may indicate either a monosomic cell or a failure of the technique to display the remaining signals. Causes of reduced hybridization efficiency have been attributed to loss of DNA during denaturation or fixation, poor probe penetration, insufficient binding of detection reagents [30,31], or overlap of chromosome-specific signals when multiple probes are used [32]. We found that poor spread of the nucleus during fixation and content of DNA per nuclei increased signal overlap [33,34]. When two signals from the same chromosome overlap a single signal is observed, therefore producing a misdiagnosis. The more the nucleus is spread during fixation, the less overlapping of signals and missing signals were found [34].

About 7.3% (89/1220) blastomeres biopsied during clinical cases were broken during the biopsy, 1.3% lost during fixation, and 6.8% did not have a nucleus after fixation. Although most broken blastomeres could still be fixed by letting the remains of the blastomere dry on top of the glass slide, their nuclei were then very condensed and the scoring of FISH signals was generally unreliable.

*Multinucleated blastomeres*

Multinucleated blastomeres (MNBs) have been described in both morphologically normal and abnormal human embryos and they occur in about one-third of the embryos [35,36, and (Winston et al., 1991)] We have shown previously that MNBs are not suitable for preimplantation diagnosis of aneuploidy because the number of chromosomes in each nuclei varies greatly [1]. However, when the MNB is dinucleated, and both nuclei are chromosomally normal, the remainder of the embryo is also normal [1].

*Loss of micronuclei during fixation*

The FISH error is higher in MNBs (11.5%, 13/113), than in mononucleated cells (3.1%, 13/415) [26,27]. This is probably due to the fact that many MNBs very often contain micronuclei, and during fixation, some of them can get lost more easily than full nucleus producing false negative FISH errors.

We found a strong correlation between types of fixation and loss of chromosomes [21]. During fixation with acid:acetic fixative the drops added before the cell breaks allow the cytoplasm to expand — the more drops added the greater the expansion is — while the drop postlysis removes cytoplasm debris, and probably some anuclear DNA. It is therefore possible that the loss of DNA is higher after adding a drop postlysis when the cell is more expanded (two drops prelysis instead of one) as was observed in this study. Currently we recommend two drops prelysis followed by no drops postlysis, which with appropriate humidity conditions (40%) allow a good spreading, few cytoplasm debris, and minimal loss of DNA.

*Polar body vs. blastomere analysis*

Preconception diagnosis was pioneered by Verlinsky and co-workers [37] for single gene defects. This approach consists of analyzing the first polar body alone or in combination with the second polar body in order to determine the genetic status of the oocyte. FISH analysis of first polar bodies in combination or not with second polar bodies has been attempted by Verlinsky and co-workers [17] and Munné et al. [15]. Since autosomal aneuploidy occurs predominantly in maternal meiosis I [38—41], aneuploidy analysis of the first polar body can detect 80—100% of autosomal aneuploidy, depending on the chromosomes studied. Since the first polar body is a mirror image of the egg, the occurrence of an extra univalent chromosome (a chromosome with two chromatids) in the first polar body would imply that the egg is nullisomic and that the resulting embryo monosomic for that particular chromosome. Similarly, the lack of a full univalent in the first polar body would imply the resulting embryo would be trisomic for that chromosome. However, this scheme assumes that aneuploidy is produced by nondisjunction of full univalents. Contrary to this hypothesis, Angell [42] has reported that predivision resulting in separate chromatids may be a significant mechanism for human trisomy. When predivision occurs at meiosis-I, aneuploid MII oocytes with 23 univalents plus 1 chromatid, and those with 22 univalents plus 1 chromatid, may recover the normal chromosome constitution (23 univalents) during the second meiotic division, if the extra or missing chromatid is favorably distributed into the oocyte and second polar body. Consequently, if predivision is a significant mechanism of aneuploidy, the second polar body should be also analyzed to prevent a misdiagnosis. Using FISH, univalent chromosomes appear as double-dotted signals, with one dot per chromatid. However, sometimes the proximity of the chromatids makes the two dots overlap appearing as a single dot. This would not be a problem if predivision was nonexistent, but may lead to misdiagnosis if its a common event. The frequency of predivision vs. nondisjunction of full univalents is still debated [42,43]. However, we have detected an extra problem. It seems that predivision of chromatids increases artefactually in both, first polar bodies and eggs, with time in culture [8,15]. Such an increase is already apparent 6 h after egg retrieval. Another disadvantage of preconception diagnosis of aneuploidy is that paternal inherited aneuploidies, polyploidy, haploidy, and some mosaics cannot be detected. Those can, however, be detected by analyzing blastomeres instead of polar bodies. On the contrary, polar body analysis is not affected by errors produced by mosaicism.

*PGD of aneuploidy results: trisomic offspring, spontaneous abortions and implantation rates*

*Reduction of trisomic offspring*

More than 500 cases of preconception diagnosis of aneuploidy and about 200 cases of preimplantation diagnosis of aneuploidy have been performed with more than 100 ongoing or delivered babies born so far. To demonstrate a decrease in trisomic offspring, from 2.6% trisomies 13, 18 or 21 detected in CVS in women 39 years old, to 0.3% after PGD (assuming a 10% error rate), at least 300 fetuses or babies should be conceived by this technique to detect a significant decrease in trisomic offspring.

Unfortunately, a misdiagnosis has recently occurred in which a spontaneous abortion after PGD of aneuploidy showed to be trisomy 21 (Munné, Cohen, Scott and Grundfeld, unpublished). After the reanalysis of the same blastomeres with only probe for chromosome 21, the same results (normal) were obtained. In addition, the signals for each chromosome 21 target were of the same size and intensity in each cell suggesting that signal overlap was unlikely. Most likely, the error was caused by mosaicism or loss of DNA during fixation.

## Increase in implantation rate

Preliminary data from our center and Verlinsky's group indicate that implantation rates do not change after embryo biopsy and PGD, but they do after polar body biopsy (unpublished). The most probable factor affecting implantation after embryo biopsy might be the embryo biopsy procedure. Although a previous study on embryo biopsy did not show a negative effect on embryo development to blastocyst [36], embryo transfer effects, if any, were not assessed. Moreover, the embryos studied were from donors and not from older patients or those with a poor prognosis. Evidence of embryo damage during transfer of zona-drilled embryos comes from assisted hatching (AHA) studies. For instance, assisted hatching has been demonstrated to increase implantation rates [5], but its potential is related to the diameter of the opening in the zona. Openings of 50–60 µm in diameter required for biopsy, instead of the recommended 20–30 µm for AHA, might eliminate any beneficial effect (Dr. Bill Schoolcraft and Terry Schlenker, personal communication), and cause embryo damage during or after embryo transfer. Another effect of embryo biopsy could be the toxicity of acidified Tyrode's solution, although the appearance of effective laser devices could make its use obsolete [44]. Polar body biopsy, although less effective in selecting abnormal embryos, does not compromise implantation since the hole in the zona is very small and the procedure is mechanical.

## Reduction in spontaneous abortions

What embryo biopsy and PGD seem to produce is a reduction in spontaneous abortions (Munné et al., unpublished). This indicates that the theory behind PGD of aneuploidy is correct and that the selection against chromosomally abnormal embryos should increase the number of babies born per embryo transfer by selecting against those that will not implant or abort spontaneously. For that to be demonstrated, alternative methods of embryo biopsy, or the use of polar body biopsy should be applied.

## Future developments

### Comparative genome hybridization

A new an promising development is the use of comparative genomic hybridization (CGH). This method, developed by Kallioniemi et al. [45], can accurately determine total or partial aneusomy by loss or gains of DNA, using a combination of PCR and FISH technology. The technique consists of:

1) The cells to test are chemically modified with an apten, i.e., with biotin.
2) Cells with normal chromosome complements are used as genomic control DNA, which is chemically modified with a different hapten, e.g., Digoxigenin.
3) Test and control DNAs are mixed, for example, in a 1:1 ratio.
4) The mixture is used as a probe for chromosomal in situ suppression hybridization, also known as chromosome painting [46,47], on metaphase spreads with normal chromosome complements of known sex.

5) Test and control DNAs are detected by different fluorochromes (e.g., biotin with green FITC and Digoxigenin with red TRITC).

6) Using an image analysis system, the resulting ratio of green/red fluorescence intensities for each chromosome should reflect the number of homologous chromosomes present in the test DNA: 0 for nullisomies, 0.5 for monosomies, 1 for normal cells, 1.5 for trisomies, etc. Similarly, partial monosomies and trisomies will also be detected in the same fashion. According to Hughes (personal communication), CGH can be applied to single cells, although presently, it takes 2–3 days to obtain a diagnosis. Once it can be done in a time frame compatible with regular IVF, CGH will allow the detection of any chromosome abnormality in single blastomeres, with the exception of balanced translocations.

*Quantitative PCR: fluorescent detection of PCR product*
Quantitative PCR could be used to detect aneuploidy or any other chromosome abnormality. The first attempts at quantitative PCR are based on simultaneous amplification of two sequences, the one to be quantitated and another that works as internal standard for the quantification. One approach has been to use the IGFI gene in chromosome 12 to quantify S100B gene in chromosome 21 [48]. This approach, however, is prone to false negatives and ambiguous results. A better approach is to use a single pair of primers to identify two genes simultaneously, the PFKM-CH1 (in chromosome 1) and the PFKL-CH21 (in chromosome 21) [49]. They found that the ratio PFKM-CH1/ PFKL-CH21 was 1.33 for disomy and 0.4 for trisomy 21. The gel intensity was measured fluorescently and the differences were very significant ($p < 0.001$). Combined with PIP it could be possible to assess multiple chromosomes simultaneously. The method, however, has the same problems as any PCR-based method, that is, risk of contamination, and allele drop out.

"PCR coupled with automated fluorescent detection of the PCR product by a highly sophisticated gene scanner also shows great potential for increasing the reliability of genetic analysis in single cells [50]. Findlay and collaborators reported using this rapid and highly discriminative automated test for single-cell diagnosis of CF mutations, with simultaneous sexing and highly informative DNA fingerprinting to exclude DNA contamination (unpublished data). The possibility of quantitative analysis by this method is being explored for PGD of aneuploidy" [51].

*Spectral imaging*
An alternative to conventional FISH is the use of 24 painting probes, one for each chromosome type, labeled in ratios of five different fluorochromes and observed with spectral imaging. The system measures all points simultaneously in the sample emission spectra, across the visible and near-infrared spectral range. Instead of measuring a single intensity, as in conventional epifluorescence

microscopy, the spectral imaging system measures the whole spectrum of emitted light allowing differentiation of overlapping multiple fluorophores. Artificial colors are then assigned to each chromosome to provide the karyotype. Display colors allow all chromosomes to be readily visualized after spectral imaging and spectra-classification colors is a chromosome classification algorithm based in spectral measurements at each pixel (Schröck et al., 1996). This technique has recently been applied to oocyte, first polar body and blastomere metaphases [52]. Since first polar bodies are found at metaphase stage shortly after retrieval [53], they could be analyzed by spectral imaging for PGD purposes.

*PNA probes*

PNAs are a DNA analog in which the phosphate backbone has been replaced by (2-aminothyl)glycine units with the nucleobases attached through methylene carbonyl linkages to the glycine amino group (Nielsen et al., 1991). This neutral backbone avoids interstrand electrostatic repulsion, allowing complementary sequences to be recognized with high affinity and selectivity relative to hybridization of analogous DNA or RNA oligomers (Egholm, 1993). Because of these advantages, PNA probes could be of use in PGD.

**PGD of structural abnormalities**

Chromosome analysis by conventional karyotyping cannot be used because an average of only 25% of blastomere nuclei show metaphase chromosomes after antimitotic treatment, and even fewer nuclei show banding-quality chromosomes [13]. Similarly, G-banding of polar body or oocyte chromosomes cannot be achieved consistently due to the poor metaphase chromosomes obtained [54].

For this reason, four approaches, all based on FISH technology have been proposed:

*Chromosome painting of polar bodies*

This method was proposed after the observation that 90% or more first polar bodies fixed 6 or less h after retrieval are at metaphase stage, and therefore the translocation can be identified using chromosome painting probes for the two chromosomes involved in the translocation [53]. This method was later improved by using telomeric probes to enhance the regions not covered by the painting probes, and also to use centromere or marker probes, desirably in a third color (blue), to distinguish chromatids and avoid the confusion between single chromatids and whole chromosomes [55]. Single chromatids have been found to occur often in degenerating polar bodies [7,14,15]. Using these modifications it was observed that the frequency of spontaneous abortions per embryo transferred in the group that became pregnant was significantly reduced ($p < 0.001$, F test), from 95% (18/19) in natural cycles to 12.5% (1/8) after PGD. The single spontaneous abortion after PGD resulted from an embryo expected to be balanced according to PGD results. Similarly, the pregnancy rate was very high, with an implantation of 50%, which is expected since most translocations of maternal origin do not produce infertility but spontaneous abortions.

One problem with this technique is the occurrence of crossing-over and predivision of chromatids. In both cases the outcome of the second meiotic division is unclear, and the second polar body or blastomeres should be analyzed. Figure 2 represents a case of predivision of chromatids, in which while balanced in the M-II egg, produced an unbalanced embryo after meiosis-Ii was finalized.

The other problem is the occurrence of interstitial crossover with subsequent segregation of balanced and unbalanced sets of chromosomes during the second meiotic division. So far we have detected one of these events (Fig. 3).

Spectral imaging, as discussed previously, has been used to analyze numerical chromosome abnormalities in polar bodies [52] and may be useful to detect simultaneously translocations and aneuploidy.

*Probes distal to the breakpoints*

For male translocations the only reliable method is to use FISH on interphase blastomeres, which requires either that specific probes be developed for each type of translocation expanding the breakpoints [56] or using probes distal to the breakpoints [57]. The exception is Robertsonian translocation (RT), for which enumerator α-satellite or locus-specific probes could be used to detect aneuploid embryos [58]. Even in cases of RT, locus specific probes cannot differentiate between balanced and normal embryos. Balanced embryos, when enough normal ones are available, should not be transferred in order prevent the perpetuation of the genetic disease in the family.

Probes distal to the breakpoints have been used by several groups, either using a probe for each distal fragment [56], or just one distal probe for one chromosome and a centromeric probe for the other chromosome involved [57]. There are several serious problems with the second approach:
1) lack of internal controls: if one probe does not work it would be interpreted as an abnormal embryo instead of a nonsense result;
2) because only two of the four chromosome types are identified, mosaic events, polyploidy and haploidy may be missed;
3) it cannot differentiate between balanced and normal embryos; and
4) it cannot detect 3:1 segregations.

*Probes spanning the breakpoints*

This approach has been recently applied to PGD of two translocations, a 46,XY,t(3;4)(p24;p15); and a 46,XY,t(6;11)(p22.1;p15.3) [56]. For example, for the first translocation, probes spanning the two breakpoints on 3p24 and 4p15 were developed by a combination of chromosome jumping (for rough breakpoint localization) and YAC walking (for probe optimization) (Fung et al., unpublished). Briefly, YAC clones that map to the short arms of chromosomes 3 and 4, respectively, were selected from the CEPH library based on data in the MIT/ Whitehead database. During the mapping process, YAC DNA isolated from overnight cultures was labeled by random priming incorporating either biotin-14-dCTP or Digoxigenin-12-dUTP [59,60]. Overnight hybridization to metaphase spreads from the translocation carrier allowed rapid "binning" of the breakpoint by mapping probes as being either proximal or distal to the breakpoints on the respective chromosomes. The binning intervals were then progressively narrowed until YAC clones were found that spanned the breakpoints. Probes prepared from these clones were then optimized using pulsed field gel electrophoresis (PFGE) and degenerate oligonucleotide-primed PCR (DOP-PCR) [59] to ensure strong signals on either side of the breakpoint. The probe spanning the breakpoint on 3p24 (YAC clone 958B5 containing markers D3S2335 and FB21H8) was labeled in green with FITC. For coverage of the breakpoint region on the short arm of chromosome 4, we isolated a four YAC contig comprised of the proximal clone 931C2 (containing markers D4S860 and D4S425), the breakpoint spanning clones 967C5 and 853C4 (both containing markers D4S425 and D4S2605) and the YAC clone 887E8 (containing markers D4S2933 and D4S972) binding distal to the breakpoint. This 4p15 contig probe was labeled with Digoxigenin by random priming, and bound probe was detected with Rhodamine-labeled anti-Digoxigenin antibodies. When the translocation occurred, each hybridization target was split in two physically separated domains of about equal intensity. Therefore, a derivative chromosome appeared as an association of a green and a red domain. To further distinguish the der(3) and the der(4) chromosomes, we added a blue fluorescent-satellite probe for the centromeric region of chromosome 3 (D3Z1, CEP-3 Spectrum Aqua®, VYSIS).

The error rate in both cases, each of which has undergone two cycles with the same method, was 3% (3/98) when analyzing control blastomeres, and 0% (0/ 14) when reanalyzing nontransferred embryos from the four PGD cycles ([56] and unpublished results). Unfortunately, only five out of 20 embryos analyzed embryos in the four cycles were found to be normal (n = 3) or balanced (n = 2) and no pregnancy resulted after either cycle.

This approach can also be used for other structural abnormalities, such inversions as previously demonstrated by Cassel et al. [61] who developed probes spanning the breakpoint of a chromosome 6p inversion.

## References

1. Munné S, Cohen J. Hum Reprod 1993;8(7):1120−1125.
2. Warburton et al. Cytogenetic abnormalities in spontaneous abortions of recognized conceptions. In: Porter IH, Willey A (eds) Perinatal Genetics: Diagnosis and Treatment. New York: Academic Press, 1986;133−148.
3. Navot et al. Fertil Steril 1994;61:97−101.
4. Keefe et al. Fertil Steril 1995;64:577−583.
5. Cohen et al. Hum Reprod 1990;5:7−13.

6.   Brenner et al. (in press).
7.   Munné et al. Am J Obs Gyn 1995a;172:1191–1201.
8.   Dailey et al. Am J Hum Genet 1996;59:176–184.
9.   Magnuson et al. J Exp Zool 1985;236:353–360.
10.  Janny L, Menezo YJR. Molec Reprod Devel 1996;45:31–37.
11.  Plachot et al. Hum Reprod 1987;1:29–35.
12.  Pellestor et al. Molec Reprod Devel 1994;39:141–146.
13.  Santaló et al. Fertil Steril 1995;64:44–50.
14.  Munné et al. Fertil Steril 1995b;64:382–391.
15.  Munné et al. Hum Reprod 1995c;10:1015–1021.
16.  Munné S, Weier U. Cytogenet Cell Genet 1996;75:263–270.
17.  Verlinsky et al. Hum Reprod 1995;10:1923–1927.
18.  Verlinsky Y, Kuliev A. Human Reprod 1996;11:2076–2077.
19.  Nederlof et al. Cytometry 1990;11:126–131.
20.  Dauwerse et al. Hum Molec Genet 1992;1:593–598.
21.  Munné et al. Hum Reprod 1998a;(In press).
22.  Benadiva CA, Kligman I, Munné S. Fertil Steril 1996;666:248–255.
23.  Harper JC, Handyside AH. Curr Obstet Gynecol 1994;4:143–149.
24.  Durm et al. Braz J Med Biol Res 1997;30:15–23.
25.  Drury et al. J Ass Reprod Genet 1997;14:436–437 (Abs.20).
26.  Munné et al. Am J Hum Genet 1994a;55(1):150–159.
27.  Munné et al. Hum Reprod 1994d;9:506–510.
28.  Munné et al. J Ass Reprod Genet 1994e;10:276–279.
29.  James RM, West JD. Hum Genet 1994;93:603–604.
30.  West et al. Lancet 1987;i:1345–1347.
31.  Pieters et al. Cytogenet Cell Genet 1990;53:15–19.
32.  Handyside AH. Reprod Med Rev 1993;2:51–61.
33.  Munné et al. J Ass Reprod Genet 1993a;10:82–90.
34.  Munné et al. J Ass Reprod Genet 1996b;13:149–156.
35.  Tesarik et al. Hum Reprod 1987;2(2):127–136.
36.  Hardy et al. Hum Reprod 1990;5(6):708–714.
37.  Verlinsky et al. Hum Reprod 1990;5:826–829.
38.  Hassold et al. J Med Genet 1987;24:725–732.
39.  Hassold et al. J Med Genet 1991a;28:159–162.
40.  Hassold TJ, Takaesu N. In: Hassold TJ, Epstein CJ (eds) Molecular and Cytogenetic Studies of
     Nondisjunction. New York: Alan Liss Inc., 1989;115–134.
41.  May et al. Am J Hum Genet 1990;46:754–761.
42.  Angel RR. Hum Genet 1991;86:383–387.
43.  Kamiguchi et al. Hum Genet 1993;90:533–541.
44.  Montag et al. Fertil Steril 1998;69:539–542.
45.  Kallioniemi et al. Science 1992;258:818–821.
46.  Lichter et al. Proc Natl Acad Sci USA 1988;85:9664–9668.
47.  Pinkel et al. Proc Natl Acad Sci USA 1988;85:9138–9142.
48.  Von Eggeling et al. Hum Genet 1993;1:567–570.
49.  Lee et al. Hum Genet 1997;99:364–367.
50.  Tully G, Sullivan KM, Gill P. Hum Genet 1993;92:554–562.
51.  Verlinsky Y, Dozortzev D, Evsikov S. J Assist Reprod Genet 1994;11:123–131.
52.  Márquez C, Cohen J, Munné S. Cytogenet Cell Genet 1998;(In press).
53.  Munné et al. Fertil Steril 1998b;69:675–681.
54.  Pellestor F. Hum Genet 1991;86:283–288.
55.  Munné et al. JARG 1998b;(In press).
56.  Munné et al. Hum Reprod 1998d;(In press).

57. Pierce et al. Molec Hum Reprod 1998;4:167—172.
58. Conn et al. Hum Genet 1998;(In press).
59. Weier et al. Genomics 1994;24:641—644.
60. Weier et al. Genomics 1995a;26:390—393.
61. Cassel et al. Hum Reprod 1997;12:2019—2027.

# Aneuploidy rates in blastomeres

Michelle Plachot
*CHI Jean Rostand, Sèvres, France*

**Abstract.** Chromosome abnormalities mostly account for the low rate of implantation of human embryos after in vivo or in vitro fertilization. They result from nondisjunctions occurring during meiosis in oocytes (21%) or spermatozoa (6%). In vitro maturation of oocytes seems to increase the incidence of diploid oocytes. Regarding spermatozoa, the rate of aneuploidy is slightly increased in infertile patients.

Abnormal fertilization such as parthenogenetic activation, polyspermy and delayed fertilization produces abnormal embryos that are usually excluded from the transfer.

Poor embryo morphology and a low rate of division are associated with a high incidence of chromosome disorders when compared with normally developing embryos. The culture of embryos to the blastocyst stage allows the selection of the most viable concepti, displaying less chromosome anomalies than earlier stages.

Chromosome anomalies in embryos may arise as a consequence of various defects such as nuclear replication without cytokinesis, fragmentation of nuclei, or defective chromosome movements at anaphase possibly linked to the formation of abnormal spindles. Damage or mutations in p53 and/ or inappropriate bcl-2 expression may reduce sensitivity to apoptosis and contribute to genetic instability.

**Keywords:** chromosome abnormalities, human embryos, in vitro fertilization.

Chromosome abnormalities are largely responsible for the low rate of implantation of human embryos. They result from abnormalities occurring during meiosis (in oocytes or spermatozoa), during fertilization (leading to parthenogenetic activation or triploidy) or during the first mitosis (leading to mosaics). Several genes have now been identified which regulate spindle formation, DNA repair and apoptosis to eliminate abnormal cells.

## Gamete abnormalities

*Oocytes* ·

Genetically abnormal oocytes are largely responsible for the high rate of chromosome abnormalities detected in preimplantion embryos. They result from nondisjunctions occurring during meiosis I and less frequently during meiosis II.

Pooling data from published studies for more than 3,000 oocytes shows that 21% are abnormal (for review see [1]). More abnormalities are detected in

---

*Address for correspondence:* M. Plachot, Laboratorie de FIV et Biologie de la Reproduction, Hospital Necker, 149 rue de Sevres, 75743 Paris, France.

oocytes from women referred to IVF clinics for tubal or idiopathic infertility than in those from fertile women, showing that ovarian pathology may cause abnormalities in the oocyte maturation process. Advanced maternal age and intrafollicular conditions (low dissolved oxygen concentration, contaminants of cigarette smoke) have been found to induce chromosome disorders.

A correlation has recently been demonstrated between the rate of diploidy in failed-fertilized oocytes and the rate of fertilization of the IVF cycle from which the oocytes were obtained [2]. The diploidy rate (11.4%) if $> 25\%$ of oocytes are fertilized is higher than that if $< 25\%$ or no oocytes are fertilized (4%), indicating that diploid oocytes may have a lower fertilizing ability.

ICSI (intracytoplasmic sperm injection), which requires the removal of cumulus-corona cells, makes it possible to determine the maturation stage of oocytes at recovery. Immature oocytes can be incubated in vitro until the metaphase II stage in order to increase the overall number of mature oocytes available. Very few pregnancies have been reported after such a procedure.

We investigated the reasons for implantation failure after in vitro maturation (IVM) of oocytes, by carrying out a cytogenetic study of IVM oocytes and comparing the results with those for in vivo matured oocytes that failed to fertilize in our ICSI program (F-ICSI).

We observed a slight increase in diploid oocytes obtained after IVM (8.4%) when compared to in vivo maturation (F-ICSI) (2.9%, $p < 0.05$). The incidence of aneuploidy (hyper + hypohaploidy) was similar for both groups. The incidence of chromosome breaks was found to be lower in IVM oocytes than in F-ICSI oocytes (Table 1).

Thus, the risk of meiotic nondisjunction resulting in monosomy or trisomy is similar for in vitro and in vivo matured oocytes. However, there were slightly more diploid oocytes after IVM which, if fertilized, will give rise to triploid eggs.

*Spermatozoa*

The development of fluorescence in situ hybridization (FISH) with chromosome-specific DNA probes has made it possible to determine the nondisjunction frequencies for most of the autosomes and the sex chromosomes in spermatozoa from cytogenetically normal men. However, there are conflicting results, mostly due to the methods of chromatin decondensation used, the number of spermato-

*Table 1.* Incidence of chromosome abnormalities in oocytes matured in vitro (IVM) or in vivo and which failed to fertilize in our ICSI program (F-ICSI).

|  | IVM | F-ICSI |  |
| --- | --- | --- | --- |
| No. of oocytes | 107 | 171 |  |
| Diploid oocytes | 8.4% | 2.9% | $p < 0.05$ |
| Aneuploid oocytes | 24% | 23.9% | ns |
| Chromosome breaks | 15.7% | 30.7% | $p < 0.02$ |

zoa and individuals studied and the scoring criteria. For control populations, the frequency of aneuploidy per haploid set in human sperm nuclei has been estimated to be 6% (for review see [3]).

Reports on chromosome abnormalities in spermatozoa from infertile men also give conflicting results. Some authors found no difference in the numbers of abnormal spermatozoa, whereas Egozcue et al. [3] found a higher incidence of abnormalities for chromosomes X, Y and 18 (2.11%) than for the control population (0.71%). Our results were consistent with those of Egozcue et al. [3] because, with dual FISH for X and Y chromosomes, there was a higher incidence of XY-bearing spermatozoa (1.26%) in semen able to fertilize oocytes only by ICSI than in semen able to fertilize oocytes by conventional IVF, 0.37% ($p < 0.001$). The incidence of XX- and YY-bearing sperm nuclei was also significantly higher in the ICSI group (0.25% XX, 0.50% YY, $p < 0.02$) than in the IVF group (0.06% XX, 0.16% YY).

We concluded that infertile men requiring ICSI treatment had a higher incidence of sex chromosome aneuploidy due to meiosis I and II nondisjunction in their spermatozoa, than men requiring IVF for reasons of predominantly female infertility [4].

**Fertilization abnormalities**

Abnormally fertilized oocytes are able to develop in vitro but development usually stops between genomic embryo activation (four to eight cells) and implantation (for review see [5]).

*1-PN oocytes*

The 1-PN oocytes usually result from a failure in the fertilization process. The karyotype of the resulting embryos in our study was the expected haploid chromosome complement in 69% of the cases. A total of 13% were diploid, due to nonextrusion of the second polar body or after spontaneous diploidization, which may occur before the first cleavage or later during embryogenesis, leading to various forms of mosaicism (18%).

The 1-PN oocytes may also result from late sperm penetration. Indeed, Sultan et al. [6] and Macas et al. [7] showed that 61.9% of zygotes resulting from 1-PN oocytes after IVF were diploid and fertilized (half with a Y chromosome) whereas nearly all of those resulting from 1-PN oocytes after ICSI were haploid, and therefore activated. The latter should be excluded from the transfer.

Levron et al. [8] demonstrated that two distinctly different types of single-pronucleated zygotes may develop after IVF. The first type is parthenogenetic, because the isolated pronuclei always had an X signal and a haploid chromosome complement and the remaining cytoplast was devoid of nuclear DNA. The second is monospermic diploid, because the isolation between the karyoplast and the cytoplasm showed diploid XY- or XX-containing pronuclei. These findings suggest that the second type of single-pronucleated zygote is produced by fusion of the paternal and maternal genomes during syngamy. This is a cellular mechanism that differs considerably from the normal one in which both male and female pronuclei remain in close contact before membrane disappearance and syngamy.

*3-PN oocytes*

Most of the 3-PN oocytes produced by IVF result from polyspermy. After ICSI of a single spermatozoon, the additional pronucleus must be of maternal origin, and in fact, most of these oocytes have not extruded the second polar body. As a consequence, in monospermic digenic embryos, a 1:1 XXX/XXY ratio is expected, whereas in dispermic embryos a 1:2:1 XXX/XXY/XYY ratio is expected.

In our study, about 13% of the 3-PN oocytes reached the blastocyst stage. This anomaly is lethal during the first weeks of development, triploidy being one of the most frequent reasons for spontaneous abortion. The detection of 3-PN zygotes and their exclusion from transfer decreases the incidence of triploid fetuses after IVF.

Cytogenetic studies on two- to eight-cell embryos derived from 3-PN oocytes unexpectedly demonstrated that very few were triploid. In our series, 24% were triploid, 32% diploid and 5% haploid, probably because of the exclusion of one or two pronuclei at the first mitotic division. About 29% of the embryos showed various forms of mosaicisms, probably caused by the chaotic migration of the chromosomes to the poles of the tripolar spindle.

The exclusion of these abnormal zygotes from the transfer decreases the overall chance of pregnancy. It would therefore be of potential value to remove the supernumerary male pronucleus from polyspermic zygotes. Feng and Gordon [9] carried out a study to test the developmental potential of polyspermic mouse zygotes corrected by manipulation. After removal of the supernumerary pronucleus, 18 out of 58 zygotes developed to the blastocyst stage and were transferred. Of these, five animals were born (two males and three females) and produced normal offspring, indicating that the abnormality really had been corrected.

Attempts to correct 3-PN oocytes in humans have been unsuccessful. Palermo et al. [10] analyzed the fertilization patterns and incidence of mosaicism in 3-PN oocytes. The rate of mosaics in monospermic (2-PN), monospermic digynic (3-PN) and corrected monospermic digynic (3-1PN) embryos was low at 18, 14 and 25%, respectively. However, the rate of mosaics in dispermic (3-PN) and corrected dispermic zygotes (3-1 PN) was high at 89 and 100%, respectively. These data show that the removal of the supernumerary male pronucleus does not restore normal chromosomal pattern despite restoring diploidy. This difference between mice and humans may be due to centrosome inheritance: in mice the centrosome is maternally inherited, whereas in humans, it is paternally inherited. The penetration of two spermatozoa (and two centrosomes) induces the formation of an abnormal spindle that is not corrected by the late removal of the extra male pronucleus.

*Delayed fertilization*

We have previously reported a correlation between the timing of fertilization and the incidence and type of chromosome abnormalities [11]. Indeed, in 1.6% of oocytes inseminated by conventional IVF, fertilization was delayed because pronuclei were observed 42 h after gamete mixing. This delayed fertilization of mature oocytes causes oocyte ageing in vitro, which is known to result in chromosome anomalies. In a series of 23 embryos resulting from late fertilized oocytes we observed a much higher incidence of chromosome disorders (87%) than with timely fertilization (29%). This was partly due to an increase in the rate of mosaics (30 vs. 10%). Such anomalies may be due to changes in the oocyte cytoskeleton and in the organization of microtubules leading to abnormal spindles. Similar observations have been reported in hamster embryos. Delayed fertilization was achieved by gradually lengthening the intervals between copulation and the estimated time of ovulation. The incidence of chromosome abnormalities increased from 0.7 to 17% when the delay increased by 3 h. In the same time, the incidence of mosaics increased from 0 to 4.3% [12].

## Cytogenetic and embryo development anomalies

*The fate of undocumented embryos*

Usually, oocytes are freed from cumulus cells 17 h after insemination to assess the normality of fertilization. In about 40% of the cases, there are no pronuclei, suggesting fertilization failure. However, 41% of these undocumented zygotes cleave the next day. We have previously assessed the viability of these embryos and the value of transferring them in utero especially because their morphological appearance and rate of division are similar to those of fertilized eggs at least until day 2 postinsemination. We observed that their capacity for further division was limited, because only 70% were able to divide on days 2—3, whereas 93% of the fertilized eggs do divide. Their viability was also low because only 5.9% were able to implant, vs. 11.1% for fertilized eggs in single transfers.

Cytogenetic analysis of these embryos showed that 55% were chromosomally abnormal (vs. 30% for fertilized eggs) with a high rate of haploidy (20%) confirming the parthenogenetic nature of some of them. The others were either triploid (9%) or mosaics (26%). Some of these embryos may result from normal fertilization with a slight modification of the timing of pronuclear growth, whereas the others may be generated from parthenogenetic activation.

Manor et al. [12] used FISH (with probes specific for chromosomes X, Y, 13, 18 and 21) to analyze the chromosome status of 23 undocumented embryos. Diploidy was confirmed in 13 (57%) embryos but the remaining embryos had various chromosome anomalies. One ongoing pregnancy was achieved following the transfer of such an embryo.

These two studies show that some of these embryos may give rise to normal pregnancies. However, a preimplantation genetic diagnosis should be carried out when only undocumented embryos are available for transfer.

*Embryo morphology*

Chromosome studies have shown that dysmorphic embryos have a higher rate of chromosome abnormalities than morphologically normal embryos. We previously observed a 78% incidence of chromosomal disorders in fragmented embryos compared to 12.5% for morphologically normal embryos [13]. Bongso et al. [14] analyzed 91 poor-quality embryos and observed 31.9% chromosome anomalies: 19.8% mosaicism, 5.5% polyploidy, 2.2% pulverized chromosomes, 2.2% aneuploidy, 1.1% prematurely condensed chromosomes and 1.1% structural rearrangements involving chromosome pair No. 2. A much higher incidence of chromosome anomalies was reported by Pellestor et al. [15] who observed 90% abnormal or aberrant chromosome complements in 118 poor-quality embryos.

FISH was used to analyze fragmented preimplantation embryos using simultaneously X-, Y-, 18- and/or 13/21-chromosome-specific probes. For these three or five chromosome pairs 56% mosaic and/or polyploid embryos were found, indicating that nearly all poor-quality embryos are abnormal when considering the entire genome [16]. This demonstrates the uselessness of both the transfer and the cryopreservation of fragmented embryos.

Other kinds of dysmorphisms are observed during the preimplantation embryo development. Cell multinucleation is a common abnormality in preimplantation embryos resulting from in vivo or in vitro fertilization [17]. Dysmorphic embryos are more likely to contain multinucleated cells. The presence of multinucleated cells in nonarrested day 2 or day 3 human embryos is indicative in 74% of the cases of extensive mosaicism and/or polyploidy [16]. The same authors have described two other groups of dysmorphic monospermic embryos chromosomally abnormal in all cases. The first refers to 13 embryos with only one large cell surrounded by smaller blastomere-sized extracellular fragments. These embryos were polyploid and frequently polyploid mosaics. Some of these embryos showed ploidies up to 20n and the single cell was multinucleated. The second group refers to six embryos which developed from larger than normal oocytes, with diameters $\geqslant 220$ µm. These embryos were invariably XXX or XXY triploids or triploid mosaics, suggesting that they were derived from diploid oocytes.

*Rate of division*

Normally developing embryos analyzed by FISH display a 28.8% incidence of chromosome disorders, comprising 2.3% polyploidy, 3.9% haploidy, 13.3% 2n-extensive mosaicism and 10.6% aneuploidy [16].

During in vitro embryo development, some embryos are considered as arrested, i.e., they do not develop beyond the eight-cell stage on their 4th day of development and do not cleave during a 24-h period. The major chromosomal abnormality detected in these embryos, derived from monospermic fertilization, is polyploidy (43.4%). Since most polyploid embryos arrest before the onset of genome activation which occurs around the four- to eight-cell stage, oocyte quality or suboptimal embryo culture conditions may be the cause of their arrest. Aneuploidy is detected less in arrested embryos (6.4%) because they are mostly mosaics (22.5%) with unexpected chromosome complements. Including 2.6% haploidy, the total incidence of chromosome anomalies in arrested embryos is 71.5%.

Selection of embryos for transfer after freezing-thawing is usually done on the basis of survival (number of intact blastomeres) and morphology. Recently, it has been shown that the selection of embryos that survive cryopreservation and continue to cleave in vitro, significantly increases the implantation rate. FISH analysis (with probes specific for chromosomes X, Y and 1) of 60 embryos that survived cryopreservation but did not cleave further after thawing, showed that 80% were abnormal with aneuploidy, nondisjunction, haploidy, polyploidy, mosaicism or chaotic divisions. These results are consistent with those obtained from nonfrozen arrested embryos in which the incidence of chromosome anomalies was 60%. They stress the need for stricter selection of embryos in freezing programs [18].

*Treatment-related chromosome anomalies*

Chromosome abnormalities observed during the preimplantation period may be due to suboptimal hormonal stimulation and/or embryo culture. Munné et al. [19] evaluated the incidence of mosaicism in the first and second mitotic division in good quality embryos from four different IVF centers. They used FISH with probes that were specific for chromosomes X, Y, 13, 18 and 21, and observed that the use of clomiphene citrate or gonadotropins for ovulation induction (before 1991), or unsuitable temperature control during culture and oocyte isolation caused a high rate of mosaicism (52—64% of the embryos). Impairment of the cytoskeleton and/or mitotic spindle, causing developmental arrest of the embryos may be responsible for the low success rate, 16.7—16.9% delivery/retrieval.

The use of downregulation (lupron-metrodin-pergonal) with appropriate temperature control when handling oocytes and embryos makes it possible to achieve a high delivery rate (30.2%) and a low rate of mosaicism (13%).

*Aneuploidy in blastocysts*

The culture of embryos to the blastocyst stage allows the selection of the most viable concepti.

We have previously cultured 1-PN oocytes (thought to result from partheno-genetic activation) to the blastocyst stage and compared the rate and nature of chromosome abnormalities at the four-cell and blastocyst stages. Most four-cell embryos were haploid. However, we did detect some diploid embryos, possibly due to asynchronous pronuclear development leading to misinterpretation of the number of pronuclei. Blastocysts, in contrast, are mostly diploid due to the early arrest of most haploid embryos (Table 2). Mosaics in early embryos were mainly n/2n due to mitotic nondisjunction whereas mosaics in blastocysts were mainly 2n/4n due to normal syncytiotrophoblastic differentiation of the blastocyst tro-phoblast.

Similar results were reported by Clouston et al. [20] for normally fertilized embryos. In total, 73 6- to 8-day-old human blastocysts were analyzed and some abnormalities were observed: polyploidy, diploid/polyploid mosaicism, nonmo-saic trisomy 16, 46, X del (X)/46, XX and several single cells with trisomies or structural anomalies in otherwise normal blastocysts. Polyploidy and diploid/polyploid mosaicism is a normal feature (the formation of the syncytiotropho-blast by fusion of trophoblast cells) so the incidence of abnormal embryos is low, about 8%. Blastocysts are a population of selected embryos when compared with 3-day-old embryos. Indeed, Menezo et al. [21] proposed an embryo selec-tion by IVF, coculture and transfer at the blastocyst stage to a woman referred for IVF, with a balanced reciprocal translocation 46, XX, t (1; 22) (p116; q112) who had experienced two early abortions. Among the seven 2-cell embryos obtained, only two reached the blastocyst stage and were transferred, resulting in the birth of a boy with the maternal balanced translocation. The five embryos that did not develop in culture were analyzed by FISH using probes for chromo-somes 1, 18 and 22. They were found to have severe lethal cytogenetic anomalies, related to the maternal translocation.

## Clinical significance

Chromosome anomalies in preimplantation embryos account for the high rate of embryo wastage. It is impossible to identify genetically abnormal embryos even with morphological or growth-rate criteria. However, the chromosome status of untransferred (spare) embryos was correlated with the probability of pregnancy after IVF. Indeed, patients who became pregnant produced a higher proportion

*Table 2.* Chromosome abnormalities in four-cell embryos and blastocysts resulting from the develop-ment of 1-PN oocytes.

|  | Four-cell embryos | Blastocysts |
|---|---|---|
| Haploidy | 69% | 22% |
| Diploidy | 13% | 56% |
| Mosaics | 18% | 22% |

of chromosomally normal spare embryos (37.5%) than those who did not achieve pregnancy (1.9%) [22]. In the same way, when analyzing morphologically normal preimplantation embryos from fertile patients (in the framework of a preimplantation genetic diagnosis for X-linked disease), it was observed that mosaic and chaotic chromosome patterns were strongly patient-dependant: some patients had chaotic embryos in several cycles whereas other patients were free from this type of anomaly [23]. This observation is of clinical relevance because such embryos are unlikely to progress beyond implantation.

## Gene regulation of nuclear division

Chromosome abnormalities may arise as a consequence of various defects such as nuclear replication without cytokinesis, fragmentation of nuclei, or defective chromosome movements at anaphase possibly linked to the formation of abnormal spindles.

The appearance of aneuploid or polyploid cells resulting from damaged spindles is presumably prevented by cell-cycle checkpoint controls, one of which is the spindle assembly checkpoint which detects defects in spindle structure or in the alignment of chromosomes on the spindle and delays anaphase until these defects are corrected [24]. p 53 is one of the best studied protein involved in cell-cycle checkpoint controls. It is the product of the p 53 gene which acts as a sequence-specific transcription factor and encodes a tumor-suppressor protein required for the DNA-damage checkpoint in vertebrate cells. This protein is able to sense damage, arrest the cycle, initiate repair or cause apoptosis in order to eliminate the abnormal cell [25]. Damage or mutations in p 53 and inappropriate bcl-2 expression may reduce sensitivity to apoptosis and contribute to genetic instability (for review see [26]).

## References

1. Plachot M. The genetics of the oocyte. In: Porcu E, Flamigni C (eds) Human Oocytes: From Physiology to IVF. Bologna: Monduzzi Editore, 1997;11–18.
2. Nakaoka Y, Okamoto E, Miharu N, Ohama K. Chromosome analysis in human oocytes remaining unfertilized after in vitro insemination: effect of maternal age and fertilization rate. Hum Reprod 1998;13:419–424.
3. Egozcue J, Blanco J, Vidal F. Chromosome studies in human sperm nuclei using fluorescence in situ hybridization (FISH). Hum Reprod 1997;3:441–452.
4. Storeng RT, Plachot M, Theophile D, Mandelbaum J, Belaisch-Allart J, Vekemans M. Incidence of sex chromosome abnormalities in spermatozoa from patients entering an IVF or ICSI protocol. Acta Obstet Gynecol Scand 1998;77:191–197.
5. Plachot M. Fertilization abnormalities. In: Ambrosini A, Melis GB, Dalla Pria S, Dessole S (eds) Infertility and Assisted Reproduction Technology. Bologna: Monduzzi Editore, 1997; 155–163.
6. Sultan KM, Munné S, Palermo GD, Alikani M, Cohen J. Chromosomal status of unipronuclear human zygotes following in vitro fertilization and intracytoplasmic sperm injection. Hum Reprod 1995;10:132–136.

7. Macas E, Imthurn B, Roselli M, Keller PJ. Chromosome analysis of single and multipronucleated human zygotes proceeded after the intracytoplasmic sperm injection procedure. J Assist Reprod Genet 1996;13:345—350.

8. Levron J, Munné S, Willadsen S, Rosenwaks Z, Cohen J. Male and female genomes associated in a single pronucleus in human zygotes. Biol Reprod 1995;52:653—657.

9. Feng YL, Gordon JW. Birth of normal mice after removal of the supernumerary male pronucleus from polyspermic zygotes. Hum Reprod 1996;11:341—346.

10. Palermo GD, Munne S, Colombero LT, Cohen J, Rosenwaks Z. Genetics of abnormal human fertilization. Hum Reprod 1995;10(Suppl 1):120—127.

11. Plachot M, Grouchy J de, Junca AM, Mandelbaum J, Salat-Baroux J, Cohen J. Chromosome analysis of human oocytes and embryos: delayed fertilization increase chromosome imbalance. Hum Reprod 1988;3:125—127.

12. Manor D, Kol S, Lewit N, Lightman A, Stein D, Pillar M, Itskovitz-Eldor J. Undocumented embryos: do not trash them, FISH them. Hum Reprod 1996;11:2502—2506.

13. Plachot M, Grouchy J. de, Junca AM, Mandelbaum J, Turleau C, Coullin P, Cohen J, Salat-Baroux J. From oocyte to embryo: a model deduced from in vitro fertilization for natural selection against chromosome abnormalities. Ann Genet 1987;30:22—32.

14. Bongso A, Ng SC, Lim J, Fong CY, Ratnam S. Preimplantation genetics: chromosomes of fragmented human embryos. Fertil Steril 1991;56:66—70.

15. Pellestor F, Dufour MC, Arnal F, Humeau C. Direct assessment of the rate of chromosomal abnormalities in grade IV human embryos produced by in vitro fertilization procedure. Hum Reprod 1994;9:293—302.

16. Munné S, Alikani M, Tomkin G, Grifo J, Cohen J. Embryo morphology, developmental rates, and maternal age are correlated with chromosome abnormalities. Fertil Steril 1995; 64:382—391.

17. Plachot M, Mandelbaum J, Junca AM, Cohen J, Salat-Baroux J, Da Lage C. Morphologic and cytologic study of human embryos obtained by in vitro fertilization. In: Feichtinger W, Kemeter P (eds) Future Aspect in Human In Vitro Fertilization. Berlin: Springer-Verlag, 1987;267—271.

18. Laverge H, Van der Elst J, De Sutter P, Verschraegen-Spae MR, De Paepe A, Dhont M. Fluorescent in situ hybridization on human embryos showing cleavage arrest after freezing and thawing. Hum Reprod 1998;13:425—429.

19. Munne S, Magli C, Adler A, Wright G, De Boer K, Mortimer D, Tucker M, Cohen J, Gianaroli L. Treatment-related chromosome abnormalities in human embryos. Hum Reprod 1997;12: 780—784.

20. Clouston HJ, Fenwick J, Webb AL, Herbert M, Murdoch A, Wolstenholme J. Detection of mosaic and nonmosaic chromosome abnormalities in 6- to 8-day-old human blastocysts. Hum Genet 1997;101:30—36.

21. Menezo YJR, Bellec V, Zaroukian A, Benkhalifa M. Embryo selection by IVF, coculture and transfer at the blastocyst stage in case of translocation. Hum Reprod 1997;12:2802—2803.

22. Zenzes MT, Wang P, Casper RF. Chromosome status of untransferred (spare) embryos and probability of pregnancy after in vitro fertilization. Lancet 1992;340:391—394.

23. Delhanty JDA, Harper JC, Ao A, Handyside AH, Winston RML. Multicolor FISH detects frequent chromosomal mosaicism and chaotic division in normal preimplantation embryos from fertile patients. Hum Genet 1997;99:755—760.

24. Rudner AD, Murray AW. The spindle assembly checkpoint. Curr Opin Cell Biol 1996;8: 773—780.

25. Minn AJ, Boise LH, Thompson CB. Expression of Bcl-xl and loss of p53 can cooperate to overcome a cell cycle checkpoint induced by mitotic spindle damage. Genes Devel 1996;10: 2621—2631.

26. Edwards RG, Beard HK. Oocyte polarity and cell determination in early mammalian embryos. Molec Hum Reprod 1997;3:863—905.

# Y chromosome and infertility

Fertility and Reproductive Medicine.
R.D. Kempers, J. Cohen, A.F. Haney and J.B. Younger, editors.

723

# Genetics of sex determination and its pathology in man

Chris Ottolenghi[1,2], Reiner Veitia[1], Manoel Nunes[1], Nicole Souleyreau-Therville[1] and Marc Fellous[1]

[1]*Laboratoire d'Immunogénétique humaine, Institut Pasteur, Paris, France; and* [2]*Dipartimento di Morfologia e Istoembriologia, Facoltà di Medicina, Università di Ferrara, Ferrara, Italy*

**Abstract.** We review data on genes known to be involved in human sex determination or early testis differentiation and suggest that, with the prominent exception of *SRY*, mutations in these genes are mainly associated with partial gonadal dysgenesis. The extensive variability of phenotypes referred to as partial gonadal dysgenesis and the recent finding that a delay of gonadogenesis is accompanied by XY sex reversal in *M33*-deficient mice, suggest that nonspecific processes, such as the gonadal growth rate, should be reappraised as a cause of sex reversal. Future studies aimed at identifying genes involved in sex reversal and at investigating genotype/phenotype correlations will shed light on the genetic and embryologic basis of mammalian sex determination.

**Keywords:** gonadogenesis, sex reversal, XX true hermaphroditism, XY gonadal dysgenesis.

## Introduction

Sex determination in mammals is distinct from sex differentiation and requires the presence of a functional testis [1]. Therefore, the impairment of either testis or ovary formation results in the development of a female phenotype. This explains the interest devoted to the physiopathology of pure and partial gonadal dysgenesis associated with 46,XY sex reversal. Indeed, establishing if these syndromes represent primarily different forms of gonadal male-to-female sex reversal or a default of testis determination may help to understand the origin of sex reversal and the associated infertility. As part of the effort to unravel this issue, we review current knowledge of the genetic bases of sex determination in humans.

### Genes mutated in sex reversal

*SRY gene: a master sex-determining gene located on Y chromosome*

*SRY* is the testis determining factor (TDF) gene, as indicated by the following facts: it is located within the minimal region of the Y chromosome that induces XX maleness when translocated on X chromosomes; it displays intragenic mutations in XY complete gonadal dysgenesis; the *SRY* orthologous counterpart

---

*Address for correspondence:* Chris Ottolenghi, Laboratoire d'Immunogénétique humaine, Institut Pasteur, 25 rue du Docteur Roux, 75724 Paris, France. Tel.: +33-1456-88888. Fax.: +33-1420-69835.

induces female-to-male sex reversal in a proportion of XX transgenic mice; and its diminished expression due to position effects is associated with XY sex reversal in both humans and mice (see [2] for recent review). It encodes a protein containing a domain (termed the HMG box) that displays DNA-binding and DNA-bending properties in vitro, suggesting that it is a transcription factor. *SRY* mutations identified in patients with XY complete gonadal dysgenesis are almost always located in the HMG box and have been shown to disrupt DNA-binding/-bending activities of the protein (reviewed [3]). Sry is expressed in pre-Sertoli cells of the male embryonic gonad [4] consistent with the central role suggested for this cell lineage in testis determination [5,6].

*SRY* is located close to the pseudoautosomal boundary of the short arm of the Y chromosome, which pairs with the homologous region on the X chromosome at meiosis and undergoes an obligatory crossing over. Following an event of illegitimate crossing over, the region containing *SRY* is susceptible to be translocated onto the X chromosome partner (Fig. 1). Despite intensive investigations,

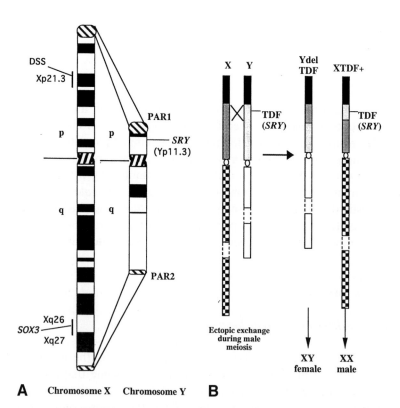

**A**  Chromosome X  Chromosome Y  **B**

*Fig. 1.* **A:** Simplified map of human sex chromosomes. The positions of *SRY,* DSS and SOX3 are indicated. PAR1 and 2: pseudoautosomal regions on the short (1) and long (2) arm of sex chromosomes. **B:** Schematic representation of an illegitimate crossing-over event leading to translocation of *SRY* onto the short arm of the X chromosome. TDF: testis determining factor.

*SRY* mutations have been found almost exclusively in patients with XY complete gonadal dysgenesis, and translocation of *SRY* on a X chromosome almost invariably leads to XX maleness (and essentially to XX maleness without sexual ambiguities [7]).

In the case of *SRY* mutations on an XY karyotype background, only three exceptions to the genotype-phenotype correlations mentioned above have been reported: a case of partial gonadal dysgenesis and a case of true hermaphrodism [8], as well as a case of transient ovarian function with initially normal menarche and development of normal secondary-sexual characteristics [9]. Two of these cases are associated with unique mutations: a deletion in the 3′ region of the gene in the patient with partial gonadal dysgenesis, and a mutation inducing a stop in the second codon of the open reading frame of *SRY* in a patient with "premature ovarian failure". On an XX karyotype background, only 20% of true hermaphrodite patients have detectable Y-material. It has been suggested that preferential inactivation of *SRY*-positive X chromosome may be responsible for *SRY*-positive, XX true hermaphrodism, whereas random X-inactivation would generate *SRY*-positive, XX males ([10], and references therein).

Mutations in *SRY* have been found in 15—20% cases of XY gonadal dysgenesis (reviewed by [11]), and translocation of *SRY* on an X chromosome is present in about 80% of XX males without genital ambiguities, and 10—20% of XX males with genital ambiguities [7]. This indicates that other genes must be involved in sex reversal.

*DAX1, a candidate gene for dosage sensitive sex reversal*
The DSS (dosage sensitive sex reversal) locus, located on Xp21.3 (Fig. 1A), is defined as a region duplicated in some XY sex-reversed patients, who have either intra-abdominal dysgenetic testes or have a streak or absent gonad, while one individual was reported to have apparently normal ovaries ([12], and references therein). Deletions of this region have no apparent effect on heterozygous XX females, whereas the phenotype of an XX true hermaphrodite, harboring an extensive deletion of the short arm of one X chromosome containing DSS, was suggested to result from the unmasking of a recessive allele on the remaining X partner [13]. This individual presented with brain, ocular and epidermal abnormalities were possibly the result of a contiguous gene syndrome. A candidate gene for the DSS phenotype is *DAX1*, an orphan steroid receptor containing a novel, putative DNA-binding domain [14]. Hemizygosity for this gene is associated with adrenal hypoplasia congenita and hypogonadotropic hypogonadism in XY males. No *DAX1* gain-of-function, intra-genic mutations have been reported in XY sex-reversed individuals. However, Dax1 is expressed in the bipotential gonad and down-regulated specifically in the embryonic testes [15]. Mice transgenic for *Dax1* display an increased frequency of XY sex reversal when placed onto the background of a natural (Y-*poschiavinus*) and an engineered Sry allele [16]. However, these alleles are known not to be fully penetrant ("weak Sry alleles"). Under the assumption that *Dax1* gene dosage sensitivity is greater

in humans than mice, these results are consistent with a role for *DAX1/Dax1* in sex determination.

*Autosomal genes implicated in testis determination/differentiation*
Deletions of the distal short arm of chromosome 9 and of the distal long arm of chromosome 10, are mainly associated with XY, partial gonadal dysgenesis ([17,18], and references therein). The locus on 9p (SRA, for sex reversal autosomal) is the most extensively studied and has been recently distinguished from another locus within the 9p monosomy contiguous gene syndrome [18]. The locus for XY sex reversal is thus assigned to 9p24.3 (Fig. 2). A candidate gene, termed *DMT1*, has been proposed for this locus, as it is 1) partly homologous (zinc-finger DM-domain) to two genes responsible for sexual dimorphism in invertebrates, *mab-3* and *dsx*, and a *DMT1* transgene can partially rescue the mab-3 (male-abnormal 3) phenotype in the nematode; 2) is expressed specifically in the testes; and 3) is located in the minimal region deleted in XY sex reversed patients (9p24.3) [19]. *Mab*-3 loss-of-function mutations are recessive and affect some traits of the nematode male sex-specific differentiation, while gonads and spermatogenesis appear unaltered. The doublesex (dsx) gene is a master regulator of the fruit fly sex determination pathway, encoding a male- and a female-specific isoform. These isoforms contain a common N-terminal DM-domain and differ in their C-terminal transactivation domain. No *DMT1* intragenic mutations have been detected so far in patients with XY gonadal dysgenesis (our unpublished observations), suggesting that another gene is responsible for 9p-associated XY sex reversal.

*WT1 and genitourinary anomalies*
Additional transcription factors are involved in XY male-to-female sex reversal in the context of more complex clinical syndromes. *WT1* (Wilms' tumor 1) is located on human chromosome 11p13 and encodes a protein containing four zinc-finger motifs near its C-terminus [20]. Some *WT1* heterozygous mutations

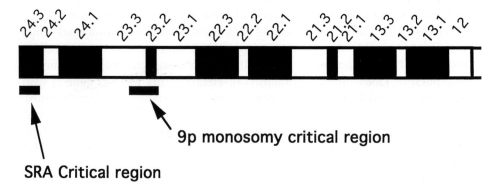

*Fig. 2.* Map of the short arm of human chromosome 9. The loci for 46,XY sex reversal (SRA) and 9p monosomy syndrome are indicated.

are associated with various degrees of XY partial gonadal dysgenesis in the context of the Denys-Drash and WAGR (Wilms' tumor, aniridia, genitourinary abnormalities, mental retardation) syndromes, and with XY, pure gonadal dysgenesis in the context of the rarer Frasier syndrome (reviewed in [21]). Missense mutations in exon 6 and in the first three zinc-fingers of the protein (exon 7–9) are detected frequently in patients presenting a complete Denys-Drash syndrome, which associates Wilms' tumor, glomerular nephropathy (characterized by diffuse mesangial sclerosis), and XY partial gonadal dysgenesis. Nonsense and frameshift mutations in N-terminal exons are apparently responsible for a syndrome related to Denys-Drash, characterized by the absence of nephropathy [21]. Alternative splicing of WT-1 produces four isoforms, which either contain exon 5 and a three amino acid motif termed KTS (lysine, threonine, serine) or not. The KTS+ isoform displays a preferential subnuclear localization, which corresponds to the position of spliceosome complexes, suggesting that it is specifically involved in RNA regulation or metabolism [22]. We have recently demonstrated that a splice site mutation in intron 9, inducing a decrease in the level of the KTS+ isoform of WT-1, was specifically found in Frasier syndrome [23]. Frasier syndrome associates a nonspecific glomerulopathy with XY, pure gonadal dysgenesis, an increased risk of gonadoblastoma and the absence of Wilms' tumor. The alternative isoform, lacking the KTS motif, appears to be involved in the transcriptional regulation of the antimüllerian hormone in cell-transfection assays [24]. In mice, Wt1 is expressed in the intermediary mesoderm and subsequently in gonads of both sexes (but with sex-specific intratissular distribution), mesonephros, metanephros, adult kidney and mesothelial tissues [25]. Knockout mice display renal and gonadal agenesis and die in utero presumably because of pericardial and pleural defects [26].

*SOX9 and M33: two closely linked genes responsible for 46, XY sex reversal*
SOX9 is located on the long arm of human chromosome 17, contains a HMG box homologous to the one described in *SRY* and regulates transcription of collagen II in chondrocytes, suggesting that it also might regulate the synthesis of testis-specific components of the extracellular matrix [27]. *Sox9* is expressed in the bipotential gonad of both XX and XY embryos and in chondrogenic cells in mice. It is upregulated in the embryonic testis and downregulated in the embryonic ovary [28]. SOX9 heterozygous mutations are found in patients affected by campomelic dysplasia and by a high frequency (70%) of XY female sex reversal [29]. Gonads and genitalia are usually unambiguously female in XY infants and fetuses, but some XY intersex patients have also been reported. Gonads of one such intersex patient contained testicular and dysplastic ovarian tissue with some germ cells [30]. Isolated XY gonadal dysgenesis is apparently not associated with mutations in SOX9 [31].

Recently, the *M33* gene, located at 5 cM from *Sox9* in a region of mouse chromosome 11 syntenic with human chromosome 17q, has been implicated in mouse XY sex reversal phenotypes. The *M33* gene is thought to be the structural and functional homologue of the fruit fly *Polycomb* (Pc) gene, as it can rescue the larval phenotype of Pc-deficient flies [32]. Pc belongs to a family of structurally diverse proteins (termed Pc-G) which repress transcriptional states of fruit fly homeobox complex genes. *M33* expression pattern is ubiquitous at 9 dpc (days postcoitum) in mouse embryos, and it is progressively restricted to a subset of tissues including the urogenital system until 15.5 dpc [33]. *M33*-deficient mice display skeletal abnormalities reminiscent of the deficiency of *Hox-d3*, and of two additional genes, *Bmi-1* and *Mel-18*, which are homologous to another member of Pc-G, the *posterior sex combs* gene [34]. While several cell types cultured from *M33* null mice display an altered proliferation pattern in vitro, growth impairment is prominent specifically in gonadogenesis in vivo and correlates with XY sex reversal [35]. XY *M33* null mice mainly display a female phenotype and ovaries containing follicles, and less frequently, true hermaphroditism. This suggests that gonadal growth retardation may be a cause of male-to-female sex reversal. Alternatively, *M33* might regulate genes upstream or downstream of Sry. Interestingly, XX *M33*-deficient females have small-sized ovaries and are apparently sterile.

## Interactions among sex-determining genes

*SRY antagonizes a suppressor of testis determination?*

It has been previously proposed of a genetic model of sex determination postulating that an autosomal or X-linked gene represses testis determination and that *SRY* acts by relieving this repression [7]. The gene repressing testis determination may be the DSS locus and perhaps *DAX1* [36]. An alternative candidate located on the X chromosome has been proposed, *SOX3* [37]. *SOX3* is positioned at Xq26-27 in humans and belongs to the family of HMG box containing transcription factors that comprises also *SOX9* and *SRY*. It is expressed in the urogenital ridge. Deletions of the gene are responsible for early testicular failure (but not sex reversal) in XY individuals, while extensive deletions of the region containing *SOX3* are associated with premature ovarian failure in XX females (reviewed by [38]).

*Genes acting upstream of SRY*

Other loci may be required for male-specific roles either upstream or downstream of *SRY* and they are expected to reproduce the effect of mutations of the primary sex-determining genes. Candidate upstream-acting genes are those expressed in the urogenital ridge and responsible for gonadal agenesis, including *WT-1* (see above) and *SF-1* (steroidogenic factor 1). *SF-1* was identified as an orphan steroid receptor regulating the promoter of cytochrome P450 hydroxylases and is expressed in the embryonic bipotential gonad of both sexes and in all steroidogenic tissues [39]. *SF-1* knockout mice display adrenal and gonadal agenesis [40]. In the mouse *SF-1* is gradually downregulated during ovary differentiation, whereas expression persists in the developing testis [41].

*Genes expressed concomitantly with SRY*

Genes expressed in the bipotential gonad (10,5-12,5 dpc in the mouse) represent possible targets of *SRY*. Namely, *SRY* might be responsible for the male-specific changes in gonadal expression pattern, including downregulation of *DAX1*, upregulation of *SOX9* and inhibition of *SF-1* downregulation (see above, and Fig. 3). This might occur through direct transcriptional control or by regulating intermediate gene targets. However, the expression patterns and molecular data can be interpreted in different ways [37,38].

*Genes acting downstream of SRY*

Although upstream flanking sequences of the antimüllerian hormone gene (*AMH*) contain a consensus site known to bind *SRY* in vitro, cotransfection

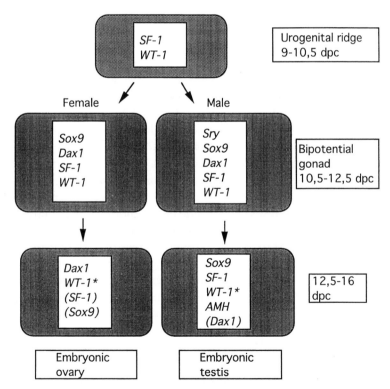

*Fig. 3.* Expression pattern of genes involved in sex reversal during mouse gonadal embryogenesis. In brackets: genes undergoing gradual downregulation in the corresponding tissue. (*)WT-1 gene expression pattern is sexually dimorphic in gonadal differentiation.

experiments do not support the hypothesis of a direct activation of the *AMH* promoter by *SRY* due to technical reasons [2]. Alternatively, *AMH* transactivation could be mediated by *SF-1*. Indeed, an SF-1-binding site in the *AMH* promoter is required for *AMH* expression in transgenic mice [42]. Although the onset of *WT-1* and *SF-1* expression precedes the onset of *AMH* expression by 2—3 days, the *WT-1* KTS-isoform apparently synergizes with *SF-1* in promoting expression of the *AMH* gene in cotransfection assays [24]. The same authors show that the *DAX1* protein inhibits the *WT1-SF1* synergism in vitro. Thus, it is possible that *SRY* may antagonize *DAX1*, relieving repression of *SF-1/WT-1*-mediated *AMH* transcription. Although recessive mutations of the *AMH* gene are responsible for male pseudohermaphroditism and not sex reversal, and thus the function of this gene is restricted to sex differentiation, the above results suggest that genes involved in gonadogenesis (*WT-1, SF-1*), and sex determination or early gonadal sex-specific differentiation (*WT-1*, perhaps *DAX1*) may be also involved in classical sex differentiation.

## Gonad histology and sex reversal: genotype/phenotype correlations?

While mutations involving *SRY* and perhaps *SOX9* are associated predominantly with pure gonadal dysgenesis, other loci induce more variable gonadal phenotypes, falling in most cases within the range of partial gonadal dysgenesis. Therefore, it is interesting to briefly present some histological results.

The appearance of gonads is similar in XY sex-reversed women with pure gonadal dysgenesis and patients presenting with Turner syndrome. This has led to the suggestion that ovarian determination takes place in XY pure gonadal dysgenesis as it does in Turner syndrome, i.e., streak gonads may be the secondary result of germ cell loss in both syndromes (reviewed by [43,44]).

Little is understood about the physiopathology of XY, partial gonadal dysgenesis. Partial gonadal dysgenesis refers to patients having any one of the following associations: bilateral dysgenetic testes with poorly organized seminiferous tubules; one dysgenetic or normal testis on one side of the abdomen and a streak gonad on the other side; ovarian-like stroma adjacent to seminiferous tubules; or areas of ovarian-like stroma next to but separate from areas of testicular tissue within the same gonad [43]. These histological findings are consistent with a pathology of the early steps of testis differentiation rather than primary sex determination, yet this would not explain why "partially dysgenetic" gonads often contain degenerated ovarian-like tissue adjacent to dysgenetic testicular tissue and why streak gonads may be found in association with testes or dysgenetic testes. The histological appearance of gonads is similar in 46, XY partial gonadal dysgenesis and 45, XO-XY mixed gonadal dysgenesis. Some evidence suggests that mixed gonadal dysgenesis may be associated with ovotestes during fetal life. For instance, in the ovarian-like tissues of some patients presenting with mixed gonadal dysgenesis, the fraction of cells bearing Y material was absent or lower than in the contralateral normal testis [45,46]. This should be compared to results obtained on XX-XY and XO-XY mouse chimaeras [5,6]. Interestingly, rare cases of XY and XO-XY true hermaphroditism have been reported in humans [8,47].

## Conclusion

Current data suggest that interactions between genes involved in the sex-determination cascade may occur at the level of transcriptional regulation, although the exact molecular relations can be interpreted in different ways. Furthermore, it is clear that cell-cell interactions are involved in sex determination, as indicated for instance by the results on mouse XX-XO and XX-XY chimaeras [5,6]. Therefore, some as yet unidentified sex-determining genes might be directly implicated in intercellular signaling.

Genotype-phenotype correlations point to the variability in the gonadal appearances associated with mutations in most genes responsible for sex reversal, with the exception of *SRY* and perhaps *SOX9*. This variability ranges from phenotypes indistinguishable from XY, pure gonadal dysgenesis to phenotypic XY intersexes with apparently normal testes. The latter finding suggests that XY, partial gonadal dysgenesis may involve a delay in testis determination in some cases [48]. A timing mismatch between the expression of *Sry* and *Sry*-interacting genes is commonly believed to cause partial or complete XY sex reversal when the Y chromosome from particular *poschiavinus* and *domesticus* mouse populations is placed onto the C57BL/6J laboratory mouse background, although this question is still not settled [49,50] (and references therein). As phenotypical variability is virtually not observed in association with *SRY* mutations in humans, it might be a derived condition and not an intrinsic feature of the sex determination process itself. However, data suggesting that a delay in gonadogenesis may be at the origin of XY sex reversal in *M33*-deficient mice suggest that the role of nonspecific processes such as the size of gonads during gonadogenesis merits a reappraisal [51]. In any case, the possibility of a pathologically derived sensitivity to nonspecific perturbations should be taken into account when the effect of genes candidate for sex-reversed phenotypes is tested. For instance, the choice of a "weak *Sry* allele" background for investigating the role of *Dax1* in mouse sex determination (see above) might prove to be unfortunate, and negative controls (transgenesis with unrelated genes) or independent experimental support in vivo are desirable.

Perhaps the most natural and most stringent test for assessing if a gene participates in determining the sex developmental switch is that it should be associated with both XY and XX sex-reversed phenotypes, depending on the nature of mutations (loss- or gain-of-function). This has been demonstrated only in the case of *SRY* so far, so that the genes determining the switch between the formation of testicular and ovarian tissues which must be invoked in a large proportion of completely or partially sex-reversed gonadal phenotypes, are yet to be identified.

732

## Acknowledgements

C.O. is supported by a fellowship of the "Associazione Italiana di Biologia Teorica", Ferrara University, Italy.

## References

1. Jost A. Problems of fetal endocrinology: the gonadal and hypophyseal hormones. Recent Prog Horm Res 1953;8:379–418.
2. Haqq CM, Donahoe P. Regulation of sexual dimorphism in mammals. Physiol Rev 1998; 78:1–33.
3. Harley VR, Goodfellow PN. The biochemical role of SRY in sex determination. Molec Reprod Devel 1994;39:184–193.
4. Rossi P, Dolci S, Albanesi C, Grimaldi P, Geremia R. Direct evidence that the mouse sex-determining gene Sry is expressed in the somatic cells of the male fetal gonads and in the germ cell line of the adult testis. Molec Reprod Devel 1993;34:369–373.
5. Palmer SJ, Burgoyne PS. XY follicle cells in the ovaries of XO/XY and XO/XY/XYY mosaic mice. Development 1991;111:1017–1019.
6. Palmer SJ, Burgoyne PS. In situ analysis of fetal, prepubertal and adult XX-XY chimaeric mouse testes: Sertoli cells are predominantly, but not exclusively, XY. Development 1991;112:265–268.
7. McElreavey K, Vilain E, Abbas N, Herskowitz I, Fellous M. A regulatory cascade hypothesis for mammalian sex determination: SRY represses a negative regulator of male development. Proc Natl Acad Sci USA 1993;90:3368–3372.
8. Braun A, Kammerer S, Cleve H et al. True hermaphrodism in an 46, XY individual, caused by a postzygotic somatic point mutation in the male gonadal sex-determining locus (SRY): molecular genetics and histological findings in a sporadic case. Am J Hum Genet 1993;52:578–585.
9. Brown S, Tu CC, Lanzano P et al. A de novo mutation (Gln2stop) at the 5′ end of the gene SRY gene leads to sex reversal with partial ovarian function. Am J Hum Genet 1998;62:189–192.
10. Fechner PY, Rosenberg C, Stetten G et al. Nonrandom inactivation of the Y-bearing X chromosome in a 46, XX individual: evidence for the etiology of 46, XX true hermaphrodism. Cytogen Cell Genet 1994;66:22–26.
11. McElreavey K. Mechanism of sex determination in mammals. Adv Genome Biol 1996;4: 305–354.
12. Bardoni B, Zanaria E, Guioli S et al. A dosage sensitive locus at chromosome Xp21 is involved in male to female sex reversal. Nature Genet 1994;7:497–501.
13. Tar A, Solyom J, Gyorvari B et al. Testicular development in an SRY-negative 46,XX individual harboring a distal Xp deletion. Hum Genet 1995;96:464–468.
14. Zanaria E, Muscatelli F, Bardoni B et al. An unusual member of the nuclear hormone receptor superfamily responsible for X-linked adrenal hypoplasia congenita. Nature 1994;372:635–641.
15. Swain A, Zanaria E, Hacker A, Lovell-Badge R, Camerino G. Mouse Dax1 expression is consistent with a role in sex determination as well as in adrenal and hypothalamus function. Nature Genet 1996;12:404–409.
16. Swain A, Narvaez V, Burgoyne P, Camerino G, Lovell-Badge R. Dax1 antagonizes Sry action in mammalian sex determination. Nature 1991;391:761–767.
17. Wilkie AOM, Campbell FM, Daubeney P et al. Complete and partial XY sex reversal associated with terminal deletions of 10q:report of 2 cases and literature review. Am J Med Genet 1993; 46:597–600.
18. Veitia RA, Nunes M, Quintana-Murci L et al. Swyers syndrome and 46, XY partial gonadal dysgenesis associated with 9p deletions in absence of monosomy 9p syndrome. Am J Hum Genet 1998;(In press).
19. Raymond CS, Shamu CE, Shen MM et al. Evidence for evolutionary conservation of sex-deter-

mining genes. Nature 1998;391:691–695.

20. Call K, Glaser T, Ito C et al. Isolation and characterization of a zinc finger polypeptide gene at the human chromosome 11 Wilms' tumor locus. Cell 1990;60:509–520.

21. Little M, Wells C. A clinical overview of WT1 gene mutations. Hum Mutat 1997;9:209–225.

22. Larsson SH, Charlieu JP, Miyagawa K et al. Subnuclear localization of WT1 in splicing or transcription factor domains is regulated by alternative splicing. Cell 1995;81:391–401.

23. Barbaux S, Niaudet P, Gubler MC et al. Donor splice site mutations in the WT1 gene are responsible for Frasier syndrome. Nature Genet 1997;17:467–470.

24. Nachtigal MW, Hirokawa Y, Enyeart-VanHouten DL et al. Wilms' tumor 1 and Dax-1 modulate the orphan nuclear receptor SF-1 in sex-specific gene expression. Cell 1998;93:445–454.

25. Armstrong JF, Pritchard-Jones K, Bickmore WA et al. The expression of the Wilms' tumor gene, WT1, in the developing mammalian embryo. Mech Devel 1992;40:85–97.

26. Kreidberg JA, Sariola H, Loring JM et al. WT-1 is required for early kidney development. Cell 1993;74:679–691.

27. Bell D, Leung KH, Wheatley SC et al. SOX9 directly regulates the type-II collagen gene. Nature Genet 1997;16:174–178.

28. Morais da Silva S, Hacker A, Harley V, Goodfellow P et al. Sox9 expression during gonadal development implies a conserved role for the gene in testis differentiation in mammals and birds. Nature Genet 1996;14:62–68.

29. Foster JW, Dominguez-Steglich MA, Giuili S et al. Campomelic dysplasia and autosomal sex reversal caused by mutations in an SRY-related gene. Nature 1994;372:525–530.

30. Cameron FJ, Hageman RM, Cooke-Yarborough C et al. A novel germ line mutation in SOX9 causes familial campomelic dysplasia and sex reversal. Hum Molec Genet 1996;5:1625–1630.

31. Kwok C, Goodfellow PN, Hawkins JR. Evidence to exclude SOX9 as a candidate gene for XY sex reversal without skeletal malformation. J Med Genet 1996;33:800–801.

32. Müller J, Gaunt S, Lawrence PA. Function of polycomb protein is conserved in mice and flies. Development 1995;121:2847–2852.

33. Schoorlemmer J, Marcos-Gutierrez C, Were F et al. Ring1A is a transcriptional repressor that interacts with the Polycomb-M33 protein and is expressed at rhombomere boundaries in the mouse hindbrain. EMBO J 1997;16:5930–5942.

34. Coré N, Bel S, Gaunt SJ, et al. Altered cellular proliferation and mesoderm patterning in Polycomb-M33-deficient mice. Development 1997;124:721–729.

35. Katoh-Fukui Y, Tsuchiya R, Shiroishi T et al. Male-to-female sex reversal in M33 mutant mice. Nature 1998;393:688–692.

36. McElreavey K, Barbaux S, Ion A, Fellous M. The genetic basis of murine and human sex determination: a review. Heredity 1995;75(Pt6):599–611.

37. Graves JAM. Interactions between SRY and SOX genes in mammalian sex determination. Bioessays 1998;20:264–269.

38. Capel B. The role of Sry in cellular events underlying mammalian sex determination. Curr Topics Devel Biol 1996;32:1–37.

39. Ikeda Y, Shen WH, Ingraham HA, Parker KL. Developmental expression of mouse steroidogenic factor 1, an essential regulator of steroid hydroxylases. Molec Endocrinol 1994;8:654–662.

40. Luo X, Ikeda Y, Parker KL. A cell-specific nuclear receptor is essential for adrenal and gonadal development and sexual differentiation. Cell 1994;77:481–490.

41. Ikeda Y, Swain A, Weber TJ et al. Steroidogenic factor 1 and Dax1 colocalize in multiple cell lineages: potential links in endocrine development. Molec Endocrinol 1996;10:1261–1272.

42. Giuili G, Shen WH, Ingraham HA. The nuclear receptor SF-1 mediates dimorphic expression of Müllerian inhibiting substance, in vivo. Development 1997;124:1799–1807.

43. Berkovitz GD. Abonrmalities of gonadal determination and differentiation. Sem Perinatol 1992;16:289–298.

44. Whitworth DJ. XX germ cells: the difference between an ovary and a testis. TEM 1998;9:2–6.

734

45. Reddy KS, Sulcova V, Ho CK et al. An infant with a mosaic 45,X/46,X,psu dic(Y) karyotype and mixed gonadal dysgenesis studied for extent of mosaicism in the gonads. Am J Med Genet 1996;66:441–444.
46. Sugarman ID, Crolla JA, Malone PS. Mixed gonadal dysgenesis and cell line differentiation. Case presentation and literature review. Clin Genet 1994;46:313–315.
47. Linskens RK, Odink RJH, van der Linden JC, Ekkelkamp S, Delemarre-van de Waal HA. True hermaphrodism in 45,X/46,XY mosaicism. Horm Res 1992;37:241–244.
48. Fuqua JS, Sher ES. Perlman EJ et al. Abnormal gonadal differentiation in two subjects with ambiguous genitalia, Mullerian structures, and normally developed testes: evidence for a defect in gonadal ridge development. Hum Genet 1996;97:506–511.
49. Lee CH, Taketo T. Normal onset, but prolonged expression, of Sry gene in the B6.YDOM sex-reversed mouse gonad. Devel Biol 1994;165:442–452.
50. Carlisle C, Winking H, Weichenhan D et al. Absence of correlation between Sry polymorphisms and XY sex reversal caused by M. m. domesticus Y chromosome. Genomics 1996;33:32–45.
51. Mittwoch U. Sex determination and sex reversal: genotype, phenotype, dogma and semantics. Hum Genet 1992;89:467–479.

# Y chromosome and male fertility genes

Peter H. Vogt[1], Angela Edelmann[1], Barbara Habermann[2], Octavian Henegariu[4], Peter Hirschmann[1], Ralf Keil[1], Franklin Kiesewetter[3], Stefan Kirsch[1] and Peter Urbitsch[1]

[1]*Reproduction Genetics, Institute of Human Genetics, University of Heidelberg, Heidelberg;* [2]*Department of Andrology, Center of Dermatology, University of Marburg, Marburg;* [3]*Department of Andrology, University of Erlangen, Erlangen, Germany; and* [4]*Department of Medical and Molecular Genetics, Medical Research and Library Building, Indianapolis, Indiana, USA*

**Abstract.** The Y chromosome has been shown to be essential for male fertility in species as different as *Drosophila* [1], mice [2] and humans [3]. In humans, the molecular analyses of Y genes believed to be functional in male infertility have now revealed two general types: Y-specific repetitive gene families expressed solely in the human testis (group I: BPY1, BPY2, CDY; PRY, TTY1, TTY2, XKRY [4]; TSPY [5]; RBM [6]; DAZ [7]); and Y genes with a homologous gene copy on the X chromosome expressed in multiple tissues (group II: DBY, DFFRY, E1F1AY, UTY [4]; DFFRY, (see also [8]), SMCY [9]). Some of the Y genes from group I (RBM, DAZ) were shown to have evolved from an autosomal homolog [10–14] and some of them from group II are reported to express testis transcripts of specific lengths as well (DBY, E1F1AY [4]).

Most of these genes were mapped to one of the three AZF (azoospermia factor) regions (AZFa, AZFb, AZFc) in the euchromatic part of the long Y arm (Yq11). These Y regions each mark the possible extension interval of at least one Y chromosomal male fertility gene as their deletion is associated with the occurrence of azoospermia and/or severe oligozoospermia [15].

Until now gene-specific mutations which are capable of inducing the same pathological phenotype as observed after deletion of the corresponding AZF region have not been reported for any of the human Y genes listed above. This has raised the question as to whether these mutations actually exist and whether the "functional unit" of a Y chromosomal male fertility gene could eventually extend possibly beyond the gene structure of one protein-encoding Y gene expressed in the human testis. This possibility has been documented for the functional units of some male fertility genes on the Y chromosome of *Drosophila* [16].

Therefore, this article is subdivided into the following chapters: a short review of the functional units of the Y chromosomal male fertility genes of *Drosophila*; a review of the analyses of AZF regions in the euchromatic part of the long arm of the human Y chromosome (Yq11), i.e., genomic DNA regions which, if deleted, induce the azoospermia phenotype (a short discussion on their possible molecular origins is included); a discussion on the clinical significance of the deletion of single STS loci in Yq11; and an overview of the structure and function of candidate male fertility genes, which until now have been mapped to the different AZF regions.

**Keywords:** AZF deletions in Yq11, *Drosophila* Y male fertility genes, idiopathic azoospermia, X-Y pairing and male fertility, Y genes expressed in human testis.

*Address for correspondence:* Peter H. Vogt, Im Neuenheimer Feld 328, D-69120 Heidelberg, Germany. Tel.: +49-6221-565050. Fax: +49-6221-565155. E-mail: peter.vogt@ukl.uni-heidelberg.de

736

## Male fertility genes on the Y chromosome of *Drosophila*

Y genes functional in spermatogenesis were first described in the genus *Drosophila* [17]. This was surprising because the Y chromosome in this species is largely heterochromatic and was long thought to be genetically inert since studies of X/O males revealed that meiosis occurs regularly and that most stages of spermiogenesis appear normal. However, the sperm degenerate before the completion of maturation. Very few sperm were found in the vasa efferentia of X/O males and these sperm were never motile. This suggests that the *Drosophila* Y chromosome expresses a germ-line-specific genetic activity probably after meiosis has occurred. Transcriptional activity of the *Drosophila* Y chromosome was observed in the primary spermatocyte [18]. This could even be seen under the microscope because, during transcription, nuclear proteins accumulate at the primary tran-

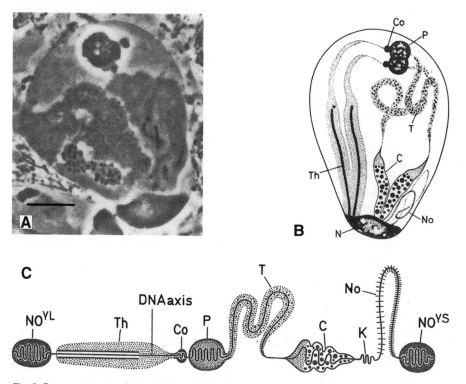

*Fig. 1.* Spermatocyte nucleus of *Drosophila hydei* with the Y chromosomal lamp brush loops displaying transcript-specific morphologies. **A:** Phase contrast; **B:** schematic drawing. The loop structures were designated according to their phenotypical appearance as: Th: threads; Co: cones; P: pseudonucleolus; T: tubular ribbons; C: clubs; No: nooses. The nucleolus (N) is attached to the nuclear membrane at this germ line stage.

The scheme of a single Y chromatid below presents the linear order of the lamp brush loops along the DNA axis (K: kinetochor). Nucleolus organizer regions (NO) are present at the tips of the long (YL) and short (YS) chromatid arms.

script structures forming granular lamp brush loops with transcript-specific morphologies (Fig. 1). Genetically, the expression of each lamp brush loop was associated with the function of one male fertility gene.

Chromatin-spreading experiments with the primary spermatocyte nucleus demonstrated extensive lengths of the various transcription units with locus-specific secondary structures [19]. Molecular analysis of the underlying DNA structures revealed complex repetitive sequence structures as their main constituents [20–22], and it was possible to show that these were locus-specific and functional parts of the Y chromosomal male fertility genes [23].

Extensive sequence analyses of the DNA structure of various lamp brush loops did not identify potential exon sequences of protein encoding Y genes but revealed a strong polarity of the repetitive sequence elements constituting the transcription unit of the lamp brush DNA structure [24]. The same repetitive sequence elements, but with a random orientation, were also present flanking these transcription units. A protein encoding gene (Dhc-Yh3) was isolated from one fertility gene locus (kl-5) of the Y chromosome of *Drosophila melanogaster* [25]. It encodes the ATP-binding domain of a presumably functional dynein gene. However, no point mutations of this dynein gene which interfered with *Drosophila* male fertility have yet been analysed. Only large deletions encompassing the total lamp brush structure and the dynein gene locus of the kl-5 fertility gene locus could be analysed in sterile male flies.

This suggested that the functional units of the Y chromosomal male fertility genes of *Drosophila* are exceptional by including not only the gene structure of a protein-encoding Y gene but also the flanking repetitive sequence structure. This view was supported by the identification of germ-line-specific proteins binding to specific lamp brush structures [26,27]. These proteins were encoded by autosomal genes and needed to constitute different parts of the sperm flagellum. So, in summary, these results match the first genetic analyses suggesting that the *Drosophila* Y chromosome has a function in spermiogenesis and they agree with the observation that male flies without a Y chromosome (X/0 males) are able to produce mature spermatozoa, but without motility [1].

## Human Y chromosome deletions in Yq11 associated with male infertility

Human Y chromosomal rearrangements that were supposed to interfere with male fertility were first analysed in the karyotypes of human male metaphase chromosomes 22 years ago [28]. Terminal deletions of the long chromosome arm were observed in six sterile men with azoospermia. Consequently, it was postulated that at least one genetic Y factor essential for male germ cell development is located in distal Yq11 (the heterochromatic chromosome region Yq12 was generally considered to be genetically inert). As these Y deletions seemed to result in "azoospermia" this Y factor was defined as azoospermia factor (AZF).

Histological analyses of testis tissue sections of sterile men with microscopically visible rearrangements of Yq11 in their karyotypes indicated different inter-

| karyotype | Yq11 anomaly | genitalia | testicular histology |
|---|---|---|---|
| 46.XYq | 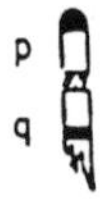 | hypoplastic testicles | testicular fibrosclerosis<br>abnormal basal lamina<br>no germ cells: no Sertoli cells<br>only Sertoli cells<br>rare spermatogonia<br>rare spermatocytes |
| 46.X.dic(Yp)<br>45.X0 | 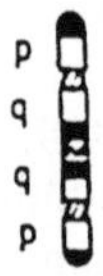 | ambiguous genitalia<br>hypospadias<br>cryptoorchidism<br>small penis | atrophic tubules<br>only Sertoli cells<br>spermatogonia<br>rare spermatocytes<br>arrest at pachytene |
| 46. X.r(Y)<br>45.X0 | 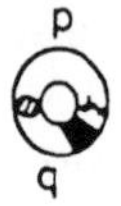 | hypoplastic testicles<br>hypospadias<br>cyrptoorchidism | only Sertoli cells<br>arrest at pachytene |
| 46.Y.t(Xp:Yq) | 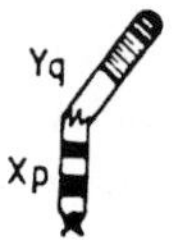 | hypoplastic testicles<br>small penis | decrease of spermatocytes |
| 46, X.Yq-,t(A:Yqh) | 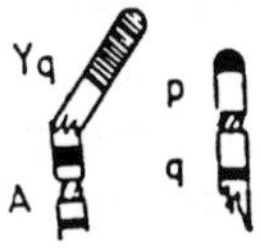 | normal or<br>hypoplastic testicles | arrest at pachytene<br>arrest during meiosis<br>spermatid diff. arrest<br>oligospermia |
| 46.X.t(A:Y) | 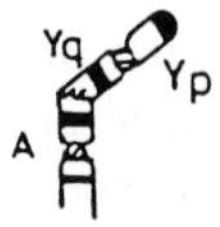 | normal or<br>hypoplastic testicles | immature seminif. tub.<br>only Sertoli cells |

*Fig. 2.* Overview on the variabilities of genitalia phenotypes and testicular histologies in men with microscopically visible anomalies of the human Y chromosome in Yq11. A 45,XO mosaic cell line is usually observed in men with a dicentric (idicYp) or ring (rY) Y chromosome (for a detailed description of these karyotypes see [29,30]).

ruption phases of germ cell development in the AZF patient group (Fig. 2, for review see also [29,30]). This suggested that not one but multiple Y genes were part of the Y chromosomal AZF locus and that these genes may be functional at different phases during human spermatogenesis. Consequently, many research groups have tried to reveal the genetic complexity of AZF by the analysis of its extension and position in Yq11 initially by means of sophisticated cytogenetic analyses of the Yq11 chromosome region (e.g., [31]). Unfortunately, however, this did not seem possible. Genetic linkage analysis commonly used for mapping a gene locus on autosomes could not be applied in Yq11 either because of the absence of crossing over events with the X chromosome in this Y region.

After the first genomic Y-DNA fragments had been cloned molecular deletion mapping therefore became the chosen method for mapping AZF in Yq11. These Y fragments were mapped in a linear order to the Y chromosomes of men with microscopically visible Yq11 deletions [32]. The most detailed map in Yq11 (14 intervals) was established by Ma et al. [33] with 39 Y-specific DNA probes. This map was sufficient to indicate the presence of different small interstitial deletions, i.e., microdeletions, in the Yq11 chromosome region of men with idiopathic non-obstructive azoospermia for the first time [34]. The patients' azoospermia was designated as "idiopathic" because the karyotypes in their lymphocytes were normal, 46,XY. These results raised the question as to whether or not at least two AZF regions exist in Yq11.

Due to the development of PCR technology it was possible to increase the number of specific genomic Y-DNA markers exponentially. Only small sequence-tagged sites (STS: oligos with 15—25 nucleotides) now need to be Y-specific in order to serve as a marker locus in Yq11. Vollrath et al. [35] established the first STS interval map of the human Y chromosome based solely on PCR. With using 110 STS loci in Yq11 and a panel of 96 individuals with cytogenetically visible Y deletions, he was able to subdivide Yq11 into 23 intervals (5A—5Q; 6A—6F; according to the nomenclature introduced by Vergnaud et al. in 1986 [32]). Each order of STS loci in deletion maps depends inherently on the genomic DNA samples used in the laboratory. Therefore, it is difficult to construct a general deletion map of the Y chromosome unless each laboratory uses the same DNA panel for all mapping experiments. Therefore, two extensive deletion maps of Yq11 exist at the moment: the Vollrath map dividing Yq11 into 23 intervals (5A—6F [35]), and the Vogt map dividing Yq11 in 25 intervals (D1—D25 [15]). They were now combined in the genome database (GDB) and are available directly at the GDB web site (http//www.gdb.org; see also the report of the 3rd international workshop on Y chromosome mapping 1997 [36]).

The Vogt map was used to map three different AZF regions in Yq11 [15]: AZFa to interval D3—D6 (corresponding roughly to interval 5C of the Vollrath map); AZFb to interval D13—D16 (corresponding roughly to interval 50—6B of the Vollrath map); AZFc to interval D20—D22 (corresponding roughly to interval 6C—6E of the Vollrath map). AZFc therefore corresponds to the AZF region as defined by Reijo et al. [7] using the Vollrath map. No AZF region was mapped in the short arm of the human Y chromosome (Yp) although molecular cloning experiments succeeded in the isolation of different genes from this Y region which are expressed in human testis (ZFY [37]; TSPY [5]). One explanation for this could be a different molecular structure of the human Y chromosome in Yp and Yq11 which produces interstitial genomic DNA deletions as a major mutation event in Yq11 but not in Yp. This view is supported presently by the results of 20 different Yq11 screening programmes published to date all pointing to the occurrence of frequent interstitial microdeletions in Yq11 [38]. Most of them were reported to overlap to one of the proposed three AZF regions. This does not rule out the possibility that even more AZF regions may exist in Yq11. However, in order to be able to analyse them, further and even more detailed screening programmes may be necessary.

## Molecular origins of the interstitial deletion events marking AZFa, AZFb, AZFc in Yq11

It is intriguing to note that the molecular extensions of the AZFa, AZFb and AZFc regions, as measured by interval mapping, were found to be similar in the Y chromosome of numerous sterile patients diagnosed in different laboratories [38]. This suggests mutational hotspots in Yq11 at the borderlines of the various AZF regions. Nothing is known about the origins and mechanisms of the molecular rearrangements preceding the different deletion events. Mutational hotspots in genomic DNA regions are frequently represented by local homologous tandem repetitive DNA blocks. Most probably deletions occur then due to intrachromosomal unequal crossing over events during meiosis of the father's spermatogenesis. This would explain why AZFc deletions are more frequent than AZFa and AZFb deletions, as local repetitive DNA blocks are enriched in distal Yq11 [32] in the neighbourhood of the highly repetitive heterochromatic Yq12 region. Physical mapping experiments with YAC (yeast artificial chromosome) clones and a series of Y-specific probes mapped to the AZFc interval in distal Yq11 revealed that this genomic Y region also includes large amplified DNA domains containing at least part of the AZFc region [39].

Stuppia et al. [40] recently reported an "oligozoospermia region" as part of the AZFc region (interval 6E). Although the same sterile phenotype was also observed in men with a complete deletion of AZFc [38] deletion of interval 6E might be considered as a premutation of AZFc. This smaller Y deletion is only associated with the phenotype of oligozoospermia but not with that of azoospermia, the major phenotype of men with an AZFc deletion. Y chromosomal rearrangements are expected to be induced during meiosis in the germ line of the patients' fathers and/or during the patients' early embryogenesis. One possible way of detecting AZF premutations in more detail may therefore be molecular deletion analysis of the Y chromosome in single spermatozoa from the patients' fathers (for further discussions see also [41]).

## Single STS deletions events in Yq11

The analysis of the deletion of single STS loci in sterile men, especially in the AZFc region is an intriguing aspect. These were found to be inherited (sY153 [42]; sY207 and sY272 [43]) and proved as "de novo" mutation events (sY153 [42]; sY134, sY138, sY139, sY147, sY152, sY155, sY167, sY158 [44]; sY146 and sY153; sY150, sY220, and sY232; sY240, sY245, sY203, sY242, and sY148 [43]). In some cases multiple deletions of one or more apparently consecutive STS loci were analysed in Yq11, most of which but not all, overlap with the AZFb and/

or AZFc regions [44—46]. Part of them were proven to be "de novo" mutation events.

Most STS loci used for deletion analysis in Yq11 represent small anonymous genomic DNA fragments [15,35]. Therefore, a causal relationship of single STS deletions to the men's infertility is generally difficult to judge even when they occur as "de novo" mutation events. In all cases where there is only one STS deletion in Yq11, it might be wise initially to regard a causal relationship to the men's infertility as questionable unless it has been shown that the deleted STS locus is part of a spermatogenesis gene structure in Yq11. However, it cannot be excluded either (at least not after it has been proved to be a "de novo" mutation event). A causal relationship of the polymorphic Y deletions: sY153, sY207 and sY272, to male infertility can probably be excluded because their occurrence is not restricted just to the infertile male population but was also found to occur in the Y chromosomes of fertile men. Systematic analyses of various Y chromosomal STS DNA markers for evolutionary and paternity studies have now revealed numerous polymorphic DNA loci on the human Y chromosome (for review see [36]). The clinical significance of single STS deletion events in Yq11 should therefore be handled with caution.

## Candidates for male fertility genes in AZFa, AZFb, AZFc

It should be possible to locate at least one functional male fertility gene in each AZF region. This gene is expected to induce the same pathological phenotype as observed after deletion of the corresponding AZF region. Various research groups have already isolated multiple candidates for this gene and these are listed in Table 1. The first Y genes that were isolated represented two gene families encoding testis specific RNA binding proteins: RBM (RNA binding motif) [6], and DAZ (deleted in azoospermia gene) [7]. A third gene family, earlier designated as SPGY (spermatogenesis gene on the Y) [3], is now known to be part of the DAZ gene family [36] and consequently, DAZ has now been renamed DAZ1 and SPGY, DAZ2 [36]. Copies of the RBM gene family are spread in Yq11 and in proximal Yp [6] but most functional RBM gene copies (RBM-I [47]) were mapped to the AZFb region [48]. All copies of the DAZ gene family are clustered in the AZFc region [15].

Both gene families seem to have evolved from an ancestral autosomal gene. The RBM-I genes share 67% sequence similarity to the HNRNPG gene [10] which was mapped to chromosome 6 and is expressed in multiple tissues [49]. RBM genes contain 12 exons, but RBM exon 8—10 is a tandem repetition of exon 7. The duplication and transposition of HNRNPG to the Y chromosome must have occurred more than 130 million years ago prior to the divergence of marsupials and eutherians [50]. The DAZ genes display 89% sequence similarity to the DAZL1 gene ([36], formerly called DAZH [11], SPGYLA [12], DAZLA [13,14]) which was mapped to chromosome 3 and is expressed only in the male germ line. Duplication and transposition of DAZL1 to the Y chromosome must

*Table 1.* Human Y genes mapped to AZFa, AZFb, AZFc in Yq11.

| Gene symbol | Gene name | Protein homolog to | Tissue expression | Yq11 interv. | X chrom. homol. |
|---|---|---|---|---|---|
| BPY2 | Basic protein Y, pI 10 | Novel | only testis | Azfc | no |
| DAZ | Deleted in azoospermia | RNA-binding RRM proteins | only testis | AZFc | no |
| DBY | DEAD-box Y | RNA helicases | multiple | AZFa | yes; DBX |
| DFFRY | *Drosophila* fat facets related Y | Ubiquitin-specific proteases | multiple | AZFa | yes; DFFRX |
| EIF1AY | Essential initiation-translation factor 1A Y | Translation initiation factor | multiple | AZFb | yes; EIF1AX |
| PRY | PTP-BL-related Y | Protein tyrosin phosphatase | only testis | AZFc | no |
| RBM | RNA binding motif | RNA binding RRM-proteins | only testis | AZFb AZFc | no |
| SMCY | Selected mouse C DNA Y | H-Y antigen HLA B7 | multiple | AZFb | yes; SMCX |
| TSPY | Testis-specific protein Y encoded | SET/NAP-1 regul. cell proliferation | only testis | AZFb | no |
| TTY1 | Testis transcript Y1 | No-protein encod. RNA | only testis | AZFc | no |
| TTY2 | Testis transcript Y2 | No-protein encod. RNA | only testis | AZFc | no |
| UTY | Ubiquitous transcribed Y | H-Y antigen HYD[b] | multiple | AZFa | yes; UTX |

have occurred before the divergence of old world monkeys (Catarrhini) and after the divergence of new world monkeys (Platyrrhini), i.e., at a time interval between 36 and 55 million years ago [12,14]. DAZ genes contain 10 exons and exon 7 is repetitive [11]. DAZ transcripts were shown to be highly polymorphic in compositions and numbers of the exon 7 unit [3,51]. It is assumed that they are created by the alternative splicing and exon skipping mechanisms of at least three DAZ gene copies [51].

Two other Y genes isolated earlier, SMCY (selected mouse CDNA on the Y) [9] and TSPY (testis-specific protein Y-encoded) [5], have now also been mapped to the AZFb region (SMCY [3]; TSPY, Urbitsch and Vogt, unpublished results). TSPY is a Y-specific gene family and, like the RBM gene family, has been conserved on the Y chromosome of mammals for more than 130 million years [50]. However, a homologous gene copy on an autosome has not yet been identified. Most of its gene copies are in the proximal part of the short Y arm. It is not known whether the TSPY and RBM gene copies in AZFb are interspersed, but as some RBM gene copies were also found in the major TSPY locus in proximal Yp [52], an interspersion pattern of both gene families in AZFb is very probable. SMCY has a homologous gene copy on the X chromosome (SMCX [9]). TSPY genes encode proteins with homology to the proto-oncogene SET and the nucleosome-assembly factor (NAP-1), suggesting that TSPY proteins serve a function related to spermatogonial proliferation [53]. The SMCY gene encodes a member of the male specific minor histocompatibility H-Y antigens (HLA-B7, identified as an 11-residue peptide in SMCY [54]).

Recently the group of X-Y homologous genes with candidate status for a Y male fertility gene increased significantly after the identification of four other X-Y gene pairs [4]: DBY/DBX (DEAD-box Y/X), DFFRY/DFFRX (*Drosophila* fat facets related Y/X), E1F1AY/E1F1AX (translation initiation factor 1A, Y isoform/ X isoform), and UTY/UTX (ubiquitous TPR motif Y/X). DFFRY and DFFRX were also isolated earlier from the group of N. Affara [8,36]. DBY and DBX belong to the DEAD-box protein family encoding ATP-dependent RNA helicases which function as key elements in the RNA metabolism of the cell [55]. DFFRY and DFFRX are homologous to the *Drosophila* faf protein which suggests that these proteins have a function in the de-ubiquitinating process of proteins which regulate their cellular stability [56]. The E1F1AX protein is involved in the translation initiation of proteins [57] and it can be assumed that its Y isoform performs a similar function. UTY encodes another male specific minor histocompatibility antigen (H-YD[b]) characterized by homology to the TPR (tetratrico-peptide-repeat) family [58]. All these genes are expressed in multiple tissues, some with an additional testis-specific transcript length (DBY, E1F1AY [4]). DFFRY, DBY and UTY were mapped to the AZFa region, E1F1AY was mapped to the AZFb region (Table 1).

Further candidates for male fertility genes were also analysed in the AZFc region: BPY2 (basic protein Y2); PRY (PTP-BL-related Y); TTY2 (testis transcript Y2) [4]. All of them were reported to belong to the Y genes with a testis specific transcription pattern and multiple copies in AZFc. PRY and TTY2 were also mapped to proximal Yp [4]. Their potential functions in human spermatogenesis have not yet been described.

A total of four other Y-specific genes with a testis-specific transcription pattern, BPY1 (basic protein Y), CDY (chromo domain Y), TTY1 (testis transcript Y1) and XKRY (XK-related Y), and one Y gene with an X homolog and a multiple tissue expression pattern, TB4Y (thymosin β4, Y isoform) were mapped outside the AZFa, AZFb, and AZFc regions in Yq11 and in proximal Yp [4]. This points to the possible existence of more AZF regions in Yq11 or in proximal Yp. However, gene-specific mutation events or their interstitial deletions associated with male infertility have not yet been reported. Most intriguing is the fact that all the AZF regions contain genes encoding proteins which probably serve different cellular functions.

## The functional unit of a Y chromosomal male fertility gene

One of the most important practical questions raised in the infertility clinic is whether indeed all of the Y genes listed above are essential for human spermatogenesis, i.e., do they cause male infertility after disruption, or is male infertility induced only after deletion of multiple genes or even only after deletion of all genes mapped to one AZF region? In addition to this (with a view to the *Droso-*

*phila* Y male fertility genes) the functional significance of the complex repetitive sequence structures especially in the AZFb and AZFc region is a source of speculation. In this context, it is remarkable that most members of the pY6H sequence family [59] were mapped to the AZFb and AZFc intervals [3,15]. This family of genomic DNA sequences was isolated by homology to dhMiF1 which is part of a male fertility gene of *Drosophila hydei* [59].

A contribution of genomic DNA sequences to a male fertility function at the chromatin level may be considered for the X-Y homologous DNA region in AZFa. The pairing structure of the X and Y chromosomes in the premeiotic synaptonemal complex structure also includes the genomic DNA region in proximal Yq11 [60] and therefore, probably the complete AZFa region as well. The functional unit of a male fertility gene in AZFa may therefore extend beyond the structure of one protein coding gene and perhaps include the whole X-Y homologous DNA region in proximal Yq11.

Possible experimental approaches towards finding an answer to the question: which of the Y genes listed above are functional for human male fertility? Are the isolation of their homologous mouse genes (in order to develop appropriate knock out animal models) and the analysis of proteins encoded from the human Y genes in the testis tissue of fertile and infertile individuals? Testis protein analysis has been performed recently for the RBM genes [48] and DAZ genes [61] by immunohistochemical experiments. To generate antibodies that are specific for RBM, the repetitive SRGY box encoded by exon 7—10 was expressed in *Escherichia coli* and the peptide used to immunize rabbits [48]. The polyclonal antiserum detected RBM proteins predominantly in the nuclei of spermatogonia, spermatocytes and round spermatids. No RBM proteins were detected in elongating spermatids. This is consistent with the role of RBM in the nuclear RNA metabolism during these germ-line phases. Antibodies that are specific for DAZ were raised in rabbits by using the specific C-terminal peptide encoded by exon 8—10 and the repetitive exon 7 part of DAZ2. The C-terminal peptide encoded by the homologous autosomal DAZL1 gene is different in length and sequence from that of DAZ [61]. Additionally, only DAZ exon 7 is amplified. The DAZ2 antiserum detects DAZ proteins predominantly in late spermatids and in the tails of mature spermatozoa (Fig. 3). This suggests a need for DAZ proteins in the storage or transport of testis-specific mRNA the translation of which is repressed until formation of mature spermatozoa [61].

RBM proteins are absent in sterile patients with deletion of AZFb [48]. This absence is probably associated with the AZFb patients' pathological testis tissue pictures which usually display a meiotic arrest of their spermatogenesis [15]. DAZ proteins are absent in sterile patients with deletion of AZFc [61]. AZFc deletions, however, do not have a distinct pathological phenotype. Assuming that DAZ proteins are functional as translational control proteins in late spermatids, testis histology of this patient class does not show a spermatid arrest as expected, and in rare cases AZFc deletions were shown to be inheritable [15,43]. Obviously, DAZ deletions do not interfere with the production of mature sperma-

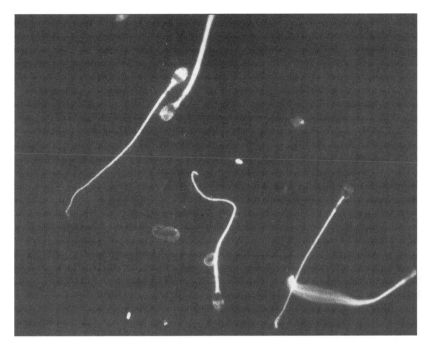

*Fig. 3.* Immunofluorescence experiment with anti-DAZ2 antiserum. A strong fluorescent signal is consistently observed on sperm tails after incubation with fluorescein isothiocyanate (FITC)-conjugated antirabbit serum as the second antibody. (Reproduced with kind permission from Oxford University Press.)

tozoa although the patients produce them only in low numbers. This suggests that DAZ proteins are not essential for the terminal differentiation of the human germ cells but required for their optimal function. A similar mutation effect was described recently for the POU protein sperm-1 in mouse spermatogenesis [62]. If this holds true, one may speculate that each Y gene mapped to the AZFc region (BPY2, DAZ, PRY, TTY2) causes subfertility but not azoospermia as the primary mutation effect. In summary, it is apparent that the Y chromosome is a sanctuary for male fertility genes in species as different as *Drosophila* and human. Our future experiments will now have to concentrate on the functional contribution of each Y gene, or perhaps multigene complexes, and on their underlying chromatin structures to human spermatogenesis in order to define the significance of their mutations for human idiopathic male infertility.

### Acknowledgements

I would like to thank Paul Burgoyne, Howard Cooke, Wolfgang Hennig, and Werner Hilscher for their numerous fruitful discussions and collaborative support in the field of research on the Y chromosomal male fertility factors. Mrs A. Jordan and Mrs H. Meng are thanked for their skillful support in preparing this manuscript, Mrs A. Wiegenstein for excellent photographic assistance. I would further like to thank the Bundesministerium für Wissenschaft, Forschung und Technologie (BMBF) for the grant 01KY 9507/4, without which my research on the analysis of the genetic complexity of AZF would not have been possible.

## References

1. Brosseau GE Jr. Genetic analysis of the male fertility factors on the Y chromosome of *Drosophila* melanogaster. Genetics 1960;55:257–274.
2. Burgoyne PS. Y chromosome function in mammalian development. Adv Dev Biol 1991;1:1–29.
3. Vogt PH. Human Y chromosome function in male germ cell development. Adv Dev Biol 1996;4:193–258.
4. Lahn BT, Page DC. Functional coherence of the human Y chromosome. Science 1997;278: 675–680.
5. Arnemann J, Jakubiczka S, Thüring S, Schmidtke J. Cloning and sequence analysis of a human Y-chromosome-derived, testicular cDNA, TSPY. Genomics 1991;11:108–114.
6. Ma K, Inglis JD, Sharkey A, Bickmore WA, Hill RE, Prosser EJ et al. A Y chromosome gene family with RNA-binding protein homology: candidates for the azoospermia factor AZF controlling human spermatogenesis. Cell 1993;75:1287–1295.
7. Reijo R, Lee T-Y, Salo P, Alagappan R, Brown LG, Rosenberg M et al. Nature Genet 1995;10: 383–393.
8. Brown GM, Furlong RA, Sargent CA, Erickson RP, Longepied G, Mitchel M et al. Characterisation of the coding sequence and fine mapping of the human DFFRY gene and comparative expression analysis and mapping to the Sxr$^b$ interval of the mouse Y chromosome of the Dffry gene. Hum Mol Genet 1998;7:97–107.
9. Agulnik AI, Mitchell MJ, Mattei M-G, Borsani G, Avner PA, Lerner JL et al. A novel X gene with a widely transcribed Y-linked homologue escapes X-inactivation in mouse and human. Hum Mol Genet 1994;3:879–884.
10. Chai N-N, Zhou H, Hernandez J, Najmabadi H, Bhasin S, Yen PH. Structure and organization of the RBMY genes on the human Y chromosome: transposition and amplification of an ancestral autosomal hnRNPG gene. Genomics 1998;49:283–289.
11. Saxena R, Brown LG, Hawkins T, Alagappan RK, Skaletsky H, Reeve MP et al. The DAZ gene cluster on the human Y chromosome arose from an autosomal gene that was transposed, repeatedly amplified and pruned. Nature Genet 1996;14:292–299.
12. Shan Z, Hirschmann P, Seebacher T, Edelmann A, Jauch A, Morell J et al. A SPGY copy homologous to the mouse gene Dazla and the *Drosophila* gene boule is autosomal and expressed only in the human male gonad. Hum Mol Genet 1996;5:2005–2011.
13. Yen PH, Chai NN, Salido EC. The human autosomal gene DAZLA: testes specificity and a candidate for male infertility. Hum Mol Genet 1996;5:2013–2017.
14. Seboun E, Barbaux S, Bourgeron T, Nishi S, Algonik A, Egashira M et al. Gene sequence, localisation, and evolutionary conservation of DAZLA, a candidate male sterility gene. Genomics 1997;41:227–235.
15. Vogt PH, Edelmann A, Kirsch S, Henegariu O, Hirschmann P, Kiesewetter F et al. Human Y chromosome azoospermia factors (AZF) mapped to different subregions in Yq11. Hum Mol Genet 1996;5:933–944.
16. Hennig W, Brand RC, Hackstein J, Hochstenbach R, Kremer H, Lankenau D-H et al. Y chromosomal fertility genes of *Drosophila*: a new type of eukaryotic genes. Genome 1989;31: 561–571.
17. Stern C. Untersuchungen über Aberrationen des Y-Chromosom von *Drosophila* melanogaster. Z Ind Abst Vererb 1929;51:253–353.
18. Meyer GF. Die Funktionsstrukturen des Y-Chromosoms in den Spermatocytenkernen von *Dro-*

*sophila Hydei*. Neohydei, D. Repleta und einigen anderen *Drosophila* Arten. Chromosoma 1963;14:207–255.

19. Glätzer KH, Meyer GF. Morphological aspects of the genetic activity in primary spermatocyte nuclei of *Drosophila hydei*. Biol Cell 1981;41:165–172.

20. Vogt P, Hennig W, Siegmund I. Identification of transcribed cloned Y chromosomal DNA sequences from a lamp brush loop of *Drosophila hydei*. Proc Natl Acad Sci USA 1982: 79:5132–5136.

21. Lifschytz E, Hareven D, Azriel A, Brodsly H. DNA clones and RNA transcripts of four lamp brush loops from the Y chromosome of *Drosophila hydei*. Cell 1983;32:191–199.

22. Bonaccorsi S, Lohe A. Fine mapping of satellite DNA sequences along the Y chromosome of *Drosophila* melanogaster: relationships between satellite sequences and fertility factors. Genetics 1991;129:177–189.

23. Hennig W. The Y chromosomal lamp brush loops of *Drosophila*. In: Hennig W (ed) Results and Problems in Cell Differentiation 14. Structure and Function of Eukaryotic Chromosomes. Heidelberg: Springer 1987;133–146.

24. Hochstenbach R, Knops M, Hennig W. Discrimination of related transcribed and nontranscribed repetitive DNA sequences from the Y chromosomes of *Drosophila hydei* and *Drosophila eohydei*. Mol Gen Genet 1994;234:54–62.

25. Gepner J, Hays TS. A fertility region on the Y chromosome of *Drosophila* melanogaster encodes a dynein microtubule motor. Proc Natl Acad Sci USA 1993;90:11132–11136.

26. Hulsebos TJM, Hackstein JHP, Hennig W. Involvement of Y chromosomal loci in the synthesis of *Drosophila hydei* sperm proteins. Dev Biol 1983;100:238–243.

27. Pisano C, Bonaccorsi S, Gatti M. The kl-3 loop of the Y chromosome of *Drosophila* melanogaster binds a tektin-like protein. Genetics 1993;133:569–579.

28. Tiepolo L, Zuffardi O. Localization of factors controlling spermatogenesis in the nonfluorescent portion of the human Y chromosome long arm. Hum Genet 1976;34:119–124.

29. Sandberg AA. Clinical aspects of Y chromosome abnormalities. In: Series: Progress and Topics in Cytogenetics. New York: Alan R Liss Inc., 1985;6.

30. Vogt P. Y chromosome function in spermatogenesis (review). In: Nieschlag E, Habenicht UF (eds) Spermatogenesis-Fertilization-Contraception. Molecular Cellular and Endocrine Events in Male Reproduction. Heidelberg: Springer, 1992;226–257.

31. Oosthuizen CJJ, Herbert JS, Vermaak LK, Brusnicky J, Fricke J, du Plessis L et al. Deletion mapping of 39 random isolated Y-chromosome DNA fragments. Hum Genet 1990;85: 205–210.

32. Vergnaud G, Page DC, Simmler M-C, Brown L, Rouyer F, Noel B et al. A deletion map of the human Y chromosome based on DNA hybridization. Am J Hum Genet 1986:38:109–124.

33. Ma K, Sharkey A, Kirsch S, Vogt P, Keil R, Hargreave TB et al. Towards the molecular localisation of the AZF locus: mapping of microdeletions in azoospermic men within 14 subintervals of interval 6 of the human Y chromosome. Hum Mol Genet 1992;1:29–33.

34. Vogt P, Chandley AC, Hargreave TB, Keil R, Ma K, Sharkey A. Microdeletions in interval 6 of the Y chromosome of males with idiopathic sterility point to disruption of AZF, a human spermatogenesis gene. Hum Genet 1992;89:491–496.

35. Vollrath D, Foote S, Hilton A, Brown LG, Beer-Romero P, Bogan JS et al. The human Y chromosome: a 43-interval map based on naturally occurring deletions. Science 1992;258:52–59.

36. Vogt PH, Affara N, Davey P, Hammer M, Jobling MA, Lau Y-FC et al. Report of the third international workshop on human Y chromosome mapping. Cytogenet Cell Genet 1997;79:1–20.

37. Page DC, Mosher R, Simpson EM, Fischer EMC, Mardon G, Pollack J et al. The sex-determining region of the human Y chromosome encodes a finger protein. Cell 1987;51:1091–1104.

38. Vogt PH. Human chromosome deletions in Yq11, AZF candidate genes and male infertility: history and update. Mol Hum Reprod 1998;4:(In press).

39. Kirsch S, Keil R, Edelmann A, Henegariu O, Hirschmann P, LePaslier D et al. Molecular analysis of the genomic structure of the human Y chromosome in the euchromatic part of its

long arm (Yq11). Cytogen Cell Genet 1996;75:197–206.

40. Stuppia L, Calabrese G, Franchi PG, Mingarelli R, Gatta V, Palka G et al. Widening of a Y-chromosome interval-6 deletion transmitted from a father to his infertile son accounts for an oligozoospermia critical region distal to the RBM1 and DAZ genes (letter). Am J Hum Genet 1996;59:1393–1395.

41. Edwards RG, Bishop CE. On the origin and frequency of Y chromosome deletions responsible for severe male infertility. Mol Hum Reprod 1997;3:549–554.

42. Kent-First MG, Skol S, Muallem A, Ofir R, Manor D, Blazer S et al. The incidence and possible relevance of Y-linked microdeletions in babies born after intracytoplasmic sperm injection and their infertile fathers. Mol Hum Reprod 1996;2:943–950.

43. Pryor JL, Kent-First M, Muallem A, van Bergen AH, Nolten WE, Meisner L et al. Microdeletions in the Y chromosome of infertile men. N Engl J Med 1997;336:534–539.

44. Stuppia L, Mastroprimiano G, Calabrese G. Microdeletions in interval 6 of the Y chromosome detected by STS-PCR in 6 of 33 patients with idiopathic oligo- or azoospermia. Cytogen Cell Genet 1996;72:155–158.

45. Najmabadi H, Huang V, Yen P, Subbarao MN, Bhasin D, Banaag L et al. Substantial prevalance of microdeletions of the Y-chromosome in infertile men with idiopathic azoospermia and oligozoospermia detected using a sequence-tagged site-based mapping strategy. JCE & M 1996; 81:1347–1352.

46. Foresta C, Ferlin A, Garolla A, Rossato M, Barbaux S, de Bortoli A. Y-chromosome deletions in idiopathic severe testiculopathies. JCE & M 1997;82:1075–1080.

47. Chai NN, Salido EC, Yen PH. Multiple functional copies of the RBM gene family, a spermatogenesis candidate on the human Y chromosome. Genomics 1997;45:355–361.

48. Elliott DJ, Millar MR, Oghene K, Ross A, Kiesewetter F, Pryor J et al. Expression of RBM in the nuclei of human germ cells is dependent on a critical region of the Y chromosome long arm. Proc Natl Acad Sci USA 1997;94:3848–3853.

49. Scoulard M, Valle VD, Siomi M, Pinol-Roma S, Codogno P, Bauvy C et al. HnRNP G: sequence and characterization of a glycosylated RNA-binding protein. Nucl Acid Res 1993;21:4210–4217.

50. Delbridge ML, Harry JL, Toder R, O'Neill RJW, Ma K, Chandley AC et al. A human candidate spermatogenesis gene, RBM1, is conserved and amplified on the marsupial Y chromosome. Nature Genet 1997;15:131–136.

51. Yen PH, Cahi NN, Salido EC. The human DAZ genes, a putative male infertility factor on the Y chromosome, are highly polymorphic in the DAZ repeat regions. Mamm Genome 1997;8: 756–759.

52. Gläser B, Hierl T, Taylor K, Schiebel K, Zeitler S, Papadopoullos K et al. High-resolution fluorescence in situ hybridization of human Y-linked genes on released chromatin. Chromosome Res 1997;5:23–30.

53. Schnieders F, Dörk T, Arnemann J, Vogel T, Werner M, Schmidtke J. Testis-specific protein, Y-encoded (TSPY) expression in testicular tissues. Hum Mol Genet 1996;5:1801–1807.

54. Wang W, Meadows LR, den Haan JM, Sherman NE, Chen Y, Blockland E et al. Human H-Y: a male-specific histocompatibility antigen derived from the SMCY protein. Science 1995;269: 1588–1590.

55. Schmid SR, Linder P. D-E-A-D protein family of putative RNA helicases. Molec Microbiol 1992;6:283–292.

56. Huang Y, Baker RT, Fischer-Vize JA. Control of cell fate by a deubiquitinating enzyme encoded by the fat facets gene. Science 1995;270:1828–1831.

57. Hershey JWB. Translational control in mammalian cells. Ann Rev Biochem 1991;60:717–755.

58. Greenfield A, Scott D, Pennisi D, Ehrmann I, Ellis P, Cooper L et al. An H-YD[b] epitope is encoded by a novel mouse Y chromosome gene (letter). Nature Genet 1996;14:474–478.

59. Vogt P, Keil R, Köhler M, Lengauer C, Lewe D, Lewe G. Selection of DNA sequences from interval 6 of the human Y chromosome with homology to a Y chromosomal fertility gene

sequence of *Drosophila hydei*. Hum Genet 1991;86:341—349.

60. Ashley T. A re-examination of the case for homology between the X and Y chromosomes of mouse and man. Hum Genet 1984;67:372—377.

61. Habermann B, Mi H-F, Edelmann A, Bohring C, Bäckert I-T, Kiesewetter F et al. DAZ (deleted in azoospermia) genes encode proteins located in human late spermatids and in sperm tails. Hum Reprod 1998;13:363—369.

62. Pearse RV II, Drolet W, Kalla KA, Hooshmand F, Bermingham JR Jr, Rosenfeld MG. Reduced fertility in mice deficient for the POU protein sperm-1. Proc Natl Acad Sci USA 1997;94: 7555—7560.

# The Y chromosome, DAZ and DAZL

Howard J. Cooke

*MRC Human Genetics Unit, Western General Hospital, Edinburgh, UK*

**Abstract.** *Background.* Multiple gene families on the human Y chromosome have been implicated in spermatogenesis. Two of these encode RNA-binding proteins RBM and DAZ.

*Methods.* Mouse genetics, transgenesis, immunocytochemistry, and ddrtPCR.

*Results.* We have shown that the autosomal ancestor of DAZ, Dazl is essential for both spermatogenesis and oogenesis in mouse and that the RBM gene is likely to be a splicing modulator.

*Conclusions.* The biochemistry and cell biology of the RNA-binding proteins Dazla and RBM are starting to be understood and may provide new insight into the processes involved in gametogenesis.

**Keywords:** RNA binding, splicing, translation.

The Y chromosome in mammals carries the gene which switches the development of the indifferent gonad from the default female pathway to the male and results in the development of the testis [1]. Despite this it has been regarded as a largely degenerate chromosome because of its small size and in some cases largely heterochromatic appearance [2]. This view of degeneracy extends to the idea that there are few genes on the Y chromosome. Whilst it is clear that there are no essential genes on the Y, because females do not have this chromosome, recent work does not support this view. The original basis for expecting few genes on the Y chromosome was the argument made about sex-chromosome evolution. This held that the Y chromosome arose from an ancestral autosomal pair, one of which acquired sex-determining properties, which then had to be isolated from recombination with its original homologue (now the X with which recombination is retained in the paring region). Isolation resulted in the loss of DNA and of functional genes from what would, in mammals, become the visually distinct Y chromosome. Lack of genes on the Y was supported by the absence of Y-linked phenotypes other than maleness.

The first challenges to this view came from the observations [3] that some males with visible deletions of the Y chromosome long arm were azoospermic leading to the naming of the azoospermia factor (AZF) originally thought of as a single gene on the human Y chromosome euchromatin/heterochromatin boundary. The Y chromosome had been thought, for evolutionary reasons, to be a favored site for genes involved in spermatogenesis [4] and it is now clear that a

*Address for correspondence:* Prof Howard J. Cooke, MRC Human Genetics Unit, Western General Hospital, Crewe Road, Edinburgh EH4 2XU, UK. Tel.: +44-131-467-8427. Fax: +44-131-343-2620. E-mail: howard@hgu.mrc.ac.uk

number of genes with either demonstrated involvement in spermatogenesis or with patterns of expression suggestive of involvement in this process exist on the mammalian Y chromosome.

## RBM and DAZ/DAZL

Using probes that map within a Y chromosome microdeletion interval found in azoospermic and severely oligozoospermic men, Ma and co-workers [5] reported the isolation and characterisation of a multigene family of about 30 members located in interval 5 and 6 of Yq11.23, the region lately defined as AZFb. These genes encode proteins with a modular structure: a single RNA-binding domain of the RRM (RNA recognition motif)-type at the N-terminus (for a review see [6]), and an auxiliary C-terminal domain containing four 37-peptide repeats. (For more detailed discussion and references on RBM see [7].) In an attempt to correlate severe spermatogenic defects with frequent and consistent de novo microdeletions of the Y chromosome, a second candidate spermatogenesis gene, DAZ (deleted in azoospermia, previously also called SPGY) has been cloned from the AZF region [8,9]. DAZ maps to the AZFc subregion, and shares with RBM many common features. DAZ is a member of a multicopy gene family of at least three members [10], and it encodes a protein with a single RNA-binding domain at the N-terminus and an auxiliary C-terminal domain containing seven repeats of a 24 amino acid unit, the so-called DAZ repeat. Like RBM, DAZ transcription is restricted to the germ line in the testis. Interestingly, the DAZ repeats are part of the DYS1 sequence DYS1, a highly polymorphic probe widely used for haplotype analysis that maps to Yq11 [11,12]. This situation is strikingly similar to that of RBM in humans, where the genes are part of a genomic region containing the Sx1 repeat [13,14]. At the moment it is not known whether the DYS1 and Sx1 repeats are actively transcribed, although it is now assumed that the DYS1 is DAZ. The DAZ transcription unit appears very complex, with the presence of pseudoexons, i.e., nonfunctional exons with degenerated 5' and 3' splice sites that are excised during the processing of DAZ pre-mRNA [10]. Moreover, it is now clear that every male contains multiple DAZ genes that vary in the population not only in the copy number of the DAZ repeats, but also in their order, and that a minimum of three DAZ genes are actively transcribed [15]. This is remarkably similar to the RBM genes in humans, for which transcripts varying in the number of copies of the SRGY repeat have been reported [16]. In both cases only a single major band could be detected by Northern blotting on human testis RNA. This raises the possibility that the different cDNAs isolated that vary in the number of repeats could be generated by alternative splicing of a common pre-mRNA. Alternatively, one type of RBM and DAZ genes could be more actively transcribed than the other, or genes with the same number of repeats could account for the vast majority of transcripts.

Unlike RBM, DAZ is found on the Y chromosome only in humans, Old World monkeys and apes [10,17]. In all the other mammals it is represented as an autosomally located, single copy gene, Dazl (DAZ-like), previously also called Dazla, Dazh, or SPGYLA. DAZL genes have been isolated independently by many groups in humans [9,18,19], mouse [17,20,21], monkey [22], frogs [23] and flies [24]. Surprisingly, while the mouse Dazl gene is located on chromosome 17B1, the human DAZL gene maps on 3p25, which represents a new region of synteny between human and mouse since no other locus on this region is known to be located on human 3p [17,19]. It is interesting to note that a number of mutations affecting spermatogenesis have been mapped to mouse chromosome 17, close or within the *t* complex [25,26] (for a review see [27]), although the phenotypic effects of homozygous mutations affecting these genes are unknown. The high degree of homology of the Dazl gene from flies to men is remarkable, and points towards a general function conserved throughout evolution. For example, a recent experiment shows that the *Xenopus* Dazl gene is able to rescue fertility in flies mutant for boule, the *Drosophila* Dazl homolog. This evidence seems to indicate that the function of Dazl is conserved between vertebrates and invertebrates [23]. The homology between DAZ and DAZL is also very high, the only major difference consisting in the presence in DAZL of only one copy of the DAZ repeat unit. On the basis of these evolutionary considerations, it is now assumed that the DAZ gene cluster on the human Y chromosome arose from transposition of a complete copy of a DAZL transcription unit from chromosome 3, tandem amplification and degeneration of the sequence encoding the DAZ repeat, and amplification of the whole Daz transcription unit after the divergence of Old World and New World monkeys 40–45 million years ago [10,19].

### What is the function of DAZ/DAZL?

Although at first it was somewhat unexpected that two candidate spermatogenesis genes on the Y chromosome both encode putative RNA-binding proteins, this is not so surprising if we consider that, together with the brain, the testis is the organ that shows the most complex pattern of RNA metabolism. If we assume that the acquisition of genes on the Y chromosome has evolutionary reasons in terms of a more efficient spermatogenesis, the presence of two gene families both encoding RRM-containing proteins may suggest that many proteins of this type could be involved in spermatogenesis. This is certainly true in *Drosophila*, where many examples of RNA-binding proteins necessary for spermatogenesis have been extensively characterised [28–32]. Recent reports describing RNA-binding proteins necessary for mouse germ cell development indicate that this is true for mammals as well [33,34].

Using a combination of genetic and biochemical approaches, we have recently shown that Dazl is a germ cell-specific protein expressed during the diploid stages of spermatogenesis from spermatogonia to spermatocytes and in the oocytes [33]. In striking contrast to RBM, Dazl is not present in the nucleus, but is localised in the cytoplasm of germ cells from the embryo to adulthood, although in developing follicles it appears to be localised to the *zona pellucida*.

The cytoplasmic localisation implies a completely different function for Dazl in RNA metabolism. Delayed translation of specific subsets of messenger RNAs through sequestration in the cytoplasm by specific RNA-binding proteins is a regulatory mechanism known to play a very important role during spermatogenesis and oogenesis [35–40]. Using targeted mutagenesis, we disrupted the Dazl gene in mice [33]. Our results show that Dazl is necessary for germ cell survival and gonadal development in both sexes. This is in contrast to the situation in *Drosophila*, where the Dazl homolog, boule, is necessary for meiotic cell cycle during spermatogenesis, but not oogenesis [24]. This implies either that the Dazl gene must have acquired an oogenesis-specific function, or a more general function in gametogenesis, during vertebrate evolution or have lost such a role in drosophila oogenesis. In the mouse the effects of the absence of Dazl start to be evident around 19 days of embryonal life. The function of Dazl is likely to be complex, since the cell types in which the protein is found in adult mice are not developed at the time in which the effects of the disruption of the gene become manifest. A possible interpretation is that the protein is essential only for the stem cell population in embryos, and simply persists during latter stages of spermatogenesis. This does not seem to be the case, since the location of the protein in adult mouse testis is consistent with RNA in situ data [41]. No information is currently available about localisation of Dazl mRNA in adult ovary, and therefore it is not known whether the localisation of the protein to the *zona pellucida* is of any functional relevance. It is possible that Dazl is simply sequestered to the zona due to the low isoelectric point of the protein components of the *zona pellucida* [42]. To elucidate this data, we favour another hypothesis, according to which Dazl might have two distinct functions in embrionic and adult gonads. A way to test this hypothesis would be to construct conditional knockout mice in which the gene can be switched off at a certain stage of spermatogenesis or oogenesis.

Many laboratories have reported microdeletions of the Y chromosome [43–52] but the frequency reported varies substantially. Forresta [53] and co-workers have reported the highest levels of 37% of azoospermic men with microdeletions of the Y chromosome. The lower levels of deletion found are difficult to estimate given the bias against publication, however, the average deletion frequency in azoospermic males is probably between 5 and 10%. The region of the Y chromosome most commonly deleted is the AZFc region but other deletions may cumulatively account for as many or more deleted chromosomes. There are a number of problems in interpreting these findings.

Firstly, the phenotype of individuals with apparently the same deletion is variable. In the case of DAZ deletions cases are known where deletions have been transmitted from father to son and in general the precise type of spermatogenic arrest is variable. The implication is that there are effects of genetic or environmental background on the penetrance of the mutation. This is also true for deletions in other regions of the Y such as those involving RBM. Secondly, the genes known to lie in the deleted regions remain candidate genes, no mutations have been found in infertile patients and it remains possible that other genes are present within these intervals. Thirdly the frequency of these deletions is relatively high and given their association with infertility they must most commonly occur de novo. This raises the possibility that germ-line mosaicism or deletions occurring during spermatogenesis could result in apparently normal fathers having sons with deleted Y chromosomes.

We do not know what other variables are involved with the repeated genes on the Y chromosome. Copy number may vary either from individual to individual or from population to population and an effect of paternal age on the frequency of deletions has been postulated.

In conclusion it is clear that despite rapid progress in the last few years in defining genes on the Y chromosome their role and importance in the spermatogenic process is not yet well-defined. Many new genes are likely to emerge and may well be found to be deleted in some members of the population. Studies on those genes for which homologies provide clues to function, such as DAZ and RBM, are underway and will hopefully provide new insights and points of intervention into the process of gametogenesis.

## References

1. Goodfellow PN, Lovellbadge R. Sry and sex determination in mammals. Ann Rev Genet 1993; 27:71—92.
2. Graves JAM. The origin and function of the mammalian Y-chromosome and Y-borne genes — an evolving understanding. Bioessays 1995;17:311—320.
3. Tiepolo L, Zuffardi O. Localisation of factors controlling spermatogenesis in the nonfluorescent portion of the human Y chromosome long arm. Hum Genet 1976;34:119—124.
4. Fisher RA. The evolution of dominance. Biol Rev 1931;6:345—368.
5. Ma K, Inglis JD, Sharkey A, Bickmore WA, Hill RE, Prosser EJ, Speed RM, Thomson EJ, Jobling M, Taylor K, Wolfe J, Cooke HJ, Hargreave TB, Chandley AC. A Y-chromosome gene family with RNA-binding protein homology — candidates for the azoospermia factor AZF controlling human spermatogenesis. Cell 1993;75:1287—1295.
6. Siomi H, Dreyfuss G. RNA-binding proteins as regulators of gene expression. Curr Opin Genet Devel 1997;7:345—353.
7. Elliott DJ, Oghene K, Makarov G, Makarova O, Hargreave TB, Chandley AC, Eperon IC, Cooke HJ. Dynamic changes in the subnuclear organisation of pre-mRNA splicing proteins and RBM during human germ cell develpoment. J Cell Sci 1998;111:1255—1265.
8. Reijo R, Lee TY, Salo P, Alagappan R, Brown LG, Rosenberg M, Rozen S, Jaffe T, Straus D, Hovatta O. Diverse spermatogenic defects in humans caused by Y chromosome deletions encompassing a novel RNA-binding protein gene. Nature Genet 1995;10:383—393.
9. Shan Z, Hirschmann P, Seebacher T, Edelmann A, Jauch A, Morell J, Urbitsch P, Vogt PH. A SPGY copy homologous to the mouse gene Dazla and the Drosophila gene boule is autosomal and expressed only in the human male gonad. Hum Molec Genet 1996;5:2005—2011.
10. Saxena R, Brown LG, Hawkins T, Alagappan RK, Skaletsky H, Reeve MP, Rejio R, Rozen S, Dinulos M, Disteche CM, Page DC. The DAZ gene cluster on the human Y chromosome arose from an autosomal gene that was transposed, repeatedly amplified and pruned. Nature Genet 1996;14:292—298.
11. Lucotte G, Ngo NY. P49f, a highly polymorphic probe, that detects taq1 rflps on the human Y-chromosome. Nucl Acid Res 1985;13:8285.
12. Ngo KY, Vergnaud G, Johnsson C, Lucotte G, Weissenbach J. A DNA probe detecting multiple haplotypes of the human Y-chromosome. Am J Hum Genet 1986;38:407—418.

756

13. Navin A, Prekeris R, Lisitsyn NA, Sonti MM, Grieco DA, Narayanswami S, Lander ES, Simpson EM. Mouse Y-specific repeats isolated by whole chromosome representational difference analysis. Genomics 1996;36:349—353.

14. Mahadevaiah SK, Odorisio T, Elliott DJ, Rattigan A, Szot M, Laval SH, Washburn LL, Mccarrey JR, Cattanach BM, Lovellbadge R, Burgoyne PS. Mouse homologues of the human AZF candidate gene RBM are expressed in spermatogonia and spermatids, and map to a Y chromosome deletion interval associated with a high incidence of sperm abnormalities. Hum Molec Genet 1998;7:715—727.

15. Yen PH, Chai NN, Salido EC. The human DAZ genes, a putative male infertility factor on the Y chromosome, are highly polymorphic in the DAZ repeat regions. Mammal Genome 1997; 8:756—759.

16. Prosser J, Inglis JD, Condie A, Ma K, Kerr S, Thakrar R, Taylor K, Cameron JM, Cooke HJ. Degeneracy in human multicopy rbm (yrrm), a candidate spermatogenesis gene. Mammal Genome 1996;7:835—842.

17. Cooke HJ, Lee M, Kerr S, Ruggiu M. A murine homolog of the human daz gene is autosomal and expressed only in male and female gonads. Hum Molec Genet 1996;5:513—516.

18. Yen PH, Chai NN, Salido EC. The human autosomal gene DAZLA — testis specificity and a candidate for male-infertility. Hum Molec Genet 1996;5:2013—2017.

19. Seboun E, Barbaux S, Bourgeron T, Nishi S, Algonik A, Egashira M, Nikkawa N, Bishop C, Fellous M, Mcelreavey K, Kasahara M. Gene sequence, localization, and evolutionary conservation of DAZLA, a candidate male sterility gene. Genomics 1997;41:227—235.

20. Reijo R, Seligman J, Dinulos MB, Jaffe T, Brown LG, Disteche CM, Page DC. Mouse autosomal homolog of Daz, a candidate male-sterility gene in humans, is expressed in male germ-cells before and after puberty. Genomics 1996;35:346—352.

21. Maiwald R, Seebacher T, Edelmann A, Hirschmann P, Kohler MR, Kirsch S, Vogt P. A human Y-chromosomal gene mapping to distal Yq11 is expressed in spermatogenesis. Cytogen Cell Genet 1996.

22. Carani C, Gromoll J, Brinkworth MH, Simoni M, Weinbauer GF, Nieschlag E. cynDazla: a cynomolgus monkey homologue of the human autosomal DAZ gene. Molec Hum Reprod 1997;3:479—483.

23. Houston DW, Zhang J, Maines JZ, Wasserman SA, King ML. A xenopus DAZ-like gene encodes an RNA component of germ plasm and is a functional homologue of Drosophila boule. Development 1998;125:171—180.

24. Eberhart CG, Maines JZ, Wasserman SA. Meiotic cell-cycle requirement for a fly homolog of human deleted in azoospermia. Nature 1996;381:783—785.

25. Kasahara M, Seboun E, Fellous M, Nadeau JH. Genetic-mapping of a male germ cell-expressed gene tpx-2 to mouse chromosome-17. Immunogenetics 1991;34:132—135.

26. Pilder SH, Oldsclarke P, Phillips DM, Silver LM. Hybrid sterility-6 — a mouse-t complex locus controlling sperm flagellar assembly and movement. Devel Biol 1993;159:631—642.

27. Silver LM. Mouse t-haplotypes. Ann Rev Genet 1985;19:179—208.

28. Karschmizrachi I, Haynes SR. The rb97d gene encodes a potential RNA-binding protein required for spermatogenesis in drosophila. Nucl Acid Res 1993;21:2229—2235 (Record - 86).

29. Matunis EL, Kelley R, Dreyfuss G. Essential role for a heterogeneous nuclear ribonucleoprotein (hnrnp) in oogenesis — hrp40 is absent from the germ-line in the dorsoventral mutant squid. Proc Natl Acad Sci USA 1994;91:2781—2784.

30. Heatwole VM, Haynes SR. Association of RB97D, an RRM protein required for male fertility, with a Y chromosome lampbrush loop in *Drosophila* spermatocytes. Chromosoma 1997;105: 285—292.

31. Zu K, Sikes ML, Haynes SR, Beyer AL. Altered levels of the drosophila hrb87f/hrp36 hnrnp protein have limited effects on alternative splicing in vivo. Molec Biol Cell 1996;7:1059—1073.

32. Haynes SR, Cooper MT, Pype S, Stolow DT. Involvement of a tissue-specific RNA recognition motif protein in Drosophila spermatogenesis. Molec Cell Biol 1997;17:2708—2715.

33. Ruggiu M, Speed R, Taggart M, Mckay SJ, Kilanowski F, Saunders P, Dorin J, Cooke HJ. The mouse Dazla gene encodes a cytoplasmic protein essential for gametogenesis. Nature 1997; 389:73—77.
34. Beck AP, Miller IJ, Anderson P, Streuli M. RNA-binding protein TIAR is essential for primordial germ cell development. Proc Natl Acad Sci USA 1998;95:2331—2336.
35. Fajardo MA, Butner KA, Lee K, Braun RE. Cell-specific proteins interact with the 3' untranslated regions of prm-1 and prm-2 messenger-RNA. Devel Biol 1994;166:643—653.
36. Nayernia K, Reim K, Oberwinkler H, Engel W. Diploid expression and translational regulation of rat acrosin gene. Biochem Biophys Res Commun 1994;202:88—93.
37. Lee K, Fajardo MA, Braun RE. A testis cytoplasmic RNA-binding protein that has the properties of a translational repressor. Molec Cell Biol 1996;16:3023—3034.
38. Kleene KC. Patterns of translational regulation in the mammalian testis. Molec Reprod Devel 1996;43:268—281.
39. Lee K, Haugen HS, Clegg CH, Braun RE. Premature translation of protamine-1 messenger-RNA causes precocious nuclear condensation and arrests spermatid differentiation in mice. Proc Natl Acad Sci USA 1995;92:12451—12455.
40. Sommerville J, Ladomery M. Transcription and masking of messenger-RNA in germ-cells — involvement of Y-box proteins. Chromosoma 1996;104:469—478.
41. Niederberger C, Agulnik AI, Cho Y, Lamb D, Bishop CE. In situ hybridization shows that dazla expression in mouse testis is restricted to premeiotic stages iv—vi of spermatogenesis. Mammal Genome 1997;8:277—278.
42. Bleil JD, Wassarman PM. Structure and function of the *zona pellucida*: identification and characterization of the proteins of the mouse oocyte's *zona pellucida*. Devel Biol 1980;76:185—202.
43. Barbaux S, Vilain E, Raoul O, Gilgenkrantz S, Jeandidier E, Chadenas D, Souleyreau N, Fellous M, Mcelreavey K. Proximal deletions of the long arm of the Y-chromosome suggest a critical region associated with a specific subset of characteristic turner stigmata. Hum Molec Genet 1995;4:1565—1568.
44. Bhasin S, Ma K, Dekretser DM. Y-chromosome microdeletions and male infertility. Ann Med 1997;29:261—263.
45. Kremer JM, Tuerlings JM, Meuleman EH, Schoute F, Mariman E, Smeets DM, Hoefsloot LH, Braat DM, Merkus HM. Microdeletions of the Y chromosome and intracytoplasmic sperm injection: from gene to clinic. Hum Reprod 1997;12:687—691.
46. Nakahori Y, Kuroki Y, Komaki R, Kondoh N, Namiki M, Iwamoto T, Toda T, Kobayashi K. The Y-chromosome region essential for spermatogenesis. Horm Res 1996;46:20—23.
47. Qureshi SJ, Ross AR, Ma K, Cooke HJ, Intyre MA, Chandley AC, Hargreave TB. Polymerase chain reaction screening for Y chromosome microdeletions: a first step towards the diagnosis of genetically-determined spermatogenic failure in men. Molec Hum Reprod 1996;2:775—779.
48. Simoni M, Gromoll J, Dworniczak B, Rolf C, Abshagen K, Kamischke A, Carani C, Meschede D, Behre HM, Horst J, Nieschlag E. Screening for deletions of the Y chromosome involving the daz (deleted in azoospermia) gene in azoospermia and severe oligozoospermia. Fertil Steril 1997;67:542—547.
49. Stuppia L, Mastroprimiano G, Calabrese G, Peila R, Tenaglia R, Palka G. Microdeletions in interval-6 of the Y-chromosome detected by sts-pcr in 6 of 33 patients with idiopathic oligospermia or azoospermia. Cytogenet Cell Genet 1996;72:155—158.
50. Vereb M, Agulnik AI, Houston JT, Lipschultz LI, Lamb DJ, Bishop CE. Absence of Daz gene mutations in cases of non-obstructed azoospermia. Molec Hum Reprod 1997;3:55—59.
51. Vogt PH. Human Y chromosome deletions in Yq11 and male fertility. [Review] [37 refs]. Adv Exp Med Biol 1997;424:17—30.
52. Yen PH, Chai NN, Salido EC. The human autosomal gene DAZLA — testis specificity and a candidate for male-infertility. Hum Molec Genet 1996;5:2013—2017.
53. Foresta C, Ferlin A, Garolla A, Rossato M, Barbaux S et al. Y-chromosome deletions in idiopathic severe testiculopathies. J Clin Endocrinol Metab 1997;82:1075—1080.

# Hormone receptor mutations

Fertility and Reproductive Medicine.
R.D. Kempers, J. Cohen, A.F. Haney and J.B. Younger, editors.

# FSH receptor defects and reproduction

Kristiina Aittomäki

*Department of Clinical Genetics, Helsinki University Central Hospital, Helsinki, Finland*

**Abstract.** Although the central role of the two gonadotropins, follicle-stimulating hormone (FSH) and luteinizing hormone (LH), as regulators of ovarian and testicular function has long been established, their role in infertility and disorders of reproduction has remained an open question. The recent development of molecular genetics that has allowed the cloning of the genes encoding these two hormones and their receptors has, however, also enabled the identification of several mutations in these genes. In comparison to many other G-protein coupled receptors, the number of mutations identified in the FSHR gene has remained low. In females, there seems to be a clear-cut phenotype caused by inactivating mutations of FSH receptor (FSHR). However, there is yet much to be learned of the action of FSH both in male and female reproduction.

## Introduction

The pituitary gonadotropins follicle-stimulating hormone (FSH) and luteinizing hormone (LH) control the production of sex steroids necessary for normal pubertal development and fertility in both sexes. In females, FSH controls the ovarian production of both mature oocytes and estrogen in the granulosa cells, the target cells of FSH, although there is evidence that not all ovarian follicular development is FSH dependent. In the testes, the target cells of FSH are the Sertoli cells, however, there are no conclusive data on the significance of FSH in the control of spermatogenesis [1]. In the granulosa and Sertoli cells, FSH action is mediated by the FSH receptor, known to be expressed in these cells [2,3]. As FSH action is dependant on the integrity of the FSH receptor (FSHR), there has been a growing interest to study the possible mutations in FSHR. Naturally occurring mutations offer the possibility to study the effects of altered FSH function in vivo without detailed knowledge of the complex network of endocrine, paracrine, and autocrine regulators of gonadal function.

### The structure of the FSH receptor and the FSH receptor gene

The FSH receptor belongs to the G-protein coupled receptors, and together with the LH receptor (LHR) and the thyrotrophic hormone receptor (TSHR) it con-

---

*Address for correspondence:* Kristiina Aittomäki MD PhD, Department of Clinical Genetics, Helsinki University Central Hospital, Haartmanink 2B, Helsinki, Finland. *Present address:* The Murdoch Institute, 10th floor Royal Children's Hospital, Flemington Road, Parkville, VIC 3052 Australia. Tel.: +61-3-9345-5045. Fax: +61-3-9345-6962.

762

stitutes the subgroup of glycoprotein hormone receptors. Like the other receptors of this family, it consists of three domains; extracellular, transmembrane and intracellular (Fig. 1). The 7-times plasma membrane piercing α-helices form the transmembrane domain and are typical of all G protein coupled receptors [4,5]. It is also the most conserved domain of the FSHR. The large extracellular domain of the glycoprotein hormone receptors, the site of hormone binding, includes several repeated leucine rich motifs [6], which have also been identified in other proteins participating in protein-protein interactions [7].

The activation of FSHR, upon FSH binding, takes place through conformational changes that allow the binding of the receptor to the stimulatory G protein (G$_s$). This results in stimulation of adenylyl cyclase and production of cAMP [8], the main intracellular secondary messenger of FSH action. Subsequently, protein kinase A (PKA) is activated by the accumulation of cAMP and the function of target proteins, such as enzymes or transcription factors, is then regulated by phosphorylation of serine/threonine residues [9]. FSH also increases the intracel-

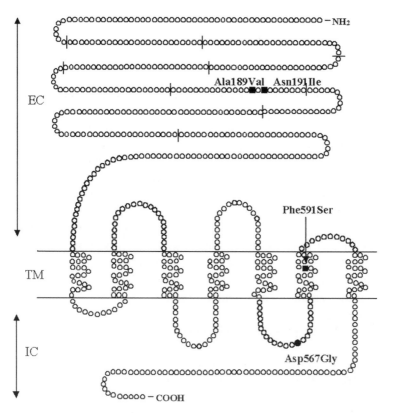

Fig. 1. A schematic presentation of the FSH receptor and gene structure. The locations of the three known inactivating mutations are designated with black squares and the location of the activating mutation is designated with a black circle. The 10 exons are separated with a short line. EC = extracellular domain; TM = transmembrane domain; IC = intracellular domain.

lular free calcium concentrations in granulosa and Sertoli cells [10,11], but the mechanisms, signalling pathways and the significance of the calcium changes as well as the role of the protein kinase C (PKC) signalling pathway [12] remain unclear.

The human FSHR gene is located in chromosome 2p [13,14] and was cloned in the early 1990s [15,16]. The gene that spans some 54 kb of genomic DNA has ten exons and nine introns, as shown in relation to the protein structure in Fig. 1 [17]. The FSHR gene shares a high degree of homology with LHR and the two genes may have arisen by duplication of one ancestral gene during evolution [6]. The length of the first nine exons of FSHR varies between 69 and 251 bp whereas the large terminal exon 10 spans 1,251 bp. The extracellular domain is encoded by exons 1−9 whereas the transmembrane, as well as the intracellular domains, are encoded by the large exon 10. The entire gene encodes 695 amino acids, a signal peptide of 17 amino acids and a protein of 678 amino acids with molecular weight of 75 kDa [17]. The FSHR gene expression is highly tissue-specific, hormone-dependent and confined to granulosa and Sertoli cells.

## FSH receptor mutations

*Inactivating mutations*

To date, only few mutations are known in the FSHR gene. The first one of these was identified as a result of a mapping study to identify the cause of primary ovarian failure and hypergonadotropic hypogonadism in Finland [18,19]. Based on a study of six multiplex families, ovarian failure was mapped to chromosome 2p, to the same chromosomal area in which both FSHR and LHR were known to reside [13,14,20]. Subsequently, these already cloned genes were studied for mutations, and a point mutation (566C→T) in exon seven of FSHR gene was identified [19]. This missense mutation predicts an Ala189Val change in protein structure. The mutation (FSHR$_{Fin}$), shown to segregate in the six families as an autosomal recessive trait, was also functionally studied. As the transfection studies showed both reduced cAMP production upon FSH stimulation and deficient FSH binding, the mutation was concluded to inactivate the function of the mutated receptor protein [19].

The phenotype caused by an inactivating mutation of FSHR has so far only been studied in the Finnish patients [21]. To date, there are 26 females known to be homozygous for FSHR$_{Fin}$, all of which have primary amenorrhea due to hypergonadotropic ovarian failure. In contrast to the patients with ovarian failure due to sex chromosome abnormalities, such as Turner syndrome, they show no other clinical features than those caused by ovarian failure. They usually seek for medical help for primary amenorrhea and not for lack of pubertal development, in which there is some variation. In hormonal studies, there are no known specific features to distinguish these patients from others with primary ovarian failure and normal female sex chromosome constitution. As expected, they have high serum FSH and LH and low estradiol concentrations [21]. However, ovarian biopsies of these patients always show ovarian follicles in contrast to the majority of patients with ovarian failure. Although the infertility of these females could not be treated in the past, the development of ovum donation programs has dramatically changed the possibilities of family planning for these females as well as for other patients with ovarian failure.

As a result of the identification of the $FSHR_{Fin}$ mutation, 25 male relatives of female patients were screened for the presence of the same mutation. Five of these men were shown to be homozygotes and were subsequently studied for a possible phenotype caused by the mutation in males [22]. This was of particular interest, as there is controversy on the role of FSH in spermatogenesis. When clinically studied, all of the males showed normal masculinization and normal serum testosterone concentration, but had relatively small testicular size (4—16 ml) and moderately elevated serum FSH concentrations (13—40 IU/l). The results of the sperm analysis were also variable with three of the five having sperm counts $< 1.0 \ 10^6$/ml and the other two having $5.6 \ 10^6$/ml and $42 \ 10^6$/ml each, thus none of the men had azoospermia. As two of them had both fathered two children as young adults, the mutation did not result in absolute male infertility in the five males, in contrast to females homozygous for the same mutation. These results suggest that FSH is not an absolute requirement for the initiation of spermatogenesis, although it is possible that the findings in the males do not represent a total lack of FSH as $FSHR_{Fin}$ might allow for some residual FSH action. They do imply, however, that very low FSH effect is sufficient for subnormal spermatogenesis with fertility in some patients.

Although relatively common in Finland, the Ala189Val mutation seems to be rare in other populations. Layman et al. studied 35 women with 46,XX ovarian failure in North America and were not able to identify this mutation in any of their patients [23]. Additionally, when four different populations were screened for this mutation, it was only identified in Finns (Jiang, personal communication). In Finland ovarian failure caused by the FSHR mutation is included in the Finnish disease inheritance with some thirty other disorders common in Finland but rare elsewhere [24]. The enrichment of the causative mutations in the Finnish population is due to population bottlenecks and both geographical and cultural isolation.

Interestingly, the second genomic mutation identified in the FSHR gene is located in the near vicinity of the $FSHR_{Fin}$ in the same highly conserved stretch of five amino acids in exon 7 [25]. It is a missense mutation (Asn191Ile) identified in a healthy heterozygous German female. The consequences of the mutation have been functionally studied and are similar to those of the Finnish mutation (Ala189Val). This suggests that the phenotype caused by this mutation in a homozygous female would most likely coincide with the phenotype caused by the $FSHR_{Fin}$.

## Constitutively activating mutations of FSHR

There is but one constitutively activating mutation of the FSHR gene identified by Gromoll et al. [26]. They studied a 28-year-old male who had been hypophysectomized for a pituitary adenoma eight years earlier. This male was able to sustain normal spermatogenesis without substitution for FSH although he had no residual pituitary function. During testosterone treatment only, four pregnancies were induced, and therefore he was hypothesized to have an activating mutation of FSHR. Indeed, a heterozygous point mutation, 1,700 A→G, predicting an Asp567Gly change in the protein, was identified in the third intracellular loop of the transmembrane domain of FSHR in this patient. In transfection studies, this mutation showed $1.5 \times$ higher basal cAMP production when compared to the wild-type FSHR and is therefore constitutively activated. It is not clear, however, whether or not this mutation would cause a phenotype in an otherwise healthy individual. Furthermore, when off the testosterone treatment, the patient showed somewhat higher serum testosterone concentrations than expected and these may have contributed to the findings. Finally, as this patient initially had normal FSH action, it is possible that FSH is needed for the initiation but not for sustaining spermatogenesis.

An inactivating mutation of FSHβ, which determines the specificity of FSH, should theoretically cause FSH deficiency corresponding to the one caused by inactivating mutations of FSHR although without resistance to exogenous FSH. Interestingly, at least four such mutations have so far been identified [27–34]. These are also inherited in the autosomal recessive fashion. The phenotype shown by the female mutation homozygotes or compound heterozygotes includes primary amenorrhea and infertility, which is treatable with exogenous FSH. The two males who were homozygous for an inactivating FSHβ mutation both had azoospermia and therefore the phenotype in these males was different from that caused by the inactivating FSHR$_{Fin.}$ [36,37]. However, the phenotype of the FSHβ knockout mouse, produced by Kumar et al. [38], was similar to the phenotype of the inactivating FSHR mutation in both sexes, that is, the females were infertile with arrested follicular development while the males had reduced testis size and some impairment of spermatogenesis but were fertile.

## FSHR mutations in ovarian tumors

Mutations in G-protein coupled receptors have been shown to occur in various tumors [27] and constitutively activating mutations of TSHR have been identified both in hyperfunctioning thyroid adenomas and thyroid carcinomas [28,29]. As many of the ovarian sex cord tumors are known to express FSHR [30] although their growth seems to be independent of FSH action [31], it has been suggested that constitutively activating mutations of FSHR may play an important role in the development of these tumors. However, the results of studies on FSHR mutations in ovarian tumors are controversial. Kotlar et al. studied 13 ovarian sex cord tumors, three small-cell carcinomas, and 116 control samples for mutations in the transmembrane domain of FSHR. They identified a point mutation (1777T→C) predicting an amino acid change of phenylalanine to serine at codon 591 in the tumor tissue [32]. The mutation was found in nine of 13 (69%) sex cord tumors and two of three ovarian small-cell carcinomas, but it was not present in control specimens. Surprisingly, a recombinant form of the mutated receptor was unable to stimulate cAMP production and therefore this mutation was not activating, as expected, but inactivating. The mutation was identified in the tumor tissue and therefore it is not known whether it was genomic or somatic. When Fuller et al. studied 15 granulosa cell tumors, the most common of ovarian sex cord tumors, for mutations in the transmembrane and intracellular domain of FSHR, they were not able to identify the Phe591Ser or other mutations in any of the tumors [33]. Therefore, as there is no evident explanation for the role of an inactivating mutation of FSHR in ovarian tumors, the significance of these two contradictory findings need to be confirmed by further studies.

**Conclusions**

In contrast to TSH and LH receptors, the mutations of FSHR seem to be rare in most populations. In Finland, however, the identification of a founder mutation has resulted in identification of more than 30 homozygous individuals. Subsequently, the phenotype caused by inactivating mutations of FSHR has been studied. A clear phenotype is caused in females homozygous for an inactivating FSHR mutation. This includes hypergonadotropic primary amenorrhea and infertility with ovaries showing mostly primordial and primary follicles. Such histological findings in an ovarian biopsy therefore suggest FSH resistance is due to an inactivating mutation of FSHR gene. Although it is evident that there are yet new mutations to be identified, they probably will not explain but a fraction of hypergonadotropic ovarian failure. However, it is already evident from the existing data that FSH is absolutely necessary for the normal cyclic ovarian function and female fertility.

As for the males, the role of FSH in spermatogenesis has been uncertain. Based on the findings of males homozygous for inactivating mutations of both FSHR and FSHβ, it does play a role in determination of testis size and both quantitatively and qualitatively contribute to spermatogenesis. At the moment, however, it is not possible to conclude whether FSH is absolutely needed for male fertility or not.

**References**

1. Zirkin BR, Awoniyi C, Griswold M, Russell LD, Sharpe RM. Is FSH required for adult spermatogenesis? J Androl 1994;15:273–276.
2. Richards JS. Hormonal control of gene expression in the ovary. Endocrine Rev 1994;15: 725–751.

3. Kangasniemi M, Kaipia A, Toppari J, Perheentupa A, Huhtaniemi I, Parviainen M. Cellular regulation of follicle-stimulating hormone (FSH) binding in rat seminiferous tubules. J Androl 1990;11:336—343.

4. Baldwin JM. Structure and function of receptors coupled to G proteins. Curr Opin Biol 1994; 6:180—190.

5. Oliveira L, Paiva ACM, Vriend GA. Common motif in G-protein-coupled seven transmembrane helix receptors. J Comput Aided Mol Design 1993;7:649—658.

6. Vassart G, Parmentier M, Libert F, Dumont J. Molecular genetics of the thyrotropin receptor. Trends Endocrinol Metab 1991;2:151—156.

7. Kobe B, Deisenhofer J. Crystal structure of porcine ribonuclease inhibitor, a protein with leucine-rich repeats. Nature 1993;366:751—756.

8. Birnbaumer L. Receptor-to-effector signaling through G proteins: roles for beta gamma dimers as well as alpha subunits. Cell 1992;71:1069—1072.

9. Lalli E, Sassone-Corsi P. Signal transduction and gene regulation: the nuclear response to cAMP. J Biol Chem 1994;269:17359—17362.

10. Flores JA, Vledhuis JD, Leong DA. Follicle-stimulating hormone evokes an increase in intracellular free calcium ion concentrations in single ovarian cells. Endocrinology 1990;127: 3172—3179.

11. Gorczynska E, Handelsman J. The role of calcium in follicle-stimulating hormone signal transduction in Sertoli cells. J Biol Chem 1991;266:23739—23744.

12. Berridge MJ. Inositol trisphosphate and calcium signalling. Nature 1993;361(6410):315—325.

13. Rousseau-Merck MF, Atger M, Loosfelt H, Milgrom E, Berger R. The chromosomal localization of the human follicle-stimulating hormone receptor gene (FSHR) on 2p21—p16 is similar to that of the luteinizing hormone receptor gene. Genomics 1993;115:222—224.

14. Gromoll J, Ried T, Holtgreve-Grez H, Nieschlag E, Gudermann T. Localization of the human FSH receptor to chromosome 2p21 using a genomic probe comprising exon 10. J Molec Endocrinol 1994;12:265—271.

15. Minegishi T, Nakamura K, Takakura Y, Ibuki Y, Igarashi M. Cloning and sequencing of human FSH receptor cDNA. Biochem Biophys Res Commun 1991;175:1125—1130.

16. Kelton CA, Cheng SVY, Nugent NP, Schweickhardt RL, Rosenthal JL, Overton SA, Wand GD, Kuzeja JB, Luchette CA, Chappel SC. The cloning of the human follicle-stimulating hormone receptor and its expression in COS-7, CHO, and Y-1 cells. Molec Cell Endocrinol 1992;89: 141—151.

17. Gromoll J, Pekel E, Nieschlag E. The structure and organization of the human follicle-stimulating hormone receptor (FSHR) gene. Genomics 1996;35:308—311.

18. Aittomäki K. The genetics of XX gonadal dysgenesis. Am J Hum Genet 1994;54:844—851.

19. Aittomäki K, Dieguez Lucena JL, Pakarinen P, Sistonen P, Tapanainen J, Gromoll J, Kaskikari R, Sankila E-M, Lehväslaiho H, Reyes Engel A, Nieschlag E, Huhtaniemi I, de la Chapelle A. Mutation in the follicle-stimulating hormone receptor gene causes hereditary hypergonadotropic ovarian failure. Cell 1995;82:959—968.

20. Rousseau-Merck MF, Mirashi M, Atger M, Loosfelt H, Milgrom E, Berger R. Localization of the human LH (luteinizing hormone) receptor gene to chromosome 2p21. Cytogen Cell Genet 1990;54:77—79.

21. Aittomäki K, Herva R, Stenman U-H, Juntunen K, Ylöstalo P, Hovatta O, de la Chapelle A. Clinical features of ovarian failure caused by a point mutation in the follicle-stimulating hormone receptor gene. J Clin Endocrinol Metab 1996;81:3722—3726.

22. Tapanainen J, Aittomäki, K, Min J, Vaskivuo T, Huhtaniemi I. Men homozygous for an inactivating mutation of the follicle-stimulating hormone receptor gene present variable suppression of spermatogenesis and infertility. Nature Genet 1997;15:205—206.

23. Layman LC, Amde S, Cohen DP, Jin M, Xie J. The Finnish follicle-stimulating hormone receptor gene mutation is rare in North American women with 46,XX ovarian failure. Fertil Steril 1998;69:300—302.

768

24. de la Chapelle A. Disease gene mapping in isolated human populations: the example of Finland. J Med Genet 1993;30:857–865.
25. Gromoll J, Simoni M, Nordhoff V, Behre HM, De Geyter C, Nieschlag E. Functional and clinical consequences of mutations in the FSH receptor. J Clin Endocrinol Metab 1996;125: 177–182.
26. Gromoll J, Simoni M, Nieschlag E. An activating mutation of the follicle-stimulating hormone receptor autonomously sustains spermatogenesis in a hypophysectomized man. J Clin Endocrinol Metab 1996;81:1367–1370.
27. Spegel AM. Genetic bases of endocrine disease: mutations in G proteins and G protein-coupled receptors in endocrine disease. J Clin Endocrinol Metab 1996;81:2434–2442.
28. Parma J, Duprez L, Van Sande J, Cochaux P. Gervy C, Mockel J, Dumont J, Vassart G. Somatic mutations in the thyrotropin receptor gene cause hyperfunctioning thyroid adenomas. Nature 1993;365:649–651.
29. Russo D, Tumino S, Arturi F, Vigneri P, Grasso G, Pontecorvi A, Filetti S, Belfiore A. Detection of an activating mutation of the thyrotropin receptor in a case of an autonomously hyperfunctioning thyroid insular carcinoma. J Clin Endocrinol Metab 1997;82:735–738.
30. Stouffer RL, Gordin MS, Davis JS, Surwit EA. Investigation of binding sites for follicle-stimulating hormone and chorionic gonadotropin in human ovarian cancers. J Clin Endocrinol Metab 1984;59:441–446.
31. Lappohn RE, Burger HG, Bouma J, Bangah M, Krams M, de Brujin HW. Inhibin as a marker for granulosa cell tumors. N Engl J Med 1989;321:790–793.
32. Kotlar TJ, Young R, Albanese C, Crowley WF Jr, Scully RE, Jameson JL. A mutation in the follicle-stimulating hormone receptor occurs frequently in human ovarian sex cord tumors. J Clin Endocrinol Metab 1997;82(4):1020–1026.
33. Fuller PJ, Verity K, Shen Y, Mamers P, Jobling T, Burger H. No evidence of a role for mutations or polymorphisms of the follicle-stimulating hormone receptor in ovarian granulosa cell tumors. J Clin Endocrinol Metab 1998;83:274–279.
34. Matthews CH, Borgato S, Beck-Peccoz P, Adams M, Tone Y, Gambino G, Casagrande S, Tedeschini G, Benedetti A, Chatterjee VKK. Primary amenorrhea and infertility due to a mutation in the beta-subunit of follicle-stimulating hormone. Nature Genet 1993;5:83–86.
35. Layman LC, Lee EJ, Peak DB, Namnoum AB, Vu KV, van Lingen BL, Gray MR, McDonough PG, Reindollar RH, Jameson JL. Delayed puberty and hypogonadism caused by mutations in the follicle-stimulating hormone beta-subunit gene. N Engl J Med 1997;337:607–611.
36. Matthews C, Chatterjee VK. Isolated deficiency of follicle-stimulating hormone re-revisited. N Engl J Med 1997;337:642.
36a. Lindstedt G, Ernest I, Nyström E, Janson PO. Fall av manlig infertilitet. Klin Kemi Nord 1997;3:81–87.
37. Philip M, Arbelle JE, Segev Y, Parvari R. Male hypogonadism due to a mutation in the gene for the β-subunit of follicle-stimulating hormone. N Engl J Med 1998;338:1729–1732.
38. Kumar TR, Wang Y, Lu N, Matzuk MM. Follicle stimulating hormone is required for ovarian follicle maturation but not male fertility. Nature Genet 1997;15(2):201–204.

Fertility and Reproductive Medicine.
R.D. Kempers, J. Cohen, A.F. Haney and J.B. Younger, editors.

# LH receptor defects

Charles Sultan[1,2] and Serge Lumbroso[1]
[1] Unité BEDR, Hôpital Lapeyronie and INSERM U439; and [2] Unité d'Endocrinologie et Gynecologie Pédiatrique, Hôpital A. de Villeneuve, Montpellier, France

**Abstract.** Mutations of the actors of the gonadotrope axis — GnRH receptor, gonadotropin β subunits or gonadotropin receptors — have been associated with several sex differentiation and reproductive diseases. This review will focus on the molecular defects of the LH receptor, which belongs to the large family of G protein-coupled receptors (GPCR). These receptors share a common structure of seven transmembrane α helices connected by three intracellular and three extracellular loops.

Heterozygous activating mutations of LH receptor are responsible for familial male-limited precocious puberty whereas they have no phenotypic consequences in females. Most activating mutations are located in the fifth transmembrane helix and in the third intracellular loop, and they lead to a constitutive production of cyclic AMP in the absence of ligand.

Homozygous or compound heterozygous inactivating mutations of LH receptor have been found in transmembrane as well as in extracellular regions. In XY individuals they cause Leydig cell hypoplasia, resulting in sex reversal or milder forms of undervirilisation. In females, these inactivating mutations lead to amenorrhea but otherwise normal pubertal development.

Identification of these molecular defects of the LH receptor in both males and females, along with knockout experiments and gene overexpression, has further improved our understanding of the contribution of LH and its receptor to male and female reproductive function.

**Keywords:** amenorrhea, male pseudo hermaphroditism, peripheral ferocious puberty, cell-receptor defects, cell-receptor activating mutations.

## Introduction

New tools of molecular biology and gene cloning and sequencing have made it possible to dissect the molecular pathology of the gonadotrope axis. Mutations have been found in the GnRH receptor [1,2], the β subunits of FSH [3,4] and LH [5], and the FSH [6,7] and LH receptors [8,9]. These findings have increased our knowledge of the physiological roles played by the different actors of the axis. In the case of LH receptor, identification of both inactivating and activating mutations in males and in women, along with knockout experiments and gene overexpression, has further improved our understanding of the contribution of LH and its receptor to male and female reproductive function.

The LH receptor (LHR) belongs to the large family of G protein-coupled receptors (GPCR). A number of different stimuli act through interaction with these receptors: photons, hormones, neurotransmitters, proteases, odorants, and

*Address for correspondence:* Prof Charles Sultan, Hospital Lapeyronie, Unite de Biochimie Endocrinienne du Developement et de la Reproduction, 34295 Monpellier Cedex 5, France. Tel.: +33-4-67-33-86-96. Fax: +33-4-67-33-83-27. E-mail: chsultan@u439.montp.inserm.fr

ions. Although there is a very large variety of receptor subtypes, GPCRs share a common structure of seven transmembrane α helices (transmembrane domains, TM1 to TM7) connected by three intracellular (IL1-3) and three extracellular (EL1-3) loops [10] (see Fig. 1). The N-terminal extracellular domain (EC), site of the hormone binding, and the C-terminal intracellular domain (IC) of the receptors are less conserved.

In the GPCR family, LHR belongs to the subfamily of glycoprotein receptors, including LH, hCG, FSH and TSH, which is characterized by a large leucine-rich N-terminal region and a relatively short intracellular portion [11].

In the past few years, mutations of different GPCRs have been identified in human diseases [10]. Interestingly, both inactivating mutations and activating mutations have been described. The inactivating mutations result in a resistance to a hormone, whereas the activating mutations cause a constitutive generation of cellular effectors. This review will focus on the molecular defects of the LH receptor.

## Structure of the LH receptor

The LH receptor gene is located in chromosome 2p21 [12]. The coding region of the gene spans over 60 kb and is composed of 10 introns and 11 exons. Exons 1 to 10 code for the most of the large N-terminal extracellular domain. Exon 11 (more than 1,200 bp) encodes for the last 50 C-terminal residues of the extracellular region, the seven transmembrane helices, the six extra- and intracellular

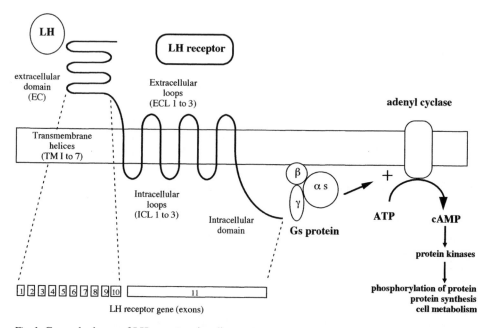

*Fig. 1.* General scheme of LH receptor signaling system.

loops and the intracellular segment (see Fig. 1). The cloning and sequencing of rat [13] and human [14] LH receptor cDNAs have led to the determination of the amino acid sequence of this receptor and the description of the general structural organization of the protein. The human LH receptor is a single polypeptide of 699 amino acids with a predicted molecular mass of 85 kDa. The large hydrophilic N-terminal region represents almost half of the protein (335 residues). It contains six N-linked glycosylation sites and also displays an internal repeat structure characteristic of members of the leucine-rich glycoprotein (LRG) family [13]. This motif is present in two copies per exon in exons 2–8 [15].

The membrane-spanning domain displays sequence homology with all members of the G protein-coupled receptor family. While the human protein is, respectively, 85 and 87% identical overall with the rat and porcine LH/hCG receptors, the most highly conserved regions are the transmembrane segments (91 and 94% similarity).

The short C-terminal domain contains several serine, threonine and tyrosine residues that are potential sites for phosphorylation.

## LH receptor defects

Since 1993, several mutations have been identified in the LHR gene (review in [9,16–18]). These mutations are associated with two disorders of sexual differentiation that have opposite clinical manifestations. Familial male-limited precocious puberty (FMPP or testotoxicosis) is due to an activating mutation of the LHR, leading to a constitutive activation of the LH transduction pathway. Conversely, Leydig cell hypoplasia (LCH) is a rare form of male pseudohermaphroditism (MPH) caused by an inactivating mutation of LHR, which is responsible for the absence or decrease of LH message delivery to target cells.

Beyond the clinical importance of these findings, in vitro experiments performed on these LHR mutants have allowed analysis of the structure-function relationship based on a physiopathological approach.

### Activating mutations of LH receptor

### Activating mutations in males
Familial male precocious puberty is an autosomal dominant disorder characterized by signs of puberty appearing most often before 4 years of age with development of external genitalia and growth acceleration [19–22]. As one form of gonadotropin-independent puberty, FMPP is characterized by adult levels of serum testosterone contrasting with low levels of LH and no response to GnRH stimulation. Testosterone production is not suppressible by GnRH agonist treatment, and it can only be reduced by ketoconazole or spironolactone/testolactone administration [21,23,24]. This situation corresponds to a continuous stimulation of Leydig cells, and it is similar to that observed for both males and females — but more frequently in females — in McCune-Albright syndrome. In this syn-

drome, autonomous gonadal hyperfunction is due to an activating mutation of the Gsa protein, which is responsible for constitutive activation of the adenylyl cyclase/cAMP pathway, and thus to target cell hyperfunction [25,26]. This observation led Kremer et al. [27] to postulate that constitutive activation of the LH receptor could be involved in FMPP. Indeed, this group identified two mutations in LH receptor that cosegregated with testotoxicosis in two families [27]. These mutations (D578G and M571I) are located in the 6th transmembrane domain (TM6) of LH receptor, close to the third intracellular loop (IL3). According to the model of the mechanism of signal transduction by the glycoprotein hormone receptors, these two domains are involved in coupling to the Gs protein that activates adenylyl cyclase [10,14,15]. Moreover, G. Cutler's group identified the same D578G substitution in affected individuals from eight different FMPP families in the USA [28]. They further demonstrated the causative role of this mutation by in vitro experiments showing that COS-7 cells, which expressed the mutant LH receptor, displayed markedly increased cyclic AMP production in the absence of ligand. These findings corroborated the hypothesis of constitutively active LH receptor as a cause of autonomous Leydig cell activity. It is important to note that these mutations are heterozygous, i.e., they concern only one allele. The expression of the wild-type allele does not affect the continuous stimulation of Leydig cells caused by the expression of the mutated allele [16].

Since these initial reports, several activating mutations of LHR have been described in the literature. The most frequent mutation is an Asp to Gly substitution at position 578. Laue et al. [29] found this mutation in 24 out of 28 families with FMPP and different groups have also reported it [30–32]. All the activating mutations of LH receptor reported thus far are listed in Table 1 and their location is shown in Fig. 2. Most of them are located in TM6 and in the C-terminal part of IL3. These mutated receptors appear to have an increased affinity for or delayed dissociation from the α subunit of the Gs protein, thus resulting in con-

*Table 1.* Activating LH receptor mutations.

| Amino acid change | Location | Proven pathogenicity in vitro | References |
|---|---|---|---|
| Ala373Val | TM1 | yes | [37] |
| Met398Thr | TM2 | yes | [34–36] |
| Ile542Leu | TM5 | yes | [29] |
| Asp564Gly | ICL3 | yes | [29] |
| Ala568Val | ICL3 | yes | [56] |
| Met571Ile | TM6 | yes | [27,57] |
| Ala572Val | TM6 | yes | [33] |
| Ile575Leu | TM6 | yes | [16] |
| Thr577Ile | TM6 | yes | [57] |
| Asp578Gly | TM6 | yes | [27–32] |
| Asp578Tyr | TM6 | yes | [29] |
| Cys581Arg | TM6 | yes | [29] |

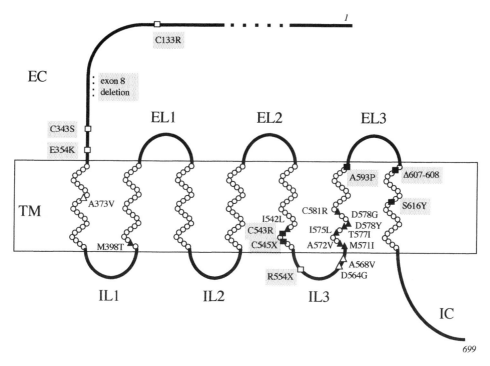

*Fig. 2.* Localization of molecular defects reported in LH receptor (see Tables 1 and 2 for references). EC = extracellular domain. IC = intracellular domain. TM = transmembrane domains (I to VII). EL = extracellular loops (1 to 3). IL = intracellular loops (1 to 3).

Activating mutations are dashed and indicated as triangles. Inactivating mutations are indicated as squares.

stitutive signal transduction cyclic AMP production [17]. Interestingly, a genotype-phenotype relationship has been shown in some cases. Laue et al. [29] reported that the LH receptor with the D578Y mutation induces a higher basal cAMP production than the D578G mutant. This difference correlated with the phenotype, since the boy carrying the D578Y mutation presented very early signs of puberty (before 1 year) [16,29].

Yano et al. [33] identified, in two unrelated Japanese patients with testotoxicosis, a heterozygous C to T transition at nucleotide 1715 leading to a Ala to Val substitution at position 572 in TM6. As the "classical" D578G mutation, the A542V mutant expressed in vitro had a high basal cAMP level, but, unlike D578G, it also modified the inositol phosphate levels, suggesting an effect on Gq protein and phospholipase C activation. In addition, the A542V mutant exhibited a higher affinity for hCG.

Two other reported mutations are located outside the TM6/IL3 segment. Kraaij et al. identified in 1995 [34] a threonine for methionine substitution at position 398 (M398T) in the N-terminal part of the second transmembrane helix (TM2). The same mutation was reported by two other groups [35,36]. M398T mutant exhibited constitutively high basal cAMP levels but maximal hormone-induced cAMP production was low compared to wild-type. As for A542V mutant, M398T modified the Gq coupling and phospholipase-C activation and also displayed a higher apparent affinity for binding hCG, suggesting changes in the conformation of the extracellular domain [35]. Surprisingly, Evans et al. found the same M398T mutation in both affected members of one family and in one unaffected sibling [36].

A mutation lying in the 5th transmembrane domain (TM5), a isoleucine to leucine substitution at position 542 (I542L), was identified in FMPP patients [16,29]. This mutant exhibited increased levels of basal cAMP production in the absence of agonist, but was ligand-unresponsive.

Very recently an activating mutation of the LHR was found in the first transmembrane helix of LH receptor [37] in a patient with testotoxicosis. Onset of puberty was at the age of 5 years. The mutation was an alanine to valine substitution at position 373. This finding suggests the involvement of TM1 in signal transduction [37].

As far as we know, no mutation in the extracellular domain has been described. Such a mutation, however, probably exists since activating mutations have been found in the extracellular domain of the TSH receptor [38,39].

### Activating mutations in females

Interestingly, activating mutations of the LH receptor seem to have no effect in females [17]. Indeed, although the hereditary pattern of these mutations is autosomal dominant, only males present precocious puberty. This insensitivity to constitutive LH receptor is puzzling, especially when comparison is made with the effect of LH overexpression in transgenic mice. These animals exhibit infertility, polycystic ovaries and ovarian tumors [40]. One would thus expect similar clinical presentation in women carrying LHR activating mutation but, to date, no fertility problems have been reported in such individuals. In a clinical study of female carriers of D578G mutation, Rosenthal et al. showed that the response to GnRH stimulation was normal, and they suggested that the negative feedback was still functioning and that the mutation did not activate LH receptor beyond the pubertal level. It is important to note in this matter that, in the majority of described mutants, the addition of hCG increases the already high basal cAMP generation [8].

Since questions about the absence of LH receptor activating mutation in females are still unresolved, the description of ovarian morphology and phenotype in females carrying more potent LH receptor mutants is awaited [17].

### Inactivating mutations of LH receptor

### Inactivating mutations in males

Male sexual differentiation depends on the determination of testis under the influence of SRY (testis determining factor) and on the production of antimüllerian hormone by Sertoli cells and of testosterone by Leydig cells. Testosterone and dihydrotestosterone then act, via the androgen receptor, on the differentiation and development of male internal and external genitalia [41]. Male pseudohermaphroditism (MPH) is defined as a defective virilization in XY individuals. MPH can be due to testis dysgenesis, androgen resistance or a defect in testosterone synthesis. This latter occurrence can be the consequence of an enzymatic defect in the steroidogenic pathway or an anomaly in Leydig cell differentiation, which is referred to as Leydig cell hypoplasia (LCH).

LCH is an uncommon and heterogeneous form of MPH (Table 2). It was initially described in 46,XY females presenting with primary amenorrhea, but a milder phenotype, characterized by undervirilization in phenotypic males, has been described [42–44]. In these patients, Leydig cells are absent, hypoplastic or unresponsive to stimulation with hCG, and analysis of testis biopsy has shown the absence of LH receptors [45]. During the fetal period of male differentiation, Leydig cell differentiation and function are regulated by placental hCG acting on LH receptor expressed in these cells. It was thus postulated early on that LH receptor inactivation (LH resistance) could be the cause of Leydig cell hypoplasia. Another, milder form of LCH has been reported to be characterized by male phenotype with micropenis and normal/low testosterone levels that do not respond normally to the hCG stimulation test. The first form of LCH (female phenotype) can be considered to be a complete resistance to LH, while the second is a partial or incomplete resistance.

*Complete resistance to LH.* The first inactivating mutation was identified by Kremer et al. [46] in two 46,XY sisters with the complete form of LH resistance. They presented with female phenotype, primary amenorrhea and no müllerian

*Table 2.* Inactivating LH receptor mutations.

| Amino acid change | Location | Proven pathogenicity in vitro | Phenotype in XY individuals | References |
|---|---|---|---|---|
| exon 8 deletion[a] | EC | yes | female | [51] |
| Cys133Arg[b] | EC | yes | micropenis | [53] |
| Cys343Ser[c] | EC | no | female | [49] |
| Glu354Lys[a,d] | EC | no | female | [50] |
| Cys543Arg[(2)] | TM5 | no | female | [49] |
| Cys545Stop[a] | TM5 | yes | female | [47] |
| Arg554Stop[a,d] | ICL3 | no | female | [52] |
| Ala593Pro[a] | TM6 | yes | female | [46,54] |
| Δ607-608[a] | TM7 | yes | female | [48] |
| Ser616Tyr[b] | TM7 | yes | female | [51] |
| Ser616Tyr[a,d] | TM7 | yes | micropenis | [52] |

Location of amino acid according to the numbering of [14]. [a]Homozygous mutations; [b] and [c]heterozygous point mutations found in same subject; [d]also identified in XX individuals with primary amenorrhea.

ducts. A homozygous mutation, A593P, was found in the C-terminal part of TM6. Testis histology revealed complete aplasia of Leydig cells. When expressed in vitro, the mutant receptor was still capable of LH binding but was unable to activate adenyl cyclase and cAMP production [46].

A nonsense mutation, Cys545Stop, in TM5 was reported by Laue et al. in two sisters with LCH [47]. This mutation leads to the expression of a truncated receptor missing IL3, TM6 and 7, and the intracellular domain, and thus it is unable to bind the Gs protein. In addition, in vitro experiments revealed that the membrane expression of the mutant was decreased, demonstrating the role played by the deleted segment of the receptor in the cell surface transfer process [47].

Another homozygous stop mutation in the IL3 domain (R554X) was found by Latronico et al. in a complete form. Although not studied in vitro, the lack of major functional domains of the receptor undoubtedly leads to an inactive receptor, as has been demonstrated for Cys545Stop.

Latronico et al. recently reported a new homozygous LHR mutation in a patient from Brazil with the complete form of LCH [48], presenting at 28 years of age as a phenotypic female with primary amenorrhea, normal pubic hair and no breast development. Sequencing revealed a 6 bp deletion responsible for the deletion of residues 608 (leucine) and 609 (valine) in the 7th transmembrane domain. In vitro experiments identified the molecular mechanisms underlying the functional defect of the mutant receptor. The total amount of receptor expressed was low and, furthermore, the receptor was retained in the intracellular compartment, leading to a very weak expression of the mutant receptor at the cell surface [48]. In addition, although binding normally to hCG, the mutant receptor was unable to activate Gsα, in comparison to wild-type with analogous cell surface expression level.

We recently identified two new heterozygous mutations in a patient with the complete form of LCH [49]. One mutation, C543R, was located in the C-terminal part of TM5, while the second substitution, C343S, was in the C-terminal part of the extracellular domain. The probable functional importance of C343 and C543 was assessed by the conservation of these residues in rat LH, human FSH and human TSH receptors (see Table 3). In vitro experiments are underway to confirm the causative role of the mutations in the LCH phenotype.

Another homozygous mutation, Glu354Lys, which lies in the extracellular domain adjacent to the first transmembrane helix, was identified by Stavrou et al. in a complete LCH [50]. This mutation has not yet been investigated in vitro.

A S616Y substitution was found, as a heterozygous defect, in a patient with a mild form of LCH. The other allele carried a deletion of exon 8 [51], which completely abolished LH receptor expression and hCG binding in vitro. In vitro studies showed that the activity of the mutant carrying the exon 8 deletion was totally impaired, whereas the S616Y mutant had a reduced, but not abolished, ligand binding and ligand-induced cAMP accumulation [51].

Table 3.

|  |  |  |  |  |  |  |  | S↑ |  |  |  |  |  |  |  |  |
|---|---|---|---|---|---|---|---|---|---|---|---|---|---|---|---|---|
| rLH-R | C | – | S | P | K | T | L | Q | **C** | **A** | **P** | **E** | **P** | **D** | **A** | **F** | **N** |
| hLH-R (336) | C | – | L | P | K | T | P | R | C | A | P | E | P | D | A | F | N |
| h-FSH-R | C | N | E | V | V | D | V | T | **C** | S | **P** | K | **P** | **D** | **A** | **F** | **N** |
| h-TSH-R | C | G | D | S | E | D | M | V | **C** | T | **P** | K | S | **D** | E | **F** | **N** |

|  |  |  |  |  |  |  |  | R↑ |  |  |  |  |  |  |  |  |
|---|---|---|---|---|---|---|---|---|---|---|---|---|---|---|---|---|
| rLH-R | N | V | V | A | F | V | V | I | C | A | C | Y | I | R | I | Y | F |
| h LH-R (536) | N | V | V | A | F | L | I | I | C | A | C | Y | I | K | I | Y | F |
| h-FSH-R | **N** | **V** | L | **A** | **F** | V | V | **I** | **C** | G | **C** | **Y** | T | H | **I** | **Y** | L |
| h-TSH-R | **N** | I | **V** | **A** | **F** | V | **I** | V | **C** | **C** | **C** | **Y** | V | **K** | **I** | **Y** | I |

Partial amino acid sequence alignment of rat and human LH receptors and human FSH and TSH receptors. Identical amino acids (bold print) are indicated relative to human LH receptor. The arrows indicate the mutated amino acids: Cys 343 to Ser and Cys 543 to Arg. Residues conserved in four family members are dashed.

*Partial resistance to LH.* Latronico et al. described the same S616Y substitution (TM7) as a homozygous mutation. The patient presented with the milder form of LCH characterized by an isolated micropenis, which responded well to testosterone treatment. Testosterone levels in serum were undetectable and did not increase after hCG stimulation. Surprisingly, the S616Y mutant was totally unable to bind to LH or activate cAMP production [52], which did not fit with the mild phenotype of the patient. This is in contrast with the in vitro activity found by Laue et al. for the same mutant [51], and probably can be explained by differences in cell type used by the two groups.

Misrahi et al. reported a homozygous mutation, C133R, located in the extracellular domain of the LH receptor, in a patient with micropenis and hypospadias [53]. Functional in vitro evaluation of the mutant receptor permitted an assessment of the role of the mutation in the inactivation of the receptor: COS-7 cells transfected with the mutant receptor exhibited a marked impairment of hCG binding, whereas some cAMP production could be observed at high hCG concentrations. Careful histological examination of the testis revealed the presence of some Leydig cells, in accordance with the incomplete male pseudohermaphroditism observed in the patient.

### Inactivating mutations in females

Four reports deal with the question of the phenotype of XX females with ovarian LH resistance [48,50,52,54]. Analysis of the LH receptor gene of XX sisters of XY individuals with LCH identified female patients with homozygous mutations. The patient reported by Latronico et al. in 1996 [52] carried the C554X mutation on both alleles. She presented at 22 years of age with normal pubertal development and female phenotype, and complete amenorrhea following one single menstrual bleeding at the age of 13. Serum LH concentration was 5 times greater than normal, but FSH and estradiol serum levels were normal. Ultrasonography revealed a small uterus and cystic ovaries of unequal size. The case reported by Toledo et al. [54] is the sister of the LCH patients reported earlier by Kremer et al., who carries a A593P mutation. She presented with similar phenotype (primary amenorrhea with normal primary and secondary sex characteristics). The hypogonadism seemed to be more pronounced than in the case described by Latronico, since the serum estradiol concentration was in the low-normal range for the follicular part of the menstrual cycle. Ovarian biopsy revealed the absence of corpora lutea and preovulatory follicles, while some collapsed antral follicles and clusters of primordial follicles were observed [16].

In her recent paper [48], Latronico reported the examination of the sister of an LCH patient with the D608-609 mutation. This XX female was evaluated at 40 years of age and presented with apparently milder phenotype than the females of the two previous reports. Pubic and breast development occurred at 13 years, followed by menarche at 15. Thereafter, menses occurred irregularly, usually every 2 months with variable periods of amenorrhea. Uterus size was normal and one ovary was enlarged and cystic. Biological data showed high levels of FSH and LH (with high LH to FSH ratio) and low-normal estradiol concentration in serum, whereas progesterone was very low.

These observations corroborate the existence of inherited LH resistance as a cause of primary amenorrhea in women. Both clinical and molecular observations are consistent with previous experimental data suggesting that, in humans, LH is necessary for ovulation but follicular maturation can occur in the presence of FSH alone. Conversely, LH does not seem to be essential for female pubertal development [52].

## Conclusion

The spectrum of molecular pathologies of sexual differentiation has been enlarged with the discovery of LH receptor mutations in Leydig cell hypoplasia. In addition to the two forms of pathology already described (complete resistance to LH/female phenotype and partial resistance to LH/male phenotype with micropenis), one can postulate the existence of other forms associated with different mutations: infertile male without genital ambiguity or female with minor degree of virilization. Indeed, this has been found to be the case in other hormone resistance syndromes such as androgen insensitivity [55].

In contrast to those mutations causing resistance to hormone, the finding of activating mutations of LH receptor has reinforced the concept of a hyperactive receptor and constitutive signal in absence of ligand. The different expressions of these activating mutations in males and females remains puzzling and requires further experiments and clinical research studies. LH receptor mutations constitute, however, a privileged model for studying the contribution of LH to pubertal development, follicular maturation and ovulation induction.

# References

1. De Roux N, Young J, Misrahi M, Genet R, Chanson P, Schaison G, Milgrom E. A family with hypogonadotropic hypogonadism and mutations in the gonadotropin-releasing hormone receptor. N Engl J Med 1997;337:1597—1602.

2. Layman LC, Cohen DP, Jin M, Xie J, Li Z, Reindollar RH, Bolbolan S, Bick DP, Sherins RR, Duck LW, Musgrove LC, Sellers JC, Neill JD. Mutations in gonadotropin-releasing hormone receptor gene cause hypogonadotropic hypogonadism (letter). Nat Genet 1998;18:14—15.

3. Layman LC, Eun-Jig L, Peak DB, Namnoun AB, Vu KV, van Lingen BL, Gray MR, McDonough PG, Reindollar RH, Jameson JL. Delayed puberty and hypogonadism caused by mutations in the follicle-stimulating hormone b-subunit gene. N Engl J Med 1997;337:607—611.

4. Phillip M, Arbelle JE, Segev Y, Parvari R. Male hypogonadism due to a mutation in the gene for the beta-subunit of follicle-stimulating hormone. N Engl J Med 1998;338:1729—1732.

5. Weiss J, Axelrod L, Whitcomb RW, Harris PE, Crowley WF, Jameson JL. Hypogonadism caused by a single amino acid substitution in the beta subunit of luteinizing hormone (see comments). N Engl J Med 1992;326:179—183.

6. Aittomaki K, Lucena JL, Pakarinen P, Sistonen P, Tapanainen J, Gromoll J, Kaskikari R, Sankila EM, Lehvaslaiho H, Engel AR, Nieschlag E, Huhtaniemi I, de la Chapelle A. Mutation in the follicle-stimulating hormone receptor gene causes hereditary hypergonadotropic ovarian failure. Cell 1995;82:959—968.

7. Gromoll J, Simoni M, Nieschlag E. An activating mutation of the follicle-stimulating hormone receptor autonomously sustains spermatogenesis in a hypophysectomized man. J Clin Endocrinol Metab 1996;81:1367—1370.

8. Themmen AP, Brunner HG. Luteinizing hormone receptor mutations and sex differentiation. Eur J Endocrinol 1996;134:533—540.

9. Simoni M, Gromoll J, Nieschlag E. Molecular pathophysiology and clinical manifestations of gonadotropin receptor defects (In Process Citation). Steroids 1998;63:288—293.

10. Shenker A. G protein-coupled receptor structure and function: the impact of disease-causing mutations. Baillieres Clin Endocrinol Metab 1995;9:427—451.

11. Milgrom E, de Roux N, Ghinea N, Beau I, Loosfelt H, Vannier B, Savouret JF, Misrahi M. Gonadotrophin and thyrotrophin receptors. Horm Res 1997;48(Suppl 4):33—37.

12. Rousseau-Merck MF, Misrahi M, Atger M, Loosfelt H, Milgrom E, Berger R. Localization of the human luteinizing hormone/choriogonadotropin receptor gene (LHCGR) to chromosome 2p21. Cytogenet Cell Genet 1990;54:77—79.

13. McFarland KC, Sprengel R, Phillips HS, Kohler M, Rosemblit N, Nikolics K, Segaloff DL, Seeburg PH. Lutropin-choriogonadotropin receptor: an unusual member of the G protein-coupled receptor family. Science 1989;245:494—499.

14. Minegishi T, Nakamura K, Takakura Y, Miyamoto K, Hasegawa Y, Ibuki Y, Igarashi M, Minegish T. Cloning and sequencing of human LH/hCG receptor cDNA (published erratum appears in Biochem Biophys Res Commun 1994 Jun 15;201(2):1057). Biochem Biophys Res Commun 1990;172:1049—1054.

15. Segaloff DL, Ascoli M. The lutropin/choriogonadotropin receptor4 years later. Endocrinol Rev 1993;14:324—347.

16. Themmen AP, Martens JW, Brunner HG. Gonadotropin receptor mutations. J Endocrinol 1997;153:179—183.

17. Conway GS. Clinical manifestations of genetic defects affecting gonadotrophins and their receptors. Clin Endocrinol Oxf 1996;45:657—663.

18. Chan WY. Molecular genetic, biochemical, and clinical implications of gonadotropin receptor mutations. Molec Genet Metab 1998;63:75—84.

19. Egli CA, Rosenthal SM, Grumbach MM, Montalvo JM, Gondos B. Pituitary gonadotropin-independent male-limited autosomal dominant sexual precocity in nine generations: familial testotoxicosis. J Pediatr 1985;106:33—40.

20. Gondos B, Egli CA, Rosenthal SM, Grumbach MM. Testicular changes in gonadotropin-independent familial male sexual precocity. Familial testotoxicosis. Arch Pathol Lab Med 1985;109:990–995.

21. Holland FJ. Gonadotropin-independent precocious puberty. Endocrinol Metab Clin North Am 1991;20:191–210.

22. Schedewie HK, Reiter EO, Beitins IZ, Seyed S, Wooten VD, Jimenez JF, Aiman EJ, DeVane GW, Redman JF, Elders MJ. Testicular Leydig cell hyperplasia as a cause of familial sexual precocity. J Clin Endocrinol Metab 1981;52:271–278.

23. Holland FJ, Fishman L, Bailey JD, Fazekas AT. Ketoconazole in the management of precocious puberty not responsive to LHRH-analogue therapy. N Engl J Med 1985;312:1023–1028.

24. Laue L, Kenigsberg D, Pescovitz OH, Hench KD, Barnes KM, Loriaux DL, Cutler GB Jr. Treatment of familial male precocious puberty with spironolactone and testolactone. N Engl J Med 1989;320:496–502.

25. Schwindinger WF, Levine MA. McCune-Albright syndrome. Trends Endocrinol Metab 1993;7:238–242.

26. Weinstein LS, Shenker A, Gejman PV, Marino MJ, Friedman E, Spiegel AM. Activating mutations of the stimulatory G protein in the McCune-Albright syndrome. N Engl J Med 1991; 325:1688–1695.

27. Kremer H, Mariman E, Otten BJ, Moll GW Jr, Stoelinga GB, Wit JM, Jansen M, Drop SL, Faas B, Ropers HH, Brunner HG. Cosegregation of missense mutations of the luteinizing hormone receptor gene with familial male-limited precocious puberty. Hum Mol Genet 1993;2: 1779–1783.

28. Shenker A, Laue L, Kosugi S, Merendino JJ Jr, Minegishi T, Cutler GB Jr. A constitutively activating mutation of the luteinizing hormone receptor in familial male precocious puberty (see comments). Nature 1993;365:652–654.

29. Laue L, Chan WY, Hsueh AJ, Kudo M, Hsu SY, Wu SM, Blomberg L, Cutler GB Jr. Genetic heterogeneity of constitutively activating mutations of the human luteinizing hormone receptor in familial male-limited precocious puberty. Proc Natl Acad Sci USA 1995;92:1906–1910.

30. Kawate N, Kletter GB, Wilson BE, Netzloff ML, Menon KM, Identification of constitutively activating mutation of the luteinising hormone receptor in a family with male limited gonadotrophin independent precocious puberty (testotoxicosis). J Med Genet 1995;32:553–554.

31. Rosenthal IM, Refetoff S, Rich B, Barnes RB, Sunthornthepvarakul T, Parma J, Rosenfield RL. Response to challenge with gonadotropin-releasing hormone agonist in a mother and her two sons with a constitutively activating mutation of the luteinizing hormone receptor — a clinical research center study. J Clin Endocrinol Metab 1996;81:3802–3806.

32. Yano K, Hidaka A, Saji M, Polymeropoulos MH, Okuno A, Kohn LD, Cutler GB Jr. A sporadic case of male-limited precocious puberty has the same constitutively activating point mutation in luteinizing hormone/choriogonadotropin receptor gene as familial cases. J Clin Endocrinol Metab 1994;79:1818–1823.

33. Yano K, Saji M, Hidaka A, Moriya N, Okuno A, Kohn LD, Cutler GB Jr. A new constitutively activating point mutation in the luteinizing hormone/choriogonadotropin receptor gene in cases of male-limited precocious puberty. J Clin Endocrinol Metab 1995;80:1162–1168.

34. Kraaij R, Post M, Kremer H, Milgrom E, Epping W, Brunner HG, Grootegoed JA, Themmen AP. A missense mutation in the second transmembrane segment of the luteinizing hormone receptor causes familial male-limited precocious puberty. J Clin Endocrinol Metab 1995; 80:3168–3172.

35. Yano K, Kohn LD, Saji M, Kataoka N, Okuno A, Cutler GB Jr. A case of male-limited precocious puberty caused by a point mutation in the second transmembrane domain of the luteinizing hormone choriogonadotropin receptor gene. Biochem Biophys Res Commun 1996;220: 1036–1042.

36. Evans BA, Bowen DJ, Smith PJ, Clayton PE, Gregory JW. A new point mutation in the luteinising hormone receptor gene in familial and sporadic male-limited precocious puberty: genotype

does not always correlate with phenotype. J Med Genet 1996;33:143−147.

37. Gromoll J, Partsch CJ, Simoni M, Nordhoff V, Sippell WG, Nieschlag E, Saxena BB. A mutation in the first transmembrane domain of the lutropin receptor causes male precocious puberty. J Clin Endocrinol Metab 1998;83:476−480.

38. Kopp P, Muirhead S, Jourdain N, Gu WX, Jameson JL, Rodd C. Congenital hyperthyroidism caused by a solitary toxic adenoma harboring a novel somatic mutation (serine281→isoleucine) in the extracellular domain of the thyrotropin receptor. J Clin Invest 1997;100:1634−1639.

39. Duprez L, Parma J, Costagliola S, Hermans J, Van Sande J, Dumont JE, Vassart G. Constitutive activation of the TSH receptor by spontaneous mutations affecting the N-terminal extracellular domain. FEBS Lett 1997;409:469−474.

40. Risma KA, Clay CM, Nett TM, Wagner T, Yun J, Nilson JH. Targeted overexpression of luteinizing hormone in transgenic mice leads to infertility, polycystic ovaries and ovarian tumors. Proc Natl Acad Sci USA 1995;92:1322−1326.

41. Sultan C, Lobaccaro JM, Lumbroso S, Poujol N. Disorders of sexual differentiation: recent molecular and clinical advances. In: Kelnar CJH (ed) Baillere's Clinical Paediatrics 4. London, 1996;221−243.

42. Berthezene F, Forest MG, Grimaud JA, Claustrat B, Mornex R. Leydig cell agenesis. A cause of male pseudohermaphroditism. N Engl J Med 1976;295:969−972.

43. Brown DM, Markland C, Dehner LP. Leydig cell hypoplasia: a cause of male pseudohermaphroditism. J Clin Endocrinol Metab 1978;46:1−7.

44. Schwartz M, Imperato-McGinley J, Peterson RE, Cooper G, Morris PL, MacGillivray M, Hensle B. Male pseudohermaphroditism secondary to an abnormality in Leydig cell differentiation. J Clin Endocrinol Metab 1981;53:123−127.

45. David R, Yoon DJ, Landin L, Lew L, Sklar C, Schinella R, Golimbu M. A syndrome of gonadotropin resistance possibly due to a luteinizing hormone receptor defect. J Clin Endocrinol Metab 1984;59:156−160.

46. Kremer H, Kraaij R, Toledo SP, Post M, Fridman JB, Hayashida CY, van Reen M, Milgrom E, Ropers HH, Mariman E et al. Male pseudohermaphroditism due to a homozygous missense mutation of the luteinizing hormone receptor gene. Nat Genet 1995;9:160−164.

47. Laue L, Wu SM, Kudo M, Hsueh AJ, Cutler GB Jr, Griffin JE, Wilson JD, Brain C, Berry AC, Grant DB et al. A nonsense mutation of the human luteinizing hormone receptor gene in Leydig cell hypoplasia. Hum Mol Genet 1995;4:1429−1433.

48. Latronico AC, Chai Y, Arnhold IJ, Liu X, Mendonca BB, Segaloff DL. A homozygous microdeletion in helix 7 of the luteinizing hormone receptor associated with familial testicular and ovarian resistance is due to both decreased cell surface expression and impaired effector activation by the cell surface receptor. Molec Endocrinol 1998;12:442−450.

49. Lumbroso S, Szarras-Czapnik M, Caubel C, Ringeard I, Romer TE, Sultan C. Novel compound heterozygous mutations of luteinizing hormone receptor gene in a patient with male pseudohermaphroditism due to Leydig cell hypoplasia. The 80th Annual Meeting of The Endocrine Society, New Orleans, 23−27 June 1998 Abstract P2-142.

50. Stavrou SS, Zhu Y-S, Cai L-Q, Katz MD, Ling Q, Herrera C, DeFillo-Ricart M, Imperato-McGinley J. A novel mutation of LH receptor presents as primary amenorrhea in (XX and XY) sisters. 1997 Proceedings of the 79th Annual Meeting of the Endocrine Society, Minneapolis, MN (Abstract OR 38-1).

51. Laue LL, Wu SM, Kudo M, Bourdony CJ, Cutler GB Jr, Hsueh AJ, Chan WY. Compound heterozygous mutations of the luteinizing hormone receptor gene in Leydig cell hypoplasia. Molec Endocrinol 1996;10:987−997.

52. Latronico AC, Anasti J, Arnhold IJ, Rapaport R, Mendonca BB, Bloise W, Castro M, Tsigos C, Chrousos GP. Brief report: testicular and ovarian resistance to luteinizing hormone caused by inactivating mutations of the luteinizing hormone-receptor gene. N Engl J Med 1996;334:507−512.

53. Misrahi M, Meduri G, Pissard S, Bouvattier C, Beau I, Loosfelt H, Jolivet A, Rappaport R, Mil-

grom E, Bougneres P. Comparison of immunocytochemical and molecular features with the phenotype in a case of incomplete male pseudohermaphroditism associated with a mutation of the luteinizing hormone receptor. J Clin Endocrinol Metab 1997;82:2159–2165.

54. Toledo SP, Brunner HG, Kraaij R, Post M, Dahia PL, Hayashida CY, Kremer H, Themmen AP. An inactivating mutation of the luteinizing hormone receptor causes amenorrhea in a 46,XX female. J Clin Endocrinol Metab 1996;81:3850–3854.

55. Sultan C, Lobaccaro JM, Lumbroso S, Poujol N. Disorders of sexual differentiation: recent molecular and clinical advances. In: Kelnar CJH (ed) Baillere's Clinical Pædiatrics 4. London, 1996;221–243.

56. Latronico AC, Anasti J, Arnhold IJ, Mendonca BB, Domenice S, Albano MC, Zachman K, Wajchenberg BL, Tsigos C. A novel mutation of the luteinizing hormone receptor gene causing male gonadotropin-independent precocious puberty. J Clin Endocrinol Metab 1995; 80:2490–2494.

57. Kosugi S, Van Dop C, Geffner ME, Rabl W, Carel JC, Chaussain JL, Mori T, Merendino JJ Jr, Shenker A. Characterization of heterogeneous mutations causing constitutive activation of the luteinizing hormone receptor in familial male precocious puberty. Hum Mol Genet 1995;4:183–188.

# Androgen receptor mutations and reproduction

L. Pinsky[1-4], L.K. Beitel[1], B. Gottlieb[1], E.L. Yong[5] and M.A. Trifiro[1,2]

[1]Lady Davis Institute for Medical Research, Departments of [2]Medicine, [3]Human Genetics and [4]Pediatrics, McGill University, Montreal, Quebec; and [5]Department of Obstetrics and Gynecology, National University Hospital, Republic of Singapore

**Abstract.** The androgen receptor (AR) protein regulates transcription of certain genes. Usually this depends upon the binding of A-AR complexes to regulatory DNA sequences near or in a target gene. The AR also has a C-terminal androgen-binding domain (ABD), and a N-terminal modulatory domain. These domains interact among themselves, and with nonreceptor proteins, to determine vectorial control over a gene's transcription rate. The precise roles of these proteins are active research areas.

Severe X-linked AR (gene) mutations cause complete androgen insensitivity (CAI); mild ones impair virilization with or without infertility (MAI); moderate ones yield a wide phenotypic spectrum, sometimes among sibs. Different expressivity may reflect variability of AR-interactive proteins. The family history must seek infertile XY maternal aunts or uncles, and heterozygous XX aunts with sparse, delayed or asymmetric pubic/axillary hair, or delayed menarche.

Mutation type and density vary along the length of the AR. N-terminal polyglutamine expansion reduces AR transactivation, causing MAI. Analysis of ABD mutations that do not impair androgen binding, or do so selectively, will illuminate its intradomain properties.

For partial AI and MAI, pharmacotherapy with certain androgens, or other steroids, may overcome some dysfunction of certain mutant ARs. Experience with this approach is limited; outcomes have been generally disappointing.

Keywords: genital ambiguity, infertility, insensitivity.

## Introduction

The androgen receptor (AR) is essential for androgen action, whether of testosterone (T) or of its 5α-reduced derivative, 5α-dihydrotestosterone (DHT). Hence, the AR is essential for normal primary male sexual development before birth (masculinization), and for normal secondary male sexual development around puberty (virilization). Androgens also participate in female sexual development around puberty, and in adult female sexual function. Therefore, androgens are involved in male and female reproduction, and AR mutations may interfere with reproduction in either sex, albeit much more subtly in females.

*Address for correspondence:* L. Pinsky, Sir Mortimer B. Davis Jewish General Hospital, Lady Davis Institute for Medical Research, Department of Medicine, McGill University, 3755 Cote Sainte-Catherine Road, Montreal, Quebec H3T 1E2, Canada. Tel.: +1-514-340-8260. Fax: +1-514-340-7502.

## The androgen receptor gene and protein

The AR is an intracellular protein encoded by a gene (AR) on the long arm of the X chromosome near the centromere (Xq11-12). Once transformed by binding an androgen molecule, the AR acquires the ability to regulate the rate of transcription of genes whose expression is subject to androgenic control (Fig. 1). To exert such regulation, a complex of an androgen and an androgen receptor (an

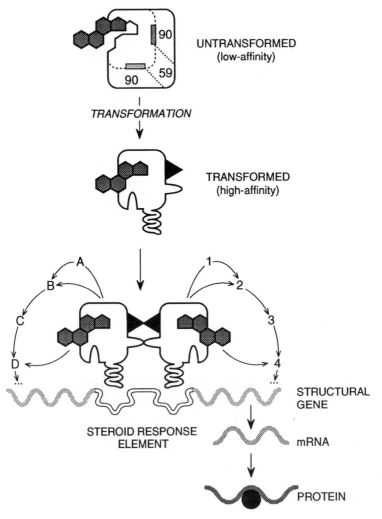

*Fig. 1.* A schematic view of androgen receptor (AR) structure and function. In its untransformed state, the AR is kept in an androgen-binding conformation by a set of chaperone proteins, the most notable of which are two molecules of heat shock protein-90. Once transformed by bound androgen, the AR acquires the ability to dimerize and to bind to a steroid response element. Some of these elements have high specificity for A-R complexes, partly by virtue of collaborative "upstream" (A—D) and/or "downstream" [1—4] coregulatory proteins; some of the latter are also DNA-binding.

A-R) must do three things: 1) dimerize; 2) bind to a sequence of regulatory nucleotides (a bipartite "androgen-response element"); and 3) interact with upstream and downstream coregulatory proteins (some also DNA-binding). These interactions, and those with basal transcription factors and core promoter elements, determine the vectorial control over the transcriptional expression of a given androgen target gene. Some of the coregulatory proteins that are able to interact with certain portions of the AR, under certain conditions, are shown in Fig. 2 with their code names.

The AR gene is about 90,000 nucleotides (nt) long (90 kb) but only $\sim 2,750$ of them, divided into eight exons, code for amino acids (aa). The variable length of the AR reflects the fact that its amino terminal transregulation modulatory portion ($\sim 537$ amino acids) contains two homopolymeric amino acid "repeats" that are polymorphic in size (Fig. 3): one is polyglutamine and its repeat size varies from n = 9 to 36 [1]; the other, polyglycine, varies from n = 10 to 31 [2]. Expansion of the polyglutamine tract beyond n = 38 is the cause of Kennedy syndrome [3], a motor neuronopathy associated with mild androgen insensitivity (MAI) that is discussed below.

There are three additional primary structure-function domains of the AR. Centrally, there is a DNA-binding domain (DBD), $\sim 557-616$ aa, encoded by exons 2 and 3. Adjacent to the DBD, C-terminally, there is a bipartite nuclear localization signal (NLS; 617–636 aa) encoded by exons 3 and 4. Finally, there is a C-terminal, $\sim 250$-aa androgen-binding domain (ABD) encoded by exons 4–8. In addition to their principal functions, the ABD, DBD and N-terminal domains embody subsidiary functions that affect dimerization, nuclear localization and transcriptional regulation (Fig. 3). Thus, the trimodular (domain) concept of AR function is a simplification; instead, domain interaction, and interac-

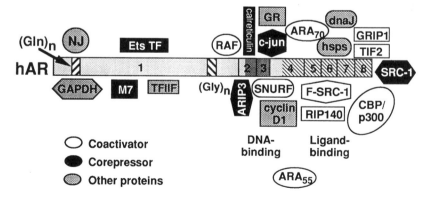

Fig. 2. A depiction of some coregulatory proteins that interact with different portions of the AR positively (coactivators), negatively (corepressors), or in an uncertain way (other proteins). The coursely hatched rectangles in the left half of the AR represent the polyglutamine and polyglycine tracts in its N-terminal transactivation domain. The portion of the AR devoted to DNA binding is darkly stippled; that devoted to ligand binding is finely hatched. (A list of references for these coregulatory proteins is available from the authors by e-mail: mc33@musica.mcgill.ca)

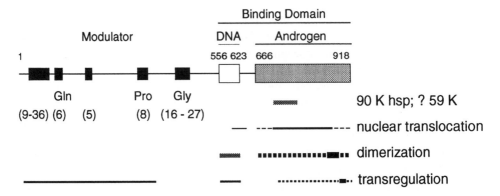

*Fig. 3.* A linear rendition of the major structure-function domains and putative subdomains of the AR. The solid portions of the interrupted lines below the androgen binding domain indicate the most likely location of a given functional subdomain. There is recent evidence [43] that a portion of the N-terminal transcriptional modulatory domain (not shown here) also serves as a dimerization interface.

tion with coregulatory proteins, hold the secrets to a full understanding of an AR's structure-function properties.

## Phenotypic aspects of AR mutations and reproduction

AR mutations that severely impair the amount, structure or function of the AR cause the phenotype of complete androgen insensitivity (CAI). Subjects are born looking unambiguously female because DHT-dependent masculinization of the external genital primordia is absent. Also, if their testes are not inguinal, they are not suspected of being abnormal until the onset of puberty, when breast development is normal, but pubic and axillary hair are not. Menarche, initially considered "late", never occurs. Müllerian duct regression, being androgen-independent, is normal. Hence, these patients usually lack a uterus, oviducts, and the cervix. In theory, they should also lack the upper, Müllerian duct-derived portion of the vagina; however, many patients with CAI have satisfactory coitus without dyspareunia. Since Wolffian duct differentiation is T-dependent, these subjects should lack vasa deferentia, epididymes, seminal vesicles, and ejaculatory ducts. Occasionally, however, rudimentary segments of the Müllerian duct or the Wolffian duct, or both, are found by ultrasonography or laparotomy.

Because all XY subjects with CAI are sterile (genetic lethals), one-third of their mutant alleles should represent new mutations. In other words, two-thirds of mothers of CAI subjects are heterozygous carriers of the mutant allele. Furthermore, because of random X-chromosome inactivation, such carriers may express their heterozygosity clinically by delayed, reduced or asymmetrical pubic and/or axillary hair, and by delayed menarche [4]. The reason for delayed menarche is not entirely clear, but females homozygous for 5α-reductase type 2 deficiency have recently been recognized to have delayed menarche also [5]. Since 5α-reductase type 2 is responsible for an important fraction of T→DHT conversion in some parts of the body, it follows that DHT deficiency or T excess, or both, contribute to the delayed menarche. However, the effect of DHT deficiency can be mimicked by DHT resistance. Furthermore, by aromatization, T excess can generate estrogen excess. The latter mimics an androgen-resistant state. Thus, pubertal resetting of the gonadostat in heterozygous females may be delayed, directly, by DHT-resistance, or indirectly, by an increased ratio of estrogen:androgen action.

Figure 4A,B are pedigrees of two families with CAI. In Fig. 4A the mutation is Arg774Cys, and heterozygosity is expressed in the mother by bilaterally reduced axillary hair, while the sister had menarche at 18 years of age. Interestingly, the diagnosis of CAI in the XY sister was delayed to 23 years of age, in the false hope that delayed menarche was a benign familial trait. In Fig. 4B, the mutation is Arg831Leu, and the mother did not have delayed menarche, but a maternal aunt did. This illustrates, dramatically, that a sophisticated family history for possible X-linked disease must include information about all maternal relatives, in pursuit of affected XY hemizygotes and XX heterozygotes. Furthermore, because of random X-chromosome inactivation, pubic and/or axillary hair in heterozygotes may be delayed or sparse, asymmetrically.

The family history becomes even more crucial when one is concerned with various degrees of partial androgen insensitivity (PAI). At one extreme ("incom-

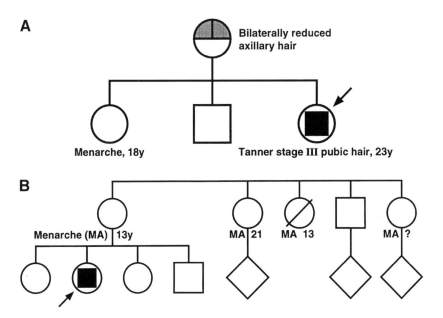

*Fig. 4.* **A:** The 46,XY proposita (arrow) has CAI due tArg774Cys in the androgen-binding domain. Her mother and sister are heterozygous. One has reduced axillary hair; the other had delayed menarche. **B:** The 46,XY proposita (arrow) has CAI due to Arg831Leu. Because of random X-chromosome inactivation, her heterozygous maternal aunt had delayed menarche; for the same reason, in the opposite direction, her heterozygous mother did not have delayed menarche.

plete"), the external genitalia are nearly normal female, except for clitoromegaly and/or posterior labial fusion; at the other extreme, MAI, the genitalia may be morphologically normal male but small, or there may be simple coronal hypo- spadias or a prominent midline raphe of the scrotum. In between these extremes are all grades of frank external genital ambiguity that require delicate decision- making in order to choose a sex-of-rearing that is compatible with surgical-ana- tomical constraints and with some predictive information concerning the prob- able balance between virilization and feminization at puberty.

MAI takes two phenotypic forms at puberty: in one, spermatogenesis and fer- tility are impaired [6,7]; in the other, spermatogenesis is normal, or sufficient, to preserve fertility [8−10]. In both, gynecomastia, high-pitched voice, sparse sex hair, and impotence may be noted. AR mutations have been described in both types, as discussed below, and in each case where the mutation has occurred in the ABD, it has impaired androgen-binding either relatively mildly or not at all. In the form where fertility is preserved, one presumes that the dysfunction of the mutant AR is sufficiently mild so that it can be overcome by collaboration with the set of coregulatory proteins that is active in Sertoli cells. Such collaboration would permit the target genes necessary for spermatogenesis to be regulated properly. In the form where fertility is not preserved, one must conclude that the mutant AR is competent to masculinize or virilize most targets of androgen action, and that its incompetence in regard to spermatogenesis cannot be recti- fied by collaboration with those coregulatory proteins that compose the tran- scriptional regulatory environment of Sertoli cells.

The great majority of families with CAI breed true; in other words affected individuals depart little from the textbook phenotype of complete testicular fem- inization (as it used to be known).

In families with PAI, on the other hand, it is not uncommon for affected indi- viduals to have frankly ambiguous external genitalia that are, nonetheless, pre- dominantly masculine, or predominantly feminine. Expectedly, this may lead to opposite sexes-of-rearing [11]. Indeed, for some mutations in the ABD, such as Met780Ile, this may be the rule, not the exception [12]. Furthermore, in rare families with PAI, the expressivity may vary markedly, from near-normal male to near-normal female.

Although experience with MAI families is limited, they appear to harbor rela- tively little phenotypic disparity. Nonetheless, between or among families, the same mutation may be responsible for MAI or PAI. One mutation that produces this situation is discussed below.

These considerations of variable expressivity within or among families have great import for taking a sophisticated family history. For instance, in the early differential diagnosis of androgen resistance as a cause of apparently isolated hypospadias or azoospermia, it would be very helpful to know if any maternally related females had delayed menarche, primary amenorrhea, delayed, and reduced or absent sex hair (symmetrically or asymmetrically), or even clitoro- megaly with or without posterior labial fusion. Of course, the reciprocal would be true in the early differential diagnosis of phenotypic females with any of the immediately preceding presenting signs.

**Phenotype-genotype correlation of AR mutation**

Figure 5 depicts all AR point mutations and small deletions or insertions that have been reported to cause CAI, PAI or MAI [13], and demonstrates an unequal distribution of these mutations along the length of the AR. It is also apparent that the types of mutations differ along the length of the AR. In particular, nearly all mutations in exon 1 (Fig. 5) cause CAI, and nearly all are of the premature translation termination variety, whether by direct mutation to a stop codon, or indirectly, by frame-shifting after small deletions or insertions.

Some mutations in the DBD cause CAI. Interestingly, however, at least as many cause PAI, but none cause MAI (Fig. 5).

In the ABD there is a striking preponderance of missense mutations, and an equally striking concentration of them in and around those exons that putatively contribute to the androgen-binding pocket of the ABD (Fig. 5).

Of greatest pertinence to the subject of this manuscript are six missense mutations in the ABD that have been proven to cause MAI. They are shown in outlined letters and numbers in Fig. 5. The Asn727Lys mutation is particularly interesting because the man bearing it did not have gynecomastia, and his oligospermia responded to two separate cycles of treatment with mesterolone (1α-methylandrostan-17β-ol-2-one) that culminated in the birth of two children [14].

In one family with Ser814Asn (numbered S813N in [15]), five maternal first cousins (including two pairs of siblings) all had a normal scrotum, a normally formed but small penis, gynecomastia and severe oligospermia or azoospermia [16]. However, a sporadic subject with the same mutation in another family had ambiguous external genitalia [17]. This is a dramatic illustration of variable expressivity of the same mutation between different families. Importantly, the genital skin fibroblasts (GSF) of subjects from both families had the same androgen-selective form of affinity defect, despite their disparate degrees of clinical severity.

The traditional explanation for such variable expressivity of an AR mutation is that the level or competence of coregulatory proteins act as genetic "background" factors in determining the overall clinical outcome.

Recently, however, it has been appreciated that somatic mosaicism (more-or-less covert), may account for some variable expressivity [18,19]. The simplest origin of such mosaicism would be forward mutation of an inherited normal allele to a mutant allele in a subject with a negative family history. However, in a family with multiple affected individuals, a relatively mild clinical outcome could reflect back-mutation of an inherited mutation to a normal allele.

One of the most interesting, and scientifically informative, MAI mutations in the ABD is Met886Val. The GSF of two apparently unrelated subjects do not

790

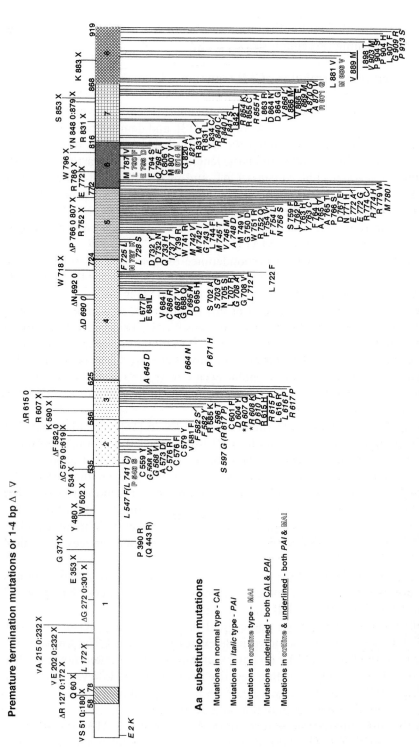

*Fig. 5.* A map of all constitutional point mutations in the *AR* including small deletions (triangle up) or insertions (triangle down) up to 4 bp. X, premature translation termination codon, either directly (e.g., E353X), or after frameshift (e.g., ▽E202 0:232X). Mutations in parentheses coexist with adjacent mutations.

have any kind of androgen-binding abnormality. Yet, the mutant A-R complexes cannot bind normally to two different androgen-response elements, and the mutant ABD does not interact normally, either with itself, or with a normal N-terminal domain (unpublished results). Thus, Met886 appears to be a rare type of amino acid in the ABD: it may, or may not contribute to androgen binding, but it is essential for the transcriptional regulatory function that is embodied within the ABD [20].

Another set of provocative MAI point mutations in the ABD are Arg788Ser (not shown in Fig. 5) [9] and Arg871Gly [21]. Both mutant receptors have normal apparent equilibrium affinity constants for one or another androgen, yet A-R complexes formed with these same androgens have increased nonequilibrium rates of dissociation. The juxtaposition of these kinetic properties implies that these mutations alter the shape of the ABD so as to increase access of the androgens to their binding site and, therefore, their rate of association. However, they also imply that the altered conformation of the ABD diminishes the ability of its binding site to retain bound androgen. Data on such mutations will be valuable for interpreting the structure-function properties of the AR's ABD, once it has been subjected to crystallographic analysis. Furthermore, the concurrence of four MAI substitution mutations in the short stretch of amino acids extending from 788 to 814 is very likely to facilitate that interpretation.

Kennedy syndrome is a spinobulbar motor neuronopathy associated with MAI. It is caused by expansion of the glutamine-coding $(CAG)_{8-35}$ CAA tract in exon 1 of the AR to a total n of $\geq 38$ (Fig. 6) [1]. The MAI component reflects a loss of AR transcriptional regulatory activity by virtue of a pathologically expanded polyglutamine (polygln) tract. This loss may be intrinsic [22–25], it may reflect decreased intracellular steady-state levels of polygln-expanded AR [26,27], or it may be both, depending on the cell type.

Gynecomastia is the single most common sign of MAI in spinobulbar muscular atrophy, and it is frequently the first [28]. Decreased libido and impotence

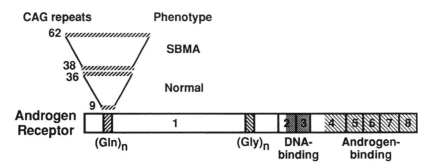

Fig. 6. Expansion of the trinucleotide repeat encoding polyglutamine (starting at residue 58 of the AR) is the cause of Kennedy syndrome (a form of spinobulbar motorneuronopathy associated with MAI). The normal number (n) of repeats varies polymorphically from 9–36. Kennedy syndrome occurs when n $\geq 38$.

usually appear next. Testicular atrophy and infertility typically appear last. Testicular atrophy represents impaired spermatogenesis and corresponds with oligospermia (reduced sperm production) or azoospermia (no sperm production) on semen analysis. Because impotence, reduced libido, and impaired spermatogenesis appear relatively late, often between 40 and 50 years of age [29], males affected with Kennedy syndrome are usually fertile. In fact, in the cases summarized by Warner et al. [30], 72% had children.

Interestingly, in Singapore otherwise normal males with 28 or more CAG repeats in their AR have been reported to have more than a 4-fold increased risk of impaired spermatogenesis, and the more severe the spermatogenic defect, the greater the frequency with a long repeat [31]. It will be interesting to see if a similar observation can be made on ethnically different populations.

Since no other AR mutation, even a complete deletion, causes spinobulbar muscular atrophy, this component of Kennedy syndrome must be due to a toxic gain-of-function by the polygln-expanded AR. At the time of writing, the most likely pathogenetic mechanism is cleavage of the polygln-expanded AR by one or more proapoptotic proteases with the release of truncated polygln-expanded "fragments" [32,33]. These fragments are presumed to aggregate with each other, or with other polygln-containing proteins, to form conjugates that are selectively motor neuronotoxic. Provocatively, androgens are known to be motor neuronotrophic in various natural [34] and experimental [35,36] situations. It is possible, therefore, that a polygln-expanded AR loses a function that is necessary but not sufficient to cause a motor neuronopathy, or that modulates the gain-of-function that is essential for the motor neuronopathy.

**The prevalence of impaired reproduction due to AR mutation**

Standard references quote rates of 2−5 per 100,000 for CAI. These estimates are derived from the frequency of otherwise normal girls whose inguinal hernias are discovered to contain normal testes.

PAI is at least as common as CAI, and essentially all subjects with PAI are infertile. Their infertility is due to impaired spermatogenesis and to impaired development of the sperm-delivery system. Interestingly, the incidence of PAI is frequently exaggerated, on the assumption that normal levels of T and luteinizing hormone postnatally, or normal testosterone biosynthetic capacity in response to human chorionic gonadotropin challenge postnatally, implies that T and DHT concentrations were normal during the critical periods of prenatal internal and external morphogenesis. In fact, it is likely that a simple delay, beyond a critical threshold, in acquiring the capacity to make sufficient T or DHT, or in the ability to respond to DHT is responsible for most cases of "isolated" hypospadias. In other words, such males should be fertile if their sperm- and semen-conduction systems are intact, and once their external genitalia have been surgically restored. "Isolated" refers to hypospadias of any degree that is not one of multiple congenital anomalies in a male newborn. When it is one component of such a multiple, its dysmorphogenesis is exceedingly unlikely to originate in deficient or defective androgen biosynthesis or androgen responsiveness.

The frequency of MAI has not been determined. However, families in which maternally related males are affected with idiopathic oligozoospermia have been rarely reported. Therefore, the infertile form of MAI must be exceedingly uncommon. On the other hand, families in which affected males have normal or near-normal spermatogenesis despite other signs of MAI, may not be rare at all. Some of these signs — decreased skeletal muscularity, increased voice pitch, erectile dysfunction — may confer a measurable reproductive disadvantage.

It would be interesting to know how many XX women with delayed menarche are heterozygotes for an AR mutation who have remained unidentified because they have not had affected XY children or maternally related relatives. The presence of delayed menarche in two or more XX relatives could represent segregation of such a mutation. Also, the coexistence of delayed, sparse, asymmetrical pubic or axillary hair should increase the index of suspicion appreciably. Of course, AR mutation screening would be necessary for a valid estimate of the prevalence of this form of delayed menarche in a given population.

An objective estimate of the prevalence of MAI in its infertile form could be determined by inserting an androgen-responsive "reporter" gene into the genital skin fibroblasts (GSF) of subjects with idiopathic oligozoospermia, and then measuring their response to androgen [25]. Such a strategy would be laborious, but it is necessary because, for unknown reasons, indigenous androgen target genes in normal GSF do not respond to androgen, despite their content of a normal AR protein. Notwithstanding this problem, the method has been shown to work well when androgen-responsive reporter genes are transfected into GSF that are known to harbor AR genes with specific point mutations, or with pathologically expanded polyglutamine tracts [25].

It is possible, of course, that the expression of androgen resistance in this test system might be due to a mutation that is not in the AR itself, but in one of its coregulatory proteins. This would lead to an overestimate of AR mutation in the infertile form of MAI, but it would be a very rewarding way of screening for mutations in AR-interactive proteins that affect overall integrity of the androgen-response apparatus.

## Prospects for the therapy and management of "reproductive" and other problems due to AR mutation

As elaborated below, it is theoretically possible to overcome the functional defects of certain mutant ARs by pharmacotherapy with appropriate androgens, or other steroids. It may even be possible to increase the concentration of deficient, but otherwise normal AR, simply by increasing the rate of its synthesis or decreasing its rate of degradation.

These statements are irrelevant for those with CAI or incomplete AI, who are irremediably infertile.

However, some missense AR mutations express androgen-binding defects that are conditional on being exposed to a particular type of androgen [16,17,21]. It follows that it may be possible to find, or design, a type of androgen (or steroid) that overcomes an androgen-binding problem that is manifested only with a natural androgen. Likewise, there is evidence from somatic AR mutations in prostatic carcinoma that certain ones of the missense variety not only permit the AR to bind unusual androgens, or other steroids [37], promiscuously, but also allow it to be activated by them [38] in a manner that allows these unorthodox steroid-receptor complexes to be effective in transcriptional regulation of certain androgen target genes.

Such strategies, if successful, could be useful for subjects with PAI reared as males, and for those with the infertile form of MAI. In PAI, phallic growth might be promoted both before surgical reconstruction, and after; and, conceivably, spermatogenesis could be promoted in testes that are brought into a reconstructed scrotum. Finally, in the absence of an intact sperm-transporting system, some form of sperm retrieval would be necessary for fertilization to occur.

In infertile subjects with MAI, promotion of spermatogenesis would be the main goal, and sperm retrieval would not be necessary in the presence of an intact sperm-delivery system.

Apart from the successful experience with mesterolone ($1\alpha$-methylandrostan-$17\beta$-ol-3-one) in promoting spermatogenesis and fertility twice in one man with MAI [14], experience with long-term natural androgen pharmacotherapy is meager, and its value unclear [39—42]. This is notably disappointing especially when laboratory studies indicate that a particular ABD mutation decreases androgen-binding affinity in a manner that should, theoretically, be normalized simply by provision of excess androgen. Failure of this therapeutic strategy implies that occupancy of the ABD by the androgen is only a superficial expression of mutant AR dysfunction: its core dysfunction is its failure to be activated to a competent transcriptional regulatory protein even when the androgen-binding pocket of the mutant AR is fully occupied.

## References

1. Andrew SE, Goldberg YP, Hayden MR. Rethinking genotype and phenotype correlations in polyglutamine expansion disorders. Hum Mol Genet 1997;6:2005—2010.
2. Lumbroso R, Beitel LK, Vasiliou DM, Trifiro MA, Pinsky L. Codon-usage variants in the polymorphic $(GGN)_n$ trinucleotide repeat of the human androgen receptor gene. Hum Genet 1997;101:43—46.
3. La Spada AR, Wilson EM, Lubahn DB, Harding AE, Fischbeck KH. Androgen receptor gene mutations in X-linked spinal and bulbar muscular atrophy. Nature 1991;352:77—79.
4. Kaufman M, Straisfeld C, Pinsky L. Male pseudohermaphroditism presumably due to target organ unresponsiveness to androgens. Deficient $5\alpha$-dihydrotestosterone binding in cultured skin fibroblasts. J Clin Invest 1976;58:345—350.
5. Katz MD, Cai L-Q, Zhu Y-S, Herrera C, DeFillo-Ricart M, Shackleton CHL, Imperato-McGinley J. The biochemical and phenotypic characterization of females homozygous for $5\alpha$-reductase-2 deficiency. J Clin Endocrinol Metab 1995;80:3160—3167.

6. Migeon CJ, Brown TR, Lanes R, Palacios A, Amrhein JA, Schoen EJ. A clinical syndrome of mild androgen insensitivity. J Clin Endocrinol Metab 1984;59:672–678.

7. Cundy TF, Rees M, Evans BAJ, Hughes IA, Butler J, Wheeler MJ. Mild androgen insensitivity presenting with sexual dysfunction. Fertil Steril 1986;46:721–723.

8. Tsukada T, Inoue M, Tachibana S, Nakai Y, Takebe, H. An androgen receptor mutation causing androgen resistance in undervirilized male syndrome. J Clin Endocrinol Metab 1994;79:1202–1207.

9. Grino PB, Griffin JE, Cushard WG Jr, Wilson JD. A mutation of the androgen receptor associated with partial androgen resistance, familial gynecomastia, and fertility. J Clin Endocrinol Metab 1988;66:754–761.

10. Pinsky L, Kaufman K, Killinger DW. Impaired spermatogenesis is not an obligate expression of receptor-defective androgen resistance. Am J Med Gen 1989;32:100–104.

11. Rodien P, Mebarki F, Mowszowicz I, Chaussain J-L, Young J, Morel Y, Schaison G. Different phenotpyes in a family with androgen insensitivity caused by the same M780I point mutation in the androgen receptor gene. J Clin Endocrinol Metab 1996;81:2994–2998.

12. Pinsky L, Beitel LK, Kazemi-Esfarjani P, Lumbroso R, Vasiliou DM, Shkolny D, Abdullah AAR, Gottlieb B, Trifiro MA. Lessons from androgen receptor gene mutations that cause androgen resistance in humans. In: Hughes IA (ed) Sex Differentiation: Clinical and Biological Aspects. Serono Symposia Series — Frontiers in Endocrinology, volume 20. Cambridge, 1996; 95–114.

13. Gottlieb B, Lehvaslaiho H, Beitel LK, Lumbroso R, Pinsky L, Trifiro M. The androgen receptor gene mutations database. Nucl Acids Res 1998;26:234–238.

14. Yong EL, Ng SC, Roy AC, Yun G, Ratnam SS. Pregnancy after hormonal correction of severe spermatogenic defect due to mutation in androgen receptor gene. Lancet 1994;344:826–827.

15. Pinsky L, Trifiro M, Kaufman M, Beitel LK, Mhatre A, Kazemi-Esfarjani P, Sabbaghian N, Lumbroso R, Alvarado C, Vasiliou M, Gottlieb B. Androgen resistance due to mutation of the androgen receptor. Clin Invest Med 1992;15:456–472.

16. Pinsky L, Kaufman K, Killinger DW, Burko B, Shatz D, Volpe R. Human minimal androgen insensitivity with normal dihydrotestosterone-binding capacity in cultured genital skin fibroblasts: evidence for an androgen-selective qualitative abnormality of the receptor. Am J Hum Genet 1984;36:965–978.

17. Pinsky L, Kaufman M, Chudley AE. Reduced affinity of the androgen receptor for 5α-dihydrotestosterone but not methyltrienolone in a form of partial androgen resistance. J Clin Invest 1985;75:1291–1296.

18. Boehmer ALM, Brinkmann AO, Niermeijer MF, Bakker L, Halley DJJ, Drop SLS. Germ-line and somatic mosaicism in the androgen insensitivity syndrome: implications for genetic counseling. Am J Hum Genet 1997;60:1003–1006.

19. Holterhus P-M, Brüggenwirth HT, Hiort O, Kleinkauf-Houcken A, Kruse K, Sinnecker GHG, Brinkmann AO. Mosaicism due to a somatic mutation of the androgen receptor gene determines phenotype in androgen insensitivity syndrome. J Clin Endocrinol Metab 1997;82:3584–3589.

20. Panet-Raymond V, Beitel LK, Abdullah AAR, Yong EL, Pinsky L, Trifiro MA. Dimerization of the androgen receptor using the yeast two-hybrid system is ligand-facilitated in normal and mutant receptors. Endocrine Society, 80th Annual Meeting, New Orleans, 1998;P1-533,229.

21. Kaufman M, Pinsky L, Gottlieb B, Schweitzer M, Brezezinski A, von Westarp C, Ginsberg J. Androgen receptor defects in patients with minimal and partial androgen resistance classified according to a model of androgen-receptor complex energy states. Horm Res 1990;33:87–94.

22. Mhatre A, Trifiro MA, Kaufman M, Kazemi EP, Figlewicz D, Rouleau G, Pinsky L. Reduced transcriptional regulatory competence of the androgen receptor in X-linked spinal and bulbar muscular atrophy. Nature Genet 1993;5:184–188.

23. Chamberlain NL, Driver ED, Miesfeld RL. The length and location of CAG trinucleotide repeats in the androgen receptor N-terminal domain affect transactivation function. Nucl Acid

Res 1994;22:3181–3186.

24. Kazemi-Esfarjani P, Trifiro MA, Pinsky L. Evidence for a repressive function of the long poly-glutamine tract in the human androgen receptor: possible pathogenetic relevance for the $(CAG)_n$-expanded neuronopathies. Hum Mol Genet 1995;4:523–527.

25. McPhaul MJ, Schweikert H-U, Allman DR. Assessment of androgen receptor function in genital skin fibroblasts using a recombinant adenovirus to deliver an androgen-responsive reporter gene. J Clin Endocrinol Metab 1997;82:1944–1948.

26. Choong CS, Kemppainen JA, Zhou ZX, Wilson EM. Reduced androgen receptor gene expression with first exon CAG repeat expansion. Mol Endocrinol 1996;10:1527–1535.

27. Brooks BP, Paulson HL, Merry DE, Salazar GE, Brinkmann AO, Wilson EM, Fischbeck KH. Characterization of an expanded glutamine repeat androgen receptor in a neuronal cell culture system. Neurobiol Dis 1997;3:313–323.

28. Beitel LK, Trifiro MA, Pinsky L. Spinobulbar muscular atrophy. In: Rubinsztein D, Hayden M (eds) Trinucleotide Repeat Diseases. Oxford; BIOS, 1998 (In press).

29. Guidetti D, Motti L, Marcello N, Vescovini E, Marbini A, Dotti C, Lucci B, Solime F. Kennedy disease in an Italian kindred. Eur Neurol 1986;25:188–196.

30. Warner CL, Servidei S, Lange DJ, Miller E, Lovelace RE, Rowland LP. X-linked spinal muscular atrophy (Kennedy's syndrome). A kindred with hypobetalipo-proteinemia. Arch Neurol 1990;47:1117–1120.

31. Tut TG, Ghadessy FJ, Trifiro MA, Pinsky L, Yong EL. Long polyglutamine tracts in the androgen receptor are associated with reduced trans-activation, impaired sperm production, and male infertility. J Clin Endocrinol Metab 1997;82:3777–3782.

32. Abdullah AAR, Trifiro MA, Panet-Raymond V, Alvarado C, de Tourreil S, Frankel D, Schipper HM, Pinsky L. Spinobulbar muscular atrophy: polyglutamine-expanded androgen receptor is proteolytically resistant in vitro and processed abnormally in transfected cells. Hum Mol Genet 1998;7:379–384.

33. Wellington CL, Ellerby LM, Hackman AS, Margolis RL, Trifiro MA, Singaraja R, McCutcheon K, Salveson GS, Propp SS, Bromm M, Rowland KJ, Zhang T, Rasper D, Roy S, Thornberry N, Pinsky L, Kakizuka A, Ross CA, Nicholson DW, Bredesen DE, Hayden MJ. Caspase cleavage of gene products associated with triplet expansion disorders generates truncated fragments containing the polyglutamine tract. J Biol Chem 1998;273:9158–9167.

34. Nordeen EJ, Nordeen KW, Sengelaub DR, Arnold AP. Androgens prevent normally occurring cell death in a sexually dimorphic spinal nucleus. Science 1985;229:671–673.

35. Perez J, Kelley DB. Trophic effects of androgen: receptor expression and the survival of laryngeal motor neurons after axotomy. J Neuroscience 1996;16:6625–6633.

36. Tanzer L, Jones KJ. Gonadal steroid regulation of hamster facial nerve regeneration: effects of dihydrotestosterone and estradiol. Exp Neurol 1997;146:258–264.

37. Culig Z, Hobisch A, Cronauer MV, Cato ACB, Hittmair A, Radmayr C, Eberle J, Bartsch G, Klocker H. Mutant androgen receptor detected in an advanced-stage prostatic carcinoma is activated by adrenal androgens and progesterone. Molec Endocrinol 1993;7:1541–1550.

38. Taplin M-E, Bubley GJ, Shuster TD, Frantz ME, Spooner AE, Ogata GK, Keer HN, Balk SP. Mutation of the androgen-receptor gene in metastatic androgen-independent prostate cancer. N Engl J Med 1995;332:1393–1398.

39. Jukier L, Kaufman M, Pinsky L, Peterson RE. Partial androgen resistance associated with secondary 5α-reductase deficiency: identification of a novel qualitative androgen receptor defect and clinical implications. J Clin Endocrinol Metab 1984;59:679–688.

40. Price P, Wess JAH, Griffin JE, Leshin M, Savage MO, Largo DM, Bu'Lock DE, Anderson DC, Wilson JD, Besser GM. High dose androgen therapy in male pseudohermaphroditism due to 5α-reductase deficiency and disorders of the androgen receptor. J Clin Invest 1984;74:1496–1508.

41. McPhaul MJ, Marcelli M, Tilley WD, Griffin JE, Isidro-Gutierrez RF, Wilson JD. Molecular basis of androgen resistance in a family with a qualitative abnormality of the androgen receptor

and responsive to high-dose androgen therapy. J Clin Invest 1991;87:1413–1421.

42. Hiort O, Huang Q, Sinnecker GHG, Sadeghi-Nejad A, Kruse K, Wolfe HJ, Yandell DW. Single strand conformation polymorphism analysis of androgen receptor gene mutations in patients with androgen insensitivity syndromes: application for diagnosis, genetic counseling, and therapy. J Clin Endocrinol Metab 1993;77:262–266.

43. Langley E, Kemppainen JA, Wilson EM. Intermolecular $NH^{2-}$/carboxyl-terminal interactions in androgen receptor dimerization revealed by mutations that cause androgen insensitivity. J Biol Chem 1998;273:92–101.

# Epidemiological controversies in reproduction

# Spontaneous and induced abortions: relationship to breast cancer

Salim Daya

*Departments of Obstetrics and Gynaecology and Clinical Epidemiology and Biostatistics, McMaster University, Hamilton, Ontario, Canada*

**Abstract.** *Background.* Results from animal studies have led to the hypothesis that only pregnancies that go to term confer protection against breast cancer. The increase in incidence of breast cancer and in the number of induced abortions in humans suggests that they may be causally linked. The purpose of this review is to evaluate the evidence from epidemiologic studies to determine whether induced and/or spontaneous abortions are associated with breast cancer.

*Methods.* The literature was searched for articles on abortion and breast cancer. Evidence from case-control and cohort studies was summarized using meta-analytic and metaregression techniques to obtain an overall estimate of risk.

*Results.* There was no significant association between spontaneous abortion and breast cancer. Case-control studies demonstrated a significant association between induced abortion and breast cancer, although the magnitude of the effect was small. In contrast, cohort studies showed no significant overall relationship, except in women undergoing induced abortion after 18 weeks' gestation.

*Conclusions.* Although the relationship between induced abortion and breast cancer is biologically plausible, the evidence suggests that there is no overall causal link except perhaps for women having late abortions (i.e., after 18 weeks' gestation). In contrast, no risk was observed with spontaneous abortion.

**Keywords:** abortion, breast cancer, epidemiology.

## Introduction

Factors associated with an increased risk of breast cancer include nulliparity, early age at menarche, late age at menopause, and late age at first full-term pregnancy. The younger a woman is at menarche, the higher her risk of breast cancer is [1]. Women with onset of menstruation at or after age 15 years had a 23% lower risk than those with an age at menarche of 12 years or younger [2]. It has been estimated that for each 2-year delay in the onset of menstruation, breast cancer risk is reduced by 10% [1]. A likely etiologic factor in this relationship is the early exposure to the hormonal mileu associated with regular ovulatory menstrual cycles [3]. In addition, some studies have reported that women with early menarche have higher estrogen levels for several years after menarche and pos-

*Address for correspondence:* Prof Salim Daya MB, ChB, MSc, FRCSC, Department of Obstetrics and Gynaecology, McMaster University, 1200 Main Street West, Hamilton, Ontario, Canada L8N 3Z5. Tel.: +1-905-525-9140 ext. 22566. Fax: 1-905-524-2911. E-mail: dayas@fhs.csu.mcmaster.ca

sibly throughout their reproductive life span [4,5].

Similarly, the older a woman is at menopause, the higher her risk of breast cancer is [1,6]. For every 5-year difference in age at menopause, the risk for breast cancer changes by about 17% [1]. In contrast, bilateral oophorectomy before menopause is associated with a reduction in risk that appears to last into older age [2,7]. For example, bilateral oophorectomy before age 40 is associated with a lifetime decrease in risk of about 50% compared to that with natural menopause [2,7].

The increased risks associated with early age at menarche and late age at menopause suggest that reproductive factors are of importance and the longer the exposure to sex hormones during the reproductive years, the higher the risk of breast cancer [8]. It has also been observed, that women who have borne children early in reproductive life have a lower risk of breast cancer than women who have never had a child [6,9]. Pregnancies that are not full-term do not show this protective effect [9,10]. These observations, and the results from animal studies, have led to the hypothesis that pregnancies that go to term protect against breast cancer because complete differentiation of breast stem cells occurs late in pregnancy, making the breast less susceptible to carcinogens; an interrupted pregnancy may not confer protection or may even increase the risk because proliferation of breast stem cells will have occurred without the protective effect of subsequent differentiation [11]. Thus, a full-term pregnancy may have opposing influences on the risk of breast cancer: a short-term increase in risk owing to the growth-enhancing properties of estrogen, and a long-term decrease in risk owing to terminal differentiation of mammary tissue [12,13]. Consequently, abortion, as an incomplete pregnancy, may increase the risk of breast cancer.

An association between induced abortion and the incidence of breast cancer was first reported in 1957 as a result of cases diagnosed between 1948 and 1952 [14]. The effect of induced or spontaneous abortion on breast cancer risk has since been evaluated by numerous epidemiologic studies and has recently been the subject of heightened attention. However, despite four decades of research on this subject, medical opinion has remained divided on the issue of a direct link between abortion and breast cancer. The approach to evaluating the possibility of a causal relationship between exposure to a putatively harmful agent and the outcome of interest involves the application of several diagnostic tests to the evidence [15]. This approach will be used to determine whether the claims of a causal relationship between abortion and breast cancer can be substantiated.

## Methodological issues

### Choice of the reference group

To determine the presence and magnitude of the risk of breast cancer associated with abortion, it is important to select the appropriate control group so that meaningful comparisons can be made. Should the reference group be nulliparous women who have never been pregnant or parous women who have never had a miscarriage or induced abortion (and who, therefore, have a lower risk than nulliparous women)? For example, in comparing groups of women who had had abortions to those who had not, regardless of parity status, the groups will consist of both nulliparous and parous women, the relative proportions of which may vary. Since nulliparous women generally have a higher risk of breast cancer and may have a higher incidence of induced abortion, the effect of parity would confound the association between breast cancer and abortion. Parity may also confound the relation between miscarriages and breast cancer because miscarriages are associated with higher parity [16].

*Ascertainment of exposure*

The utilization of retrospective study designs in the evaluation of the association between abortion and breast cancer is fraught with inaccuracies resulting from recall bias, especially when personal and sensitive information about distant events is sought. Abortion history particularly is prone to misclassification. Spontaneous abortions frequently go unnoticed because they often occur early and may not have been confirmed. Clinically recognized miscarriages are sometimes not reported and are less often remembered [17]. Such misclassification leads to underestimation of the association between abortion and breast cancer.

Induced abortions are likely to be under reported [18] because of their highly sensitive nature, the threatening actions of antiabortion crusaders [19], and the practice remaining illegal in some countries. Even when the procedure is legal, the social and religious stigma associated with induced abortion may cause reporting bias.

*Confounding*

Among parous women, those with an abortion before their first live birth tend to have a later age at first birth than those with no abortion. Failing to adjust for age at first birth might lead to an overestimation of the association between abortion and breast cancer. Other confounding factors include early menarche (which is associated with subsequent spontaneous abortions [20]), use of oral contraceptives (which might reduce the number of abortions) and nulliparity, low parity and late age at first birth, all of which may indicate the presence of infertility, which has been reported to be associated with breast cancer [6,21,22].

*Effect modification*

Any association between abortion and breast cancer may be modified by parity at abortion, timing of abortion in relation to other pregnancies, duration of pregnancy, age at abortion, time since abortion and number of abortions [23].

*Spontaneous and induced abortions*

Spontaneous and induced abortions should be studied separately. The hormonal changes in an induced abortion are similar to those in a normal pregnancy up to the time of the abortion. In contrast, spontaneous abortions are often associated with an inadequate rise of pregnancy hormones. Also, in a large number of spontaneous abortions, a nonviable fetus with chromosomal abnormalities is present. Induced and spontaneous abortions, therefore, are systematically different from each other except for the gestational age at pregnancy termination. Consequently, qualitative differences are likely to be found when evaluating a possible association with breast cancer, and any influence of these two conditions on breast cancer risk should be evaluated separately.

## Diagnostic tests for causation

*Is there evidence from true experiments in humans?*

The ideal method of gathering evidence on causation is through random allocation, whereby individuals exposed to the putative causal factor, and those not exposed, are followed over time to determine how frequently the outcome of interest occurs in each group. Clearly, such evidence linking abortion to breast cancer is not available and can not be obtained. Consequently, there is no evidence from true experiments in humans implicating abortion in causing breast cancer.

*Is the association consistent from study to study?*

The demonstration by different investigators of an association between abortion and breast cancer in different setting provides evidence that is consistent, thereby strengthening the inference of a causal link. In the study of a disease with a long induction or latency period, such as malignancy, the case-control design is generally preferred to the cohort design primarily because of the shorter duration of time required to gather the information [24]. However, it is readily acknowledged that case-control studies are more likely to reach conclusions that are biased owing to faulty recall. Such bias would result in some of the data being unreliable, especially exposure data collected through interviews or questionnaires. It is likely that a woman, responding to a diagnosis of breast cancer, would reflect more intently on the possible causes of her illness and would remember and report an induced abortion more readily and consistently than would a healthy control. In addition, to recall bias that results in differential misclassification, response bias may be introduced by inconsistent interview techniques that, in part, may reflect the interviewer's belief that exposure and outcome are (or are not) causally linked.

Most of the published studies have used the case-control design and have been reviewed and subjected to meta-analysis [25]. These data will be reviewed and the findings compared with those from a more recent large cohort study [26].

*Review of evidence from case-control studies*
Published studies were located using several search strategies. The Medline (National Library of Medicine, USA) database from 1966 to 1996 and the Embase fertility database from 1986 to 1996 were searched using the subject search terms "breast", "cancer" and "abortion". Bibliographies of relevant publications and review articles were scanned for additional references. A total of 21 publications of case-control studies was identified wherein data were available for cases and controls (list of references available from author). In some publications, spontaneous and induced abortions were grouped together. Each study provided one or more estimates of relative risk for breast cancer in relation to abortion history. Statistical techniques were used to combine the published risks, weighted according to their sample size and the precision of their risk estimates. Where adjusted estimates were unavailable, the adjusted relative risk was calculated from the raw odds ratio (OR) and a study-specific adjustment factor. Meta-regression analysis [27], using the logarithm of the weighted adjusted relative risks as the dependent variable, assessed the effects on the risk of breast cancer of abortion (induced, spontaneous and combined).

There were 10 studies contributing 15 risk estimates for breast cancer with induced abortion, 14 studies with 21 risk estimates with spontaneous abortion, and seven studies with 11 risk estimates with induced and spontaneous abortion grouped together. The overall relative risk (RR) for breast cancer with induced abortion was 1.17 (95% confidence interval (CI) = 1.07−1.27) indicating a statistically significant risk. For spontaneous abortion, the RR was not significant at 0.99 (95% CI 0.95−1.04). Among studies which did not differentiate between induced and spontaneous abortions, the RR for breast cancer was statistically significant but the overall estimate was lower than for studies with only induced abortion, i.e., 1.07 (95% CI 1.02−1.12).

The role of induced abortion as an independent risk factor for breast cancer was recently evaluated by other investigators who conducted a comprehensive review and meta-analysis of the evidence [25]. The literature review identified 28 original published reports of 23 independent studies on the subject. The meta-analysis summarized the data according to several categories. The risk of breast cancer for women with a history of one or more induced abortions was calculated using data from 21 studies. The overall pooled OR was 1.3 (95% CI = 1.2−1.4). The OR for breast cancer in women with a history of one or more induced abortions before a first full-term pregnancy was 1.4 (95% CI 1.2−1.6). Among this group of studies, a subgroup analysis demonstrated that in nulliparous women, the pooled OR was 1.3 (95% CI 1.0−1.6) compared to 1.5 (95% CI 1.2−1.8) in parous women. In parous women with a history of one or more induced abortions after the first full-term pregnancy, the OR was 1.3 (95% CI 1.1−1.5). All these estimates were statistically significant. For each category, a majority of the studies exhibited an OR that was greater than unity. Furthermore, the studies with a positive result outnumbered those with a negative result. In particular, there were 10 studies with significantly positive findings and only one with negative finding out of the 21 independent studies reviewed. Thus, in general, the findings were reasonably consistent from study to study. However, in none of the studies was the methodology strong.

Studies of spontaneous abortion and breast cancer were summarized in another review in which no important association was observed in the majority of the case-control studies included in the review [23].

*Evidence for recall bias*
As previously discussed, one of the problems with case-control studies is that of recall bias which arises when individuals with a particular adverse health outcome remember and report their previous exposure experience differently from those who are not similarly affected. A unique opportunity to examine the effect of recall bias became available in a Dutch case-control study of abortion and breast cancer by comparing the risks between two geographic areas that differed in the prevalence of, and attitude toward, induced abortion [28]. The data analyzed in this study were obtained from 918 women (20–54 years of age at diagnosis) who were diagnosed with invasive breast cancer during the period from 1986 to 1989, and who had been initially enrolled in a population-based, case-control study investigating oral contraceptive use and breast cancer risk. The women resided in one of four geographic areas. Each case patient was pair-matched, on the basis of age (within 1 year) and region, with a control subject who was randomly selected from municipal registries of the whole Dutch population. Structured questionnaires were administered by a trained interviewer during home interviews of the subjects. Reporting bias was examined indirectly by comparing the risks of breast cancer between the western and the southeastern regions of the country, wherein differences exist in the prevalence and attitude toward induced abortion. In the conservative, predominantly Roman Catholic, southeastern region of the country people are more opposed to terminating pregnancy, whereas the western region is more liberal with more tolerant attitudes towards induced abortion which is performed more commonly.

A significant association was observed between induced abortion and breast cancer (adjusted RR = 1.9, 95% CI = 1.1–3.2). The association was stronger in the more conservative southeastern region (RR = 14.6, 95% CI 1.8–120.0), than in the more liberal western region (RR = 1.3, 95% CI = 0.7–2.6). This difference was statistically significant (p = 0.017) suggesting the presence of reporting bias. Support for this notion was found in data supplied by the subjects and their physicians on the use of oral contraceptives. In the southeastern region, when duration of contraceptive use reported by physicians was compared to that reported by control subjects, an underreporting by more than 6.3 months was found compared to subjects in the western region (p = 0.007).

Thus, the evidence from this study suggests that the increased risk for breast cancer following induced abortion is largely attributable to poorer recall (resulting in underreporting of abortion) by healthy control subjects. Almost all the reported induced abortions in this study took place before abortions were legalized in The Netherlands. Consequently, the control subjects from the southeastern region were more likely to have withheld information on previous abortions during the interview.

The higher likelihood of underreporting with in-person interviews compared with written questionnaires has been observed in other studies. For example, in a representative sample of US women aged 15—44 years of age participating in the National Survey of Family Growth, data on abortions obtained from interviews and questionnaires were compared with national abortion data [18]. Although no more than 60% of all induced abortions were reported, underreporting was more pronounced in data obtained by interviews compared with questionnaires.

*Evidence for response bias*
The use of retrospective data collection methods for evaluating a possible causal association between breast cancer and induced abortion may be influenced by a heightened ability during an interview to recall events that may have produced disease in those affected by breast cancer (i.e., response bias). Thus, a recent diagnosis of breast cancer would make it more likely for a woman to remember and report to the interviewer an induced abortion than a healthy control would. Response bias could also result from inconsistent interview techniques between cases and controls.

The issue of response bias was evaluated in a study that compared information about induced abortion from two independent Swedish epidemiologic studies of breast cancer in young women [29]. In the first study, a case-control design was employed and data were collected through interviews [30]. In the second study, a cohort record linkage design was used, wherein data were obtained from an abortion registry [31]. The two studies overlapped the same abortion period and all women in the case-control study had been included in the registry. Cases included all women with histologically confirmed invasive breast cancer diagnosed in Sweden from May 1984 to May 1985. Controls were chosen from a nationwide population register. In addition, for each woman less than 40 years of age, a second control was chosen from a nationwide fertility register. Cases and matched controls were interviewed in their homes by the same professional female interviewer using a standard format.

From 1939 to the end of 1974, abortion reporting to the Swedish National Board of Health and Welfare was mandatory. Computerized records which provided objectively documented information on abortions performed were available on all abortions (n = 166,840) performed from January 1966 to December 1974.

The data sets from the two studies were compared for concordance (i.e., abortion or no abortion identified by interview and on abortion register from 1996 to 1974) and discordance (abortion identified by interview but not on register or vice versa). The information from the two studies was concordant for 800 women, but discordant for 29 women. The crude OR for breast cancer for women with a history of abortion was 0.95 from data in the case-control study and 0.63 from data in the abortion register. The ratio (Q) between these OR was 1.5 (95% CI = 1.1—2.1). In contrast the value for Q in the discordant cases was 22.4 (i.e., ratio between underreporting of previous-induced abortions among controls relative to underreporting among cases) which was significantly different from the expected value of unity ($p < 0.007$).

The results of this study suggested that there was a statistically significant bias in underreporting of induced abortions among healthy controls compared with women newly diagnosed with breast cancer. No evidence of selective forgetfulness among the cases was found. Furthermore, the value of Q indicated that data from the case-control study produced an apparent 50% increase in breast cancer risk. The liberal abortion laws during the period studied made it unlikely that the additional abortions reported during the interviews were misclassifications of illegal abortions.

Thus, response bias may be a source of significant error in case-control studies regarding malignant diseases based on retrospective interviews or questionnaires when sensitive and personal issues are studied. This bias may, in part, explain the tendency toward increased risk of breast cancer associated with induced abortion in many case-control studies.

*Review of evidence from a cohort study*

The varying estimates, ranging from moderately elevated to significantly lowered of the risk of breast cancer associated with induced abortion, are in large part the result of bias inherent in case-control studies owing to their retrospective nature. Although the cohort design is more appropriate to investigate the possibility of a causal link between abortion and breast cancer, it is more difficult to execute and is time consuming. However, the results of such a study recently completed in Denmark, where a policy of mandatory reporting of all induced abortions is in place, were published adding new information to the debate [26]. In this study, data from the Civil Registration System (CRS) were linked with those from the National Registry for Induced Abortions and the Danish Cancer Registry (DCR). Linkage was possible through unique identification numbers that are assigned by CRS to all Danish residents. Also, reporting of induced abortions has been mandatory since 1939, and since 1973, information on all induced abortions, including the gestational age and date when the procedure was performed, has been computerized. In addition, the DCR contains information on all cases of cancer diagnosed in the country since 1943.

The research database comprised all Danish women born between 1 April 1935 and 31 March 1978. Follow up for breast cancer for all the women began on 1 April 1968, or on their 12th birthday, whichever came later. The period at risk was extended until the diagnosis of breast cancer, death, emigration, loss to follow up, or 31 December 1992, whichever came first. The possible effect of the gestational age at the time of the induced abortion was investigated using a log-linear Poisson regression model.

Overall, out of 1,529,512 women who were included in the cohort, 280,965 (18.4%) had had at least one induced abortion (78.8, 17.1 and 6.1% had had one, two and three or more abortions, respectively). There were 8,908 cases of breast cancer among 25,850,000 person-years of follow up in women without a history of induced abortion compared with 1,338 cases among 2,697,000 person-years of follow up in women with a history of induced abortion. These observations translated into an adjusted (for age, parity, age at delivery of first child and calendar period) RR of 1.00 (95% CI = 0.94−1.06) for breast cancer with induced abortion.

Female age at the time of the induced abortion did not significantly influence the overall risk, nor did the number of induced abortions or whether or not the woman had given birth to a live infant. The RR increased with gestational age, with the highest risk being for induced abortion > 18 weeks (RR = 1.92, 95% CI 1.13−3.26).

The results of this population-based control study demonstrate that the overall risk of breast cancer is not increased in women with a history of induced abortion. These observations are in line with the results of previous retrospective cohort studies [16,31−33].

Thus, although both the metaregression analysis and meta-analysis of the case-control studies demonstrated an increased risk of breast cancer with induced abortion, the results of the individual studies are inconsistent. In contrast, the cohort studies do not show an increased risk of cancer. The main reason for this discrepancy is that case-control studies lead to a biased estimate of risk because of methodologic problems, which are avoided in cohort studies.

*Is the association strong?*

The strength of association, summarized by the point estimate and its 95%-confidence interval, is highly dependent on the type of study performed. Inferences drawn from the point estimate can be enhanced if the precision of this estimate is high, and the study design and methods used are valid. In the meta-analysis of case-control studies the overall estimate of risk of breast cancer with induced abortion was found to be OR = 1.3 (95% CI 1.2−1.4). Thus, although this estimate had high precision, its magnitude was low. In contrast, the risk using a cohort design was RR = 1.00 (95% CI 0.94−1.06) indicating that the overall risk was not increased. However, in women with induced abortion in the second trimester (i.e., > 18 weeks) the risk was much higher (RR = 1.92, 95% CI 1.13−3.26), but the precision of this estimate is low and reflects the small number of cases from which this estimate was derived.

*Is the temporal relationship correct?*

A consistent sequence of events in which induced abortion in disease-free women is subsequently followed by breast cancer supports the temporal requirement for causation. By definition, such a requirement can be fulfilled with certainty only by prospective studies. Most of the published literature on breast cancer and induced abortion is based on the case-control design in which absence of disease prior to the induced abortion can not be verified making it difficult to confirm a temporal relationship between exposure and outcome. In contrast, cohort studies begin with a disease-free state among subjects followed by exposure (i.e., induced abortion) in one group and no exposure in the other. The data from the cohort studies indicate that in general, induced abortion is not associated with breast cancer, except in women undergoing abortion in the second trimester (i.e., > 18 weeks of gestation) in whom the risk appears to be increased.

*Is there a dose-response gradient?*

This is an important test of causation and, if satisfied, provides good evidence for a causal link between induced abortion and breast cancer. The "dose-effect" can be evaluated from two perspectives: the number of abortions and the duration of pregnancy at the time of abortion.

*Number of previous abortions*
The effect of the number of previous induced abortions on breast cancer risk was investigated in the Danish population-based cohort study [26]. Although the majority of women in this study had had only one abortion, 23.2% of them had had two or more abortions. When compared to the group of women with one previous abortion as the reference group, the RR for breast cancer with two induced abortions was 1.08 (95% CI 0.92−1.26) and the RR for three or more abortions was 0.99 (95% CI 0.73−1.35). Thus, no dose effect from the number of abortions was observed on the risk of developing breast cancer.

*Duration of pregnancy*
Induced abortions can be performed at various gestational ages. Consequently, the exposure risk indicated by the length of time the pregnancy was allowed to continue may vary depending on when it was terminated. Reliable information on gestational age was not available from either the case-control studies or in most of the cohort studies. However, the Danish study was able to take advantage of Denmark's policy of mandatory reporting of the date and the week of gestation of all induced abortions, to determine whether a dose-response relationship with breast-cancer could be ascertained using gestational age as a measure of the dose of exposure.

Although induced abortions had no overall effect on the risk of breast cancer, a linear relationship with gestational age was observed. With each 1-week increase in the gestational age of the fetus, there was a 3% increase in the risk of breast cancer [26]. The RR increased from 0.81 (95% CI 0.58–1.13) among women whose most recent induced abortion was at less than 7 weeks' gestation, to 1.38 (95% CI 1.00–1.90) among women whose most recent abortion was more than 12 weeks' gestation. Furthermore, a significant linear trend (p = 0.016) was observed for gestational ages greater than 12 weeks: the relative risks were 1.13 (95% CI 0.51–0.53) for gestational age 13–14 weeks, 1.23 (95% CI 0.76–2.00) for 15–18 weeks' gestation and 1.89 (95% CI 1.11–3.22) for > 18 weeks' gestation. The fact that such an increase did not affect the overall result clearly indicates that it is based on small numbers and, therefore, requires cautious interpretation.

*Does the association make biologic sense?*

Although the cause of breast cancer is not known, observations from epidemiologic studies indicate that there are both protective and stimulating factors that influence the development of breast cancer. Among the protective factors are a first full-term pregnancy before 30 years of age and a late menarche [6]. Among the risk factors are nulliparity, late pregnancy, early menarche and late age at menopause [6]. The rise in breast cancer incidence follows an exponential pattern until age 50 years, and then becomes linear for about 20 years thereafter. This incidence pattern implies that cancer cells arise during the reproductive years and become clinical cancers in later years.

The mammary gland is not fully developed at birth and undergoes dramatic changes in size, shape and function during growth, puberty, pregnancy and lactation. Four different lobular structures have been characterized in the breast of postpubertal women, each one representing a sequential developmental stage [34]. The breasts of nulliparous women contain more undifferentiated structures than those of parous women.

The use of an experimental system involving the induction of mammary gland carcinoma by administration of 7,12-dimethylbenz(a)anthracene (DMBA) to young virgin rats, has provided some insights into the role of pregnancy in the susceptibility to carcinogenesis [11]. It has been shown that full-term pregnancy renders the mammary gland less susceptible to DMBA carcinogenesis, and that, although lactation is not required for complete protection, animals that have not lactated are more prone to develop benign tumors [11]. In order to avoid the occurrence of cancer, the development of the mammary gland must be complete. Pregnant or lactating rats treated with chemical carcinogens respond with a significant reduction in the incidence of mammary tumors, whereas pregnancy interruption gives no protection at all [11]. This observation is explained by the fact that the mammary glands of animals, in which pregnancy has been terminated, contain some areas with completely differentiated structures and others in which undifferentiated structures prevail.

The parallelism between the DMBA-induced rat mammary carcinoma model

812

and the human situation is remarkable. In human pregnancy, the secretion of prolactin, estrogen and progesterone is increased. These hormones act synergistically to promote breast growth and differentiation. Abortion would interrupt this process, leaving undifferentiated structures in the breast that could render the gland susceptible to carcinogenesis [11]. Thus, by forestalling the late protective effect of differentiation by abortion, the breast is placed at a higher risk of developing cancer, especially if the abortion is performed later rather than earlier in pregnancy. Although this theory is biologically plausible, further research is required to confirm whether the recently observed increased risk of breast cancer with induced abortion performed later in pregnancy is consistently maintained.

## Conclusions

Despite intense study, the causes of breast cancer remain unknown. Based largely on animal models, it has been proposed that pregnancies that go to term have a protective effect against breast cancer because complete differentiation of cells in the breast occurs late in pregnancy, making them less susceptible to carcinogens. Consequently, an interrupted pregnancy may not confer protection and may even increase the risk because proliferation of breast cells would occur without the protective effect of subsequent differentiation.

The increasing incidence of both breast cancer and induced abortions suggests that they are causally linked. However, epidemiological evidence has failed to produce a consensus on this issue. In this paper, the evidence for causation is reviewed using several diagnostic tests. Meta-analysis and meta-regression analysis of case-control studies indicate that the relationship between induced abortions and breast cancer is statistically significant. However, the magnitude of the association is small. In contrast, there is no risk associated with spontaneous abortion. Case-control studies are fraught with bias owing to their retrospective nature. In particular, it has been determined that both recall bias and response bias are likely to result in an overestimation of the risk. Using a methodologically better approach with a cohort design, the data suggest that, overall, there is no risk of breast cancer with induced abortion. However, in a subgroup of women having abortion after 18 weeks of gestation, the risk appears to be significantly increased, but these conclusions should be interpreted cautiously because of the small number of cases from which this estimate has been derived.

## References

1. Hsieh C-C, Trichopoulos D, Katsouyanni K, Yuasa S. Age at menarche, age at menopause, height and obesity as risk factors for breast cancer: associations and interactions in an international case-control study. Int J Cancer 1990;46:796—800.
2. Brinton LA, Schairer C, Hoover RN, Fraumeni JF Jr. Menstrual factors and risk of breast cancer. Cancer Invest 1988;6:245—254.
3. Apter D, Vihko R. Early menarche, a risk factor for breast cancer, indicates early onset of ovulatory cycles. J Clin Endocrinol Metab 1983;57:82—86.

4. MacMahon BB, Trichopoulos D, Brown J, Andersen AP, Cole P, deWaard F, Kauraneiemi T, Polychronopoulou A, Ravnikar B, Stormby N, Westlund K. Age at menarche, urine estrogens and breast cancer risk. Int J Cancer 1982;30:427—431.

5. Apter D, Reinila M, Vihko R. Some endocrine characteristics of early menarche, a risk factor for breast cancer, are preserved into adulthood. Int J Cancer 1989;44:783—787.

6. Kelsey JL, Gammon MD, John EM. Reproductive factors and breast cancer. Endocrine Rev 1993;15:36—47.

7. Irwin KL, Lee NC, Peterson HB, Rubin GL, Wingo PA, Mandel MG. Hysterectomy, tubal sterilization, and the risk of breast cancer. Am J Epidemiol 1988;127:1192—1201.

8. Henderson BE, Ross RK, Judd HL, Krailo MD, Pike MC. Do regular ovulatory cycles increase breast cancer risk? Cancer 1985;56:1206—1208.

9. Bain C, Willett W, Rosner B, Speizer FE, Belanger C, Hennekens CH. Early age at first birth and decreased risk of breast cancer. Am J Epidemiol 1981;114:705—709.

10. Salber EJ, Trichopoulos D, MacMahon B. Lactation and reproductive histories of breast cancer patients in Boston 1965—66. J Natl Cancer Inst 1969;43:1013—1024.

11. Russo J, Russo IH. Susceptibility of the mammary gland to carcinogenesis. II Pregnancy interruption as a risk factor in tumor incidence. Am J Pathol 1980;100:497—512.

12. Janerich DT, Hoff MB. Evidence for a crossover in breast cancer risk factors. Am J Epidemiol 1982;116:737—742.

13. Hsieh C-C, Pavia M, Lambe M, Lan SJ, Colditz GA, Ekbom A, Adami HO, Trichopoulos D, Willett WC. Dual effect of parity on breast cancer risk. Eur J Cancer 1994;30A:969—973.

14. Segi M, Fukushima I, Fujisaku S. An epidemiological study on cancer in Japan. GANN 1957; 48(Suppl):1—63.

15. Department of Clinical Epidemiology and Biostatistics, McMaster University Health Sciences Centre: how to read clinical journals: IV To determine etiology or causation. Can Med Assoc J 1981;124:985—990.

16. Calle EE, Mervis CA, Wingo PA, Thun MJ, Rodriguez C, Health CW. Spontaneous abortion and risk of fatal breast cancer in a prospective cohort of United States women. Cancer Cause Conrol 1995;6:460—468.

17. Wilcox AJ, Horney LF. Accuracy of spontaneous abortion recall. Am J Epidemiol 1984;120: 727—733.

18. Jones EF, Forrest JD. Underreporting of abortions in surveys of US women: 1976 to 1988. Demography 1992;29:113—126.

19. Chavkin W. Topics for our times: Public health in the line — abortion and beyond. Am J Pub Health 1996;86:1204—1206.

20. Liestøl K. Menarcheal age and spontaneous abortion: a causal connection? Am J Epidemiol 1980;111:753—758.

21. Cowan LD, Gordis L, Tonascia JA, Jones GS. Breast cancer incidence in women with a history of progesterone deficiency. Am J Epidemiol 1981;114:209—217.

22. Ron E, Lunenfeld B, Menczer J, Blumstein T, Katz L, Oelsner G, Serr D. Cancer incidence in a cohort of infertile women. Am J Epidemiol 1987;125:780—790.

23. Michels KB, Willet WC. Does induced or spontaneous abortion affect the risk of breast cancer? Epidemiol 1996;7:521—528.

24. Daya S. Understanding clinical research. II Study design. J Soc Obstet Gynaecol Can 1992;14: 69—83.

25. Brind J, Chinchilli VM, Severs WB, Summy-Long J. Induced abortion as an independent risk factor for breast cancer: a comprehensive review and meta-analysis. J Epidemiol Commun Health 1996;50:481—496.

26. Melbye M, Wohlfart J, Olsen JH, Frisch M, Westergaard T, Helweg-Larsen K, Andersen PK. Induced abortion and the risk of breast cancer. N Engl J Med 1997;336:81—85.

27. Greenland S. Quantitative methods in the review of epidemiologic literature. Epidemiol Rev 1987;9:1—30.

814

28. Rookus MA, van Leeuwen FE. Induced abortion and risk for breast cancer: reporting (recall) bias in a Dutch case-control study. J Natl Cancer Inst 1996;88:1759—1764.
29. Lindefors-Harris B-M, Eklund G, Adami H-O, Meirik O. Response bias in a case-control study: analysis utilizing comparative data concerning legal abortions from two independent Swedish studies. Am J Epidemiol 1991;134:1003—1008.
30. Meirik O, Lund E, Adami H-O, Bergström R, Christoffersen T, Bergsjö P. Oral contraceptive use and breast cancer in young women. A joint national case-control study in Sweden and Norway. Lancet 1986;2:650—654.
31. Lindefors-Harris B-M, Eklund G, Meirik O, Rutqvist LE, Wiklund K. Risk of cancer of the breast after legal abortion during first trimester: a Swedish register study. Br Med J 1989;299: 1430—1432.
32. Kvåle G, Heuch I, Eide GE. A prospective study of reproductive factors and breast cancer. I. Parity. Am J Epidemiol 1987;126:831—841.
33. Sellers TA, Potter JD, Severson RK, Bostick RM, Nelson CL, Kushi LH, Folsom AR. Difficulty becoming pregnant and family history as interactive risk factors for postmenopausal breast cancer: the Iowa Women's Health Study. Cancer Cause Control 1993;4:21—28.
34. Russo J, Russo IH. Development of the human mammary gland. In: Neville MC, Daniel C (eds) The Mammary Gland. New York: Plenum, 1987;67—93.

# Ovarian cancer, infertility and infertility therapy

David L. Healy

*Monash University, Department of Obstetrics and Gynaecology, Monash Medical Centre, Melbourne, Victoria, Australia*

**Abstract.** *Cancer risks related to infertility treatment.* Appropriate evaluation of long-term health effects of infertility treatments must understand the methodological problems and difficulties encountered in this area of research. The question of whether infertility drugs are associated with an increased risk of cancer remains largely unresolved. The challenge facing epidemiologists, fertility societies and individual fertility clinics, is to conduct studies which have large enough numbers of patients with both the exposure and the outcome of interest. Key issues include selecting appropriate study populations, defining and measuring the exposures and outcomes of interest, estimating the effects of bias, and defining the role of chance in producing the findings. Australia is currently undertaking a cohort study of 30,000 patients following IVF (in vitro fertilization) and other assisted reproductive technologies. Even with a cohort of this size, only 14 cases of invasive ovarian cancer and 144 cases of breast cancer are expected from general population incidence rates. National collaborations of this type, and even international collaboration, perhaps with reanalysis or pooled original data such as that used to examine the relationship between oral-contraceptive use and breast cancer may assist in more rapid answers to these questions at an international level.

**Keywords:** infertility, infertility therapy, ovarian cancer.

## Introduction

No drug is safe when used for infertility treatment. No operation is safe when used for infertility treatment. Media allegations that drugs used in infertility treatment caused cancer in women has probably been the greatest threat to the trust between infertility couples and their doctors in the past 10 years. The crisis in infertility therapy introduced very clearly to all patients and their doctors the concept of risk and, in particular, the concept of epidemiological risk. It reinforced for many of us that no medical treatment is completely safe.

Quantitative assessment of health risks for informed consent with any medical or surgical treatment is still in its infancy. The aim of this chapter is to give our current approach in providing this information to the infertile woman. We also review current knowledge of cancer risk with drugs in infertility treatment.

## Material risk

A material risk is, in the circumstance of the particular case, a risk that a reason-

*Address for correspondence:* Prof David L. Healy, Monash University, Department of Obstetrics and Gynaecology, Level 5, Monash Medical Centre, 246 Clayton Road, Clayton, 3168 Vic, Australia.

able person in the patient's position, if warned of the risk, would be likely to attach significance to [1].

In dealing with these issues of informed consent and material risk, we have found it useful to attempt to provide infertile patients with information about their proposed medical and surgical treatments which are related to the general risks of death in community activities. For example, all infertile couples are interested in having a pregnancy and a baby. Nevertheless, even in Western democracies, there is a risk of death from pregnancy. In most developed countries this risk is about one in 14,000 in urban communities as indicated in Table 1. We found that a risk of one in 14,000 of a woman dying in pregnancy is still difficult for many infertile couples to put into context of other life risks [1].

The Perinatal Society of Australia identified in 1995 (Table 1) that even normal couples have a risk of miscarriage of about one in seven in the general community [2]. Quite clearly, some infertile couples will have a significantly higher risk than this. Nevertheless, a risk of one in seven is understandable by most infertile patients. The risk of preterm birth, again in the general community, is about one in 15. It surprises many patients in Australia to know that the rate of notifiable birth defect in the Australian community is one in 20, as indicated by the Royal Australian College of Paediatricians. Although the risk of any couple having a baby with cerebral palsy is one in 400, most infertile couples are relieved to know that their risks are so low, and that, conversely, they have 399 chances out of 400 of having a baby without cerebral palsy [3].

A similar approach can be taken to a woman's lifetime risk of developing of cancer. In industrialized societies, the lifetime risk of the development of breast cancer is about one in 14. In women aged 50 years, with no known family history, the chance of the development of breast carcinoma over the next 12 months is about one in 500. Ovarian carcinoma will occur in about one woman in 90 in our general community. Once again, it is possible to put such risks into some sort of general community reference as indicated in Table 2. The Australian Bureau of Statistics data indicate that a fit and health 40-year-old woman has a one in 1,000 chance of dying within the next year. At 50 years of age, this risk is one in 500 in 1 year, and at 60 years of age the risk is one in 170.

Risks associated with ovulation-induction treatment, laparoscopy and various

*Table 1.* Information sheet of risks for pregnancy for an infertile couple.

| Event | Material risk |
| --- | --- |
| Miscarriage | 1 in 7 |
| Premature birth | 1 in 15 |
| Birth defect in the baby | 1 in 20 |
| Death of the baby | 1 in 100 |
| Cerebral palsy in the baby | 1 in 400 |
| Death of the mother | 1 in 14000 |

Adapted from Medical Journal of Australia 1995;162;86—91 [3].

*Table 2.* Material risks related to a woman's age.

| Activity | Chance of death in 1 year |
| --- | --- |
| Fit and healthy at 40 years | 1 in 1000 |
| Fit and healthy at 50 years | 1 in 500 |
| Fit and healthy at 60 years | 1 in 170 |

Adapted from the Australian Bureau of Statistics.

IVF-related procedures can also be addressed in this general matter [4]. Table 3 indicates some of those risks; we incorporated these into the general risks of death from a range of community and personal activities which most of use have undertaken at some time or another. We provide such a Material Risk Information Sheet to our infertile patients. Many are greatly relieved to know that risk of death from laparoscopy or related procedures is so low! Most are amazed to learn that sexual intercourse can actually kill a woman from subsequent acute pelvic inflammatory disease!

**The material risk of cancer**

The use of fertility drugs in women with ovulation disorders has held an important place in infertility treatment for 30 years [5–7]. The aim is to stimulate the production of a limited number of oocytes, preferably one per cycle. However, the use of fertility drugs with assisted conception such as IVF and gamete intra-fallopian transfer (GIFT) is different. In IVF, combinations and different dosages of fertility drugs are given to stimulate production of multiple oocytes to improve

*Table 3.* Material risks with various events and community activities.

| Activity | Chance of death in 1 year |
| --- | --- |
| Motor cycling | 1 in 1000 |
| Hysterectomy | 1 in 1600 |
| Driving a car | 1 in 6000 |
| Power boating | 1 in 6000 |
| Rock climbing | 1 in 7500 |
| Continuing pregnancy | 1 in 14000 |
| Playing football | 1 in 25000 |
| Laparoscopy | 1 in 67000 |
| Canoeing | 1 in 100000 |
| Having sexual intercourse (PID) | 1 in 100000 |
| RU486 use | 1 in 200000 |
| Using tampons | 1 in 300000 |
| Legal termination of pregnancy: < 9 weeks | 1 in 500000 |
| Jumbo jet flight | 1 in 2000000 |

Adapted from [4] and Australian Bureau Statistics.

the chances of fertilization in any given treatment cycle [8].

Two important studies suggested an association between exposure to fertility drugs and an increased risk of ovarian cancer. A pooled analysis of three case-controlled studies showed an odds ratio (OR) of 2.8 (95% CI 1.3—6.1) for ovarian cancer in infertile women treated with fertility drugs compared with women with no diagnosis of infertility or fertility drug treatment [9]. In 1994, Rossing and colleagues [10], using record linkage with a population-based cancer registry, identified an increased incidence of ovarian cancer (invasive or borderline malignant tumors) with a standardized incidence rate (SIR) of 2.5, (95% CI 1.3—4.5) in a cohort of infertile women compared with age standardized general population rates. An increased relative risk (RR = 11.1, 95% CI 1.5—82.3) was also found in women, with or without ovarian abnormalities, who had been treated with the fertility drug clomiphene citrate for more than 1 year compared with infertile women who had not taken the drug.

Studies of cancer after infertility and infertility treatment are difficult to undertake. A common problem is the limitations placed upon the conclusions of the study by low statistical power. Other problems are the difficulties in distinguishing possible effects of fertility drug exposure from the underlying ovulation disorder they were used to treat. Important contributions in this area were the publications of Ron and colleagues, Brinton and associates and Gammon and Thompson [11—13].

More recently, Shushan and associates (1996) [14] undertook a case-controlled study of ovarian cancer by examining self-reported fertility drug use in 200 women with epithelial ovarian tumors. Invasive ovarian malignancy was present in 164 patients, and 36 had borderline ovarian cancers. There were 408 controls. They found no significant association between fertility drug use and epithelial ovarian tumors (OR = 1.31, 95% CI 0.63—2.74). Fertility drug use was significantly associated with borderline tumors in this study (OR = 3.52, 95% CI 1.23—10.29). The strongest association was seen in women who had used human menopausal gonadotrophins (OR = 9.38, 95% CI 1.66—52.08). This study shows the difficulties, strengths and weaknesses of these methods in trying to provide the best data about risks from the use of drugs in infertility treatment. For example, women who had died of ovarian cancer were not included in this study. Their families were not approached. Such studies were further limited by the lack of verification of medical records of fertility drug use.

At Monash, we have taken a different approach with a cohort study [15]. Since ovulation disorders are not in themselves an indication for IVF, and because most patients exposed to ovarian stimulation for IVF have normal ovulatory cycles, studies of cancer incidence after IVF enable any effect of fertility drug exposure to be distinguished from underlying ovulation disorders. We studied a cohort of women who were referred for IVF to examine whether exposure to fertility drugs to induce multiple folliculogenesis was associated with an increased cancer rate.

Our cohort was 10,358 women registered with the Monash IVF program in

Melbourne, Australia. To be eligible for the study, patients were known to have been treated or referred for IVF treatment. They were normally resident in Australia at the time of registration with a known date of birth or age and a known time of entry into the cohort between 1 June 1978 and 31 December 1992. Women resident outside the state of Victoria (11.9% of the cohort) were included if their date of entry was up to 31 December 1 year before the end of complete data collection for their state's cancer registry. From 11,129 women identified as being treated or referred for IVF in the time period, 771 were excluded because of overseas residence, unknown date of birth, unknown age or unknown date of entry into the cohort.

### Data collection

Data were retrieved from computerized records kept by Monash IVF from August 1990 onwards. Data for patients who registered or were treated before that time were retrieved manually from medical histories or registration forms kept by the clinic. Data items collected included: name and date of birth, husband's name, address, type of infertility, date of registration (unexposed), date of first stimulated treatment cycle (exposed), and total number of stimulated treatment cycles (exposed). Infertility was classified as tubal, male factor, endometriosis, ovarian disorders (ovulation disorders, polycystic ovary syndrome, donor egg recipients for premature menopause, and oophorectomy), unexplained, or other (cervical factors, other uterine abnormalities, donor egg recipients for genetic disease, and altruistic egg donors). Women could be included in more than one cause-of-infertility group, however, unexplained infertility was a unique classification.

### Exposure ascertainment

Women who had had one or more IVF treatment cycles with ovarian stimulation to induce multiple folliculogenesis were allocated to the exposed group (n = 5,564), including women who had started but not completed a stimulated IVF cycle. The drug regimens used for ovarian stimulation were similar to those used in other IVF programs around the world. Until 1987 most stimulated IVF cycles used clomiphene citrate in combination with human menopausal gonadotrophins (HMG) to induce multiple folliculogenesis, followed by human chorionic gonadotrophin (HCG) for oocyte maturation before retrieval. From 1987 the gonadotrophin-releasing hormone (GnRH) agonists leuprolide and buserelin were introduced to replace clomiphene and to prevent untimely surges of luteinizing hormone. From 1990 to 1992 the main drug regimen was a GnRH agonist in combination with HMG or follicle stimulating hormone followed by HCG. With this regimen oocytes retrieved per stimulated cycle averaged nine; with clomiphene-HMG-HCG the average had been six.

Information on fertility drug exposures outside the Monash IVF program was not available, except for those women who had also attended the other major IVF program in Victoria at the Royal Women's Hospital and Melbourne IVF clinic (RWH/Melbourne IVF). The two Victorian programs were the first to be established in Australia and have provided most IVF services to women in the state. Record linkage showed that 414 women had registered with both programs, and data were adjusted to include exposure to stimulated cycles on the RWH/Melbourne IVF program. The number of women who attended Monash IVF and other Australian IVF programs was not known, but was expected to be small. Exposure to fertility drugs outside IVF programs was also not known but was expected to have occurred for only those women in the cohort who had ovulation disorders and who might have had prior exposure to conventional ovulation induction.

Women in the unexposed group (4,794) were those who had registered for IVF but had not received treatment (93.4%) or who had "natural cycle" treatment only, without ovarian stimulation (6.6%). Women who did not receive treatment withdrew of their own accord. Their reasons were not usually recorded, but included: pregnancy while on the waiting list, other treatment options pursued (e.g., tubal surgery), financial or relationship difficulties, and change of mind due to perceived discomforts and risks or other personal reasons.

**Follow up and case ascertainment**

Ascertainment of cancer cases was by record linkage with the population-based Victorian Cancer Registry (VCR) for Victorian residents (88.1% of the cohort) and the National Cancer Statistics Clearing House (NCSCH), which compiles data from all Australian state cancer registries, for residents of other states. Data collection at the VCR was complete from 1982 to the end of 1993, with over 90% notification between 1978 and 1982 from the major Victorian hospitals. The NCSCH had complete data from 1982 to the end of 1988–93, depending on the state. Follow up was from the time each woman entered the cohort until 31 December for the year of complete cancer data for her state of residence. All women had at least 1 year of follow up. Cancers of all types were identified from the VCR for Victorian residents, and invasive breast cancers (ICD-9 code 1740–1749) and ovarian cancers (ICD-9 code 1830) from the NCSCH for residents of other States.

Attempts were made to locate women to do a sensitivity analysis of the possible effect of loss to follow up. Loss to follow up was expected to occur mainly due to name change and migration. There was no contact with women in the study. Location searches were based on woman's name, husband's name and last known address, used 1993 Australian electoral roll listings on microfiche and electronic telephone listings. The electoral roll has compulsory enrolment for Australian citizens aged 18 or over.

## Statistical methods

Expected numbers of cancers were calculated from the person-years in exposed and unexposed groups assuming the age specific rates for the Victorian female population 1982—91. From these it was estimated that the study had 80% power at the 5% level, to detect SIRs of 1.7 for breast cancer in both exposed and unexposed groups and an SIR of 4.0 for ovarian cancer in both groups. The study had also had 80% power at the 5% level to detect an RR of 2.15 for breast cancer in the exposed group and an RR of 5.05 for ovarian cancer.

All women registered in cohort were included for the SIR estimation of breast and ovarian cancer risk. For analysis of other cancers, only those women whose original address was Victoria were included, since linkage was not made with other than Victorian registries for those cancers. Sensitivity analyses for the SIRs estimated were performed for breast and ovarian cancers. Using only those women who were located in a 1993 address or who had died from cancer (and an adjustment to the denominator to account for the number of women expected to have died from all causes) an upper limit of association was estimated. To allow for a possible latency period, further SIR estimates were made using only those women with at least 5 years follow up.

The proportional hazards models, including age at diagnosis or (censored) time to end of follow up and type of infertility as covariates, were fitted to estimate the relative risk for the exposed group for various cancers. Relative risks were also estimated for each type of infertility, with absence of that type of infertility as the reference group.

The DATAB and PEANUTS modules of the EPICURE software package were used for the SIR and RR calculation.

## Results

The median age at entry into the cohort was 32 for the exposed group (range 18—49) and 31 for the unexposed group (19—51). At the end of follow up, the median age was 38 (21—57) in the exposed group and 38 (22—59) in the unexposed group. The median length of follow up for the exposed group (5.2 (range 1—15.1)) was less than that in the unexposed group (7.6 (1—15.5)). More women in the unexposed group entered the cohort in the earlier years when waiting times for IVF treatment were as long as 3 years. The figure shows the person-years distribution by age group for women in the exposed and unexposed groups. The total person-years contributed was 31,272 for the exposed group and 33,655 for the unexposed group.

### Standardized incidence rate

Table 4 shows the observed number of cases identified, the expected number, and SIR estimates for the exposed group, the unexposed, and both groups combined.

Table 4. Observed and expected cases, SIRs and confidence intervals by cancer and exposure to IVF treatment.

| Cancer | ICD-9 code | Exposed | | | | Unexposed | | | | Combined | | | |
|---|---|---|---|---|---|---|---|---|---|---|---|---|---|
| | | Obs | Exp | SIR | 95% CI | Obs | Exp | SIR | 95% CI | Obs | Exp | SIR | 95% CI |
| Breast | 1740-1749 | 16 | 17.90 | 0.89 | 0.55-1.46 | 18[a] | 18.29 | 0.98 | 0.62-1.56 | 34 | 36.19 | 0.94 | 0.67-1.31 |
| Ovarian | 1830 | 3 | 1.77 | 1.70 | 0.55-5.27 | 3 | 1.85 | 1.62 | 0.52-5.02 | 6 | 3.62 | 1.66 | 0.75-3.69 |
| Body of uterus | 1820-1828 | 2 | 0.90 | 2.22 | 0.55-8.87 | 3 | 0.86 | 3.48 | 1.12-10.8 | 5 | 1.76 | 2.84 | 1.18-1.75 |
| Melanoma | 1720-1729 | 7 | 7.36 | 0.95 | 0.45-1.99 | 9 | 7.55 | 1.19 | 0.62-2.29 | 16 | 14.92 | 1.07 | 0.66-1.75 |
| Colorectal | 1530-1549 | 1 | 2.75 | 0.36 | 0.05-2.58 | 3 | 2.66 | 1.13 | 0.36-3.50 | 4 | 5.41 | 0.74 | 0.28-1.97 |
| Cervix | 1800-1809 | 5 | 5.03 | 0.99 | 0.41-2.39 | 1 | 5.16 | 0.19 | 0.03-1.38 | 6 | 10.19 | 0.59 | 0.26-1.31 |
| Other[b] | | 8 | 8.79 | 0.91 | 0.45-1.82 | 12 | 7.87 | 1.53 | 0.87-2.69 | 20 | 16.66 | 1.20 | 0.77-1.86 |
| All cancers[c] | 1400-2089 | 42 | 44.51 | 0.94 | 0.70-1.28 | 48 | 44.24 | 1.08 | 0.82-1.44 | 90 | 88.75 | 1.01 | 0.82-1.25 |
| CIS cervix | 2331 | 18 | 30.52 | 0.59 | 0.37-0.94 | 16 | 33.99 | 0.47 | 0.29-0.77 | 34 | 64.51 | 0.53 | 0.38-0.74 |

Sensitivity analysis

Including only women located in electoral roll, electronic telephone directory, or who had died

| Cancer | ICD-9 code | Obs | Exp | SIR | 95% CI | Obs | Exp | SIR | 95% CI | Obs | Exp | SIR | 95% CI |
|---|---|---|---|---|---|---|---|---|---|---|---|---|---|
| Breast | 1740-1749 | 13 | 13.53 | 0.96 | 0.56-1.65 | 13 | 11.51 | 1.13 | 0.66-1.95 | 26 | 25.04 | 1.04 | 0.71-1.53 |
| Ovarian | 1830 | 3 | 1.34 | 2.25 | 0.72-6.97 | 2 | 1.17 | 1.72 | 0.43-6.86 | 5 | 2.50 | 2.00 | 0.83-4.80 |

Including only women with at least 5 years follow up

| Cancer | ICD-9 code | Obs | Exp | SIR | 95% CI | Obs | Exp | SIR | 95% CI | Obs | Exp | SIR | 95% CI |
|---|---|---|---|---|---|---|---|---|---|---|---|---|---|
| Breast | 1740-1749 | 12 | 14.46 | 0.83 | 0.47-1.46 | 15 | 16.99 | 0.88 | 0.53-1.46 | 27 | 31.45 | 0.86 | 0.59-1.25 |
| Ovarian | 1830 | 3 | 1.40 | 2.14 | 0.69-6.63 | 3 | 1.71 | 1.75 | 0.57-5.44 | 6 | 3.11 | 1.93 | 0.87-4.29 |

[a]1 Breast cancer case not resident in Victoria, therefore, not included in "all" cancer category, see methods, follow up, and case ascertainment. [b]Other cancers not including those above or CIS. [c]Sum of above.

There was no evidence of an increase in breast cancer incidence in the exposed or unexposed groups compared with the female population of Victoria. The median time to diagnosis from time of registration (unexposed) or first-stimulated treatment cycle (exposed) was 3.5 years (range 0.7—6.7) for the exposed group, and 4.7 (0.8—11.0) years for the unexposed group. The median time between the last stimulated cycle and diagnosis for the exposed group was 3.1 (0.1—5.3) years. The median age at diagnosis was 39.7 (33—49) for the unexposed group. Seven women were known to have died.

Invasive ovarian cancer occurred in six women (three exposed, three unexposed). SIR estimates suggested an increased incidence of ovarian cancer in the cohort, irrespective of exposure status, which was not significant. The ovarian tumors were serous and mucinous adenocarcinomas. Women were aged 28—42 at diagnosis and three were known to have died. The times to diagnosis were 3.4, 6.6, 7.5 years in the exposed group and 1.9, 6.5, and 7.6 years in the unexposed group. Three additional ovarian tumors (ICD-9 code 2362) were identified (two exposed, one unexposed) and all were mature cystic teratomas, which were benign. The times to diagnosis were 0.7 and 2.4 years in the exposed group and 0.2 years in the unexposed group. Combining invasive ovarian cancers and mature cystic teratomas gave SIR estimates of 2.17 (0.90—5.20) for the exposed group, 1.65 (0.62—4.39) for the unexposed group, and 1.90 (0.99—3.65) for the groups combined. No borderline ovarian tumors were identified.

The incidence of other cancers identified in the VCR (Table 4) showed an increased incidence of cancer of the body of the uterus (ICD-9 code 182), irrespective of exposure status, with an SIR for the groups combined of 2.84 (1.18—6.81). Of the five tumors, four were endometrial adenocarcinomas and one (unexposed to IVF treatment) was leiomyosarcoma. It was not possible to obtain morphology-specific population cancer rates for these two types of uterine cancer. Removal of the leiomyosarcoma gave an SIR of 2.27 (0.85—6.04) which was not significant. The times to diagnosis were 0.7 and 3.4 years in the exposed group and 0.1, 2.1, and 9.2 years in the unexposed group. Women were aged 35—48 at diagnosis. Melanomas and colorectal cancer (the most common cancers in Victorian women after breast cancer) showed similar incidence to the general population. The incidence of invasive cervical cancer and that of all cancers (excluding in situ cancers) in the exposed and unexposed groups was found to be not significantly different from age-standardized general population rates. However, the incidence of carcinoma in situ of the cervix was significantly less in both the exposed and unexposed groups than in the general population (SIR for groups combined 0.53 (0.38—0.74)).

**Exposure dosage: number of stimulated IVF treatment cycles**

Table 5 shows, for the exposed group, the distribution of the number of stimulated cycles and the cancer incidence. The median number of cycles with ovarian stimulation was two (range 1—22). Seventy-seven percent of women had three or

*Table 5.* Distribution of exposed group and incident cancers in that number of IVF cycles.

| | Number of IVF cycles | | | | | | | |
| | 1 | 2 | 3 | 4 | 5 | 6 | 7 | 8+ |
|---|---|---|---|---|---|---|---|---|
| | 2052 (37%)[a] | 1362 (24%) | 869 (16%) | 469 (8%) | 299 (5%) | 191 (3%) | 122 (2%) | 200 (4%) |
| Breast | 6[b] | 5 | 2 | 2 | | 1 | | |
| Ovarian | 1 | 1 | | | 1 | | | |
| Other | 10 | 10 | 1 | 1 | | 1 | | 1 |
| All cancers | 17 | 16 | 3 | 3 | 1 | 2 | 0 | 1 |

[a]Number exposed (% of total exposed); [b]number of cancers, excluding CIS.

fewer stimulated cycles; 1.9% (104 women) had 10 or more cycles. 74% of incident cancers occurred in women having only one or two stimulated cycles. There was no apparent increase in risk associated with level of exposure to stimulated treatment cycles. For breast cancer the SIR was 1.02 (0.46—2.27) for women exposed to one stimulated cycle, and 0.83 (0.45—1.55) for women exposed to more than one. For all cancers these SIRs were 1.13 (0.69—1.84) and 0.86 (0.58—1.26), respectively. There was no evidence for a trend effect with dose ($\chi^2$ = 0.5 for breast cancer and 0.8 for all cancers). Other cancers had too few numbers for a dose effect to be studied.

## Type of infertility

Infertility for both groups was classified as tubal 43.4%, male factor 23.2%, endometriosis 13.2%, ovarian disorders 6.2%, unexplained infertility 18.7%, and other causes 3.5%. Information on type of infertility was missing for 8.4% of women in the cohort. Some women had more than one type of infertility recorded, but unexplained and missing were unique classifications. Table 6 shows the distribution of type of infertility by breast cancer incidence and exposure status, and, for the groups combined the SIR and 95% CI. There was no association between infertility type and breast cancer or exposure to IVF. None of the women with ovarian cancer were recorded as having ovarian disorders as their cause of infertility. For both ovarian and body of the uterus cancers an unexpectedly high number of women had unexplained infertility recorded. For those with unexplained infertility, the SIR for ovarian cancer was 6.98 (2.90—16.7) and for cancer of the body of the uterus 8.30 (2.77—25.7).

## Adjusted RR assessment

Cancers of the breast, ovary, body of the uterus and all cancers combined were not associated with exposure to stimulated IVF cycles. The RRs of these four cancer groups, estimated by proportional hazards modelling and adjusting for

*Table 6.* Observed and expected and SIRs for combined groups by certain cancers by type of infertility.

| Site and type of infertility | Observed | | | Expected | SIR | CI 95% |
|---|---|---|---|---|---|---|
| | Exposed | Un-exposed | Com-bined | | | |
| **Breast cancer** | | | | | | |
| Tubal | 6 | 7 | 13 | 19.28 | 0.67 | 0.39—1.16 |
| Male factor | 3 | 8 | 7 | 6.57 | 1.06 | 0.51—2.23 |
| Endometriosis | 2 | 0 | 2 | 3.99 | 0.50 | 0.13—2.00 |
| Ovarian disorders | 1 | 2 | 3 | 1.66 | 1.81 | 0.58—5.60 |
| Unexplained | 2 | 4 | 6 | 7.16 | 0.84 | 0.38—1.87 |
| Other | 0 | 0 | 0 | 0.48 | 0.00 | — |
| Missing | 1 | 2 | 3 | 1.86 | 1.62 | 0.52—5.01 |
| **Ovarian cancer** | | | | | | |
| Ovarian disorders | 0 | 0 | 0 | 0.17 | 0.00 | — |
| Unexplained | 3 | 2 | 5 | 0.72 | 6.98 | 2.90—16.8 |
| **Cancer of body of uterus** | | | | | | |
| Ovarian disorders | 0 | 0 | 0 | 0.08 | 0.00 | — |
| Unexplained | 1 | 2 | 3 | 0.36 | 8.30 | 2.68—25.7 |
| **All cancers** | | | | | | |
| Ovarian disorders | 1 | 4 | 5 | 4.19 | 1.19 | 0.50—2.86 |
| Unexplained | 12 | 12 | 24 | 18.10 | 1.33 | 0.89—1.98 |

*Table 7.* For various cancers, shown are: relative risk estimates for IVF exposure adjusted for age and infertility type, and relative risk estimates for unexplained infertility vs. known causes of infertility, and adjusted for age and IVF exposure.

| | RR adj | 95%CI | p |
|---|---|---|---|
| **Breast cancer** | | | |
| IVF exposure | 1.11 | 0.56—2.20 | 0.8 |
| Unexplained infertility | 0.77 | 0.19—3.10 | 0.07 |
| **Ovarian cancer** | | | |
| IVF exposure | 1.45 | 0.28—7.55 | 0.7 |
| Unexplained infertility | 19.19 | 2.23—165 | 0.007 |
| **Cancer of body of uterus** | | | |
| IVF exposure | 0.65 | 0.11—3.94 | 0.6 |
| Unexplained infertility | 6.34 | 1.06—38.0 | 0.04 |
| **All cancers** | | | |
| IVF exposure | 0.96 | 0.62—1.47 | 0.8 |
| Unexplained infertility | 2.01 | 0.84—4.78 | 0.11 |

age at diagnosis or end of follow up (depending on disease status) and infertility type, were 1.11 (0.56—2.20), 1.45 (0.26—7.55), 0.65 (0.11—3.94), and 0.96 (0.62—1.47), respectively (Table 7). Also shown are RRs adjusted for exposure, of unexplained infertility (with all other types of infertility as the reference group). For ovarian and body of the uterus cancers the effect of unexplained infertility was independent of exposure status and gave significant adjusted RRs of 19.19 (2.23—165, p = 0.0007) and 6.34 (1.06—38, p = 0.04), respectively.

### Cancers diagnosed before cohort entry

Ninety-eight tumors (invasive cancers, mature cystic teratomas, and CIS of the cervix), identified by record linkage with the VCR, had been diagnosed before the women registered or received IVF treatment (58 exposed, 40 unexposed). These included two breast cancers, four mature cystic teratomas, and four invasive cervical cancers, with equal numbers of each cancer in the exposed and unexposed groups. There were no prior cancers of the body of the uterus. There were 64 prior diagnoses of CIS of the cervix (42 exposed, 22 unexposed, compared with the expected 41 and 23, respectively).

There was one case of Hodgkin's lymphoma in the exposed group and four in the unexposed group and there were two cases of chronic myeloid leukaemia in the unexposed group. For five of these six women, treatment had caused ovarian failure and infertility, as noted in their clinic records.

### Sensitivity analyses

Analysis based on only those women who were located in 1993 (79% of exposed group and 66% of the unexposed) gave estimates of SIRs for breast cancer of 0.96 (0.56—1.65) for the exposed group and 1.13 (0.66—1.95) for the unexposed. For invasive ovarian cancer SIRs were 2.25 (0.72—6.97) exposed, and 1.72 (0.43—6.86) unexposed. The adjusted RRs calculated from the located cohort were 1.06 (0.48—2.31) for breast cancer in the exposed group relative to the unexposed group, and 2.09 (0.33—13.2) for ovarian cancer. A further sensitivity analysis, which included only women with at least 5 years follow up (51% of exposed group and 78% of the unexposed group) gave SIRs for breast cancer in the exposed group of 0.83 (0.47—1.46) and in the unexposed group 0.88 (0.53—1.48). For ovarian cancer the SIRs were 2.14 (0.69—6.63) and 1.75 (0.57—5.44), respectively (Table 4). The adjustment RR for breast cancer was 1.27 (0.58—2.77) and for ovarian it was 1.81 (0.35—9.70).

### Conclusions and future directions

Our results showed that the incidence of breast cancer in women who have had IVF treatment with ovarian stimulation was no different from the incidence in women referred for IVF but not treated. The incidence in breast cancer in women who have had infertility was also no different than the incidence of this malignancy in the general population.

This cohort study showed the limitations of this type of epidemiological approach. Our study had limited power to detect differences in the incidence of gynecological cancers. It did suggest that the incidence of cancer of the body of the uterus appeared significantly higher, irrespective of whether IVF treatment was undertaken or not. An increased risk of endometrial adenocarcinoma has been associated with the unopposed action of estrogens, postmenopausal status, obesity, polycystic ovary syndrome and nulliparity.

We found that the incidence of ovarian cancer in the cohort was higher than that in the general population. However, this increase was not significant. Once again, the findings were limited by the low power of the study and the rarity of ovarian cancer in this age group. In contrast to Rossing and colleagues, we found no evidence to suggest an increased risk of borderline ovarian tumors associated with exposure to fertility drugs.

An unexpected finding from our study was the significant association between unexplained infertility and both invasive ovarian cancer as well as invasive cancer of the body of the uterus. This was independent of exposure status (Tables 6 and 7). It is unlikely that early cancer was a cause of infertility for women in our exposed group with unexplained infertility, since endometrial sampling was common practice in the diagnostic work up and all cancers were diagnosed at least 3 years after the first IVF treatment.

Our study also showed a reduced incidence of in situ and invasive carcinoma of the cervix. This finding has subsequently been confirmed by Rossing and colleagues (1996) [16]. These authors studied the incidence of cancer in a cohort of 3,837 women evaluated for infertility between 1974 and 1985 in Seattle, USA. The incidence of cancer was determined by record linkage with a population-based cancer registry. The incidence of in situ and invasive carcinoma of the cervix was less than expected (36 cases observed, 67 expected) giving a standardized incidence ratio of 0.5 (95% CI 0.4–0.7). Women with tubal causes of infertility had relatively more cervical carcinoma than women with other causes. By contrast, we did not observe a relatively increased incidence in women with tubal infertility. We suggested that the higher levels of screening for cervical abnormalities in the infertile women may account for the lower incidence of cervical carcinoma observed.

An Australian multicenter study of cancer after infertility and IVF is currently being undertaken. Our study will allow for larger numbers of patients (approximately 30,000) as well as a longer latency effect between exposure to fertility drugs and the possible later development of cancer. This study shall also include a nested case control study. We hope to contact patients who may have developed cancer, or their relatives, after infertility or IVF treatment.

## References

1. Healy DL, Petrucco O. Effective Gynaecological Day Surgery. London: Thompson Scientific, 1998.
2. Consensus statement: Cerebral Palsy.
3. Med J Austr 1995;162:86—91.
4. Hatcher RD, Stewart F, Trusell J et al. Contraceptive Technology. New York: Irvington, 1990—1992.
5. McDougall MJ, Tan SL, Jacobs HS. In vitro fertilisation and the ovarian hyperstimulation syndrome. Hum Reprod 1992;7:597—600.
6. McClure N, Healy DL, Rogers PAW, Sullivan J, Beaton L, Heaning RV, Connelly DT, Robertson DM. Vascular endothelian growth factor as capillary permeability agent in ovarian hyperstimulation syndrome. Lancet 1994;344:235—236.
7. Healy DL, Trounson AO, Andersen AN. Female Infertility: pathogenesis and management. Lancet 1994;343:1539—1544.
8. Trounson AO, Leeton JF, Wood EC, Webb J, Wood J. Pregnancies in humans by fertilisation in vitro and embryo transfer in the controlled ovulatory cycle. Science 1981;212:616—619.
9. Whittemore A, Harris R, Itnyre J, the Collaborative Ovarian Cancer Group. Characteristics related to ovarian cancer risk; collaborative analysis of 12 US case-control studies. II: Invasive epithelial cancer in white women. Am J Epidemiol 1992;136:1184—1203.
10. Rossing MA, Daling JR, Weiss NS, Moore DE, Self SG. Ovarian tumors in a cohort of infertile women. N Engl J Med 1994;331:771—776.
11. Ron E, Lunenfeld B, Menczer J. Cancer incidence in a cohort of infertile women. Am J Epidemiol 1987;125:780—790.
12. Brinton LA, Melton J, Malkasian GD, Bond A, Hoover R. Cancer risk after evaluation for infertility. Am J Epidemiol 1989;129:712—722.
13. Gammon MD, Thompson WD. Infertility and breast cancer; a population-based case-controlled study. Am J Epidemiol 1990;132:708—716.
14. Shushan A, Paltiel O, Oiscovich J, Elchalal U, Peretz T, Schenker JG. Human menopausal gonadotrophin and the risk of epithelial ovarian cancer. Fertil Steril 1996;65:13—18.
15. Venn A, Watson L, Lumley J, Giles G, King C, Healy DL. Breast and ovarian cancer incidence after infertility and in vitro fertilisation. Lancet 1995;346:995—1000.
16. Rossing MA, Daling JR, Weiss NS, Moore DE, Self SG. In situ and invasive cervical carcinoma in a cohort of infertile women. Fertil Steril 1996;65:19—22.

# Polycystic ovary syndrome: medical implications and cardiovascular complications

Daniela Jakubowicz

*Hospital de Clinicas Caracas, Department of Endocrinology and Reproductive Medicine, Caracas, Venezuela*

**Abstract.** It is becoming clearer that women with polycystic ovary syndrome (PCOS) commonly have associated insulin resistance accompanied by compensatory hyperinsulinemia. It also seems likely that this pathophysiological pattern begins to translate into complications ranging from cosmetic concerns to hypertension, dislypidemia, premature atherosclerosis, cardiovascular disease (CVD), non-insulin-dependent diabetes mellitus (NIDDM) and cancer.

The increasing knowledge that the metabolic consequences of PCOS can potentially end in premature cardiovascular disease has shifted the clinical focus from a short-term and symptom-driven method to a recognition that these conditions are chronic with long-term complications. It is therefore reasonable to assume that interventions that reduce circulating insulin levels in women with PCOS by diet and or adjuvant therapy with "insulin sensitizing" agents should decrease serum androgens and, perhaps beneficially influence reproductive function. Moreover, insulin-sensitizing agents have the added theoretical advantage of perhaps favorably affecting those complications of PCOS, which may be attributable in part to hyperinsulinemic insulin resistance — namely glucose intolerance, dyslipidemia, hypertension, atherosclerosis, NIDDM and CVD.

This article will review: 1) evidence of the presence hyperinsulinemia in PCOS; 2) the effects of hyperinsulinemia on ovarian androgens; 3) short- and long-term medical complications, namely obesity, NIDDM, gestational diabetes mellitus, dyslipidemia, impaired fibrinolytic system, hypertension and coronary artery disease; and 4) therapeutic considerations.

**Keywords:** cardiovascular disease (CVD), non-insulin-dependent diabetes mellitus (NIDDM), polycystic ovary syndrome (PCOS).

## Introduction

Polycystic ovary syndrome (PCOS) is the most common endocrine disorder affecting up of 15% of women of reproductive age. It is a heterogeneous clinical entity that is defined as the association of hyperandrogenism with chronic anovulation, abnormal gonadotropin concentration, enlarged cystic ovaries and obesity [1,2]. The syndrome is responsible for over 73% of cases of anovulatory infertility and at least 85% of women with hirsutism [3]. The fact is that up to 75% of women with secondary amenorrhea will fulfill diagnostic criteria for PCOS [4].

There is now increasing evidence that PCOS is followed not only by several psychological and physical android characteristics, but also by the risk of devel-

*Address for correspondence:* Dr Daniela Jakubowicz, P.O. Box 025323, Miami FL 33102-5323, USA.
E-mail: jak@ccs.internet.ve

oping glucose intolerance, dyslipidemia, hypertension, and premature athero-sclerosis, (CVD) and (NIDDM) [5—8].

## Hyperinsulinemia in PCOS

It has been recognized that women with PCOS have a greater frequency and degree of insulin resistance [8] and compensatory hyperinsulinemia [9], and increasing evidence suggests that hyperinsulinemia plays an important role in the pathogenesis of PCOS and may have important implications for long-term health [10]. Both lean and obese women with PCOS have shown to be more insulin-resistant than controls, and that this difference was even more dramatic when there is an interaction between obesity and the syndrome [11].

Burghen, Givens and colleagues noted in 1980 [12] that PCOS was associated with hyperinsulinemia, basally and during an oral glucose tolerance test, compared with appropriately age- and weight-matched control women [12]. After this report, the presence of hyperinsulinemia in PCOS was confirmed by many other studies and now is a general consensus that most of women with PCOS are insulin resistant [1,2,10,13].

It has been also found that obese PCOS women had significantly increased glucose levels during an oral glucose tolerance test compared with age- and weight-matched control women [9,12,14] and a substantial decrease by 35—40% in insulin-mediated glucose disposal (IMGD) has been observed in both lean and obese PCOS women [14]. This decrease in IMGD is of a similar magnitude to that seen in NIDDM, and correlates with the presence of peripheral insulin resistance and with the increased insulin secretion by β-cells in a compensatory fashion [14]. Family studies have shown that some first-degree relatives of PCOS women are insulin resistant or NIDDM including brothers, suggesting that insulin resistance is a genetic defect in PCOS [15]. Insulin resistance appears to be feature of PCOS in women of many racial and ethnic groups including Japanese, Caribbean and Mexican Hispanics, non-Hispanic Whites, and African Americans [16].

Many women with PCOS are obese (50—80%) and it seems likely that obesity, which itself induces insulin resistance and hyperinsulinemia, contributes to the development of PCOS in some women, adding an obesity-specific form of insulin resistance, on to the pre-existing insulin resistance that is unique to PCOS [10,17].

## Effects of hyperinsulinemia on ovarian androgens

Several lines of evidence suggests that hyperinsulinemia precedes and is causative to the hyperandrogenism in PCOS rather than vice versa [1,2,14,18].

Burghen and Givens at al. in 1980 noted a significant positive linear correlation between insulin and androgen levels and suggested that this might have etiological significance [12]. Insulin appears to affect androgen secretion and metabolism by direct stimulation of its own receptor in the ovary [19,20], and is highly correlated with testosterone in obese and nonobese patients with PCOS as is the correlation of insulin with ovarian vein testosterone levels (r = 0.88) [21].

No changes in insulin resistance were observed in studies in which androgen levels have been significantly suppressed using gonadotropin-releasing hormone analogues (GnRHa), suggesting that the insulin resistance is adequate and fundamental to the androgen excess [22].

In contrast, studies of PCOS women in which insulin levels have been lowered with agents that either decrease insulin secretion, diazoxide [23] or somatostatin [24], or that improve insulin sensitivity: metformin [25] or troglitazone [26], resulted in a significant decrease of circulating androgen levels.

Recently we reported [25] that hyperinsulinemia increases ovarian cytochrome P450cl7α activity in obese PCOS women, either by directly stimulating ovarian steroidogenesis and/or indirectly by stimulating gonadotropin release, which results in excessive androgen production [25] (Fig. 1).

Collectively these observations suggest that hyperinsulinemia is highly correlated with androgen levels in patients with PCOS [1].

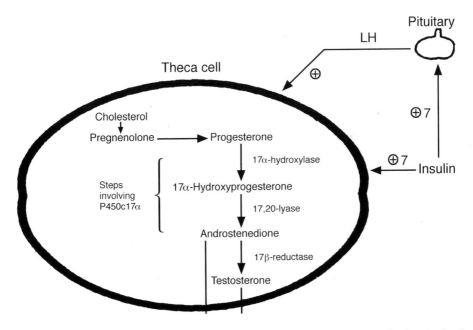

*Fig. 1.* Postulated schema of how insulin might stimulate ovarian androgen production. In the theca cell, insulin may directly stimulate (+ signs) ovarian cytochrome P450cl7α, resulting in increased 17α-hydroxylase and to a lesser extent, 17,20 lyase activities. This would lead to increased production of androstenedione, which is then converted to testosterone by the enzyme 17β-reductase. Alternatively or in conjunction with, insulin may stimulate ovarian androgen production indirectly by enhancing the amplitude of serum luteinizing hormone pulses, and luteinizing hormone then stimulating ovarian cytochrome P450cl7α activity. LH denotes luteinizing hormone. (Reprinted with permission from [25].)

## Short- and long-term medical complication of PCOS

Insulin resistance and hyperinsulinemia play a major role in the pathogenesis of PCOS, thus women with PCOS would be predicted to be at high risk for the insulin-resistance-associated complications, such as type II diabetes mellitus (NIIDDM) obesity, increase of the waist-to-hip ratio (WHR), dyslipidemia, hypertension, impaired fibrinolytic activity, premature atherosclerosis, and increased risk for CVD [5].

## Obesity in PCOS

In many studies it has been shown that PCOS is frequently associated with obesity. One of these studies has reported that between PCOS women 38.4%, had a body mass index (BMI) above 25 kg/m$^2$. The prevalence of obesity in women with PCOS, depends on how the condition is diagnosed, since in some schema obesity is seen as an essential diagnostic feature [17,27].

Given the important and universally adverse effects of obesity on the PCOS, the question arises as to its origin. With the development of adolescence, a degree of insulin resistance occurs normally, presumably as a reflection of the increased secretion of growth hormone that induces the pubertal growth spurt. In girls with polycystic ovaries this is compounded by a propensity to obesity, presumably inherited as a complication of the defect in transduction of the insulin signal [28]. As weight increases, obesity itself provokes further insulin resistance and hypersecretion of insulin and, therefore, further deterioration in the clinical status [28]. Disorders of the leptin-neuropeptide-Y axis may be anticipated in some of these patients and may contribute to the reproductive defect through a putative disturbance of hypothalamic control of pituitary gonadotropin secretion [29]. Obesity-mediated hyperinsulinism, is also the most probable mediator of the oligomenorrhoea that characterizes overweight women with PCOS, since there is an inverse relation of serum insulin concentrations with the interval between menstrual cycles [30]. A clinical perspective of these observations is that obesity contributes to the deterioration of the PCOS clinical status as patients become obese, and its improvement as they lose weight. Both exercise and dietary caloric restriction improve the biochemical and clinical manifestations of insulin resistance and should therefore feature in clinical management programs of women with PCOS [17,31].

## PCOS and risk for NIDDM

Insulin resistance is an important defect in the pathogenesis of NIDDM. Data based on prevalence estimates of PCOS and glucose intolerance, and studies on postmenopausal women within history of PCOS all suggest that PCOS-related insulin resistance confer significantly increased risk for NIDDM [31,34]. Furthermore, according the National Diabetes Data Group Criteria, 20% of the obese PCOS women had impaired glucose tolerance or frank NIDDM. When the less stringent World Health Organization (WHO) criteria are used the prevalence rates of glucose intolerance were as high as $-40\%$ in obese PCOS women [22,31,33,34].

Glucose intolerance of PCOS women usually manifests during the third decade of life, but can appear even during the second decade; similarly NIDDM in PCOS has a substantially earlier age of onset (third or fourth decade) than it does in the general population (sixth to seventh decades) [22]. The prevalence of both impaired glucose tolerance and NIDDM is increased (more than 35%) in women with PCOS. The association of insulin resistance and hyperinsulinemia with PCOS is linked with a 7-fold increase in risk for NIDDM [32]. The study in postmenopausal women with a history of PCOS found a 15% prevalence of NIDDM. It is thus clear that PCOS is a major risk factor for NIDDM in women regardless of age [34]. Insulin resistance of PCOS is unique in that it is independent of obesity and fat-free body mass; the magnitude of the insulin resistance in PCOS is similar to that observed in NIDDM. Thus increased risk of NIDDM in women with PCOS has usually been attributed to the associated insulin resistance [5,10,33].

Although a high proportion of women with PCOS ultimately develop NIDDM, this is not a universal outcome. It seems reasonable to postulate that only those women with PCOS having an additional defect such as $\beta$-cell secretory function actually go on to develop NIDDM. Recent studies have suggested that the defects in insulin sensitivity and secretion in woman with PCOS, may be related to genetic factors, since glucose intolerance is most common among those PCOS women, who have a family history of NIDDM. PCOS thus promises to be a commonly encountered subphenotype of NIDDM with intrinsic abnormalities of insulin action [14,35—37]. Insulin sensitivity, as assessed by the hyperinsulinemic euglycemic clamp technique, was lower in women with PCOS. The incremental insulin secretory response to meals was markedly reduced in women with PCOS. This reduction in postprandial responses resulted from a reduction in the relative amplitude of meal-related secretory pulses. This pattern resembles that of NIDDM more than that of simple obesity [14,33,38].

Women with PCOS had normal first-phase insulin secretion in absolute terms when compared with women without PCOS. However, when first-phase insulin secretion was analyzed in relation to the basal insulin secretion, we found that it is substantially reduced [36]. The ability of the $\beta$-cell to adjust the insulin secretion in response to a graded glucose infusion was significantly reduced in the PCOS subjects with a family history of NIDDM compared with those without such a family history [33].

Taken together, these results suggest that a history of NIDDM in first-degree relatives define a subset of PCOS subjects who may be at greatest risk for secretory defects and for the development of NIDDM. Additional studies in this population suggest that interventions that attenuate hyperinsulinemia may have a salutary effect on both insulin action and $\beta$-cell function. Studies are ongoing to examine whether insulin-sensitizing agents will ameliorate the hormonal and metabolic sequelae of PCOS.

## Gestational diabetes mellitus

Women with a history of gestational (GDM) are insulin resistant, have an increased risk of developing NIDDM, and have defects in the $\beta$-cell function that can be detected in the absence of glucose tolerance [39].

PCOS women share these traits, and it would he expected that they would be at an increased risk of developing GDM, if GDM is yet another manifestation of insulin resistance. However, two small studies of this phenomena have yielded conflicting results: one study found no increase in GDM while another detected an increased risk for GDM in PCOS women [40]. A large prospective study of PCOS women containing appropriately matched control women is required to address this issue further. Until such a study has been completed, it is thus prudent to advise PCOS women contemplating pregnancy that they may be at an increased risk of developing GDM.

## Dyslipidemia

Insulin resistance is characterized by impaired insulin action on glucose metabolism in skeletal muscle, adipose tissue, and liver. There is also abnormal insulin activation of antilipolysis, lipoprotein lipase, and hepatic lipase. The activities of these two major enzyme systems influence circulating lipoprotein lipid concentrations in an opposing fashion [5].

Women with PCOS have lower HDL levels, higher LDL/HDL ratios, and higher triglyceride levels than regularly menstruating women with no evidence of androgen excess [22,41,42]. Some investigators have found that LDL and HDL changes in PCOS can he accounted for by obesity and that only modest increases in total triglyceride levels appear secondary to PCOS-related insulin resistance [36]. In order to confirm that these more male-like patterns of lipoprotein lipid concentrations were not due solely to differences in body weight, lipid and androgen profiles were measured in another group of PCOS women and compared vs. non-PCOS women, who were matched for percent ideal body weight. After controlling for percent ideal body weight, age and other confounding variables, differences in total cholesterol, total HDL, $HDL_2$, LDL- cholesterol, and triglycerides, were still significant between case and control subjects [22,41,42].

Percent ideal body weight correlated with triglyceride and HDL-cholesterol levels only in the control group, but the correlation just missed significance for the women with PCOS [42]. These studies suggest that excess weight alone does not readily explain the differences in lipoprotein lipid profiles observed in PCOS women. It is in keeping with the notion that a factor or factors in the PCOS patients may alter circulating lipoprotein. Both the influence of androgen excess and of hyperinsulinemia on lipoprotein lipids profile need to be evaluated in greater depth [42].

It is of interest that in PCOS patients, as opposed to the other women, triglyceride levels and cholesterol/HDL ratio correlated positively with age. This suggests that some factor or factors are magnifying the influence of age in patients with PCOS and that the phenomenon is more likely to be seen in older patients with the disorder [22,42].

In an attempt to clarify the influence of insulin resistance vs. endogenous sex steroids, namely testosterone, on lipoprotein lipid levels in hirsute hyperandrogenic women, a group of hirsute and normal women were tested with GnRHa over 3 months to remove the possible effects of endogenous gonadal hormones [22]. Hirsute women were heavier and had higher systolic and diastolic blood pressures, more menstrual irregularities, and higher waist/hip ratios. Furthermore, they were more hyperandrogenic than controls. They also had higher triglyceride, VLDL cholesterol, and lower HDL-cholesterol concentrations. After administration of GnRHa, there was a significant suppression of androgen and estrogen levels, but there were no significant changes in average lipid, lipoprotein cholesterol and apolipoprotein concentration [22]. In contrast to significant changes of gonadal hormones, the insulin resistance remained unaltered. Insulin correlated with apolipoprotein lipid abnormalities. Insulin rather than androgen levels correlated best with lipid abnormalities, and suppressing androgen levels did not alter lipid profiles in PCOS [22].

One of the most important observations is that the differences in risk factors between PCOS women and control subjects are generally stronger at earlier ages [41]. This is probably due to an early onset of hormonal changes and obesity and possibly to the distribution of intra-abdominal fat among PCOS patients. These observations provide answers regarding the chances in risk factors over time, especially among the younger PCOS women [41].

One can argue that PCOS represents one of the best examples of syndrome X as defined by Reaven [41]. The risk factors in the PCOS women are probably elevated at an earlier age than among, non-PCOS women. If the central obesity, hyperinsulinemia, and low HDL-cholesterol and high triglyceride levels noted in the PCOS cases are really a unique profile of risk factors of atherosclerosis and subsequent coronary heart disease in women, then women with PCOS should have much more atherosclerosis than control subjects, especially at younger ages. If the risk of atherosclerosis is primarily related to elevated LDL-cholesterol, then there is an alternative reason for a higher prevalence of atherosclerosis in PCOS patients. A comparison of the evaluation of the risk of atherosclerosis in relation to these different risk factors may provide an estimate of the independent contributions of LDL-cholesterol compared with the syndrome X profile [41].

PCOS women in many ways present risk-factor characteristics found in younger men and also among older obese postmenopausal women. It will be important in the subsequent follow-up study and evaluation to determine whether the clinical presenting characteristics of PCOS women are related to changes in risk factors or to the development of atherosclerosis [41].

**Impaired fibrinolytic system.**

PCOS women also have impaired fibrinolytic activity with increased circulating levels of plasminogen activator inhibitor, PAI-1 [43,44]. Elevated PAI-1 levels are associated with insulin resistance and are considered to be an independent cardiovascular risk factor by increasing the risk of intravascular thrombosis [44]. In PCOS increased PAI-1 levels are also associated with insulin resistance, and these levels decrease with improvements in insulin sensitivity mediated by weight loss [57] or insulin-sensitizing agents [45].

**Hypertension**

It has been suggested that insulin resistance causes hypertension; thus PCOS women would be expected to be hypertensive [46]. Significant increases in systolic blood pressure, albeit within the normal range, have been reported in obese PCOS women, but this study did not include a weight-matched control group [47]. Moreover, lean PCOS women in the study were not hypertensive, consistent with an effect of obesity rather than PCOS on blood pressure. Most women with significant insulin resistance, including those with PCOS, have higher blood pressure or overt hypertension [46,47].

Careful studies of 24-h blood pressures and left ventricular mass have failed to find evidence for hypertension in PCOS women in their second to fourth decade of life [47]. This has been confirmed in another recent study [56]. The studies in postmenopausal PCOS women, however, have found a significant increase in prevalence of hypertension [34]. It may be that hypertension is not manifested until later in life in PCOS women.

**Coronary artery disease risk in PCOS**

Evidence is accumulating indicating that women with PCOS are more likely to suffer from cardiovascular events, because of unfavorable alterations in insulin action and/or production, accompanying altered apolipoprotein metabolism and altered androgenicity and/or estrogenicity. All these metabolic and hormonal abnormalities can be translated into increased CVD risk and decreased longevity [5,48,49].

A number of CVD risk factors, including central obesity, insulin resistance (with associated hyperinsulinemia), high triglyceride levels, low high-density lipoprotein cholesterol (HDL-c) levels, and/or diabetes mellitus, tend to cluster in these women [5,22,46,48]. There are several intriguing cross-sectional studies that suggest those PCOS women may indeed be at increased risk for cardiovascular disease. It has been demonstrated that in PCOS women, the android pattern of fat distribution, characterized by excessive abdominal adiposity and a high waist-to-hip ratio (threshold ratio of 0.85), is associated with insulin resistance, hyperandrogenism, hirsutism, hypertension and diabetes, are strongly linked with excessive mortality from CVD [22,46,49,50]. Compared with control subjects PCOS patients (mean age 50 years), had a higher prevalence of central obesity diabetes and hypertension, and had higher basal serum insulin concentrations. Thus the increase CVD and diabetes among PCOS patients should be viewed not only as a condition requiring treatment for anovulation and infertility but also as a metabolic syndrome requiring ongoing medical surveillance [49—51]. Vague et al. [50], have reported that increased concentrations of hemostatic variables, principally PAI-1, accompany hyperinsulinemia, hypertriglyceridemia, hypertension, and obesity, all of which are associated with insulin resistance. This syndrome is associated with the development of CVD as measured by angiography [22,44,46,50]. It has been shown that women with well-defined PCOS who are followed for 15—20 years are more likely to develop hypertension and diabetes than same-age non-PCOS patients [52]. These conditions are well known to lead to premature myocardial infarction, stroke and death. Furthermore, a number of prospective studies have established that hyperinsulinism, both fasting and postprandial, is a risk factor for the development of CAD in nondiabetic subjects [5,53,54]. Hyperinsulinemia independent of obesity and of hyperandrogenism, may play a role in the lipid disturbances that increase the risk of CVD in women with PCOS, and the lipoprotein abnormalities appeared to be associated more with insulin than with endogenous androgen or estrogen [5,46,47,51,54,55].

Although all of these data suggested that women with androgen excess are at an increased risk of coronary artery disease, definitive results linking them with CVD were still lacking. To try to elucidate this relationship further, another study assessed 102 consecutive women who were to undergo cardiac catheterization, (mean ages were 63.6 and 60.5 years for case and control subjects, respectively), and were correlated by self administered questionnaire for waist-to-hip ratio and for problems related to androgen excess earlier in life. A positive correlation was found between complaints of extra facial hair and acne early in life, with confirmed coronary artery disease later in life [22]. The waist-to-hip ratio was found to be significantly associated with both hirsutism and CAD, and the strongest relationships were found in older women (aged ±60 years), indicating that androgen excess may be a signal of increased risk for coronary artery disease, even in younger women [17,22,50,52,55].

In another study it was also reported that women who had a history of symptoms of hyperandrogenism also had an increased prevalence of coronary artery disease [5]. Those postmenopausal women with a history of ovarian wedge resection for PCOS had a significantly increased frequency of cardiovascular events compared with age-matched control women [5,34,56]. It is unknown whether women with more extensive coronary artery disease are more likely to have PCOS ovaries. The extent of coronary artery disease assessed by quantitative angiography was compared with the presence or absence of polycystic ovaries. Pelvic ultrasonography was carried out without knowledge of the extent of coronary artery disease. Polycystic ovaries were found in 42% of 143 women studied and were associated with hirsutism, higher testosterone, trigliceride and C-peptide levels, and lower HDL-c levels [51].

Women with PCOS ovaries had more extensive coronary artery disease than women with normal ovaries (number of segments with $> 50\%$ stenosis). The extent of coronary artery disease and family history of heart disease were predictors of the presence of polycystic ovaries.

The PCOS women were more hirsute and had higher triglycerides, testosterone levels, Apo B, C-peptide, and fibrinogen levels than normal women suggesting that they both had the endocrine and the metabolic derangement of PCOS [51,52].

Finally, increased carotid wall thickness measured by ultrasonography was found in PCOS women compared with case controls [48,56]. The carotid wall thickness was significantly and positively correlated with fasting insulin levels and body mass index, after adjustment for possible confounding variables [56]. Preliminary evidence therefore suggests that PCOS women may be at increased risk for coronary vascular events.

## Therapeutic considerations

Treatment is symptom-driven, and this approach neither corrects the defects nor addresses the long-term sequelae [5]. The increasing knowledge that the metabolic consequences of PCOS can potentially end in premature cardiovascular disease has shifted the clinical focus from short-term and symptom-driven method to recognition that these conditions are chronic with long-term complications.

Agents that exacerbate insulin resistance should probably be avoided in PCOS, particularly in women who are also obese. Further worsening of insulin resistance is an inevitable risk of treatment of PCOS with glucocorticoids, medroxyprogesterone and oral anticontraceptives [57—60], which for all of that reasons implicit, should be escheved [57,58,60]. There are several therapeutic agents for hyperandrogenism that do not worsen and may even improve insulin sensitivity in PCOS. These are spironolactone, GnRHa, and flutamide [59]. Furthermore, reduction of hyperinsulinemia through weight loss in obese PCOS women is associated with a reduction in androgens and restoration of ovulatory menstrual cycles despite an unchanged gonadotropin profile as measured by luteinizing hormone (LH) level, pulsatility and amplitude [1,17,35,36,61]. It now appears that a reduction in circulating insulin levels is the mechanism for weight-loss-associated reproductive benefits [17,61], since lowering insulin levels by other modalities has similar results [17,25,26,61,63].

Pharmacological interventions, which reduce serum insulin concentrations, may prove useful in the clinical management of women with PCOS. It is probable that the use of some of these agents, particularly those classified as "insulin-sensitizing" may become standard (and perhaps second-line after diet) therapy of PCOS [17].

Recently, an uncontrolled study reported that troglitazone treatment of women with PCOS-reduced serum insulin decreased circulating androgens, and improved reproductive status [26].

Metformin, which is a biguanide that appears to enhance peripheral tissue sensitivity to insulin and inhibit hepatic glucose production [62], was used in another uncontrolled study of PCOS women. Reduced circulating insulin after metformin treatment was also associated with concurrent decreases in total and free testosterone, a rise in SHBG, and a reduction in serum LH. Moreover, seven women experienced resumption of normal menses, and three additional women became pregnant. Hence, 38% of the women experienced improved reproductive function during treatment with metformin [53].

In our previous study [25] we have shown that the reduction of fasting serum insulin and the insulin response to a glucose challenge achieved by metformin therapy, was also associated with significant reduction of P450c17α as assessed by the reduction in basal serum 17α-hydroxyprogesterone concentrations and peak serum 17α-hydroxyprogesterone responses to stimulation by the GnRHa [25]. Notably, basal serum LH decreased and its response to leuprolide tended to be reduced, serum-free testosterone fell by 44% and SHBG rose 3-fold. This suggests that reducing serum insulin with metformin can substantially ameliorate the hyperandrogenism of PCOS [25] (Fig. 1).

More recently [63] we found that insulin reduction achieved by metformin treatment of PCOS women, was associated with a significant increase in spontaneous ovulation as well as in the ovulation induced by clomiphene [63]. Moreover, insulin-sensitizing agents have the added theoretical advantage or perhaps favorably affecting those complications of PCOS, which may be attributable in part to hyperinsulinemic insulin resistance, namely glucose intolerance, dyslipidemia, hypertension, and atherosclerosis.

Insulin resistance is a forerunner of PCOS, diabetes and premature coronary heart disease. When a woman becomes a diabetic, her selective female advantage against premature cardiovascular death disappears. Improving insulin sensitivity through diet or drug [25,26] normalizes insulin and testosterone and increases sex hormone-binding globulin and might be preventive to the long-term sequelae such as obesity, dyslipidemia, hypertension, glucose intolerance, NIIDM and thus diminish the cardiovascular risk. Although the later stages of this syndrome are likely to involve diabetes and CVD, two of the most common disorders affecting older women, the time to prevent them is very early in life, before irreversible thresholds are crossed.

## Acknowledgements

The author wishes to thank Dr John Nestler for his encouragement and expert advice in the preparation of this manuscript.

# References

1. Nestler JE. Role of hyperinsulinemia in the pathogenesis of the polycystic ovary syndrome, and its clinical implications. Sem Reprod Endocrinol 1997;15(2):111—122.
2. Franks S. Polycystic ovary syndrome. N Engl J Med 1995;333:853—861.
3. Waterworth DM, Bennett ST, Gharani N, McCarthy MI, Hague S, Batty S,Conway GS,White D,Todd JA, Franks S,Williamson R. Linkage and association of insulin gene VNTR regulatory polymorphism with polycystic ovary syndrome. Lancet 1997;349:986—990.
4. Hull MGR. Epidemiology of infertility and polycystic ovarian disease endocrinological and demographic studies. Gynecol Endocrinol 1987;1:235—245.
5. Wild RA. Obesity, lipids, cardiovascular risk, and androgen excess. Am J Med 1995;98:27S.
6. Per Bjorntorp. The android woman — a risky condition. J Int Med 1996;239:105—110.
7. Rittmaster RS. Hyperandrogenism what is normal? N Engl J Med 1992;327:1946.
8. Nestler JE, Powers LP, Matt DW, Steingold KA, Plymate SR, Rittmaster RS, Clore JN et al. A direct effect of hyperinsulinemia on serum sex hormone binding globulin levels in obese women with the polycystie ovary syndrome. J Clin Endocrinol Metab 1 1991;72:83—89.
9. Nestler JE. Editorial. Sex hormone-binding globulin: a marker for hyperinsulinemia and/or insulin resistance? J Clin Endocrinol Metab 1993;76:273—274.
10. Dunaif A, Futterweit W, Segal KR, Dobransky A. Profound peripheral insulin resistance, independent of obesity, in the polycystic ovary syndrome. Diabetes 1989;38:1165—1174.
11. Zawadzki JK, Dunaif A. Diagnostic criteria for polycystic ovary syndrome: towards a rational approach. In: Dunaif A, Givens JR, Haseltin FP, Merriam GR (eds) Polycystic Ovary Syndrome. Oxford, UK: Blackwell Scientific, 1992;377—384.
12. Burghen GA, Givens JR, Kitabchi AE. Correlation of hyperandrogenism with hyperinsulinism in polycystic ovarian disease. J Clin Endocrinol Metab 1980;50:113—116.
13. Pasquali R,Venturoli S, Paradisi R, Capelli M, Parenti N, Melchionda N. Insulin and C- peptide levels in obese patients with polycystic ovaries. Horm Metab Res 1982;14:284—287.
14. Dunaif A, Segal KR, Shelley DR, Green G, Dobransky A, Licholai T. Evidence for distinctive and intrinsic defects in insulin action in polycystic ovary syndrome. Diabetes 1992;41: 1257—1266.
15. Norman RJ, Masters S, Hague W. Hyperinsulinemia is common in family members of women with polycystic ovary syndrome. Fertil Steril 1996;66:942—947.
16. Carmina E, Koyama T, Chang L, Stanczyk FZ, Lobo RA. Does ethnicity influence the prevalence of adrenal hyperandrogenism and insulin resistance in polycystic ovary syndrome? Am J Obstet Gynecol 1992;167:1804—1812.
17. Kiddy DS, Hamilton-Fairley D, Bush A, Short F, Anyaoku V, Reed Mj, Franks S. Improvement in endocrino and ovarian function during dietary treatment of obese women with polycystic ovary syndrome. Clin Endocrinol Oxf 1992;36:105—111.
18. Nestler JE, Clore JN, Blackard WC. Effects of insulin on steroidogenesis in vivo. In: Dunaif A, Civeru IR, Haselline FP, Merriam CR (eds) Polycystic Ovary Syndrome. Cambridge: MA Blackwell Scientific Publications, 1992.
19. Willis D, Franks S. Insulin action in human granulosa cells from normal and polycystic ovaries is mediated by the insulin receptor and not the Type-1 insulin-like growth factor receptor. J Clin Endocrinol Metab 1995;80:3788—3790.
20. Nestler JE, Jakubowicz DJ, Falcon de Vargas A, Brik C, Quintero N, Medina F. In the polycystic ovary syndrome insulin stimulates human thecal testosterone production via its own receptor by using inositolglycan mediators as the signal transduction system. J Clin Endocrinol Metab 1998;80:2001—2005.
21. Nagamani M, Dinh TV, Kelver ME. Hyperinsulinemia in hyperthecosis of the ovaries. Obstet Gynecol 1986;54:384—389.
22. Wild RA, Alaupovic P, Parker IJ. Lipid and apolipoprotein abnormalities in hirsute women. Am J Obstet Gynecol 1992;166:1191.

23. Nestler JE, Barlascini CO, Matt DW. Suppression of serum insulin by diazoxide reduced serum testosterone levels in obese women with polycystic ovary syndrome. J Clin Endocrinol Metab 1989;68:1027.

24. Prelevic GM, Wurzburger MI, Balint-Peric L, Nesic JS. Inhibitory effect of sandostatin on secretion of luteinizing hormone, ovarian steroids in polycystic ovary syndrome. Lancet 1990; 336:900—903.

25. Nestler JE, Jakubowicz DJ. Decreases in ovarian cytochrome P450cl7c activity and serum free testosterone after reduction of insulin secretion in polycystic ovary syndrome. N Engl J Med 1996;335:617—623.

26. Dunaif A, Scott D, Finegood D, Quintana B, Whitcomb R. The insulin sensitizing agent Troglitazone: a novel therapy for the polycystic ovary syndrome. J Clin Endocrinol Metab 1996;81: 3299—3306.

27. Balen AH, Conway GS, Kaitsas G, Techatraisak K, Manning P, West C, Jacobs HS. Polycystic ovary syndrome: The spectrum of the disorder in 1741 patients. Human Reprod 1995;10: 2107—2111.

28. Amiel SA, Sherwin RS, Simonsen DC, Lauritano AL, Tamboriane WV. Impaired insulin action in puberty. A contributing factor to poor glycemie control in adolescents with diabetes. N Engl J Med 1986;315:215—219.

29. Scott J. New chapter for the fat controller. Nature 1996;379:113—114.

30. Conway GS. Polycystic ovary syndrome: clinical aspects. Baillieres Clin Endocrinol Metab 1966;10:263—280.

31. Dunaif A, Graf M, Mandeli J, Laumas V, Dobransky A. Characterization of groups of hyperandrogenie women with acanthosis nigricans, impaired glucose tolerance and/or hyperinsulinemia. J Clin Endocrinol Metab 1987;65:499—507.

32. Ehrmann DA, Bames RB, Rosenfield RT. Polycystic ovary syndrome as a form of functional ovarian hyperandrogenisni due to dysregulation of androgen secretion. Endocrinol Rev 1995; 16:322—353.

33. Ehrmann DA, Sturis J, Byme MM, Karrison T, Rosenfield RL, Polonksy KS. Insulin secretory defects in polycystic ovary syndrome. Relationship to insulin sensitivity and family history of non-insulin-dependent diabetes mellitus. J Clin Invest 1995;96:520—527.

34. Dahlgren E, Johansson S, Lindstedt G, Knutsson F, Oden A, Janson PO, Mattson L, Crona N, Lundberg P. Women with polycystic ovary syndrome wedge resected in 1956 to 1965: a long-term follow-up focusing on natural history and circulating hormones. Fertil Steril 1992;57: 505—513.

35. Lobo RA, Goebelsmann U, Horton R. Evidence for the importance of peripheral tissue events in the development of hirsutism in polycystic ovary syndrome. J Clin Endocrinol Metab 1983; 57:393—397.

36. Holte J, Bergh T, Beme C, Wide L, Lithell H. Restored insulin sensitivity but persistently increased early insulin secretion after weight loss in obese women with polycystic ovary syndrome. J Clin Endocrinol Metab 1995;80:2586—2593.

37. Ciraldi TP, El Roely A, Madar Z, Relchart D, Olefsky IM, Yen SSC. Cellular mechanism of insulin resistance in polycystic ovary syndrome. J Clin Endocrinol Met 1992;75:577—883.

38. Polonsky KS, Given BD, Van Cauter E. Twenty four hours profiles and pulsatile patterns of insulin secretion in normal and obese subjects. J Clin Invest 1988;81:442—448.

39. Ryan EA, O'Suilivan MJ, Skyler JS. Insulin action during pregnancy: studies with the euglycemic clamp technique. Diabetes 1985;34:380—389.

40. Lanzone A, Caruso A, DiSimone N, DeCarolis S, Fulghesu AM, Mancuso S. Polycystic ovary disease. A risk factor for gestational diabetes? J Reprod Med 1995;40:312—316.

41. Talbott E, Guzick D, Clerici A, Berga S, Detre K, Weimer Kuller L. Coronary heart disease risk factors in women with polycystic ovary syndrome. Arter Throm Vas Biol 1995;15:821—826.

42. Wild RA, Bartholomew MJ. The influence of body weight on lipoprotein lipids on patients with polycystic ovary syndrome. Am J Obstet Gynecol 1988;159:423—427.

842

43. Sampson M, Kong C, Patel A, Unwin R, Jacobs HS. Ambulatory blood pressure profiles and plasminogen activator inhibitor (PAI-1) activity in lean women with and without the polycystic ovary syndrome. Clin Endocrinol Oxf 1996;45:623—629.
44. Andersen P, Seljeflot I, Abdelnoor M, Amesen H, Dale PO, Lovik A, Birkeland K. Increased insulin sensitivas and fibrinolytic capacity after dietary intervention in obese women with polycystic ovary syndrome. Metabolism 1995;44:611—616.
45. Ehrmann DF, Schneider DJ, Sobel BE, Cavaghan JI, Rosenfield RL, Polonslty KS. Troglitazone improves defects in insulin action, insulin secretion ovarian steroidogenesis, and fibrinolysis in women with polycystic ovary syndrome. J Clin Endocrinol Metab 1997;82:2108—2116.
46. DeFronzo RA, Ferrannini E. Insulin resistance. A multifaceted syndrome responsible for NIDDM, obesity, hypertension, dyslipidemia, and atherosclerotic cardiovascular disease. Diabetes Care 1991;14:173—194.
47. Zimmerman S, Phillips RA, Wikenfeld C, Dunaif A, Finegood D, Ardeljan M, Wallenstein S, Gorlin R, Krakoff L. Polycystic ovary syndrome: lack of hypertension despite insulin resistance. J Clin Endocrinol Metab 1992;75:508—513.
48. Adams MR, Nakagomi A, Keech A et al. Carotid intim-media thickness is only were correlated with the extent and severity of coronary artery disease. Circulation 1995;92:2127—2134.
49. Holienbauch DC, Pavek TJ, Crampton MJ, Laxson DD. Hyperglycemia impairs coronary microvascular endothelium-dependent vasodilation [abstract 2156]. Circulation 1995;92: 1—451.
50. Vague J. Bjontrop P. In: Vague P (ed) Metabolic Complications of Human Obesities. Amsterdam: Elsevier Scientific Publishers, 1985;115—130.
51. Birdsall MA, Farquhar CM, White HD. Association between polycystic ovaries and extent of coronary artery disease in women having cardiae catheterization Ann Intern Med 1997;126:32—35.
52. Moller DE, Flier JS. Insulin resistance-mechanisms, syndromes, and implications. N Engl J Med 1991;325:938—948.
53. Velazquez EM, Mendoza 5, Hamer T, Sosa F, Glueck CJ. Metformin therapy in polycystic ovary syndrome reduces hyperinsulinemia, insulin resistance, hyperandrogenemia, and systolic blood pressure, while facilitating normal menses and pregnancy. Metabolism 1994;43:647—654.
54. Knopp RH, Zhu X-D, Lau J, Walden C. Sex hormones and lipid interactions: implications for cardiovascular disease in women. Endocrinology 1994;4:286—301.
55. Dahlgren E, Janson PO, Johansson S, Lapidus L, Oden A. Polycystic ovary syndrome and risk for myocardial infarction. Acta Obstet Gynecol Scand 1992;71:599—603.
56. Guzick DS, Talbott EO, Sutton-Tyrrell K, Herzog HC, Kuller LH, Woifson SK. Carotid atherosclerosis in women with polycystic ovary syndrome: initial results from a case-control study. Am J Obstet Gynecol 1996;174:1224—1232.
57. Godsland IF, Walton C, Feiton C, Proudler A, Patel A, Wynn V. Insulin resistance, secretion, and metabolism in users of oral contraceptives. J Clin Endocrinol Metab 1992;74:64—70.
58. Korytkowski MT, Mokan M, Horwitz MJ, Berga SL. Metabolic effects of oral contraceptives in women with polycystic ovary syndrome. J Clin Endocrinol Metab 1995;80:3327—3334.
59. Elkind-Hirsch KE, Valdes CT, Malinak LR. Insulin resistance improves in hyperandrogenic women treated with Lupron. Fertil Steril 1993;60:634—641.
60. Elkind-Hirsch KE, Shemian ID, Malinak R. Hormone replacement therapy alters insulin sensitivity in young women with premature ovarian failure. J Clin Endocrinol Metab 1993;76: 472—475.
61. Jakubowicz DJ, Nestler JE. 17-$\alpha$-hydroxyprogesterone responses to leuprolide and serum androgens in obese women with polycystic ovary syndrome after dietary weight loss. J Clin Endocrinol Metab 1987;82:556—560.
62. DeFronzo RA, Barzilai N, Simonson DC. Mechanism of metformin action in obese and lean non-insulin-dependent diabetic subjects. J Clin Endocrinol Metab 1991;73:1294—1301.
63. Nestler JE, Jakubowicz DJ, Evans WS. Pasquali R. Effect of metformin on spontaneous and clomiphene-induced ovulation in the polycystic ovary syndrome. N Engl J Med 1998;336(2): 1876—1880.

# Index of authors

# Keyword index